Open MRI

Open MRI

Edited by

Peter A. Rothschild, M.D.

Adjunct Assistant Professor of Radiology
University of California, San Francisco, School of Medicine
San Francisco, California
Medical Director, Open MRI
Hayward, California
Medical Director, Open MRI
Louisville, Kentucky

Debra Reinking Rothschild, M.D.

Anesthesiologist
Open MRI
Hayward, California
Summit Medical Center
Oakland, California

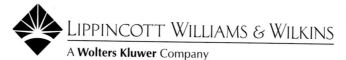

LIPPINCOTT WILLIAMS & WILKINS
A **Wolters Kluwer** Company
Philadelphia • Baltimore • New York • London
Buenos Aires • Hong Kong • Sydney • Tokyo

Acquisitions Editor: Joyce-Rachel John
Developmental Editor: Selina M. Bush
Production Editor: Allison Spearman, Silverchair Science + Communications
Manufacturing Manager: Kevin Watt
Cover Designer: Mark Lerner
Compositor: Silverchair Science + Communications
Printer: Maple Vail

© 2000 by LIPPINCOTT WILLIAMS & WILKINS
227 East Washington Square
Philadelphia, PA 19106-3780 USA
LWW.com

Printed in the USA

Library of Congress Cataloging-in-Publication Data
Open MRI / [edited by] Peter Rothschild, Debra Reinking Rothschild.
p. cm.
Includes bibliographical references and index.
ISBN 0-7817-2173-3
1. Magnetic resonance imaging. I. Rothschild, Peter. II. Rothschild, Debra Reinking.
[DNLM: 1. Magnetic Resonance Imaging--instrumentation. 2. Magnetic Resonance Imaging--methods. WN 185 O615 1999]
RC78.7.N83 O65 1999
616.07'548 21--dc21
99-042876

Care has been taken to confirm the accuracy of the information presented and to describe generally accepted practices. However, the authors, editors, and publisher are not responsible for errors or omissions or for any consequences from application of the information in this book and make no warranty, expressed or implied, with respect to the currency, completeness, or accuracy of the contents of the publication. Application of this information in a particular situation remains the professional responsibility of the practitioner.

The authors, editors, and publisher have exerted every effort to ensure that drug selection and dosage set forth in this text are in accordance with current recommendations and practice at the time of publication. However, in view of ongoing research, changes in government regulations, and the constant flow of information relating to drug therapy and drug reactions, the reader is urged to check the package insert for each drug for any change in indications and dosage and for added warnings and precautions. This is particularly important when the recommended agent is a new or infrequently employed drug.

Some drugs and medical devices presented in this publication have Food and Drug Administration (FDA) clearance for limited use in restricted research settings. It is the responsibility of health care providers to ascertain the FDA status of each drug or device planned for use in their clinical practice.

10 9 8 7 6 5 4 3 2 1

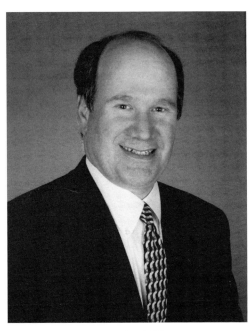

Peter A. Rothschild, M.D.

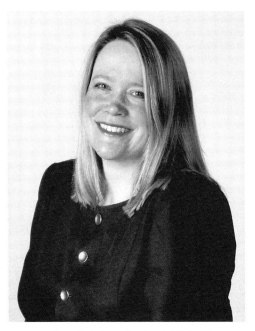

Debra Reinking Rothschild, M.D.

To our children, Annie, Cynthia, and Karen,
and to our parents, Nyra and Wilbert Reinking and
Frances and Edward Rothschild

Contents

III. CLINICAL IMAGING

IV. FUTURE DIRECTIONS

V. APPENDIX

Contributing Authors

Yoshimi Anzai, M.D.
Assistant Professor of Radiology
University of Michigan Medical School
Ann Arbor, Michigan

Robert Berkenblit, M.D.
Assistant Professor of Radiology
Albert Einstein College of Medicine
  of Yeshiva University
Montefiore Medical Center
Associate Medical Director
Montefiore Imaging Center
Bronx, New York

Jack Chen, M.D.
Clinical Instructor
Department of Radiological Sciences
University of California, Los Angeles,
  UCLA School of Medicine
Los Angeles, California

Lawrence E. Crooks, Ph.D.
Research Fellow
Radiologic Imaging Laboratory
Toshiba America MRI, Inc.
South San Francisco, California

Elizabeth J. DuBose, M.D.
Staff Radiologist
Open MRI
Hayward, California
Open MRI
Louisville, Kentucky

Terry Duggan-Jahns, R.T.(R)(M)(CT)(MR)
Center Manager/ Technical Director
Union Avenue Open MRI/ Tacoma Magnetic
  Imaging
Tacoma, Washington

Sean R. Evers, Ph.D.
Evers Psychological Associates, P.C.
Manasquan, New Jersey

William H. Faulkner, Jr., R.T.(R)(MR)(CT)
MRI Education and Operation Consultant
William Faulkner & Associates, LLC
Chattanooga, Tennessee

Joy D. Foster, M.D.
Staff Radiologist
Open MRI
Hayward, California
Open MRI
Louisville, Kentucky

Blaine L. Hart, M.D.
Associate Professor of Radiology
University of New Mexico School of Medicine
Albuquerque, New Mexico

Leon Kaufman, Ph.D.
Chief Scientist and Vice President, Engineering
Radiologic Imaging Laboratory
Toshiba America MRI, Inc.
South San Francisco, California

John Koveleski, R.T.(R)(MR)
Chief Technologist
Magnetic Imaging Center
Mechanicsburg, Pennsylvania

Robert Lufkin, M.D.
Professor of Radiology
University of California, Los Angeles,
  UCLA School of Medicine
Los Angeles, California

Kevin R. Moore, M.D.
Clinical Instructor of Radiology
Neuroradiology Section
University of Utah School of Medicine
Salt Lake City, Utah

Kim Nguyen, M.D.
Department of Radiology
University of California, San Francisco,
  Medical Center
San Francisco, California

William W. Orrison, Jr., M.D.
Professor and Chairman
Department of Radiology
University of Utah School of Medicine
Salt Lake City, Utah

Louis Paladino
Executive Director
Business Development
InSight Health Services Corporation
Myrtle Beach, South Carolina

R. Craig Platenberg, M.D.
Medical Director
Wide Open MRI
Med-Ted International Corporation
McLean, Virginia

V. G. Raaj Prasad, M.S.
Vice President of Research and Development
Image Enhancement System, Inc.
Hayward, California

Karen Procknow, R.T.(R)
Advanced Applications Specialist
Mid-Field and Open Products
General Electric Medical Systems
Milwaukee, Wisconsin

Debra Reinking Rothschild, M.D.
Anesthesiologist
Open MRI
Hayward, California
Summit Medical Center
Oakland, California

Peter A. Rothschild, M.D.
Adjunct Assistant Professor of Radiology
University of California, San Francisco, School
    of Medicine
San Francisco, California
Medical Director, Open MRI
Hayward, California
Medical Director, Open MRI
Louisville, Kentucky

Frank G. Shellock, Ph.D., FACSM
Adjunct Clinical Professor of Radiology
University of Southern California School
    of Medicine
Shellock R & D Services, Inc.
Los Angeles, California

John L. Sherman, M.D.
Medical Director
Open MRI of Colorado
Colorado Springs, Colorado
Associate Clinical Professor of Radiology
University of Colorado School of Medicine
Denver, Colorado

Shantanu Sinha, Ph.D.
Associate Professor of Radiological Sciences
University of California, Los Angeles, UCLA
    School of Medicine
Los Angeles, California

Usha Sinha, Ph.D.
Assistant Professor of Radiological Sciences
University of California, Los Angeles, UCLA
    School of Medicine
Los Angeles, California

Lawrence N. Tanenbaum, M.D.
Assistant Professor of Neuroscience
Seton Hall University School of Graduate
    Medical Education
South Orange, New Jersey
Staff Radiologist and Section Chief
Neuroradiology, Head and Neck Radiology,
    Magnetic Resonance Imaging, and Computed
    Tomography
New Jersey Neuroscience Institute at John F.
    Kennedy Medical Center
Edison, New Jersey

Joseph Triolo, M.D.
MRI Director
Ocean Medical Imaging Center
Community Medical Center
Toms River, New Jersey

Mark L. Winkler, M.D.
Professor of Health Sciences
University of Nevada, Las Vegas
Las Vegas, Nevada
Director of MRI
Steinberg Diagnostic Medical Imaging
Las Vegas, Nevada

Foreword

In magnetic resonance imaging (MRI), patient comfort and economics matter. Open MRI was once scorned as a triumph of marketing over science. The fact that patients liked it, but radiologists and their referring physicians often did not, made it suspect. The attitude of many academic investigators was to go for the most horsepower MRI had to offer. The magic number has long been 1.5 tesla, as though Nikola Tesla himself ordained it as a natural law of magnetism.

Today, we know better. There remains a majority of academics for whom high-field systems are the *sine qua non*. They have worked exclusively on 1.5-tesla machines for their entire careers and understand their strengths, which are considerable. The machismo that was once exhibited at MRI symposia by high-field advocates is no longer so conspicuous, however. Everyone understands that mid and even low-field MRI scans have their place in diagnostic medicine. In the evolutionary march of MRI, the technology has divided, and the branch supporting open systems is flourishing.

Gradually, those who toiled relatively anonymously to advance open systems have been vindicated. They have proven that lower-field MRI can be patient-friendly and diagnostically potent. Like all of radiology, optimizing open MRI requires a degree of artistry; those secrets are being shared, with this text being an example. As academics become more involved with open systems, image quality will improve, and the variety of applications will multiply. Intraoperative MRI is but a sliver of potential patient volume; this use of open systems alone is proof of its maturity.

Patient comfort and economics matter, now more than ever. Open MRI has officially arrived.

Peter Ogle
Editor
Diagnostic Imaging

Preface

Open MRI was created in response to the explosion of interest and demand for clear, straightforward information about this trend in medical imaging. We created a text to explain what the term means and how best to use the technique. The goal was to create a resource that explained, technically and clinically, what open magnetic resonance imaging (MRI) *is* and what it *is not.*

The term *open MRI* was coined in the late 1980s. At that time, some of my colleagues thought that it meant "open for business," whereas others joked that it meant "open 24 hours a day." Despite the initial questionable definitions, today there is no mistaking that the term is synonymous with patient comfort, accurate diagnosis, and pristine image quality.

Although numerous excellent books on MRI cover certain clinical areas in depth, no single source of information on open magnets has been available—the reader who needed to learn specifically about open MRI had nowhere to turn. *Open MRI* not only represents a complete resource with a clinical and practical basis, it also features many topics (e.g., how best to handle anxious and claustrophobic patients, the physics of open MRI, and technical information on optimizing open MRI image quality) not covered in other volumes.

As more health care providers considered open magnet systems, the need for a text that translated and summarized the current and future status of open MRI became clear. This text is more than an extension of the educational process regarding the benefits of this type of imaging; it is also intended as a "how-to" guide for every person who is, will be, or is considering working with open magnets. Therefore, it was decided early in this book's development to incorporate the experience of many contributors, including a number of clinical radiologists, so that their common, everyday experiences could be shared.

Open MRI is organized into four logical sections and an appendix. The first section has chapters of interest to anyone even peripherally curious about open MRI. Chapter 1 explains why open MRI has taken off in popularity. Chapter 2 delves into the sometimes mysterious psychological issues that our patients face and offers succinct, easy to follow, practical advice to help our patients successfully undergo their scans. Chapter 4 presents the latest knowledge about MRI safety from the world's leading expert on MRI safety. Finally, Chapter 5 provides details of basic issues involved in setting up a sedation program.

Because the optimal usage of open MRI is so heavily dependent on user comprehension of the underlying theory, the second section is devoted entirely to the physics of open MRI. Chapter 6 is a must read for anyone who is considering an open magnet. Chapter 7 was written by Leon Kaufman and Larry Crooks, who developed the first commercially available open magnet. Chapters 8 and 9 explain, in easily understood language, these critical techniques. Chapter 10 details how to maximize image quality and tailor sequences.

The third section, Clinical Imaging, includes thirteen practical chapters describing open MRI (from head to toe) as it is clinically used today. The emphasis is on disease processes that routinely present for an open MRI system. The common examinations, detailing technical approaches and clinical interpretations, are thoroughly explained. A strong foundation is laid so that the reader can apply the basic open MRI principles to unusual types of examinations and readily identify even rare pathologic processes.

Advances in open MRI and new developments are the focus of the fourth section. These new techniques and sequences offer a glimpse into the future of open MRI. Chapter 23 discusses an area that distinguishes open MRI from closed MRI. The freedom of open magnets allows greater ranges of motion and the ability to perform biopsies with real time imaging. Chapter 24 discusses the potential for this noninvasive technique to replace angiography, especially in extremely anxious and large patients—the same patients in whom it is difficult to perform invasive testing such as angiography. Chapter 25 details open MRI's enormous potential, as this technique blurs the distinction between radiology and microscopy, making the diagnostic ability of the radiologist edge even closer toward that of the pathologist. Chapter 16 explains the use of the Internet to efficiently transfer images to off-site locations. This raises the concept of virtual radiology, in which a single radiologist can interpret MRIs at numerous centers quickly and efficiently.

The clinical applications of open MRI continue to accelerate with technical developments and greater availability. Progress in open MRI will dominate the field of MRI. *Open MRI* is a culmination of patient demand and advances in technical developments.

Peter A. Rothschild

Acknowledgments

We wish to express our deepest appreciation to those who made this, the first book on open magnetic resonance imaging (MRI), possible. First, we thank the editors and staff at Lippincott Williams & Wilkins, who enthusiastically supported the concept of an open MRI book, including Joyce-Rachel John, Dennis Teston, Selina M. Bush, James D. Ryan, and Michael Stoneking, as well as Allison Spearman of Silverchair Science + Communications.

We also would like to extend our sincere appreciation to Drs. Murray Solomon and Alex Margulis, who sparked and supported my interest in MRI. Also, thanks go to the referring physicians who believed in open MRI: Drs. Michael Krinsky, Warren King, Richard Nolan, Gregg Pottorff, Douglas Abeles, Warren Strudwick, and Grant Gauger; and, most important, to all of our open MRI patients.

We wish also to thank the staff of Open MRI of Hayward, California, and Louisville, Kentucky, who have assisted with this text: Millie Kenna, Shannon Estill, Scott Clark, Tina Lewis, Robin Graham, Robert Smith, Nikki Ferreira, Chris Allen, Jarrett Arbogast, Angela Krause, and Elizabeth Bisconer. We are also grateful to Michael Cragin, Suzanne Martin, and InSight Health Services for their support. A special thanks to Margaret Omaque for her secretarial assistance.

Peter A. Rothschild

SECTION I

General Considerations

Open MRI,
edited by Peter A. Rothschild and Debra Reinking Rothschild.
Lippincott Williams & Wilkins, Philadelphia © 2000.

CHAPTER   1

Why Open Magnetic Resonance Imaging?

Peter A. Rothschild

Medicine consists of essentially two parts: diagnosis and treatment. The diagnostic part of medicine has gone through a revolution in the last few decades, primarily because of the improvements in computer technology, which have culminated in magnetic resonance imaging (MRI). MRI has replaced very invasive and less diagnostic methods such as pneumoencephalography, myelography, and nuclear medicine brain scans. Due to its highly accurate diagnostic ability combined with its minimal risk and noninvasive nature, the use of MRI has skyrocketed. The term *MRI* has come into common usage even within the nonmedical population. For example, over the course of a year, the sports section of most newspapers has numerous articles describing the MRI findings of local or national sports figures. MRI is able to diagnose neurologic and musculoskeletal pathology earlier and more accurately than any other modality. MRI is beginning to approach the "tricorder" of Dr. McCoy in the popular television series *Star Trek*.

NEED FOR OPEN MAGNETIC RESONANCE IMAGING

As use of MRI has proliferated, significant limitations have appeared: Claustrophobia and anxiety-related reactions, restrictions on patient size and weight, and lack of access to the patient undergoing the examination have surfaced as problems facing traditional closed MRI scanners. When I began working with MRI in the 1980s, I faced these problems and realized the need for an MRI to accommodate these patients. I joined a research laboratory that was developing just such a patient-friendly magnet. To differentiate this new type of magnet, I coined the term *open MRI* and named my first imaging center *Open MRI*. At that time, however, most radiologists believed that only traditional closed MRI scanners

held promise for the future. The simple descriptive term caught on quickly with patients and referring doctors. A decade later, many of the same radiologists who previously shunned "open" technology have become converted, a fact reflected in the soaring popularity of open magnets. Several explanations for this evolution exist.

Advancements in Magnetic Resonance Imaging Technology

MRI technology has advanced at a whirlwind pace, allowing the once unthinkable to become reality. Improved computer hardware, software, gradients, and magnets have dramatically advanced the performance and functionality of all MRI systems. Today, lower field strength open magnets can readily outperform the higher field strength magnets of just a few years ago.

Patients Resistant to Traditional Magnetic Resonance Imaging

In the past, radiologists clearly underestimated the number of claustrophobic and anxious patients. Most radiologists simply looked at rejection rates from closed-tube MRI and extrapolated this number to the general population. In so doing, they came up with extremely low numbers, indicating that only 1% to 2% of the population is claustrophobic. However, this method overlooks the simple fact that patients who come to an MRI center are already preselected. Many claustrophobic and anxious patients are never scheduled for MRI, "forget" their appointments, or may simply be no-shows. Determining how many patients are anxious or claustrophobic by looking at the rejection rates of patients who come to the MRI center and refuse to get into the scanner is analogous to trying to determine what percentage of the general population is afraid to fly by counting the number of ticketed passengers at an airport who refuse to board the airplane. The fact is that, just as people who are afraid to fly usually do not go

P. A. Rothschild: Department of Radiology, University of California, San Francisco, San Francisco, California; Open MRI, Hayward, California; Open MRI, Louisville, Kentucky

to the airport to board an airplane, people who are afraid of MRI usually do not go to an MRI center.

To understand the demand for open MRI, we must first understand these so-called claustrophobic patients. These patients are actually experiencing something much more complex than simple claustrophobia. Many psychiatrists and psychologists believe that the claustrophobia associated with MRI is really a form of posttraumatic stress syndrome; my own clinical experience supports this conclusion.

A clear example of this hypothesis is submariners. The U.S. government spends thousands of dollars on one thing when screening possible submariners: making sure that these individuals are not claustrophobic. Many of these submariners, who are not claustrophobic by standardized, rigorous testing and who successfully have completed long periods in very small quarters, refuse to submit to tube-type MRI.

In my practice, several other patients reluctant to undergo traditional MRI have related stories of being trapped as children. One patient told me that when she was a child, her parents routinely punished her by locking her in a closet. Another patient told of an episode when, as a child, she had been lying on a mattress on the floor. Another mattress, from an overlying bunk bed, fell onto her and nearly suffocated her. These patients are experiencing much more than simple claustrophobia: I feel that they have a type of posttraumatic stress syndrome.

Furthermore, I have found that the largest class of patients referred for open MRI are those who have successfully completed a tube-type, closed MRI examination but who found the experience so intense that they refused to undergo a second closed MRI. These patients frequently state that they did not know they were claustrophobic, but they just could not tolerate another closed MRI. When questioned, patients describe being "shoved" into the tube, and frequently state that it was not only the tube but also the overall experience of isolation and loss of control that prompted their subsequent refusals to undergo repeat MRI examinations in a tube-type MRI. This population has been growing, reflecting the increasing number of patients who have undergone MRI scanning.

The exact number of claustrophobic patients is unclear and probably irrelevant. What is relevant is that when patients are given a choice, I have found that 30% to 40% prefer the comfort of an open MRI. As the public becomes increasingly sophisticated regarding their medical care, these patients are less likely to simply do what their doctors tell them. These new, assertive patients think and act like well-informed consumers of any other goods or services. Therefore, I prefer to call them health care *consumers* instead of *patients*. If these consumers want their MRI examinations performed in an open magnet, they will likely find an open magnet and demand to have their scans performed in the magnet of their choice.

Other Groups That Benefit from Open Magnetic Resonance Imaging

Open MRI has also enabled the examination of other types of patients unable to undergo conventional closed MRI. Large patients and patients with wide shoulders who either exceed the table weight limit or simply do not fit into the tube-type gantry can usually fit into an open MRI with ease. The open architecture and quieter operation allow direct visual and auditory patient monitoring. Electronic and life support equipment can be brought much closer to the patient, because fringe fields are generally much lower in open magnets.

The direct access to the patient provided by open MRI is advantageous for newer techniques such as interventional MRI procedures and kinematic joint studies.

CONCLUSION

The medical and patient communities have become accustomed to the advantages of open MRI and will not go back. As the technology improves over the next 5 to 10 years, even high field strength magnets will be open. The market is demanding open magnets. Open MRI, therefore, is not only here to stay; open magnets are also the future of MRI.

Open MRI,
edited by Peter A. Rothschild and Debra Reinking Rothschild.
Lippincott Williams & Wilkins. Philadelphia © 2000.

CHAPTER 2

Claustrophobic Anxiety and Magnetic Resonance Imaging: A Clinician's Perspective

Sean R. Evers

Magnetic resonance imaging (MRI), like no other medical test, has become closely linked with the psychological response it elicits. In many patients, the MRI procedure—despite its technological sophistication and efficacy—elicits fears and anxieties that are primitive in origin, such as the fight-or-flight response. Although usually associated with claustrophobia, MRI can trigger or exacerbate many psychological conditions.

Claustrophobia, "the dread of closed places" (1), is the popular psychological term associated with MRI, but what actually occurs is much more complex and differs from patient to patient. What has been called *claustrophobia* when describing the patient response to MRI may instead be a class of anxiety responses caused by the MRI procedure rather than a specific phobia of its own. The term *claustrophobic anxiety* might be used more accurately to refer to a condition in its own right, claustrophobia, and more generally to an anxiety stimulus for other psychological issues that may be just beneath the surface. Based on this terminology, a patient's anxiety in response to the MRI procedure can be considered both an immediate reaction, labeled correctly or incorrectly as claustrophobia, and a potentially significant stimulus (stressor) aggravating other psychological conditions, either preexisting or heretofore unelicited.

Psychological issues that have become commonplace with the use of traditional closed MRI units must also be considered with the use of short-bore and open MRI scanners. Short-bore units—in which the cavity is shallower—allow the patient to be somewhat less enclosed but still maintain the closed cavity design and potentially all or most of the psychological limitations of the standard tube MRI. The open units, which by their very design and name seek to avoid

claustrophobia, may still precipitate psychological issues similar to those elicited during closed MRI but often for different reasons. Quieter, less restrictive, and more patient friendly, these units offer obvious psychological benefits. Unfortunately, open scans generally take more time to complete, and the patient is thus asked to lie motionless for a longer period than is generally required with a traditional scanner. Additionally, whether in a closed, short-bore, or open MRI unit, a patient must have a radiofrequency coil placed around the body part being imaged. This coil can make the procedure, regardless of the unit type, feel less open. Open units also appear to attract individuals who have avoided the more restrictive closed units. Due either to personal or vicarious experience, MRI patients have become more aware of open MRI and have begun to request it more frequently. The combination of the increased popularity of MRI as a diagnostic test and the anxious patient's desire for open units require the professional in the open MRI field to become more sensitive to the patient's subjective experience and his or her psychological evaluation of that experience. Offering a state of the art open diagnostic procedure is not enough; the individual is lost sight of all too easily. Beyond offering the best quality open MRI scans, it is also necessary to address the patient's psychological response to the entire experience.

Medical technologies in general and MRI technology in particular have evolved rapidly since the late 1980s. Tests once available in only a few large medical centers are now in standard use, and discoveries presented as breakthroughs on the evening news have become standard outpatient procedures. Rapid advances in technology can come into direct conflict with the human psyche that has evolved over many centuries. Irrational fears of suffocation, claustrophobia, helplessness, and the unknown all echo in the collective unconscious of MRI patients. Potentially ill and vulnerable when they present for

S. R. Evers: Evers Psychological Associates, P.C., Manasquan, New Jersey

MRI, patients may find that their less rational selves surface under the pressures of the MRI examination.

As a psychologist and a clinician, my first awareness of MRI came from stories told to me by my patients. The stories have become increasingly frequent and have come from patients with a wide variety of psychological diagnoses. The psychological responses they describe have not been limited to a few truly claustrophobic responses but have precipitated anxiety that is multifaceted (2,3). The important issue is that MRI can trigger many different psychological conditions. In response to my growing population of MRI patients and at the request of a local MRI facility, I became involved in direct staff-sensitivity training focusing on the anxious and claustrophobic patient. This training eventually led to similar sensitivity presentations for corporate and management personnel who shape patient care policy for MRI centers. These experiences, heavily colored by my clinical focus, shape this chapter. This chapter provides a basic introduction to the psychology of the MRI patient. This overview is by no means exhaustive, nor is it directed at an audience of mental health professionals. Rather, it is designed for those personnel in the MRI field who, although experts in their own specialty, are still learning to manage the psychological responses of patients to MRI technology, which they themselves feel so comfortable with. That psychotherapy patients and those who seek mental health services tend to show a pattern of high use of medical services such as MRI only underscores the importance of understanding the psychology of these patients.

To put the MRI in psychological context, this chapter is divided into four sections. First, I briefly discuss the rapid growth of MRI usage and technology, which has precipitated the inclusion of MRI as part of our modern medical mythology. Second, I present an overview of the theory of how anxiety and stress act on patients. Also explored is how this claustrophobia and stress can cause anxiety, which can interact with a patient's preexisting psychological condition or perhaps even elicit a new one. These subjective feelings of the patient with regard to the MRI experience becomes the psychological focus more than are the specifics of the test and the results. Third, individual patient responses to MRI are discussed in more detail, based on specific psychological conditions, with case vignettes that detail several popular conditions. Finally, the chapter concludes with a proposal for a staff training model that addresses the psychological needs of the patient, with an eye toward clinical practicality and efficiency. With appropriate training, MRI personnel can meet the immediate psychological needs of the patient, helping him or her cope with the imaging process and meet the needs of the medical and technical staff with whom they interact.

MAGNETIC RESONANCE IMAGING AND MEDICAL MYTHOLOGY

MRI has rapidly become a staple among the tools of diagnostic testing. It is estimated that in 1996 alone, 9.8 million scans were done. Statistics for 1997 and 1998 were not available for inclusion here, but with the increased sales of MRI units and their growing availability we can only imagine the number of scans will be well over 10 million per year. Estimates of 1998 MRI unit sales show that more than half of the approximately 500 to 600 new units sold could be described as *open*. Along with this substantial growth in the number of scans, there has been an increase in the number of patients who experienced the procedure for the first time. That is, for the first time they had to face their fears and depend on MRI personnel to be sensitive to their needs and to address their irrational anxieties with understanding, confidence, and empathy.

This increase in MRI usage has led to its inclusion in our modern medical mythology. At one time, the idea of a heart transplant was unique—almost magical—and the surgeons who performed the procedure were mythic in stature. In the collective consciousness of the medically uninformed public, the procedure seemed like magic. Medical breakthroughs often gain this quasi-mythical state when they are new or unique. Many other medical technologies developed in the last few decades became part of this mythology for a time. Listening to or watching the evening news, we commonly hear about new medical procedures, findings, and research. The *New England Journal of Medicine* has even become a common news source. Heart-lung transplants, hand reattachments, laser surgery to allow vision without glasses, and laparoscopic procedures through tiny incisions have become commonplace. Each new technology goes through a period of almost mythologic proportion before it becomes accepted and eventually expected. MRI appears to be going through this same evolution, but uniquely it has become associated as much with its psychological responses as it has been with its diagnostic efficacy.

As I began to research this chapter, I did an Internet search using a popular search engine. When I searched for "claustrophobia," the first suggested Web site was that of a center offering the new open MRI. In fact, the most represented issues in the first 500 entries were different MRI sites and technologies designed to address or prevent the claustrophobia generated by the procedure. Many of the Web sites even seemed to guarantee that their open system would eliminate the issue of claustrophobia simply by design. This approach primarily focused on the open descriptor of the MRI unit while avoiding the possibility of a patient's subjective response. By virtue of the number of Web sites addressing the issue of MRI-related claustrophobia, we can see how linked the MRI procedure is to its psychological sequelae.

A popular television program that included an off-handed comment about claustrophobia and MRI in an episode further echoes this popular equation: When a patient walked out of the hospital against medical advice, one of the characters commented that "she was scheduled for an MRI, and people often get claustrophobic and leave." The MRI has become a popular topic of conversation, whether during a brief discussion over lunch or on a popular talk show. Along with this popularity, the equation of the MRI and its uncomfortable psychological consequences seems ubiquitous.

The association of a negative psychological consequence with MRI addresses the subjective nature of the psychological response. Often, our responses to events and situations are not necessarily related to the events themselves but to our subjective perception of the events. "The situation itself does not directly determine how they feel; their [the patients'] emotional response is mediated by their perception of the situation" (4). Not only are our personal experiences and preexisting psychological issues shape our expectations, they are also shaped by the popular media and our unique subjective interpretations and perceptions. These subjective interpretations can be formed by third-person comments from television shows or friends, such as "Aunt Martha had one of those MRIs and became magnetized for life. Yeah, she could never wear a watch again!" One patient commented to me after visiting some MRI-related Web sites on the Internet in preparation for his scheduled scan, "I guess there is something to worry about with all this talk of claustrophobia. I really never thought of it before."

CLAUSTROPHOBIC ANXIETY

Understanding a patient's psychological responses to MRI requires an understanding of several concepts:

1. We need to understand what anxiety is, how it feels, and how it is manifested in an individual. Anxiety is a basic fact of life, but as a concept it is often misused and has been popularized to the point that its meaning has become confused.
2. We need to become familiar with the concept of stress, how stress impacts the individual, and how our sensitivity to stress can be cumulative. Stress is also a term that is subject to overuse in common conversation, but it still is useful in understanding how we function and cope.

A combined understanding of these two basic concepts allows us to look at the specific anxiety usually attributed to the MRI, claustrophobic anxiety.

Anxiety

Fight-or-Flight Response

Centuries ago, when our ancestors lived in caves, there were many threats to their lives. Living was hard, and survival was the only rule. When a threat surfaced, only two choices existed—to fight or to run. Both called for a vast expenditure of energy. Those who did not have the energy probably ended up as dinner for some saber-toothed tiger (Fig. 2-1). Those who won the fight or ran the fastest

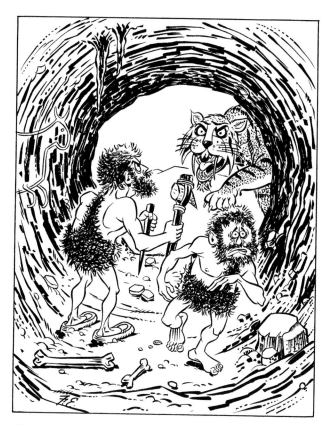

FIG. 2-1. Primitive origins of the fight-or-flight response.

became our forefathers. The fight-or-flight response was very adaptive. This response causes a massive release of adrenaline and corticosteroids, and these stress hormones trigger numerous bodily responses. They alter blood flow, causing peripheral capillary constriction. (That is the source of the old saying about getting "cold feet" when one is afraid.) The massive release of stress hormones causes hyperventilation; this rapid breathing, along with the increased activation of muscle tissue, gave our ancestors an extra edge for survival. This once adaptive response, however, has become the root of many psychological problems, specifically anxiety. The threat of saber-toothed tigers no longer exists, but the fight-or-flight mechanism persists. Now, the threats that trigger it are often psychological in nature, as our perception of a situation as threatening elicits the once appropriate coping mechanism. Unfortunately, with no one to fight and nowhere to run, we are stuck. We experience the gamut of disturbing and uncomfortable symptoms and often feel as if our very lives are threatened.

Anxiety versus Fear

One easy way to understand anxiety and put it in a more personal context is to think of a situation in which we are really afraid. Fear and anxiety are related in that we can see in a fear response the same mental and physical activation that occurs in anxiety. Consider the following example:

Imagine you are on vacation. It has been much too long since your last break, and you have been looking forward to the sun, the sand, and the quiet. You get into your hotel room and look out the window to see the beautiful beach, and you just can't wait to lie in the sun, sip a cool drink, and relax. You then open your suitcase to take out your bathing suit and feel something crawling on the back of your hand. Looking down, you see a spider. In a flash, you recall something in the travel brochure about the indigenous poisonous insects to be avoided, and you become afraid. Your heart begins to race, you begin to sweat, and you have the overwhelming urge to run out of the room, but you are convinced that if you move you're done for. In the seconds it takes the spider to walk off your hand you feel you have lived a lifetime. You have written your own obituary, rewritten your will, and thought of a hundred different ways to get rid of the spider and negated each one as impossible.

That is a classic fear response. It is a complex psychological and physical set of behaviors set in motion by a genuine stimulus.

Anxiety is similar to fear, but no real observable stimulus (e.g., the spider in the example above) exists. Rather than a real observable stimulus, anxiety is triggered by our perception of a situation or event as dangerous. Our perception of the situation and our evaluation of its level of threat elicit the fear response. To repeat our above example:

Imagine you are on vacation. It has been much too long since your last break and you have been looking forward to the sun, the sand, and the quiet. You get to your hotel room and look out the window to see the beautiful beach and you just can't wait to lie in the sun, sip a cool drink, and relax. Before you open your suitcase to take out your bathing suit you recall the travel brochure, and you freeze. You are sure that a poisonous spider is waiting to jump on your hand. You begin to sweat and hyperventilate, and you want to run away. You experience all the same feelings and emotions you would if the spider were real and on your hand, yet it is nowhere to be found.

The take-home lesson of this example is that anxiety can be triggered at any time and in any situation, because it is not the reality of the threat that causes the response. Rather, it is our perception of the situation and our evaluation of the threat.

Panic Attack

Panic attack, for those who have experienced one, is one of the most frightening events that can happen. In a matter of seconds and usually without significant warning, a flood of anxiety-related symptoms overwhelms one's ability to cope. These symptoms are the same as for fear and anxiety, only much more intense, and they usually follow a pattern of rapid escalation that reaches a peak in just a few minutes. A *panic attack* is defined as "a discrete period of intense fear or discomfort" that is accompanied by at least four of the following symptoms: palpitations, sweating, trembling, shortness of breath, choking feelings, chest pain, nausea, dizziness, derealization, fear of losing control, fear of dying, paresthesias, and chills or hot flashes (5). A panic attack is the most intense form of the anxiety response. It brings the primitive fight-or-flight mechanism to a new level. It is often one of the most frightening events in a person's life and can actually shape the behavior of a person who has one for years after the attack. It is not uncommon for someone to have just one full-blown panic or anxiety attack and seek treatment, often living in fear that the next attack will happen at any time and that he or she might not survive the next panic attack.

Phobias

With an understanding of fear, anxiety, and panic attack, we can look more specifically at phobias. *Phobias* are defined as persistent, marked fears and anxieties that are excessive or unreasonable. They can be triggered by a specific object or situation and may take the form of a panic attack (5). In essence, when we have a phobia, we have evaluated a situation, object, or event and labeled it as threatening—so threatening that it must be avoided at all costs. The stimulus we have labeled as threatening and become afraid of makes us want to fight or flee. It triggers the symptoms of fear and anxiety and the belief that only by avoiding the stimulus will we be able to escape the overwhelming, uncomfortable feelings we are having. People can have anxiety and develop phobias triggered by any stimulus. Claustrophobia is the specific phobia of closed spaces.

The definition of claustrophobia is specific, and although it successfully describes some MRI-induced anxiety responses, it does apply to all. The traditional tube-type, the short-bore, and even the open MRI unit can be perceived as closed in and confining. Furthermore, it is the perception—not necessarily the fact—that can trigger the anxiety and claustrophobia. As a patient lies in the confined space and is told not to move, he or she can evaluate the situation as threatening. This evaluation can then trigger the same response that our imaginary spider triggered in the previous scenario. The truly claustrophobic patient believes it when he or she says, "If I don't get out of here right away, I'm going to die." Not all patients with claustrophobic anxiety have true claustrophobia. For many, if not most, the claustrophobic anxiety triggers other psychological and emotional conditions.

Beyond those patients who have a genuine claustrophobic response to MRI, many others present whose response does not follow the pattern of a full-fledged claustrophobia but who are nonetheless troubled by the procedure. These patients may experience the fight-or-flight response to some degree and may also exhibit some of the symptoms of anxiety, but their response is less intense. Instead, their responses may involve increased generalized anxiety, such as increased restlessness, difficulty concentrating, irritability, unexplained fatigue, muscle tension, and a feeling of being on edge. Also involved are other psychological symptoms, secondary to the MRI-related increased anxiety, that exacerbate preexisting psychological conditions.

Stress

An understanding of the concept of stress is also critical to the consideration of MRI-related claustrophobic anxiety. Stress as a working concept in psychology began with the pioneering work of Hans Selye, who discussed how, in addition to a physical response, every demand on a person evokes a nonspecific stress response (6). This nonspecific stress response involves many different body systems and causes a person to use energy—energy that is in limited supply—to cope with the stressor. *Stressor*, therefore, is the term used to describe anything that a person uses energy to deal with. The following are all relevant examples of stressors: being ill or potentially ill and needing an MRI, being asked to lie still for an extended period in an unfamiliar device, being positioned to a head coil. As is illustrated in the example below, the entire experience of being ill, seeking care, and undergoing a scan involves many different stressors that must be coped with. In an evaluation of claustrophobic anxiety and MRI, it is important to be aware that the patient who presents for a scan may well be under extreme stress. A patient who has been sick for some time and who is asked to undergo yet another test to elicit possibly alarming information about his or her condition may already be exhausting his or her emotional reserves simply to cope with the existing stressors.

Stress seeks the weakest link: Just as a piece of metal being bent eventually breaks at its weakest spot, a patient's ability to cope with stress shows at his or her psychological weak spot. The patient can perceive the stressors (in this case, preexisting illness and an upcoming MRI procedure) negatively and consider them a threat. This patient may not have a history of claustrophobia, claustrophobic anxiety, or panic attacks. He or she may not have previously conceived of an MRI as a threat or as an anxiety-inducing circumstance. The accumulating stressors and resulting weakened ability to cope, however, combine to increase the likelihood of a difficult anxiety response, such as a direct panic response, a more generalized anxiety response, or an exacerbation of preexisting psychological issues. The simple fight-or-flight response that once saved us from the saber-toothed tiger can precipitate unwanted effects as well.

Hypothetical Case Example

The following hypothetical scenario draws on the foregoing discussion of the psychology of stress and the anxiety

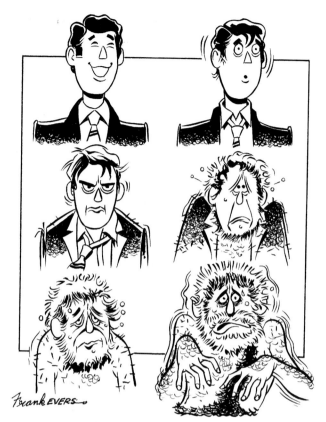

FIG. 2-2. Mounting stressors combine, increasing a less-than-rational response to the magnetic resonance imaging as the more primitive fight-or-flight response becomes evident.

response to put these factors in perspective. Note how each stressor depletes Bob's energy (i.e., ability to cope) and increases his susceptibility to experiencing a problem with his MRI scan. Bob has never really had claustrophobic fears or feelings before. Sure, Bob had read or heard about claustrophobic feelings, but he had never felt any of those feelings. He had been in crowded elevators and visited theme parks on school vacations without incident.

Consider the following set of stressors facing Bob:

1. Bob wakes up on Monday morning and feels ill. He calls work and talks to his new supervisor, who is not very sympathetic when Bob tells him he will not be coming in to work. Bob then calls his family doctor and is told that the doctor is no longer covered by his insurance and that he must call the 800 number on the back of his insurance card to find a new doctor. After waiting for what seems like hours in a voice-mail maze, he is given the number of a physician across town and told to call to make an appointment. Detailing his insurance information and medical history to several anonymous voices, Bob's appointment is scheduled for Wednesday.

2. Bob has to call work back and tell them he will be out until at least Wednesday. After procrastinating for a while, he

makes the call. This time, he is lucky and leaves a message on his supervisor's voice-mail, hoping he won't call back.

3. After a few days of feeling sick, he finds himself in the doctor's office on Wednesday. The waiting room is full of strangers, who look much sicker than he feels. After standing for half an hour, he finds a chair. As he sits down, the nurse calls his name. After sitting in a tiny examining room for some time, he is finally seen by the doctor and in 90 seconds is referred for an MRI. He has trouble validating the insurance card on the way out of the office, and he finally returns home to await the scheduling of his scan.

4. On Thursday, he calls work again and is given the "cold shoulder." Seeking support from friends, he makes a few phone calls, only to be greeted with new horror stories about MRI experiences.

5. On Friday he presents at the MRI center. Although he may not have been claustrophobic or anxious at the beginning of the week, his level of stress has risen and he is now much more vulnerable to claustrophobic anxiety (Fig. 2-2).

CASE VIGNETTES

Case vignettes from actual patients accompanied by discussion of the psychological conditions in evidence can better elucidate the varied impact an MRI can have. In discussing these cases, I point to some of the possibilities, focusing only on the trigger of claustrophobic anxiety. Diagnostic criteria for the psychological conditions discussed are provided. The staff training proposal outlined in the section that follows these case vignettes addresses these cases and has been shaped by my patients' own feedback as well as by research findings.

Classic Claustrophobia

Mr. J was a 71-year-old father of two. In World War II, he served in the invasion of Europe and landed in France on D-Day plus 1 as an army combat medic. In addition to his medic training, he was trained and licensed as an x-ray technologist. He had an involved medical history that included heart disease, diabetes, partially detached retina, and hypertension. His heart condition had been the result of childhood rheumatic fever and he had undergone many medical procedures throughout his life, beginning in childhood and including a quadruple cardiac bypass. Although he did not like medical testing and treatment, he had no prior difficulties with any medical test. When he was referred for an MRI, he didn't even question the nature of the test. He later commented that it was the shortest MRI on record: He lasted approximately 20 seconds in the MRI chamber. As soon as the technologist began to slide the table into the machine, he panicked and began to yell. He was immediately pulled out of the MRI chamber. "I just stood up and walked. They are going to have to find some other way to see what's wrong."

DIAGNOSTIC CRITERIA: Specific Phobia (5)

- Excessive or unreasonable fear cued by the presence or anticipation of a specific object
- Exposure to the feared stimulus causes anxiety
- Fear is recognized as excessive and unreasonable
- Feared situation is avoided
- Marked distress about the phobic reaction

Mr. J's response follows the classic claustrophobia/panic pattern. He did not anticipate any problems with the procedure and, because of his medical training and history, was very familiar with diagnostic testing. On discussion after the scan, he commented that he needed to get out because he felt that he could not breathe. This statement is typical of one of the most popular claustrophobic fears, suffocation (7). Mr. J did not undergo another MRI even when he was offered open MRI. Although he did not show a generalization of his phobia and did not have problems in other closed-in or tight areas, the phobic response to the MRI continued. He did not seek further treatment for this phobia, but he avoided the MRI, and his physician was forced to look into other diagnostic tools to address his condition.

Mr. J's response and failure to complete his MRI point to several important psychological issues. The incidence of persistent claustrophobia resulting from the MRI procedure was reported as early as 1988 (2). As recently as 1996, this incidence was echoed by the findings that 92% of patients who could not complete MRI experienced panic attacks and that most (83%) also reported having panic attacks 1 month after the MRI (8). The importance of these statistics lies in the fact that, in essence, the testing for a medical condition has become the cause of a psychological condition that can be persistent and require treatment in its own right.

Generalized Anxiety Disorder

Ms. C is a 41-year-old married mother of four. She works part-time and manages her duties as mother and employee relatively successfully. She was referred for treatment because of an increased feeling of anxiety that she felt came on suddenly and for no reason. During the initial phase of her treatment, it became apparent that she had an unusual fear of cancer. She had lost her mother and a very close aunt to the disease. It was eventually learned that, in the month before her psychological referral, she had had a cancer scare, which was the result of her experience during an MRI procedure. She had been having some lower back pain and was referred for an MRI to assist in diagnosis. Although she reported no trouble with the procedure, she was unprepared for the time it took, and during the testing she was a bit anxious that she would miss her daughter's school bus. What bothered her and became the cause of her anxiety was the fact that as she lay in the MRI she thought she had begun to hear sounds. At first, she dismissed them as part of the apparatus or the technologists talking. Over time, however, they began to sound like "bone scan, bone scan, bone scan . . ." and she became sure that they had discovered cancer and just weren't telling her. Ms. C believed that "You only need a bone scan when you have cancer." Even with medical reassurance she continued to have troubling fears of cancer and reported hearing the "bone scan" chant days after the test was done.

DIAGNOSTIC CRITERIA: Generalized Anxiety Disorder (5)

- Excessive worry and anxiety
- Worry and anxiety that are difficult to control
- Three or more of the following symptoms: restlessness, easy fatigability, difficulty concentrating, irritability, muscle tension, sleep difficulties

DIAGNOSTIC CRITERIA: Obsessive Features (5)

- Recurrent and persistent thoughts
- Recognition that the thoughts are self-generated
- Thoughts are not simply excessive worries about real-life problems

Ms. C's condition showed a generalized pattern of anxiety. She did not feel any anxiety at the time of the MRI and reported that the scan went well except for the sounds. Although the sounds made by MRI units have been commented on by many of my other patients, her comments are unique. Ms. C began treatment as a result of the MRI procedure and continued for some time after her anxiety began. Her anxiety began with the MRI, then extended to her family's medical history, and then her perception of her medical risk seemed to free float over different topics, which is the usual course of this condition until it is resolved. She also had an obsessive pattern of thinking—the replaying in her mind of the "bone scan" sound. Treatment lasted for approximately 9 months, first on a weekly basis and then twice monthly for the last 2 months.

Ms. Y is a 46-year-old white woman. She is the mother of two adult children and has been married for more than 23 years. She is overweight and has been diagnosed as having a generalized anxiety disorder. She was referred for an MRI subsequent to a minor stroke. Her mother had had several strokes beginning in Ms. Y's childhood and spent most of her adult life bedridden. When Ms. Y learned that she was to have yet another medical test, she was not concerned. She had had numerous medical tests over the years since a minor heart attack, and because she was recovering well from the stroke, she felt confident that this test would be no problem. In her next psychotherapy visit after the MRI she related the following about the experience: "When I went into the room where the MRI was, I was surprised. No one had told me that I would have to get into something like that. I looked around for the Vaseline because the only way I was going to fit into that hole was if they greased me up and slid me in. I really thought they were kidding until they told me to lie down. Then

the test seemed to take forever. The whole time I was worrying: Could they get me out?" Subsequent to the testing she reported that her anxiety was heightened for several days and that, although things were fine now, she would not want to have another MRI examination any time soon, especially if she would have time to think about it in advance—now that she knew what it was. She commented that the next time, if there were a next time, she would get an "open" one. When asked, she couldn't say what that meant except that it sounded new, fast, and open, "like sitting in this office."

Ms. Y presents another case of generalized anxiety disorder but with a unique twist. She is overweight and quite sensitive about it. During the course of treatment, she revealed that, in addition to being afraid that she would get stuck in the MRI chamber, she was afraid that everyone would laugh at her. She built up a strong aversion to the closed MRI system after her experience and held out the anticipatory hope that the "open MRI" by its very title would be open, "like sitting in this office." Although she has not yet had to undergo another MRI, work needs be done to correct her perception before she receives another scan. Ms. Y continues in therapy at this time and has recognized that an open MRI is not like sitting in my office. She has been shown pictures of several open devices and has reframed her thinking. This case highlights the importance of patient education before an MRI and especially before a second procedure if the first caused anxiety.

Posttraumatic Stress Disorder

Mr. M is a 72-year-old, recently widowed father of two. He is a World War II navy veteran who was highly decorated for his service in the Pacific. He has been diagnosed with posttraumatic stress disorder and depression. He was referred for his first MRI because of a shoulder injury. He reportedly slipped on the ice and landed on his arm and shoulder. The MRI was part of the diagnostic testing required to evaluate the need for surgery. Mr. M showed no anxiety before the testing and even mentioned that he was going to have an open MRI. He wasn't sure what that was, but he said that the nurse who told him about it made it sound special. At his next therapy session after the open MRI, he reported that everything went pretty well with the scan, although it was very long. He was afraid that his ride wouldn't wait for him because he had expected to be there only 15 to 20 minutes. He also stated that he was glad that the test wasn't any longer than it was (approximately 40 minutes) because the "longer you are in that thing, the closer the top and bottom get. It's like the top comes down slowly. If I had been in there any longer I would have been squashed."

DIAGNOSTIC CRITERIA: Posttraumatic Stress Disorder (5)

- Exposure to a traumatic event that involves actual or threatened death or serious injury and evoked intense fear, helplessness, or horror

- Persistent reexperiencing of the traumatic event
- Persistent avoidance of stimuli associated with the trauma
- Persistent autonomic arousal

Mr. M's response was unique in that it added a new dimension to the popular fear of suffocation: that of confinement (7). His naval career put him in numerous battles in the Pacific Campaign. He often talks about how small the ships seem when out on the ocean. He also discusses the time he was locked up by mistake for a breach of discipline. The experience of being locked below decks during a potential combat encounter made him feel trapped. The trapped feeling was the subject of his next few sessions and precipitated vivid nightmares and heightened daytime anxiety for several weeks. Another interesting facet of his response to the open-MRI procedure was his perception that the top of the unit moves down over time. Although this is not the case, it is a good example of the importance of understanding a patient's subjective response to the MRI procedure.

Mr. D is a 51-year-old, married father of three. He was referred for a psychological evaluation and treatment after his first MRI. He served in the U.S. Army during the Vietnam War. Mr. D reported that he had fallen on a flight of stairs while going into his basement carrying some boxes. He developed significant back pain after the fall and went to his doctor. He was referred for MRI. He reported that he was a little anxious at the time of the test, but that overall it was just uncomfortable to lie there for so long. In the nights after the testing he began to be plagued by nightmares of his wartime duty, which involved exploring and often fighting in the dark of the enemy tunnel complexes. These recollections began to intensify and became intrusive thoughts and flashbacks that were spontaneously occurring during the day when he eventually sought treatment. He was diagnosed with posttraumatic stress disorder, delayed onset, with his military duty as the initial stressor and the MRI procedure as the proximate trigger.

Like Mr. M, Mr. D suffers from posttraumatic stress disorder, but in Mr. D's case the MRI procedure precipitated a preexisting condition that had been dormant for many years. Posttraumatic stress disorder cannot uncommonly be hidden and its onset delayed. The tight space, the stress of his back pain, and the feelings of helplessness that resulted from having to lie still for the scan all played a part in his posttraumatic recall. Using the concept of coping with stress, we can postulate that the stress of the scan and the similarity of the scanner gantry to the close quarters he experienced in combat led to the aggravation of his underlying condition. Mr. D became involved in individual psychotherapy and joined a veterans' discussion group. His treatment is ongoing.

Depression

Ms. R is a 53-year-old, twice-married mother of two. Her first husband, the father of her children, died a number of years ago. She sought treatment for depression subsequent to the death of her 12-year-old daughter in an auto accident and her own medical complications resulting from that accident. Ms. R is employed as a yoga instructor. Sensitized as she was by the medical treatment of her daughter, she was quite anxious about the need for MRI. She commented, however, "I can do anything for 20 minutes." A friend had told her of her own experience with the procedure, which was approximately that long. When she was told at scheduling that the open procedure would take more than 45 minutes, she became extremely agitated and refused to undergo the test until it could be rescheduled for only 20 minutes.

DIAGNOSTIC CRITERIA: Depression (Selected Symptoms) (5)

- Depressed mood most of the day, nearly every day
- Marked diminished interest or pleasure in almost all activities
- Fatigue
- Feelings of worthlessness
- Difficulty concentrating

Ms. R's case is interesting for several reasons. Her depression had a specific trigger. The reality of her loss is difficult to cope with, so she has made psychological deals with herself to make it through the day. Each new stressor is coped with by an internal compromise and a concrete agreement. She can make it through the day only minute by minute. Although the open system is more patient-friendly and quieter than are closed MRI systems and it seems to be the unit of choice, her ability to cope depends on the length of the procedure. Therefore, in Ms. R's case, the length of the procedure is much more important that the increased openness of the scanner. A feeling of helplessness is one of the subjective components of depression. Patient education and prescreening would have helped her cope with the procedure more successfully. Realizing that she could have chosen a high-field or open MRI and understanding in advance the duration of the scanning procedure would have enabled her to create a more successful internal contract that most likely would have resulted in a more successful scan.

Substance Abuse

Mr. B is 31 years old. He was married once and divorced. He has no children. He describes himself as "in recovery" from years of alcohol and substance abuse and as a dedicated Alcoholics Anonymous (AA) member. He was referred for treatment because of a dysthymia (i.e., chronic minor depression) that became evident after his substance abuse ceased. He was referred for MRI because of an upper-back injury that occurred at work and had become part of a workers' compensation issue. He was very anxious about tight or closed spaces and often commented that he liked construction work because he could be outside. When he learned of the necessity for an MRI, he was anxious. Recognizing this anxiety, his doctor scheduled an open procedure. When Mr. B called to schedule the procedure, he was reassured that he shouldn't worry, because "things would be fine." He arrived for the test and was told that he would be given something to alleviate his anxiety about the procedure. Although he acknowledged his claustrophobic tendencies and anxiety about the test, he was more concerned that he would violate his sobriety by taking a "mood-altering" drug, a direct violation of the AA program that had, in his opinion, saved his life. He was unable to stay for the test, and he now refuses to return for an MRI until he can do so without medication.

Mr. B's case addresses another issue in MRI: the use of premedication. Although premedication is reported to be effective at alleviating patient anxiety and, if used appropriately, in facilitating a successful scan, it can pose other problems. Mr. B eventually returned for an open MRI after several relaxation training and systematic desensitization sessions. *Systematic desensitization* is the graded exposure of a patient to progressively more anxiety-producing situations that approximate the feared situation. This successive exposure to mental images that gradually increase anxiety while the patient is in a controlled, relaxed state is a classic treatment method for phobias and has been shown to work in some cases to facilitate the successful completion of an MRI examination (9).

Mr. B's substance abuse is in remission, and thus he no longer meets the criteria for that diagnosis. He, like many other successful AA and NA members, has become a believer in the tenets of the program and adheres to them religiously. Although there may be no medical reason he cannot take the premedication, his fervent belief that it could cause him to relapse became the problem.

STAFF TRAINING MODEL

Understanding the subjective nature of the psychological experience and recognizing the pressure of delivering high-quality, efficient medical treatment makes the issue of radiology staff training more important than ever before. With more MRI scanners in use every year and more scans being done every day, the demand for efficient use of the technology is high. A new MRI machine can cost between $800,000 and $1.5 million, and with build out and installation the cost rises to between $1 million and $2 million. An investment of this amount places a certain pressure on the staff of a facility to make maximum use of the equipment. Cancelled appointments and failed scans due to psychological issues are unwelcome developments.

A training model should address the range of patient needs. I have organized a model based on the points of contact each patient has with the medical system in the course of preparing for and completing an MRI examination.

Points of Contact

Staff training for each point of contact should be with the expressed aim of positively shaping the patient's subjective expectations of the MRI, whether open or closed. The first step is to identify those patients with a history of anxiety and claustrophobia or at risk due to overwhelming stress. Next, every member of the staff is trained to be sensitive to the signals that an anxious patient may give and aware of immediate interventions that can thwart a bad experience. When anxiety or fear responses are noted, the staff can intervene to minimize the damage and either complete the scan or make an appropriate referral. A mental health professional, if no one on staff is so trained, can often treat and desensitize the unsuccessful patient to MRI so that he or she is able to complete the next attempted procedure. The use of medication is also a topic that may be discussed between the patient and the MRI facility's medical staff at the point of contact or with the initial referring physician.

Referral for Magnetic Resonance Imaging

Often, the first point of contact in the MRI referral process is the primary care doctor. The physician or specialty provider who makes the initial referral can have a significant influence on the potential patient's psychological response to the MRI. Optimally, the referring physician is calm, supportive, and concerned when discussing the referral and serves to start the patient off on a positive note. However, this optimal handling is often *not* seen. I have had a patient come into my office and ask me what an MRI was. At his referring doctor's office, no one had offered to explain the procedure to him. As we discussed MRI, he did not know whether he was scheduled for an open or closed scan. After further explanation of the two options, he stated, "I think I want one of them [open MRI]." At the first point of contact, the procedure could have been discussed, and the patient could have been given a brochure describing open MRI. The first information a patient receives shapes his or her subjective evaluation of the entire experience, and the initial point of contact may be one of the most important moments before an MRI is undertaken, because it can set the tone for all that follows. An informative, positive brochure describing the nature of the procedure, the time it takes, and what can be expected goes a long way toward creating positive and realistic expectations. Such literature also serves as the first piece of official, tangible, or medically valid information that can counteract the commonly encountered equation of MRI with claustrophobia.

Appointment Scheduling

The next point of contact is the scheduling department or secretarial staff. Training here needs to focus on the need to provide realistic, positive descriptions. Patients' psychological expectations are shaped by casual comments and attitudinal nuances. Given that patients calling to schedule an appointment may be in a heightened state of stress and thus more vulnerable than usual, the tenor and content of the scheduling conversation influence patients' subjective perception of the scan they are about to undergo. This need for positive interactions seems self-evident, but the importance of training staff in this regard is underscored by the following actual conversation from a staff training meeting I conducted: A facility manager told of a new patient who had recently called the facility to schedule an MRI examination. The patient told the staff member making the appointment that she had chosen that open facility because, when she had called another MRI center to schedule an appointment, the receptionist described the scanning procedure as follows: "If you think you'd have no trouble lying in a coffin you won't have any problems with the MRI." Realistic, optimistic descriptions that do not negate patients' fears can be important in making them more comfortable with the upcoming MRI. Lying to patients, even about minor issues, can have serious consequences. Just as the MRI gantry should not be described as a coffin, we do patients a disservice when we dismiss the procedure by saying, "It's nothing." Even well-intentioned lies can cause stress and lead patients to question our credibility.

Noting Specific Patient Concerns

The initial scheduler can also make note of a patient's concerns and append such notes to the patient's chart. Doing so allows these concerns to be addressed by the technical staff when the patient arrives. One way to reduce a patient's stress is to take a personal approach, for example: "When you called to schedule your MRI, you commented that you are afraid of loud noises, so before we start your scan let me show you what it will sound like." A simple reassurance from a forewarned technologist can make the process much more smooth. Many anxious patients find it comforting to bring a family member to the facility; this option can be suggested if a concern is voiced.

Case Example

The following example underscores the importance of the patient-staff interaction and the need for realistic information when an appointment is made. A patient of mine who underwent open MRI recounts his experience as follows:

I'm a big guy (6 ft 3 in., 345 lb), and I had heard that these MRI things were kind of tight to fit in, so I asked the girl when I was scheduled. She said that I shouldn't worry because I was scheduled for an open one. When I heard "open," I thought OPEN. When I got there I felt that I had been spoken to by a car salesman who tells you there is a lot of room in the back seat.

The scan was successful but the feeling that developed when he saw the MRI equipment made him more tense. We had been working on self-hypnosis, and he used that technique to remain relaxed and calm during the scan (10).

Presentation for the Appointment

Without even realizing it, patients presenting for their scans offer a wealth of information to the technical staff. Beyond the fears they may voice directly, their body language and presentation also provide clues. Fears that are directly voiced should be answered just as directly. For example, "I'm afraid of closed spaces," is a common patient comment that may need to be explored immediately. As discussed, anticipatory anxiety and subject expectation contribute much of what the patient brings to the scanning session. These feelings manifest in different ways in different people. Although we are all subject to the same fight-or-flight mechanism, it sometimes manifests directly as tension and fear, whereas at other times it manifests as irritability. Often, the difficult patient is merely anxious. With the pressures placed on staff to make efficient use of MRI units, staff members may occasionally pressure irritable, anxious patients to proceed, in an effort to move patients through the procedure as quickly as possible. In so doing, staff may overlook the fact that the patient is merely afraid. One of my patients described his experience as follows:

I walked out. They tried to push me down the hall. I think they were running late or something. No one pushes me! I felt like a cow going to the slaughter. When I tried to ask a question, they seemed distracted and you know I never had one of those things before.

When staff members are sensitive to the symptoms of anxiety and panic discussed earlier, under Claustrophobic Anxiety, they are more likely to understand the information that anxious patients often unconsciously convey when presenting for an MRI. Cold hands, clammy palms, stiff muscles, hesitancy in walking down the hall to the scanner suite, excessive slowness not based on a medical condition, overly dilated pupils, rapid heart rate, and unexplained sweating are all signs of an anxious patient. The difficulty in addressing the needs of patients exhibiting such symptoms lies in the sheer breadth of possible manifestations of anxiety. For many people, cold hands and chills are a direct manifestation, and a blanket may help reduce the discomfort. For those with a claustrophobic fear of suffocation (7), increased airflow during the scan may allay their fear. Claustrophobic patients often comment that "there doesn't seem to be enough air in the room," and although irrational, this belief precipitates their panic. When staff members carefully listen to and observe patients as they prepare for the examination, it is often possible to correctly assess and meet patients' needs, thus reducing the number of concomitant stressors and improving patients' abilities to cope with the MRI process.

During the Scanning Procedure

Central to the training model outlined here is the assertion that each step of the process is a point at which medical personnel can intervene to reduce patients' anxiety and fear. Because stress often builds gradually, each step that MRI personnel facilitate and each symptom that is addressed reduce the likelihood of serious problems stemming from the scan. Once scanning begins, personnel can continue to have a positive impact on patients' subjective perception of the process. Some of my patients underwent MRI at facilities that have a technologist stay with the patient in the scanning room, offering a caring touch as the scan progresses, a technique that seems quite effective. One patient described his experience with this technique, which also places additional stress on the staff:

When I got there, I told them I was kind of afraid. The technologist told me she would be with me the whole time, and I felt better. Once she slid me under the top, she asked if I was okay. I said, "Yes." Then I asked what was going to happen next and she wasn't there. I panicked and said, "Get me out of here!"

This scan was over before it began. Apparently, the staff member had to leave momentarily for some reason. A brief comment to the patient would have probably helped. Unfortunately, staffs' familiarity with the scanning process can cause them, despite the best intentions, to occasionally lose focus on the patient, often with negative results.

A variety of interventions can help allay a patient's growing claustrophobic discomfort. The technologist's ongoing dialogue with the patient keeps the personal touch alive. Music and other individualized types of intervention already in use in many facilities help make the process less stressful. Several patients of mine have asked for relaxation tapes custom made for them and found them very helpful. Further work with this method seems indicated, given that successfully trained patients can address their anxiety without medication and without putting additional stress on the technical staff. It has also been suggested that a staff member at each facility be identified and trained in specific skills to assist these anxious patients. Simple relaxation training at the time of the scan and positive visualization can also contribute a more positive overall experience.

The Personal Touch

The value of the personal touch cannot be overemphasized. Whether it is a family member in the room or a staff member with a reassuring voice addressing individual concerns, any intervention that reduces patient stress reduces the likelihood of a claustrophobic anxiety event overwhelming the patient.

Premedication

Premedication is a popular and effective means of addressing patients' claustrophobic and anxious fears. For several reasons, this approach is not always as simple as it may first appear. The earlier case vignette dealing with substance abuse and recovery described one possible barrier to premedication. Many anxious patients fear loss of control, and although a minor tranquilizer may seem to make the scan easier, it may also exacerbate patients' "I'm not myself" feeling and backfire. Additionally, the complex medication regimens of some patients can make it difficult to avoid the larger problem of a negative drug interaction.

The primary care physician who is familiar with the patient's history may best handle premedication. He or she is also most likely to be appraised of a patient's current medications and previously unsuccessful drugs. This physician may also be able to premedicate before the scheduled scan. The following example points to the need for this type of procedure:

A claustrophobic patient presented for her scan and, having identified her anxious state, she was assured that she would be given medication. When she arrived, and after a brief wait in the reception area, she was given what she described as a Valium tablet. Within minutes, she was moved to the scanning suite and the scanning began. Although she completed the scan, she later said, "I don't think the medication worked 'til I got home." She also had some trouble driving home after the procedure and wished that she had been told to bring someone with her to drive, because she felt that the medication had an impact on her driving.

Had she been medicated before the scan by taking a minor tranquilizer 1 or more hours in advance and brought a friend or family member to drive her, her overall experience would have been more positive and less stressful.

Children may offer an added complication with regard to MRI imaging. Although premedication is often used, it can produce problematic side effects (11–13). Special care must be taken, and detailed information should be given to parents before and after the procedure to reduce traumatic anxiety. Parents' preexisting beliefs and evaluations of MRI will also color their children's responses. In addition, children need an explanation of the procedure that is geared to their intellectual level. It may be especially difficult for them to lie still for the scan, especially in an open scanner, with its longer acquisition times. Rescheduling and rescanning a traumatized child can be very difficult.

Ongoing Training

Staff and sensitivity training should be an ongoing process. As with many other endeavors, although it is often easy to generate initial enthusiasm, the difficulty is in keeping that enthusiasm alive and fresh over time. Because much of the work with anxious and claustrophobic patients is in the interpersonal arena and because the professional staffs of MRI centers are also subject to financial stressors and time pressures, training needs to be ongoing. Many of the skills developed to address the needs of anxious patients may help relax less anxious patients more effectively as well. A calmer patient usually results in a more successful scan.

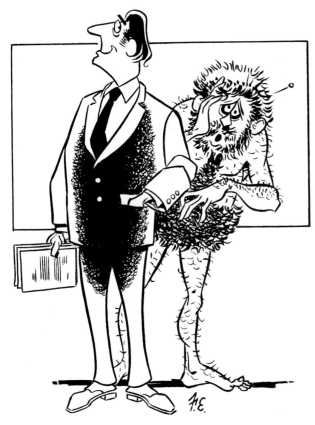

FIG. 2-3. Beneath the surface of every twenty-first–century human lies the less than rational psychological fears that are our emotional heritage.

I have found that initial training followed by periodic refresher courses keep the skills of MRI center personnel sharp and enhances patient success.

DIRECTIONS FOR THE FUTURE

Little formal psychological research has been undertaken in the area of open MRI. Due to its relative newness and the nature of the publishing process, few articles have directly addressed patients' responses to this new technology. Claustrophobic anxiety is a common response to closed scanners and may well be seen with short-bore units, owing to their similar designs. The recognition that open MRI scanners, by their very design, may reduce the incidence and severity of claustrophobia and claustrophobic anxiety, however, does not eliminate the need to address patients' psychological reality. Further research continues to be needed to explore this concept, although anecdotal reports indicate that the open design has helped significantly. Continued improvements in technology will attempt to address the anxiety of the claustrophobically sensitive patient. However, owing to the nature of the human condition and the subjective psychological world each of us inhabits, these improvements can only go so far. Humans are all subject to a psychology that is subject to irrational thoughts and fears, anxiety, and panic, as well as the stressors that increase susceptibility to them. Medical personnel always should be aware of the psychological responses of patients and, with awareness and sensitivity, medical providers can deliver less threatening and more effective medical treatment. Beneath the surface of every twenty-first–century human lies the less than rational psychological fears that are our emotional heritage (Fig. 2-3).

REFERENCES

1. Kaplan H, Sadock B. *Comprehensive textbook of psychiatry*, 4th ed. Baltimore, MD: Williams & Wilkins, 1985.
2. Fishbain D, Goldberg M, Labbe E, et al. Long-term claustrophobia following magnetic resonance imaging. *Am J Psychiatry* 1988;145: 1038–1039.
3. Katz R, Wilson L, Frazer N. Anxiety and its determinants in patients undergoing magnetic resonance imaging. *J Behav Ther Exp Psychiatry* 1994;25:131–134.
4. Beck J. *Cognitive therapy: basics and beyond*. New York: Guilford, 1995.
5. American Psychiatric Association. *Diagnostic and Statistical Manual of Mental Disorders*, 4th ed. Washington: American Psychiatric Association, 1994.
6. Charlesworth E, Nathan R. *Stress management: a comprehensive guide to wellness*. New York: Atheneum, 1984.
7. Harris H, Robinson J, Menzies R. Evidence for fear of restriction and fear of suffocation as components of claustrophobia. *Behav Res Ther* 1999;37:155–159.
8. Koechling U, Spevack M, Gerstein S, et al. Panic attacks while undergoing the magnetic resonance imaging scan (MRI). Paper presentation August 12, 1996, Metro Toronto Convention Center. http://www.apa.org/releases/mri.html.
9. Klonoff E, Janata J, Kaufman B. The use of systematic desensitization to overcome resistance to magnetic resonance imaging (MRI) scanning. *J Behav Ther Exp Psychiatry* 1986;17:189–192.
10. Friday P, Kubal W. Magnetic resonance imaging: improved patient tolerance utilizing medical hypnosis. *Am J Clin Hypn* 1990;33:80–84.
11. Greenberg SB, Faerber EN, Aspinall CL, Adams RC. High-dose chloral hydrate sedation for children undergoing MR imaging: safety and efficacy in relation to age. *AJR Am J Roentgenol* 1993;161:639–641.
12. Greenberg SB, Faerber EN, Radke JL, Aspinall CL, Adams RC, Mercer-Wilson DD. Sedation of difficult to sedate children undergoing MR imaging: value of thioridazine as an adjunct to chloral hydrate. *AJR Am J Roentgenol* 1994;163:165–168.
13. Rosenberg D, et al. Magnetic resonance imaging of children without sedation: preparation with stimulation. *J Acad Child Adolesc Psychiatry* 1997;36:853–859.

Open MRI,
edited by Peter A. Rothschild and Debra Reinking Rothschild.
Lippincott Williams & Wilkins. Philadelphia © 2000.

CHAPTER 3

Open Magnetic Resonance Imaging: A Practical Perspective

Terry Duggan-Jahns

A challenging new technology, open magnetic resonance imaging (MRI), has become quite popular. Patients as well as referring physicians now ask for and demand this technology as an alternative to a conventional MRI examination on a closed MRI system. It has become a specialized area of MRI, with its own considerations and concerns. Setting up a successful open MRI practice requires consideration of many factors, including equipment selection, protocol selection and imaging capabilities, marketing, suite design, staffing and staff training, patient concerns and assumptions, and available sedation methods. Each of these considerations is discussed in the sections that follow.

EQUIPMENT SELECTION

Choosing the correct equipment for your practice is essential. Although often less expensive than closed, open MRI systems are very expensive to purchase and maintain. A host of diverse questions must be answered before an open MRI system can be selected.

Role and Focus of the Equipment and Facility

The selection of low- versus mid-field strength, magnet configuration, and magnet type (permanent or resistive) needs to be taken into account. Will this system be placed in a stand-alone imaging center or within a hospital? Will this be an additional or secondary system to an already established MRI center, or will this purchase be for a primary MRI system in an imaging center? The costs associated with these options are factors in decisions reached.

What is your primary focus for this purchase? Attracting obese, claustrophobic, or special needs patients? Muscu-

loskeletal imaging or neuroimaging? What imaging capabilities do you need: fast spin echo, fluid attenuated inversion recovery, magnetic resonance angiography, kinematic, interventional, phase array capabilities, and so forth? What image resolution factors are important to your practice: gradient strength, small fields of view and small slice-thickness capabilities? What types of coils are available and come with the system, and which types must be purchased separately? Are the coils themselves restrictive, and do they create further discomfort to the already anxious patient? How many patients will you need to scan per day, and what is the economic break-even point? The answers to these questions determine the qualities and capabilities to be evaluated as you investigate the purchase of an open MRI system.

Practical, Day-to-Day Considerations

Site visits during the evaluative process are extremely important. They allow radiologists to evaluate image quality in a clinical setting. Site visits also provide an opportunity to talk with technologists who have experience working with a particular equipment vendor. It is extremely beneficial to include your chief technologist in a site visit because it is important to gain the technologist's perspective on the equipment's ease of operation, patient and coil positioning, and through-put capabilities.

The following questions may also require consideration: Can larger or elderly patients easily get on and off the table? What is the recommended table weight limit? How big is the opening of the scanner, and what is the magnet configuration? Is the scanner truly an open system?

Longer-Term Considerations

Accessory equipment maintenance issues, such as any additional electrical or air conditioning needs or the costs of additional equipment required for the system to operate, should be investigated. When comparing service maintenance contracts,

T. Duggan-Jahns: Union Avenue Open MRI/Tacoma Magnetic Imaging, Tacoma, Washington

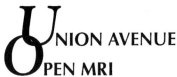

UNION AVENUE OPEN MRI

Your feelings are important to us.

Please take a moment to complete this questionnaire. Your assessment can help us to provide you with the excellent service you deserve.

Your examination date_____

Your referring provider_____

Your name (optional)_____

We'd like to know.

1. My registration (and/or scheduling) by the reception staff was handled courteously and efficiently.
   1-strongly disagree   2   3   4   5-strongly agree

2. The surroundings were pleasant and comfortable.
   1-strongly disagree   2   3   4   5-strongly agree

3. On the day of my examination, the waiting time was reasonable.
   1-strongly disagree   2   3   4   5-strongly agree

4. The information used to explain my procedure was helpful and adequate.
   1-strongly disagree   2   3   4   5-strongly agree
   I received a brochure about my examination from my health care provider prior to my test.   yes   no

5. The technical/medical staff were professional and caring.
   1-strongly disagree   2   3   4   5-strongly agree

6. I was satisfied with my overall care and treatment at Union Avenue Open MRI.
   1-strongly disagree   2   3   4   5-strongly agree

7. I would recommend Union Avenue Open MRI to others.
   1-strongly disagree   2   3   4   5-strongly agree

8. How was Union Avenue Open MRI selected for your examination?
   ____my doctor
   ____my request
   ____my health plan coverage
   ____other_____

Could we have done something to have made your examination a more pleasant experience?

_____
_____
_____
_____
_____
_____
_____
_____
_____
_____
_____

Thank you for choosing us.
#8654 • 7/30/98

FIG. 3-1. A patient satisfaction survey can pinpoint areas that need improvement and improve your marketing efforts.

seek answers to the following questions: What is the cost per year for a service contract? What services are covered under the contract? What is the equipment guaranteed up-time percentage for this particular vendor? Is the service engineer readily available, and what is the vendor's guaranteed service response time? What are the additional charges for hours not covered within the service contract, such as weekend and after-hours coverage? And perhaps most important, what is the penalty to the vendor if the vendor breaches the contract?

The open scanner you choose should provide inexpensive pathways for future software and hardware upgrades to improve image quality and through-put. The service maintenance contract agreement should provide for any additional training of technical staff as these improvements become available.

PROTOCOL SELECTION AND IMAGING CAPABILITIES

High-field protocols do not work on open or low-field scanners. The radiologist and the technical staff must be aware of the physics and technical aspects of open MRI. Image quality and resolution can be improved if the technologist and radiologist truly understand the technical aspects of this technology. Scan times are longer in an open scanner, and through-put may not be as good as that seen with a high-field scanner. Owing to the types of patients attracted to these scanners (e.g., claustrophobic and anxious patients), a significant amount of time is devoted to counseling the patient to begin and complete the examination.

MARKETING

Before a marketing plan can be developed, the types of patients you want to attract to this new technology should be identified. Do you hope to attract patients that are obese or claustrophobic? Determination of your competition is critical. What other types of open systems exist in your area? How will your center distinguish itself in terms of improved services or new types of services? What methods do you have to evaluate or measure the services you provide, and which additional services should you provide?

UNION AVENUE OPEN MRI

Referring Provider Satisfaction Survey

Referring Provider Name_____ Specialty_____

We are dedicated to the highest quality care and service. We value your opinion. We would appreciate your taking the time as a referring provider to complete this questionnaire. Your response is postage paid.

Thank you.

1. Compared to other open MRI services, how do you rate the quality of our radiologist's reports?
   1-inferior   2   **3-about the same**   4   **5-superior**

2. How do you rate our report turnaround time?
   1-poor   2   3   4   **5-exceeds expectations**

3. What is the average report turnaround time you are experiencing with Union Avenue Open MRI?
   _____**two hours** _____**same day** _____**next day** _____**longer, how many days?**_____

4. Do you prefer same day faxed reports? _____**yes** _____**no**

5. How do you rate the accessibility of our radiologists for consultative purposes?
   1-poor   2   3   4   **5-exceeds expectations**

6. Compared to other open MRI services, how do you rate the quality of Union Avenue Open MRI services?
   1-inferior   2   **3-about the same**   4   **5-superior**

7. Compared to other open MRI services, how do you rate our effort to accommodate and schedule patients quickly?
   1-inferior   2   **3-about the same**   4   **5-superior**

8. How do you or your office personnel rate the service commitment of our staff and physicians?
   1-poor   2   3   4   **5-exceeds expectations**
   _____Schedulers/Receptionists
   _____Technologists
   _____Radiologists
   _____Couriers
   _____Service Coordinators

9. How satisfied are your patients with open MRI services provided by Union Avenue Open MRI?
   1-not satisfied   2   **3-satisfied**   4   **5-exceeds expectations**

10. How do you rate the value of our patient information (Low Field Open MRI brochure)?
    1-poor   2   3   4   **5-exceeds expectations**

11. Would you be interested in attending educational presentations related to open MRI applications and interpretation?
    _____**yes** _____**no**   **If yes, what are your areas of interest?**_____

12. What suggestions do you have for changes, improvements or additions to our open MRI services?

    _____

    _____

13. How often do you refer to Union Avenue Open MRI?   **daily**   **weekly**   **monthly**

#738 4 • 5/20/97

FIG. 3-2. A referring doctor satisfaction survey can determine how the referring providers can be better served.

Feedback

You should elicit feedback from referring physicians and their staff as well as from patients on how well your center provides these services. These could include but may not be limited to periodic physician and patient satisfaction questionnaires (Figs. 3-1 and 3-2). Feedback can help you evaluate your present services, areas that need improvement, and possible additional areas of service.

Database

A database can be developed to track the sources of referrals to your center, volumes per referral, and types of examinations per month. This database can provide important information that can be a key to your practice's success and development. It will enable you to see immediately when a referral source suddenly falls below historical or typical volume. Such information can be a key to your practice's success and development, because it can help you analyze your practice and determine your future path.

Educational Materials

Developing patient and referring physician educational materials, with information such as your center's scheduling procedures, services offered, radiologist specialties, operational hours, and patient brochures, will be required to help market your open MRI services. Having sufficient staff is essential to maintain ease of scheduling and appointment availability and thus ensuring that your referrals are not lost to another center. Some sites that also have a high-field scanner

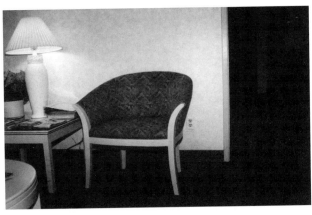

FIG. 3-3. Large and sturdy, yet attractive, chairs should be provided for the large and overweight patients often attracted to an open MRI center.

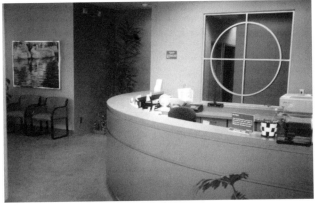

FIG. 3-5. An attractive reception area welcomes patients.

have a dedicated phone line just for calls related to open scanner procedures.

Dedicated Service Coordinator

A dedicated service coordinator who routinely visits and calls referring physicians and their staff can be very beneficial to your practice. This person can help develop a professional relationship between the referring physicians and your center, which can help ensure that referring physicians are satisfied with the services you provide. Such contact also keeps referring physicians aware of new services as they become available. A service coordinator also works to ensure that referrals are not lost to other centers owing to communication problems.

RECEPTION AREA AND SCAN ROOM DESIGN

The reception area should project a relaxed atmosphere. It should appear as friendly and spacious as possible. Comfortable, roomy chairs should be available (Fig. 3-3). Patients

should have easy access to your front-desk staff and should be greeted by name when they arrive for their appointments (Figs. 3-4 and 3-5).

The scan room itself should also appear spacious and nonthreatening to the anxious or phobic patient. The decor, lighting, and colors should be subdued. Windows or skylights often make the room appear more spacious and less sterile and allow more natural light. Positioning the technologist's window in view of the patient may alleviate patients' fears of being left alone in the room (Fig. 3-6). Plants, carpeting, framed prints, and comfortable chairs for accompanying family or friends provide warmth. Soothing background music provides a less threatening and more relaxing atmosphere. Extra large gowns for larger patients are a must to ensure that their dignity is protected and respected. Larger dressing rooms and doorways may be needed to accommodate larger patients (Fig. 3-7). In facilities with more than one scanner, a common technologist's control area can be beneficial when sharing of staff is required.

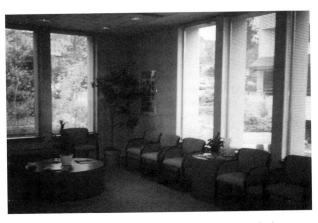

FIG. 3-4. A pleasant and spacious waiting room helps anxious patients relax. Windows contribute to an open feeling.

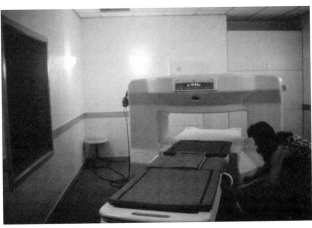

FIG. 3-6. Placement of the technologist's window near the patient's head, instead of at the patient's feet, enhances communication between the technologist and patient. A large scanning room can minimize a patient's claustrophobic anxieties.

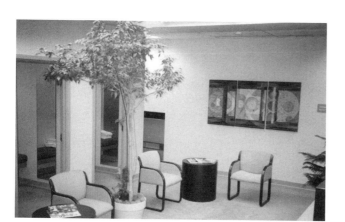

FIG. 3-7. Extra large dressing rooms (mirrored doors) maximize large patients' comfort and minimize their self-consciousness. An adjacent small, secluded waiting area is ideal.

STAFF SELECTION AND TRAINING CONSIDERATIONS

Open MRI patients include conventional MRI patients, but open scanners often attract patients who have special needs. Patients with special needs require more of your staff's time and patience. They can be demanding and extremely uncooperative. They will place new burdens on your staff. Choosing the right employees is therefore critical. Additional training by a professional counselor experienced in working with phobic patients may be beneficial for all members of your staff.

Your staff should be professional, friendly, outgoing, compassionate, willing to listen to the patient, and be able to put the patient at ease. The staff will be challenged daily! They should be extremely dedicated, because they play a key factor in the overall success of your practice by setting the tone and pursuing the mission of your practice.

Front Office and Receptionist Staff

The front office and receptionist staff members are the first contact referring physicians and their patients have with your facility. The front office staff members are the front runners in setting the tone and mission of your practice. They must understand the goals of your practice and the services your facility provides. Customers include the referring physicians, insurance providers, and the patients themselves. Staff members must be sensitive and compassionate to patients' needs. They should call patients by name as they arrive at your office, to put the patient at ease. They need to be able to recognize potential problems or patient concerns that may be due to physical or mental limitations or possible communication barriers. These concerns should be communicated to the technologists or other staff members who will be involved with the patient's examination. Your front desk staff should be prepared to go the extra mile to provide the services needed.

Technical Staff

MRI technologists are another key factor in the success of your center. Not only will they be learning a new technology and new equipment, they will need to develop new methods and skills to manage patients with special needs. Technologists should be educated about the power of fear and its influence on patient behavior. Of all staff members, technologists are with the patient for the largest portion of the office visit. Technologists should be willing to do whatever is necessary to alleviate patients' fears and guide patients to successful completion of the MRI examination. The technologist's role is changing because of the types of patients scheduled for open MRI. Fifty percent of the technologist's job is technical; the remaining 50% is spent counseling the patient. Your technical staff must be sympathetic to patients' needs, demonstrate their concern for patients, be accommodating, allow the patient to feel in control, and be able to truly listen to the patient. Technologists must seek to gain patients' trust and confidence.

The expanded population that open MRI attracts will require additional staff training for the management of phobic and very anxious patients. Training for the management of these patient groups includes crisis intervention techniques, understanding patient fears, patient relaxation techniques, methods for handling abusive patients, and staff communication skills.

Having enough properly trained technical staff members to manage these types of patients is critical to the success of your practice. These patients demand more time and patience than do traditional MRI patients. In fact, these patients' demands can increase technologists' work-related stress. Working with special needs patients can be both mentally and physically draining at times. It can be a difficult and challenging task to undertake on a daily basis. In a multi-imaging facility, consider cross-training your technologists in this technology and rotating their responsibilities, to avoid "burn out."

Patient Advocate Position

Some centers use a patient advocate whose responsibility is to assist patients through the entire process. For example, the advocate calls patients the day before their examination, answers questions to alleviate any concerns or fears, and may even stay with the patient during the procedure. This position reduces the pressures placed on the technologists, freeing them to focus on the performance of accurate and efficient examinations.

PATIENT CONCERNS AND ASSUMPTIONS

Patients requesting an open MRI may have been unable to complete an MRI in a closed system, may have been too large to fit in a closed system, or may be unwilling to undergo MRI in anything other than an open scanner. Patients who are unable to undergo closed MRI expect your

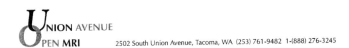

2502 South Union Avenue, Tacoma, WA (253) 761-9482 1-(888) 276-3245

Patient Plan for Safe Use of Sedating Medication

I _____ (patient name),

understand that my physician, _____ has prescribed the administration
of _____, an oral sedative medication at _____ dosage prior to my MRI
examination at **Union Avenue Open MRI**.   I have discussed, or had the opportunity to discuss with my physician the
risks and effects of sedation.

**I understand that this medication can cause drowsiness
and impair my physical and mental abilities. I agree:**

1.   To arrange for a supportive partner to drive me to and from my examination.

2.   For at least <u>24</u> hours following my examination to **not**:

   (a)   operate a motor vehicle, boat or other machinery or equipment;
   (b)   engage in any activity involving any degree of risk;
   (c)   make any important decisions or commitments, or;
   (d)   consume any alcoholic beverages or other drugs or medications unless specifically
          instructed by my physician.

I understand that drivers impaired by sedating medication can be cited for driving under the influence in Washington
State (RCW 46.61.502).

Appointment Date   _____

Patient Name   _____

Signature   _____

Driver Name   _____

Signature: _____

Witness: _____

A copy of this form is available to you upon request.

FIG. 3-8. Use of a sedation consent form can help to minimize the facility's liability.

staff to be compassionate and understanding of their often unexpressed needs. Their abusive behavior or unrealistic demands may be fear motivated. These patients need to feel that all members of your staff are ready to listen and to accommodate any and all of their needs. They may assume that your staff has counseling skills and unlimited time to complete their MRI examination. These patients may need constant reassurances and encouragement during the procedure. They need to feel that they are in control and that your staff is truly concerned about them. Patient appointment times should be adjusted to reflect these increased time demands. Anxious patients cannot and should not be rushed if you hope to complete a successful examination.

SEDATION CONSIDERATIONS AND PROTOCOL

Most patients undergoing open MRI do not require sedation when the staff effectively manages anxious or phobic patients. Using relaxation techniques, encouraging the patient during the examination, and reassuring the patient can alleviate the need for sedation.

Despite the openness of the scanner, some patients may still require some type of sedation to successfully complete an MRI examination. You must determine whether conscious sedation or deep sedation methods will be offered at your facility. It is extremely important to follow the recommendations and guidelines of the American College of Radiology for each of these methods.

Patients receiving sedation need to sign a sedation consent form (Fig. 3-8). A risk management attorney should be consulted in the preparation of your facility's sedation consent form. For deep sedation, additional MRI-compatible monitoring equipment is required. A properly trained staff (anesthesiologist and nurse) should be on site during the procedure.

CONCLUSION

You have been provided some items to consider before setting up an open MRI facility. As a Center Manager or Administrator of an open practice, you must have a realistic expectation of the efforts necessary to succeed with this technology and its most-challenging patients.

Open MRI,
edited by Peter A. Rothschild and Debra Reinking Rothschild.
Lippincott Williams & Wilkins. Philadelphia © 2000.

CHAPTER 4

Magnetic Resonance Imaging: Bioeffects and Safety

Frank G. Shellock

During the performance of magnetic resonance imaging (MRI), the patient is exposed to three different forms of electromagnetic radiation: a static magnetic field, gradient magnetic fields, and radiofrequency (RF) electromagnetic fields. Each may cause significant bioeffects if applied at sufficiently high exposure levels.

Numerous investigations have been conducted to identify potentially adverse bioeffects of MRI (1–83). Although none of these has determined the presence of any substantial or unexpected hazards, the data are not comprehensive enough to presume absolute safety.

This chapter discusses the bioeffects and safety of static, gradient, and RF electromagnetic fields and provides an overview of other safety considerations related to the use of MRI, particularly open MRI.

BIOEFFECTS OF STATIC MAGNETIC FIELDS

A relative lack of data exists concerning the effects of static magnetic fields on human subjects. Some of the original investigations involving humans exposed to static magnetic fields were performed by Vyalov (84,85), who studied workers in the permanent magnet industry. These subjects were exposed to static magnetic fields ranging from 0.0015 to 0.3500 T and reported feelings of headache, chest pain, fatigue, vertigo, loss of appetite, insomnia, itching, and other more nonspecific ailments. Of note is that exposure to other potentially hazardous environmental working conditions (e.g., elevated room temperature, airborne metallic dust, chemicals) may have been partially responsible for the reported symptoms in these study subjects. Because this investigation lacked an appropriate con-

trol group, it is difficult to ascertain whether a definite correlation exists between the exposure to the static magnetic field and the reported abnormalities. Subsequent studies performed with more scientific rigor have not substantiated many of these findings (86–89).

Temperature Effects

Reports in the literature conflict regarding the effect of static magnetic fields on body and skin temperatures of mammals, including humans. Reports have indicated that static magnetic fields either increase or increase and decrease tissue temperature, depending on the orientation of the organism in the static magnetic field (19,66). Other articles state that static magnetic fields have no effect on the skin and body temperatures of mammals (55,61,88,90).

None of the investigators that identified a static magnetic field effect on temperatures proposed a plausible mechanism for this response, nor has this experimental work been supported by subsequent studies. In addition, investigations that reported static magnetic field–induced skin or body temperature changes used either laboratory animals known to have labile temperatures or measurement instrumentation that was likely affected by the static magnetic fields (19,66).

Several investigations indicated that exposure to high static magnetic fields does not alter skin and body temperatures (55,61,90). These studies were performed using a special fluoroptic thermometry system demonstrated to be unperturbed by high-intensity static magnetic fields. Therefore, skin and body temperatures of human subjects are believed to be unaffected by exposure to static magnetic fields of up to 1.5 T (55,61).

Electrical Induction and Cardiac Effects

Induced biopotentials may be observed during exposure to static magnetic fields and are caused by blood, a conductive

F. G. Shellock: University of Southern California School of Medicine, Los Angeles, California; R & D Services, Inc., Los Angeles, California

fluid, flowing through a magnetic field. The induced biopotential is exhibited by an augmentation of T-wave amplitude as well as by other nonspecific waveform changes that are apparent on the electrocardiogram and have been observed at static magnetic field strengths as low as 0.1 T (86,91,92).

The increase in T-wave amplitude is directly related to the intensity of the static magnetic field, such that at low static magnetic field strengths the effects are not as predominant as they are at higher field strengths. Other portions of the electrocardiogram may also be altered by the static magnetic field; these alterations vary with the placement of the recording electrodes. Alternate lead positions can be used to attenuate the static magnetic field–induced electrocardiographic (ECG) changes to facilitate cardiac gating studies (93). Once the patient is no longer exposed to the static magnetic field, these ECG voltage abnormalities revert to normal. Because no circulatory alterations appear to coincide with the ECG changes, no bioeffects are believed to be associated with exposure to static magnetic fields of up to 2.0 T (86,91,92).

Neurologic Effects

Theoretically, electrical impulse conduction in nerve tissue may be affected by exposure to static magnetic fields. However, the bioeffects literature on this topic contains inconclusive information. Some studies have reported remarkable effects on the function and structure of those portions of the central nervous system that were associated with exposure to static magnetic fields, whereas others have failed to show any significant changes (14,20,34,68,69,76–79,94–99). Further investigations of potential unwanted bioeffects are needed because of the relative lack of clinical studies in this field that are directly applicable to MRI. At present, exposures to static magnetic fields of up to 2.0 T do not appear to significantly influence bioelectric properties of neurons in humans (97–99).

Summary

In summary, no evidence exists of irreversible or hazardous bioeffects related to short-term exposures of humans to static magnetic fields of strengths up to 2.0 T. However, as of 1999, several 3.0- and 4.0-T, whole-body MRI systems and one 8.0-T MRI system are in operation at various research sites around the world. At least one study has indicated that health care workers and volunteer subjects exposed to a 4.0-T MRI system have experienced vertigo, nausea, headaches, a metallic taste in their mouths, and magnetophosphenes (i.e., visual flashes) (50). Therefore, considerable research is required to study the mechanisms responsible for these bioeffects and to determine possible means, if any, to counterbalance them.

BIOEFFECTS OF GRADIENT MAGNETIC FIELDS

MRI exposes the human body to rapidly varying magnetic fields during the imaging sequence. Gradient magnetic fields can induce electrical fields and currents in conductive media (including biological tissue) according to Faraday's law of induction. The potential for interactions between gradient magnetic fields and biological tissue is inherently dependent on the fundamental field frequency, maximum flux density, average flux density, presence of harmonic frequencies, waveform characteristics of the signal, polarity of the signal, current distribution in the body, and electrical properties and sensitivity of the particular cell membrane (97–99).

For animals and human subjects, the induced current is proportional to the conductivity of the biological tissue and the rate of change of the magnetic flux density (98–101). In theory, the largest current densities will be produced in peripheral tissues (i.e., at the greatest radius) and will linearly diminish toward the body's center (98–101). The current density is enhanced at higher frequencies and magnetic flux densities and is further accentuated by a larger tissue radius with a greater tissue conductivity. Current paths are affected by differences in tissue types, such that tissues with low conductivity (e.g., adipose and bone) will change the pattern of the induced current.

Bioeffects of induced currents can be due to either the power deposited by the induced currents (thermal effects) or direct effects of the current (nonthermal effects). The thermal effects associated with switched gradients used in MRI are negligible and are not believed to be clinically significant (96,98,99).

The production of magnetophosphenes is considered one of the most sensitive physiologic responses to gradient magnetic fields (96–99). Magnetophosphenes are supposedly caused by electrical stimulation of the retina and are completely reversible with no associated health effects (96–99).

BIOEFFECTS OF RADIOFREQUENCY ELECTROMAGNETIC FIELDS

RF radiation is capable of generating heat in tissues as a result of resistive losses. Therefore, the main bioeffects associated with exposure to RF radiation are related to the thermogenic qualities of this electromagnetic field (96–99,102–110). Regarding RF power deposition concerns, investigators have typically quantified exposure to RF radiation by means of determining the specific absorption rate (SAR) (102–106,110–113). SAR is the mass normalized rate at which RF power is coupled to biological tissue, expressed as watts per kilogram. Measurements or estimates of SAR are not trivial, particularly in human subjects, and several methods exist for determining this parameter for RF energy dosimetry (102–106,113).

The SAR produced during MRI is a complex function of numerous variables including the frequency (which, in turn, is determined by the strength of the static magnetic field), type of RF pulse (i.e., 90° or 180°), repetition time, pulse width, type of RF coil used, volume of tissue within the coil, resistivity of the tissue, configuration of the anatomical region imaged, as well as other factors (96–99). Typically,

RF power deposition is not a primary safety issue for low- or mid-field strength open MRI systems. The actual increase in tissue temperature caused by exposure to RF radiation is dependent on the subject's thermoregulatory system (e.g., skin blood flow, skin surface area, sweat rate) (97–99).

The efficiency and absorption pattern of RF energy are determined primarily by the physical dimensions of the tissue in relation to the incident wavelength: If the tissue size is large relative to the wavelength, energy is predominantly absorbed on the surface; if it is small relative to the wavelength, little absorption of RF power occurs (102–106).

Little quantitative data have been previously available on thermoregulatory responses of humans exposed to RF radiation before the studies performed with MRI. The few studies that existed did not directly apply to MRI because these investigations examined either thermal sensations or therapeutic applications of diathermy, usually involving only localized regions of the body (102–104,108).

Several studies of RF power absorption during MRI have yielded useful information about tissue heating in human subjects (28,58–60,62,63,65). During MRI, tissue heating results primarily from magnetic induction with a negligible contribution from the electric fields, so that ohmic heating is greatest at the surface of the body and approaches zero at the center of the body. Predictive calculations and measurements obtained in phantoms and human subjects support this pattern of temperature distribution (58–60,109,110).

Although one paper reported significant temperature rises in internal organs produced by MRI (65), this study was conducted on anesthetized dogs and is unlikely to be applicable to conscious adult human subjects because of factors related to the physical dimensions and dissimilar thermoregulatory systems of these two species. However, these data may have important implications for the use of MRI in pediatric patients because this patient population is typically sedated or anesthetized for MRI examinations.

An investigation using fluoroptic thermometry probes that are unperturbed by electromagnetic fields (111) demonstrated that human subjects exposed to MRI at SAR levels up to 4.0 W/kg have no statistically significant increases in body temperatures and elevations in skin temperatures that are not believed to be clinically hazardous (62). Additional studies are needed, however, to assess physiologic responses of patients with conditions that may impair thermoregulatory function. These patient groups include elderly patients; patients with underlying health conditions such as fever, diabetes, cardiovascular disease, or obesity; and patients taking medications that affect thermoregulation (e.g., calcium channel blockers, beta blockers, diuretics, vasodilators).

Temperature-Sensitive Organs

Certain human organs that have reduced capabilities for heat dissipation, such as the testis and eye, are particularly sensitive to elevated temperatures. Therefore, these are primary sites of potential harmful effects if RF radiation exposures during MRI are excessive. Laboratory investigations have demonstrated detrimental effects on testicular function (e.g., a reduction or cessation of spermatogenesis, impaired sperm motility, degeneration of seminiferous tubules) caused by RF radiation–induced heating from exposures sufficient to raise scrotal or testicular tissue temperatures up to 42°C (112).

Scrotal skin temperatures (i.e., an index of intratesticular temperature) were measured in volunteer subjects undergoing MRI at a whole-body averaged SAR of 1.1 W per kg (63). The largest change in scrotal skin temperature was 2.1°C, and the highest scrotal skin temperature recorded was 34.2°C. These temperature changes were below the threshold known to impair testicular function. However, excessively heating the scrotum during MRI could exacerbate certain preexisting disorders associated with increased scrotal and testicular temperatures (e.g., acute febrile illnesses, varicocele) in patients who are already oligospermic and lead to temporary or permanent sterility (63). Additional studies designed to investigate these issues are needed, particularly if patients are scanned at whole-body averaged SARs higher than those previously evaluated.

Dissipation of heat from the eye is a slow and inefficient process owing to the eye's relative lack of vascularization. Acute near-field exposures of RF radiation to the eyes or heads of laboratory animals have been demonstrated to be cataractogenic as a result of the thermal disruption of ocular tissues if the exposure is of sufficient intensity and duration (102,104). An investigation conducted by Sacks et al. (53) revealed no discernible effects on the eyes of rats were produced by MRI at exposures that far exceeded typical clinical imaging levels. However, it may not be acceptable to extrapolate this data to human subjects considering the coupling of RF radiation to the anatomy and tissue volume of the laboratory rat eyes compared to those of humans.

Corneal temperatures have been measured in patients undergoing MRI of the brain using a send/receive head coil at local SARs of up to 3.1 W per kg (59). The greatest corneal temperature change was 1.8°C, and the highest temperature measured was 34.4°C. Because the temperature threshold for RF radiation–induced cataractogenesis in animal models has been demonstrated to be between 41° and 55°C for acute near-field exposures, it does not appear that clinical MRI using a head coil has the potential to cause thermal damage in ocular tissue (59). The effect of MRI at higher SARs and the long-term effects of MRI on ocular tissues remain to be determined.

Radiofrequency Radiation and Hot Spots

Theoretically, RF radiation hot spots caused by an uneven distribution of RF power may arise whenever current concentrations are produced in association with restrictive conductive patterns. It has been suggested that RF radiation hot spots may generate thermal hot spots under certain conditions during MRI. Because RF radiation is primarily absorbed by peripheral tissues, thermography has been used to study the heating pattern associated with MRI at high whole-body SARs (57). This study demonstrated no evidence of surface thermal hot spots related to MRI of human subjects. The thermoregulatory system apparently responds to the heat challenge by distributing the thermal load, producing a "smearing" effect of the surface temperatures. However, it is possible that internal thermal hot spots may develop from MRI (65).

MAGNETIC RESONANCE IMAGING AND ACOUSTIC NOISE

The acoustic noise produced during MRI represents a potential risk to patients. Acoustic noise is associated with the activation and deactivation of electrical current that induces vibrations of the gradient coils. This repetitive sound is enhanced by higher gradient duty cycles and sharper pulse transitions. Therefore, acoustic noise tends to increase with the strength of the static magnetic field of the MRI system and decrease in section thickness, fields of view, repetition times, and echo times. Notably, acoustic noises associated with low- or mid-field strength open MRI systems are relatively minor.

Gradient magnetic field–related noise levels measured on several commercial MRI scanners were in the range of 65 to 95 dB, which is within the recommended safety guidelines set forth by the U.S. Food and Drug Administration (FDA) as well as other governmental agencies (114). However, it has been reported that acoustic noise generated during MRI has caused patient annoyance, interference with oral communication, and reversible hearing loss in patients who did not wear ear protection (9,115). A study of patients undergoing MRI without earplugs resulted in temporary hearing loss in 43% of the subjects (9). Furthermore, the possibility exists that significant gradient coil–induced noise may produce permanent hearing impairment in patients who are particularly susceptible to the damaging effects of relatively loud noises (9,115).

The safest and least expensive means of preventing problems associated with acoustic noise during clinical MRI is to encourage the routine use of disposable earplugs (9,115). The use of hearing protection has been demonstrated to successfully avoid the potential temporary hearing loss sometimes associated with clinical MRI. MR-safe headphones that significantly muffle acoustic noise are also commercially available.

An acceptable alternative strategy for reducing sound levels during MRI is to use an "antinoise" or destructive interference technique that not only effectively reduces noise but also permits better patient communication (116). This technique consists of a real-time Fourier analysis of the noise emitted by the MRI system. A signal possessing the same physical characteristics but opposite phase than the sound generated by the MRI system is produced. The two opposite-phase signals are combined, resulting in a cancellation of the repetitive noise, while allowing other sounds such as music and voices to be transmitted to the patient. One investigation demonstrated no significant degradation of image quality when MRI is performed with MRI systems that use this antinoise method (116). Although this technique has not yet found widespread clinical application, it has considerable potential for minimizing acoustic noise and its associated problems.

MAGNETIC RESONANCE IMAGING AND ELECTRICALLY, MAGNETICALLY, AND MECHANICALLY ACTIVATED OR OTHER IMPLANTS, DEVICES, MATERIALS, AND OBJECTS

In general, any patient or individual with an electrically, magnetically, or mechanically activated or other implant, device, material, or object should be excluded from the MRI environment unless it has been demonstrated to be unaffected by the electromagnetic fields of the MRI system (117–150). Certain electrically, magnetically, mechanically activated or other implants or devices may be specially designed to be safe or compatible with the MRI environment. However, the federal agencies responsible for the safe operation of MRI systems generally indicate whether the implant or device is acceptable for exposure to the MRI environment. This information is usually indicated in the product insert for the object (not in the marketing materials or other promotional information). In lieu of this information, MRI users may rely on the peer-reviewed literature to guide them with respect to the safety of performing MRI procedures when a patient has an implant or device (150). A compilation of implants, devices, materials, and devices is updated on an annual basis (see MRIsafety.com).

According to information issued by the Society for Magnetic Resonance Imaging Safety Committee (115), individuals with electrically, magnetically, or mechanically activated or electrically conductive devices should be excluded from MRI procedures unless it has been previously shown (i.e., usually by *ex vivo* testing procedures) that the particular device is unaffected by the electromagnetic fields used for clinical MRI and no possibility of injuring the individual exists. During the screening process for MRI, individuals with these objects should be identified before their examination and before being exposed to the electromagnetic fields of the MRI system.

MRI is contraindicated for individuals who have certain ferromagnetic implants, materials, or foreign bodies, primarily owing to the possibility of movement or dislodgement of these objects (97–99). Other problems may also occur in individuals with ferromagnetic implants, materials, or foreign bodies who undergo MRI, including the induction of electrical current in the object, excessive heating of the object, and the misinterpretation of an artifact produced by the presence of the object as an abnormality

(97,99,125–128). These latter potentially hazardous situations, however, are encountered infrequently or are insignificant in comparison with movement or dislodgement of a ferromagnetic implant or foreign body by the magnetic fields of the MR system.

Numerous investigations have evaluated the ferromagnetic qualities of a variety of metallic implants, materials, or foreign bodies by measuring deflection forces or movements associated with the static magnetic fields used by MRI (128–147, 150). These studies were conducted to determine the relative risk of performing MRI on an individual with a metallic object with respect to whether the magnetic attraction was strong enough to produce movement.

A variety of factors require evaluation when establishing the relative risk of performing an MRI procedure in an individual with a ferromagnetic implant, material, device, or foreign body, such as the strength of the static and gradient magnetic fields, the relative degree of ferromagnetism of the object, the mass of the object, the geometry of the object, the location and orientation of the object *in situ*, and the length of time the object has been in place (98,99). Each of these factors should be considered before allowing an individual with a ferromagnetic object to enter the electromagnetic environment of the MR system. The information in the subsequent sections pertains to all individuals without regard for the specific type of MR system being used.

Magnetic Resonance Imaging and Electrically Activated Implants and Devices

Patients and other individuals who enter the MRI environment may have implants, devices, or materials that present problems for MRI examinations (117–150). In general, the FDA requires labeling of MR systems to indicate that patients with electrically activated implants or devices should not undergo MRI, because the electromagnetic fields used by MR systems may interfere with the operation of the devices and patient injury is a possibility. Examples of electrically activated implants and devices include cardiac pacemakers, implantable cardioverter defibrillators (ICDs), external hearing aids, cochlear implants, neurostimulators, bone-growth stimulators, and implantable electronic drug-infusion pumps. In addition, several experimental implants and devices currently undergoing clinical trials incorporate electrically activated mechanisms. Several implants and devices have been tested with regard to MRI safety and, as a result, specific guidelines and recommendations have been developed to permit the safe use of MRI in patients with certain electrically activated implants and devices.

Cardiac Pacemakers

Cardiac pacemakers are crucial implanted devices for many patients with heart conditions and have maintained quality of life and substantially reduced morbidity for these individuals. The first cardiac pacemaker was implanted in 1958. Since then, more than 2 million patients have had cardiac pacemakers implanted. Each year, more than 100,000 patients in the United States and an additional 100,000 in other parts of the world receive pacemakers for treatment of heart rhythm disturbances.

Cardiac pacemakers are the most common electrically activated implants found in patients who may be referred for MRI. Unfortunately, the presence of a cardiac pacemaker is considered a strict contraindication for MRI (150). The effects of MR systems on the function of a cardiac pacemaker are variable and dependent on several factors, including the type of cardiac pacemaker, the static magnetic field strength of the MR system, and the specific type of imaging conditions being used (e.g., the anatomic region imaged, the type of surface coil used, the pulse sequence) (150).

A commonly posed question is whether MRI may be safely performed under any conditions in patients with implanted cardiac pacemakers. Cardiac pacemakers present potential problems to patients undergoing MRI from several mechanisms, including movement of the pacemaker due to the strong static magnetic field of the MR system, modification of the function of the pacemaker by the static magnetic field of the MR system, heating induced in the pacemaker leads owing to the time-varying magnetic fields of the MR system during the imaging process, and voltages and currents induced in the pacemaker leads or myocardium during the MRI procedure by the RF or the gradient magnetic fields, or both. In consideration of the potential cardiac pacemaker–related problems in the MRI environment, it is generally considered unsafe to permit any patient with a cardiac pacemaker to enter the MRI environment. However, this may change as more knowledge is acquired about this issue and as more information becomes available defining which patients may be safely imaged with MR systems and under what conditions.

Various theories suggest that it may be possible to perform MRI safely in certain patients (e.g., patients who are not pacemaker-dependent) with certain pacemakers. For example, for MRI in which the body coil is not used for RF excitation and in which continuous physiologic monitoring is performed throughout the examination, an MRI examination may be acceptable.

Most of the previous studies on MRI-related pacemaker interactions were performed with older MR systems (i.e., virtually a decade ago) using weaker RF transmitter and gradient subsystems. Therefore, there may be reason for hesitation regarding the substantially stronger RF transmitters and gradient magnetic fields more commonly used in many present-day MR systems. This is especially so for the echo-planar MR systems with gradient fields that may be five to ten times more powerful than those available 15 years ago. Perhaps at these gradient magnetic field levels the issue of induced arrhythmias secondary to change in gradient magnetic fields needs to be reexamined.

In the event of exposure (inadvertent or intentional) of a patient with an implanted cardiac pacemaker to the static or time-varying magnetic fields of an MR system, it is prudent to have the functionality of the pacemaker checked and verified by a cardiologist. Furthermore, if possible, it is advisable to have the functionality affirmed by the manufacturer of the particular cardiac pacing device (150).

Implantable Cardioverter Defibrillators

ICDs are implantable medical devices designed to automatically detect and treat episodes of ventricular fibrillation, ventricular tachycardias, and bradycardia. When an arrhythmia is detected, the device can deliver defibrillation, cardioversion, antitachycardia pacing, or bradycardia pacing therapy. Each year, more than 35,000 ICDs are implanted in patients throughout the world. ICDs are most often used to treat patients with sustained arrhythmias that are refractory to antiarrhythmic pharmacologic treatment (150).

An ICD uses a programmer that has an external magnet to test the battery charger and to activate and deactivate the system. Deactivation of an ICD is accomplished by holding a magnet over the device for approximately 30 seconds and has occurred accidentally as a result of patients' encountering the magnetic fields in the home and workplace. For example, deactivation of ICDs has occurred in patients from exposure to the magnetic fields found in stereo speakers, bingo wands, and 12-V starters (150).

Magnetic fields of MR systems would have a similar effect on ICDs and, therefore, patients with these devices should avoid exposure to the MR environment. In addition, ICDs have electrodes that are placed in the myocardium, and patients should not undergo MRI because of the previously mentioned risks related to the presence of these conductive materials.

Hearing Aids and Cochlear Implants

External hearing aids are included in the category of electrically activated bioimplants that may be found in patients referred for MRI procedures. The magnetic fields used for MRI can easily damage these devices. Fortunately, external hearing aids can be readily identified and removed from the patients or individuals to allow them to safely enter the MRI environment or to undergo MRI.

Some types of cochlear implants use a relatively strong magnet in conjunction with an external component to align and retain an RF transmitter coil on the patient's head (150). The magnet may also be used to provide sufficient transmission quality between the external transmitter and internal receiver. Other types of cochlear implants are electronically activated. Consequently, MRI procedures are typically contraindicated in patients with this classification of implant because of the possibility of injuring the patient or damaging or altering the function of the cochlear implant. In general, visitors or other individuals should be prevented from entering the MRI environment if they have a cochlear implant.

Implanted Neurostimulators

The incidence of patients receiving implanted neurostimulators for treatment of various forms of neurologic disorders is increasing. Because of the specific design and intended function of neurostimulators, the electromagnetic fields used for MRI may produce problems with the operation of these devices. Malfunction of a neurostimulator owing to exposure to the electromagnetic fields of an MR system may cause discomfort or pain to the patient (150). In extreme cases, damage to the nerve fibers at the site of the implanted electrodes of the neurostimulator may also occur. Therefore, the present policy regarding patients with neurostimulators is that patients with these devices should not undergo MRI for reasons similar to those indicated for patients with cardiac pacemakers and ICDs.

Six different models of implantable neurostimulators have been evaluated in an *ex vivo* manner in conjunction with 0.35- and 1.50-T MR systems (150). The authors of this study reported that "patients with certain types of implanted neurostimulators can be scanned safely under certain conditions." However, this investigation had several limitations, including the fact that it did not assess the effects of the variety of pulse sequences used for MRI that may substantially alter the function of an implantable neurostimulator and an *in vivo* evaluation was not performed (150).

Implantable pulse generators also are used for suppression of upper-extremity tremors in patients diagnosed with essential tremor or parkinsonian tremor not adequately controlled by medications or in whom the tremor constitutes a significant functional disability. For example, the Medtronic Activa Tremor Control System (Medtronic Neurological, Minneapolis, MN) is an implantable, multiprogrammable quadripolar system that delivers electrical stimulation to the thalamus to control tremor. It consists of the Itrel II Model 7424 Implantable Pulse Generator that has electronic circuitry and a battery, which are hermetically sealed in a titanium case. The operation of this device is supported by a console programmer and a control magnet (product information, 1997).

The product insert information for the Medtronic Activa Tremor Control System indicates that patients with this system should not be exposed to the electromagnetic fields produced by MRI. Besides possible dislodgement, heating, and induced voltages in the pulse generator or lead, an induced voltage through the pulse generator or lead may cause uncomfortable jolting or shocking levels of stimulation for the patient in the MRI environment. Of note are two anecdotal reports from patients using deep brain stimulation for the treatment of chronic pain who experienced speech problems, temporary sensation of visual light, dizziness, and nausea when exposed to MRI (product information, Medtronic Neurological, 1997). Owing to the obvious associated problems, MRI procedures are not recommended in patients with this or a similar device. Furthermore, the FDA indicates that the presence of this implantable neurostimulator is a contraindication for MRI. Therefore, MRI should not be performed in patents with implantable neurostimulators until the FDA reviews the available safety data and provides the proper approval or recommendations.

The neurostimulator NeuroCybernetic Prosthesis, Pulse Generator, Model 100 (Cyberonics, Webster, TX) has received approval of an MR-safe labeling claim from the FDA, allowing MRI to be conducted in patients according to the following strict guidelines (product label):

1. MRI should not be done with the MR system's body coil.
2. Static magnetic fields should be 2.0 T or less.
3. The whole-body averaged SAR must be less than 1.3 W/kg for a 70-kg patient.
4. The time-varying field should be less than 10 T/second.
5. Magnetic and RF fields produced by MRI may change the pulse generator settings (e.g., change to reset parameters), activate the device, and injure the patient.

Implantable Bone Fusion Stimulators

The implantable spinal fusion stimulator (Electro-Biology, Inc., Parsippany, NJ) is designed for use as an adjunct therapy to a spinal fusion procedure. The implantable spinal fusion stimulator consists of a direct current generator with a lithium iodine battery and solid-state electronics encased in a titanium shell, partially coated with platinum that acts as an anode. The generator weighs 10 g and has the following dimensions: 45 mm × 22 mm × 6 mm. Two nonmagnetic silver and stainless steel leads insulated with silastic provide a connection to two titanium electrodes that serve as the cathodes. A continuous 20-µA current is produced by this device. The cathodes comprise insulated wire leads that terminate as bare wire leads, which are embedded in pieces of bone grafted onto the lateral aspects of fusion sites. The generator is implanted beneath the skin and muscle near the vertebral column and provides the full-rated current for approximately 24 to 26 weeks.

Studies using excessively high electromagnetic fields under highly specific experimental conditions and modeling scenarios for the lumbar/torso area (e.g, high-field strength MR system, excessive exposures to RF fields, excessive exposures to gradient magnetic fields) have demonstrated that the implantable spinal fusion stimulator does not present a hazard to patients undergoing MRI with respect to movement, heating, or induced electric fields (150). Additionally, no evidence was found of malfunction of the implantable spinal fusion stimulator based on *in vitro* and *in vivo* experimental findings (150). Notably, these studies addressed the use of conventional pulse sequences and parameters with an acknowledgement that echo-planar techniques or imaging parameters that require excessive RF power have different implications and consequences for the patient with an implantable spinal fusion stimulator.

MRI examinations have been performed in more than 120 patients (conceivably, using MRI conditions that involved a wide variety of imaging parameters and conditions) with implantable spinal fusion stimulators, with no reports of substantial adverse events (based on review of data obtained through the Freedom of Information Act and unpublished observations, Simon BJ, Electro-Biology, Inc., Parsippany, NJ, 1998). Furthermore, the manufacturer of this implant and the FDA have not received complaints of injuries associated with the presence of this device in patients undergoing MRI.

Recommended guidelines for conducting an MRI examination in a patient with the implantable spinal fusion stimulator are as follows (product label, 1999):

1. The cathodes of the implantable spinal fusion stimulator should be positioned a minimum of 1 cm from nerve roots to reduce the possibility of nerve excitation during an MRI procedure.
2. Plain films should be obtained before MRI to verify that there are no broken leads present for the implantable spinal fusion stimulator. If this cannot be reliably determined, the potential risks and benefits to the patient requiring MRI must be carefully assessed in consideration of the possibility of the potential for excessive heating in the leads of the stimulator.
3. MRI should be performed using MR systems with static magnetic fields of 1.5 T or less; conventional techniques including spin-echo, fast spin-echo, and gradient-echo pulse sequences should be used. Pulse sequences (e.g., echo-planar techniques) or conditions that produce exposures to high levels of RF energy (i.e., exceeding a whole-body averaged SAR of 1.0 W/kg) or exposure to gradient fields that exceed 20 T/second or any other unconventional MRI technique should be avoided.
4. Patients should be continuously observed during MRI and instructed to report any unusual sensations, including any feelings of warming, burning, or neuromuscular excitation or stimulation.
5. The implantable spinal fusion stimulator should be placed as far as possible from the spinal canal and bone graft because doing so decreases the likelihood that artifacts will affect the area of interest on MRI scans.
6. Special consideration should be given to selecting an imaging strategy that minimizes artifacts if the area of interest for MRI is in close proximity to the implantable spinal fusion stimulator. The use of fast spin-echo pulse sequences minimizes the amount of artifact associated with the presence of the implantable spinal fusion stimulator.

Electronically Activated, Implantable Drug-Infusion Pump

A programmable, implantable drug-infusion pump (SynchroMed, Medtronic) used for automatic delivery of antineoplastic agents, morphine, or antispasticity drugs was tested for compatibility with MR systems. This device has ferromagnetic components and a magnetic switch and is programmed by telemetry. The presence of these features in a device is usually considered reason for the device being designated as contraindicated for patients undergoing MRI (150). Nevertheless, the function and integrity of this implantable drug-infusion pump were evaluated for compatibility with a 1.5-T MR system. The investigators concluded that MRI was safe as long as the area of interest is at least 10 cm from the pump and medical personnel are aware that a temporary cessation of infusion (i.e., the roller pump rotor appeared to be frozen when the infusion pump was inside the MR system) occurs during MRI (150).

Several limitations of the assessment performed to determine compatibility of the electronic SynchroMed drug-infusion pump (note that there is also a vascular access port named Synchromed that is an osmotic, passive device that is acceptable for patients undergoing MRI) with MR systems were noted. For example, only a *single* volunteer was examined by MRI and the infusion pump was placed *externally* on this subject (150). It is possible that substantially different test results would have been obtained with an implanted infusion pump.

Additionally, only conventional T1-weighted, proton density–weighted, and T2-weighted pulse sequences were evaluated using a single type of MR system. Different MR systems operating with different static magnetic field strengths and different RF fields or using pulse sequences that require higher levels of RF energy (i.e., fast spin-echo) or more severe gradient magnetic fields (i.e., fast gradient-echo or echo-planar techniques) were not assessed. Therefore, it is probably premature, considering the limited testing procedures conducted to date, to recommend that MRI may be performed safely on patients with the electronic SynchroMed infusion pump.

Magnetic Resonance Imaging and Magnetically Activated Implants and Devices

Various types of implants and devices incorporate magnets as a means of activating the implant. The magnet may be used to retain the implant in place (e.g., certain prosthetic devices), to guide a ferromagnetic object into a specific position, to change the operation of the implant, or to program the device (150). Because there is a high likelihood of perturbing the function of magnetically activated implants, demagnetizing the implants, or displacing the implants, MRI typically should not be performed in patients with these implants or devices (150). In some cases, however, patients with magnetically activated implants and devices may undergo MRI as long as certain precautions are followed (150).

Implants and devices that use magnets (e.g., certain types of dental implants, magnetic sphincters, magnetic stoma plugs, magnetic ocular implants, otologic implants, and other similar prosthetic devices) may be damaged by the magnetic fields of the MR systems which, in turn, may necessitate surgery to replace or reposition them (150). For example, the MRI procedure is capable of demagnetizing

the permanent magnet associated with an otologic implant (i.e., the Audiant magnet). Obviously, this has important implications for the patient undergoing MRI.

Whenever possible and if this can be done without risk to the patient (i.e., from the retained magnetic "keeper" or similar component), a magnetically activated implant or device (e.g., an externally applied prosthesis or magnetic stoma plug) should be removed from the patient before the procedure. Doing so permits the examination to be performed safely. Knowledge of the specific aspects of the magnetically activated implant or device is essential to recognize potential problems and to guarantee that MRI may be performed on a patient without problems or an injury.

Extrusion of an eye socket magnetic implant in a patient imaged with a 0.5-T MR system has been described (147). This type of magnetic prosthesis is used in a patient after enucleation. A removable eye prosthesis adheres with a magnet of opposite polarity to a permanent implant sutured to the rectus muscles and conjunctiva by magnetic attraction through the conjunctiva (147). This magnetic linkage enables the eye prosthesis to move in a coordinated fashion with that of normal eye movement. In the reported incident, the static magnetic field of the MR system produced sufficient attraction of the ferromagnetic portion of the magnetic prosthesis to cause it to extrude through the tissue, resulting in injury to the patient.

Magnetic Resonance Imaging and Mechanically Activated or Other Implants, Devices, Materials, and Objects

Aneurysm Clips

The surgical management of intracranial aneurysms and arteriovenous malformations by the application of aneurysm clips is a well-established procedure. The presence of an aneurysm clip in a patient referred for an MRI is a situation that requires the utmost consideration because of the associated risks. Certain types of intracranial aneurysm clips (e.g., those made from martensitic stainless steels, such as 17-7PH or 405 stainless steel) are an absolute contraindication to MRI procedures because excessive magnetically induced forces can displace these clips and cause serious injury or death (150).

By comparison, aneurysm clips classified as nonferromagnetic or weakly ferromagnetic [e.g., those made from Phynox (Evanston, IL), Elgiloy (Triangle Park, NJ), austentitic stainless steels, titanium alloy, or commercially pure titanium] are safe for patients undergoing MRI procedures (150). [For the sake of discussion, *weakly ferromagnetic* refers to metal that may demonstrate some extremely low ferromagnetic qualities using highly sensitive measurement techniques (e.g., vibrating sample magnetometer, superconducting quantum interference device, or SQUID, magnetometer) and as such, may not be technically called *nonferromagnetic*. It is further recognized that all metals possess some degree of magnetism, such that no metal is considered entirely nonmagnetic or nonferromagnetic.]

No injuries have been reported in a patient or individual in the MRI environment related to the presence of an aneurysm clip made from a nonferromagnetic or weakly ferromagnetic material. In fact, in some cases (unpublished observations, F. Shellock, 1998) patients with ferromagnetic aneurysm clips (based on the extent of the artifact seen during MRI or other information) have undergone MRI procedures at 1.5 T without any injuries. In these cases, the aneurysm clips were exposed to magnetically induced translational and torque forces associated with MR systems that had static magnetic fields of up to 1.5 T. Although these cases do not prove or suggest safety, they do demonstrate the difficulty of predicting the outcome for patients with ferromagnetic aneurysm clips undergoing MRI.

In view of the current knowledge about aneurysm clips, the following guidelines (150) are recommended for careful consideration before performing an MRI procedure in a patient with an aneurysm clip or before allowing any other individual with an aneurysm clip into the MRI environment:

1. Specific information (i.e., manufacturer, type or model, material, lot and serial numbers) about the aneurysm clip must be known, especially with respect to the material used, so that only patients or individuals with nonferromagnetic or weakly ferromagnetic clips are allowed into the MRI environment. This information is provided in the labeling of every aneurysm clip by the manufacturer. The implanting surgeon is responsible for properly noting this information in the patient's or individual's records.
2. An aneurysm clip in its original package and made from Phynox, Elgiloy, MP35N, titanium alloy, commercially pure titanium, or another material known to be nonferromagnetic or weakly ferromagnetic does not need to be evaluated for ferromagnetism. Aneurysm clips made from nonferromagnetic or weakly ferromagnetic materials in original packages do not require testing of ferromagnetism because the manufacturers ensure the pertinent MRI safety aspects of these clips and, therefore, should be held responsible for the accuracy of the labeling.
3. If the aneurysm clip is not in its original package and properly labeled, it should undergo testing for magnetic field interaction.
4. The radiologist and implanting surgeon should be responsible for evaluating the available information about the aneurysm clip, verifying its accuracy, obtaining written documentation, and deciding to perform the MRI procedure after considering the risk versus benefit aspects for a given patient.

Hemostatic Clips

None of the various hemostatic vascular clips that has been evaluated was attracted by static magnetic fields up to 1.5 T (150). These hemostatic clips are made from nonferromagnetic materials such as tantalum and nonferromagnetic

forms of stainless steel. Injury to a patient in association with the presence of a hemostatic vascular clip in the MRI environment has not been reported. Notably, patients with nonferromagnetic hemostatic clips may undergo MRI procedures immediately after these clips are placed surgically.

Halo Vests and Cervical Fixation Devices

Halo vests or cervical fixation devices may be constructed from ferromagnetic, nonferromagnetic, or a combination of metallic components and other materials (150). Although some commercially available halo vests or cervical fixation devices are composed entirely of nonferromagnetic materials, there is a theoretical hazard of inducing electrical current in the ring portion of any halo device made from conductive materials according to Faraday's law of electromagnetic induction. Additionally, the patient's tissue could potentially be involved in part of this current loop, resulting in the possibility of a burn or electrical injury to the patient. The induced current within such a ring or conductive loop is of additional concern because of eddy current induction and potential image degradation effects (150).

No reports have been made of injuries associated with MRI procedures performed in patients with halo vests or cervical fixation devices. Owing to safety and image quality issues, MRI procedures should only be performed on patients with specially designed halo vests or cervical fixation devices made from nonferromagnetic and nonconductive materials that have little or no interaction with the electromagnetic fields generated by MR systems (150).

Heart Valve Prostheses

Many heart valve prostheses have been evaluated for the presence of attraction to static magnetic fields of MR systems at field strengths as high as 2.35 T (150). Of these, the majority displayed measurable yet relatively minor attraction to the static magnetic field of the MR system used for testing. Because the actual attractive forces exerted on these heart valves were minimal compared to the force exerted by the beating heart (i.e., approximately 7.2 N) (150), MRI is not considered hazardous for a patient who has any of the heart valve prostheses that have been tested. This includes the Starr-Edwards Model Pre-6000 (American Edwards Laboratories, Santa Ana, CA) heart valve prosthesis, which was previously suggested to be a potential hazard for patients undergoing an MRI procedure. With respect to clinical MRI procedures, no patient incidents or injuries related to the presence of a heart valve prosthesis have been reported.

Intravascular Coils, Filters, and Stents

Various types of intravascular coils, filters, and stents have been evaluated for safety with MR systems (150). Several of these demonstrated magnetic field interactions associated with exposures to MR systems. These particular devices typically become incorporated securely into the vessel wall primarily owing to tissue ingrowth within approximately 6 weeks after their introduction. Therefore, it is unlikely that any of them would move or become dislodged as a result of being attracted by static magnetic fields of MR systems up to 1.5 T (150). Other similar devices made from nonferromagnetic materials, such as the LGM IVC filter (Vena Tech, Phynox) used for caval interruption or the Wallstent biliary endoprosthesis [Schneider (USA), Inc., Plymouth, Massachusetts] used to treat biliary obstruction, are safe for patients undergoing MRI procedures (150). It is unnecessary to wait for a period after surgery to perform an MRI procedure in a patient with a metallic implant made from a nonferromagnetic material.

Ocular Implants and Devices

Of the different ocular bioimplants and devices tested, the Fatio eyelid spring, the retinal tack made from martensitic (i.e., ferromagnetic) stainless steel (Western European), the Troutman magnetic ocular implant, and the Unitech round wire eyelid spring were attracted by a 1.5-T, static magnetic field (150). A patient with a Fatio eyelid spring or round wire eyelid spring may experience discomfort but probably would not be injured as a result of exposure to the magnetic fields of an MR system. Patients have undergone MRI procedures with eyelid wires after having a protective plastic covering placed around the globe along with a firmly applied eye patch.

Orthopedic Implants, Materials, and Devices

Most of the orthopedic implants, materials, and devices evaluated for ferromagnetism are made from nonferromagnetic materials and, therefore, are safe for patients undergoing MRI (150). Only the PerFix interference screw used for reconstruction of the anterior cruciate ligament has been found to be highly ferromagnetic. Because this interference screw is firmly embedded in bone for its specific application, it is held in place with sufficient force to counterbalance it and prevent movement or dislodgement (150).

Pellets and Bullets

The majority of pellets and bullets tested for MRI safety are composed of nonferromagnetic materials (150). Ammunition that is ferromagnetic tends to be manufactured in foreign countries or used for military applications (150). Because pellets, bullets, and shrapnel may be contaminated with ferromagnetic materials, the risk-benefit ratio of performing an MRI procedure should be carefully considered, as should whether the metallic object is located near a vital anatomic structure, with the assumption that the object is likely to be ferromagnetic. Shrapnel typically contains steel and, therefore, presents a potential hazard for patients undergoing MRI.

Penile Implants

Several types of penile implants and prostheses have been evaluated for MRI safety. Of these, two [i.e., the Duraphase (American Medical Systems, Minneapolis, MN) and Omniphase (Dacomed, Minneapolis, MN) models] demonstrated substantial ferromagnetic qualities when exposed to a 1.5-T static magnetic field of an MR system (150). Although it is unlikely that a penile implant would severely injure a patient undergoing MRI because of the relative strength of the magnetic field interactions and the manner in which this type of device is used, it would undoubtedly be uncomfortable for the patient. Thus, subjecting a patient with one of these implants to an MRI procedure is inadvisable.

SCREENING INDIVIDUALS WITH SUSPECTED METALLIC FOREIGN BODIES

All individuals with a history of metallic foreign bodies, such as slivers, bullets, shrapnel, or other types of metallic fragments, should be carefully screened before being allowed into the MRI environment. The relative risk of exposing individuals to the magnetic fields of the MRI setting depends on the ferromagnetic properties of the object, the geometry and dimensions of the object, and the strength of the static and gradient magnetic fields of the MR system. Also important are the strength with which the object is fixed within the tissue and whether it is positioned in or adjacent to a potentially hazardous site of the body such as a vital neural, vascular, or soft tissue structure.

An individual who encounters the static magnetic field of an MR system with an intraocular metallic foreign body is at a particular risk for significant eye injury. The single reported case of an individual who experienced a vitreous hemorrhage resulting in blindness underwent MRI in a 0.35-T system and had an occult intraocular metal fragment (2.0 mm × 3.5 mm) dislodge during the procedure (148). This incident emphasizes the importance of adequately screening individuals with suspected intraocular metallic foreign bodies before MRI.

Research has demonstrated that small intraocular metallic fragments as small as 0.1 mm × 0.1 mm × 0.1 mm are detected using standard plain-film radiographs (149). Although thin-slice (i.e., ≤3 mm) computed tomography has been demonstrated to detect metallic foreign bodies as small as approximately 0.15 mm, it is unlikely that a metallic fragment of this size would be dislodged during MRI, even with a static magnetic field of up to 2.0 T (149). Metallic fragments of various sizes and dimensions ranging from 0.1 mm × 0.1 mm × 0.1 mm to 3.0 mm × 1.0 mm × 1.0 mm have been examined to determine whether they moved or were dislodged from the eyes of laboratory animals during exposure to a 2.0-T MR system (149). Only the largest fragment (3.0 mm × 1.0 mm × 1.0 mm) rotated, but it did not cause any discernible damage to the ocular tissue. The use of plain-film radiography may be an acceptable technique for identifying or excluding an intraocular metallic foreign body that is a potential hazard to the individual undergoing MRI (115).

Individuals in whom an intraocular metallic foreign body (e.g., a metal worker exposed to metallic slivers with a history of an eye injury) is strongly suspected should have plain-film radiographs of the orbits to rule out the presence of a metallic fragment before exposure to the static magnetic field. If an individual with a suspected ferromagnetic intraocular foreign body has no symptoms and plain-film series of the orbits do not demonstrate a radiopaque foreign body, the risk of performing MRI is minimal (115).

The use of plain-film radiography to search for metallic foreign bodies is a sensitive and relatively inexpensive means of identifying individuals who are unsuitable for MRI. Plain-film radiography can also be used to screen individuals who may have metal fragments in other potentially hazardous sites of the body (115).

Each MRI site should establish a standardized policy for screening individuals with suspected foreign bodies. The policy should include guidelines as to which individuals require workup by radiographic procedures and the specific procedure to be performed (e.g., number and type of views, position of the anatomy), and each case should be considered on an individual basis. These precautions should be taken with individuals referred for MRI in any type of MR system, regardless of the field strength, magnet type, and the presence or absence of magnetic shielding (115).

MAGNETIC RESONANCE IMAGING AND THE PREGNANT PATIENT

Although MRI is not believed to be hazardous to the fetus, only a few investigations have examined the teratogenic potential of this imaging modality. By comparison, literally thousands of studies have been performed to examine the possible hazards of ultrasound during pregnancy, and controversy still exists concerning the safe use of this nonionizing-radiation imaging technique.

Most of the earliest studies conducted to determine possible unwanted bioeffects during pregnancy showed negative results (17,22,26,31,41,47,82). One study examined the effects of MRI on mice exposed midgestation (22). No gross embryotoxic effects were observed; however, a reduction in crown-rump length was noted (22). In another investigation, exposure to the electromagnetic fields used for a simulated clinical MRI examination caused eye malformations in a genetically prone mouse strain (74). Therefore, it appears that the electromagnetic fields used for MRI have the ability to produce developmental abnormalities.

A variety of mechanisms exist that could produce deleterious bioeffects with respect to the developing fetus and the use of electromagnetic fields during MRI (86,88,89,102, 103,112,151). In addition, it is well known that cells undergoing division, as in the developing fetus during the first trimester, are highly susceptible to damage from different types of physical agents. Owing to the limited data available,

a cautionary approach is recommended for the use of MRI in pregnant individuals.

The current guidelines of the FDA require labeling of MRI devices to indicate that the safety of MRI when used to image the fetus and infant "has not been established" (150). In Great Britain, the acceptable exposure limits for clinical MRI recommended by the National Radiological Protection Board in 1983 specify that "it might be prudent to exclude pregnant women during the first three months of pregnancy" (150).

According to the Safety Committee of the Society for Magnetic Resonance Imaging (115) (this information has also been adopted by the American College of Radiology), MRI is acceptable for use in pregnant women if other non-ionizing forms of diagnostic imaging are inadequate or if the examination provides important information that would otherwise require exposure to ionizing radiation (e.g., x-ray, computed tomography). It is recommended that pregnant patients be informed that, to date, no indication exists that the use of clinical MRI during pregnancy has produced deleterious effects. As noted by the FDA, however, the safety of MRI during pregnancy has not been demonstrated (114).

Patients who are pregnant or suspect they are pregnant must be identified before undergoing MRI to assess the risks versus benefits of the examination. Because the spontaneous abortion rate in the general population during the first trimester of pregnancy is high (i.e., >30%), particular care should be exercised with the use of MRI during this time owing to associated potential medicolegal implications relative to spontaneous abortions.

MAGNETIC RESONANCE IMAGING AND CLAUSTROPHOBIA, ANXIETY, AND PANIC DISORDERS

Claustrophobia and a variety of other psychological reactions, including anxiety and panic disorders, may be encountered by as many as 3% to 10% of the individuals undergoing MRI. These sensations are proposed to originate from several factors, including the restrictive dimensions of the interior of the scanner, duration of the examination, gradient-induced noises, and ambient conditions within the bore of the scanner (152–161). Notably, no prior investigation of the incidence of claustrophobia in patients undergoing MRI procedures in mid- and low-field open MR systems versus conventionally designed MR systems has been undertaken to substantiate that a more open configuration improves the individual's tolerance of the examination. However, adverse psychological responses to MRI are usually transient and are easily handled by experienced MRI technologists.

MAGNETIC RESONANCE IMAGING SAFETY CONSIDERATIONS FOR THE EXTREMITY SYSTEM

In 1993, a specially designed low-field-strength (0.2-T MR system, Artoscan, Lunar Corp., Madison, WI/ Esaote,

Genoa, Italy) MR system became available for MRI of extremities. This MR system uses a small-bore permanent magnet to image feet, ankles, knees, hands, wrists, and elbows. The ergonomic design of the extremity MR system is such that the body part of interest is placed inside the magnet bore, with the patient positioned in a seated or supine position (depending on the body part being imaged).

The entire extremity MR system weighs approximately 800 kg and has a built-in RF shield, multiple body part–specific extremity coils, and 10-mT/m magnetic gradients. A major advantage of this extremity MR system is that it can be sited in a relatively small space (e.g., approximately 100 sq ft) without the need for a special power source, magnetic field shielding, or RF shielding. This is the only commercially available extremity MR system approved for use in the United States by the FDA. Of note is that MRI using the extremity MR system has been demonstrated to provide a sensitive, accurate, and reliable assessment of various forms of musculoskeletal pathology (162–165).

Because of the unique design features of the extremity MR system (which includes a low-field strength static magnetic field with a relatively small fringe field) and in consideration of the positioning of patients for MRI procedures using this device (i.e., only the body part imaged is placed within the magnet bore, while the rest of the body remains outside), it was suggested that it may be possible to safely image patients with aneurysm clips, even if they are made from ferromagnetic materials. Furthermore, it may be possible to perform extremity MRI in patients with cardiac pacemakers or ICDs. Therefore, investigations were conducted to specifically evaluate these safety issues (166,167).

Patients with Ferromagnetic Aneurysm Clips

A study was performed to assess the magnetic field interaction for a variety of aneurysm clips exposed to the 0.2-T extremity MR system (161–165). Twenty-two types of aneurysm clips were evaluated, including those made from nonferromagnetic, weakly ferromagnetic, and ferromagnetic materials [i.e., a Heifetz (Triangle Park, NJ) aneurysm clip made from 17-7PH and a Yasargil Model FD aneurysm clip (Aesculap, Inc, South San Francisco)]. The results indicated that none of the aneurysm clips tested displayed substantial magnetic field interaction in association with the 0.2-T extremity MR system (167).

Because of unique design features of the extremity MR system and in consideration of how patients are positioned for MRI procedures using this device (i.e., the head does not enter the magnet bore), it is considered safe to perform MRI in patients with the specific aneurysm clips that have been evaluated. These findings effectively permit an important diagnostic imaging modality to be used to evaluate the extremities of patients with suspected musculoskeletal abnormalities using the Artoscan MR system. By comparison, various studies have reported that patients with Heifetz (17-7PH) and

Yasargil Model FD aneurysm clips (i.e., two of the clips evaluated in the study using the Artoscan) should not undergo MRI using MR systems with conventional designs because of the strong attraction shown by these aneurysm clips, which would pose a potential hazard to patients (167).

Patients with Cardiac Pacemakers and Implantable Defibrillators

As previously indicated, patients with cardiac pacemakers and ICDs are generally not permitted to undergo MRI procedures. However, because of the design of the Artoscan extremity MR system, it may be possible to safely perform MRI in patients with these devices (166). Because the magnetic fringe field of the extremity MR system is in close proximity to the 0.2-T magnet and this system has an integrated Faraday cage, only the patient's extremity is predominantly exposed to the MRI-related electromagnetic fields. Of note is that it is not possible for the MR system's gradient or RF electromagnetic fields to induce currents in a pacemaker or ICD, because the patient's thorax (i.e., in which the pacemaker or ICD is typically placed) remains outside the MR system (166). Therefore, *ex vivo* experiments were conducted on seven different cardiac pacemakers and seven different ICDs manufactured by Medtronic, Inc. (166). The following devices were tested:

Device	*Name*	*Model*
Pacemaker	Elite II	7086
Pacemaker	Thera D	7944
Pacemaker	Thera D	7960I
Pacemaker	Thera DR	7962i
Pacemaker	Thera SR	8940
Pacemaker	Kappa	400
Pacemaker	Kappa	700
ICD	PCD	7217D
ICD	Jewel	7219D
ICD	Jewel Plus	7220C
ICD	Micro Jewel	7221Cx
ICD	Micro Jewel II	7223Cx
ICD	Prototype	7250G
ICD	Prototype	7271

Magnetic field attraction was assessed relative to the 0.2-T static magnetic field of the extremity MR system. Additionally, the cardiac pacemakers and ICDs were operated with various lead systems attached while immersed in a tank containing physiologic saline. This apparatus was used to simulate the thorax and was oriented in parallel and perpendicular positions relative to the closest part of the MR system to which a patient undergoing MRI would be positioned. MRI studies were performed on a phantom using T1-weighted spin-echo and gradient echo sequences. Various functions of the pacemakers and ICDs were evaluated before, during, and after MRI.

The results of these tests indicated that magnetic field attraction did not present problems for the devices (166).

The activation of the pacemakers and cardioverter defibrillators did not substantially affect image quality during MRI. Most important, the operation of the extremity MR system produced no alterations in the function of the cardiac pacemakers and ICDs. Given these data and patient positioning during MRI using the extremity MR system (i.e., the thorax does not enter the magnet bore), it should be safe to perform MRI in patients with the specific cardiac pacemakers and ICDs evaluated in this study.

Other Types of Dedicated Extremity Magnetic Resonance Imaging Systems

In 1998, a new dedicated extremity MR system was developed jointly by Esaote and Siemens Medical Systems (Iselin, NJ). This new device allows MRI studies to be conducted on each of the aforementioned body parts as well as the shoulder. Understandably, this particular type of MR system does not have the same inherent design features as the previously described dedicated extremity system and, as such, this new system should not be used to conduct MRI procedures in patients with ferromagnetic aneurysm clips or cardiac pacemakers and ICDs. Studies are required to determine whether this particular dedicated extremity system may be used to perform MRI examinations safely in patients with ferromagnetic implants or other similar typically contraindicated devices.

Additional ongoing work is being done by various manufacters to develop specialized MR systems that are also extremity or niche (i.e., designed for MRI of one or more specific body parts) scanners. Accordingly, bioeffects and safety issues specific to the use of these new types of MR systems will exist.

REFERENCES

1. Adzamli IK, Jolesz FA, Blau M. An assessment of blood–brain barrier integrity under MRI conditions: brain uptake of radiolabeled Gd-DTPA and In-DTPA-IgG. *J Nucl Med* 1989;30:839.
2. Barber BJ, Schaefer DJ, Gordon CJ, et al. Thermal effects of MR imaging: worst-case studies in sheep. *AJR Am J Roentgenol* 1990;155:1105–1110.
3. Bartels MV, Mann K, Matejcek M, et al. Magnetresonanztomographie und Sicherheit: Elektroenzephalographische und neuropsychologische Befunde vor und nach MR-Untersuchungen des Gehirns. *Fortschr Rontgenstr* 1986;145:383–385.
4. Besson J, Foreman EI, Eastwood LM, et al. Cognitive evaluation following NMR imaging of the brain. *J Neurol Neurosurg Psychiatry* 1984;47:314–316.
5. Bore PJ, Galloway GJ, Styles P, et al. Are quenches dangerous? *Magn Reson Imaging* 1986;3:112–117.
6. Bourland JD, Nyenhuis JA, Mouchawar GA, et al. Physiologic indicators of high MRI gradient–induced fields. In: *Book of abstracts.* Berkeley, CA: Society of Magnetic Resonance in Medicine, 1990:1276.
7. Brody AS, Sorette MP, Gooding CA, et al. Induced alignment of flowing sickle erythrocytes in a magnetic field. A preliminary report. *Invest Radiol* 1985;20:560–566.
8. Brody AS, Embury SH, Mentzer WC, et al. Preservation of sickle cell blood flow patterns during MR imaging. An *in vivo* study. *AJR Am J Roentgenol* 1988;151:139–141.
9. Brummett RE, Talbot JM, Charuhas P. Potential hearing loss resulting from MR imaging. *Radiology* 1988;169:539–540.
10. Budinger TF, Fischer H, Hentschel D, et al. Physiological effects of fast oscillating magnetic field gradients. *J Comput Assisted Tomogr* 1991;15:909–914.
11. Carson JJL, Prato FS, Drost DJ, et al. Time-varying fields increase cytosolic free Ca^{2+} in HL-60 cells. *Am J Physiol* 1990;259:C687–C692.
12. Cohen MS, Weisskoff R, Rzedzian R, et al. Sensory stimulation by time-varying magnetic fields. *Magn Reson Med* 1990;14:409–414.
13. Cooke P, Morris PG. The effects of NMR exposure on living organisms. II. A genetic study of human lymphocytes. *Br J Radiol* 1981;54:622–625.
14. Doherty JU, Whitman GJR, Robinson MD, et al. Changes in cardiac excitability and vulnerability in NMR fields. *Invest Radiol* 1985;20:129–135.
15. Fischer H. Physiological effects of fast oscillating magnetic field gradients. *Radiology* 1989;173:382.
16. Garber HJ, Oldendorf WH, Braun LD, et al. MRI gradient fields increase brain mannitol space. *Magn Reson Imaging* 1989;7:605–610.
17. Geard CR, Osmak RS, Hall EJ, et al. Magnetic resonance and ionizing radiation: a comparative evaluation *in vitro* of oncogenic and genotoxic potential. *Radiology* 1984;152:199–202.
18. Gore JC, McDonnell MJ, Pennock JM, et al. An assessment of the safety of rapidly changing magnetic fields in the rabbit: implications for NMR imaging. *Magn Reson Imaging* 1982;1:191–195.
19. Gremmel H, Wendhausen H, Wunsch F. Biologische Effekte statischef Magnetfelder bei NMR-Tomographie am Menschen. Wiss, Radiologische, Klinik, Christian-Albrechts-Universitat zu Kiel, 1983.
20. Gulch RW, Lutz O. Influence of strong static magnetic fields on heart muscle contraction. *Phys Med Biol* 1986;31:763–769.
21. Hammer BE, Wadon S, Mirer SD, et al. *In vivo* measurement of RF heating in Capuchin monkey brain. In: *Book of abstracts.* Berkeley, CA: Society of Magnetic Resonance in Medicine, 1991;1278.
22. Heinrichs WL, Fong P, Flannery M, et al. Midgestational exposure of pregnant balb/c mice to magnetic resonance imaging. *Magn Reson Imaging* 1988;6:305–313.
23. Hong CZ, Shellock FG. Short-term exposure to a 1.5 Tesla static magnetic field does not effect somato-sensory evoked potentials in man. *Magn Reson Imaging* 1989;8:65–69.
24. Innis NK, Ossenkopp KP, Prato FS, et al. Behavioral effects of exposure to nuclear magnetic resonance imaging: II. Spatial memory tests. *Magn Reson Imaging* 1986;4:281–284.
25. Jehenson P, Duboc D, Lavergne T, et al. Change in human cardiac rhythm by a 2 Tesla static magnetic field. *Radiology* 1988;166:227–230.
26. Kay HH, Herfkens RJ, Kay BK. Effect of magnetic resonance imaging on *Xenopus laevis* embryogenesis. *Magn Reson Imaging* 1988;6:501–506.
27. Keltner JR, Roos MS, Brakeman PR, et al. Magnetohydrodynamics of blood flow. *Magn Reson Med* 1990;16:139–149.
28. Kido DK, Morris TW, Erickson JL, et al. Physiologic changes during high field strength MR imaging. *AJNR Am J Neuroradiol* 1987;8:263–266.
29. LaPorte R, Kus L, Wisniewski RA, et al. Magnetic resonance imaging (MRI) effects on rat pineal neuroendocrine function. *Brain Res* 1990;506:294–296.
30. McRobbie D, Foster MA. Cardiac response to pulsed magnetic fields with regard to safety in NMR imaging. *Phys Med Biol* 1985;30:695–702.
31. McRobbie D, Foster MA. Pulsed magnetic field exposure during pregnancy and implications for NMR foetal imaging: a study with mice. *Magn Reson Imaging* 1985;3:231–234.
32. Messmer JM, Porter JH, Fatouros P, et al. Exposure to magnetic resonance imaging does not produce taste aversion in rats. *Physiol Behav* 1987;40:259–261.
33. Montour JL, Fatouros PP, Prasad UR. Effect of MR imaging on spleen colony formation following gamma radiation. *Radiology* 1988;168:259–260.
34. Muller S, Hotz M. Human brainstem auditory evoked potentials (BAEP) before and after MR examinations. *Magn Reson Med* 1990;16:476–480.
35. Niemann G, Schroth G, Klose U, et al. Influence of magnetic resonance imaging on somatosensory potential in man. *J Neurol* 1988;235:462–465.
36. Ngo FQH, Blue JW, Roberts WK. The effects of a static magnetic field on DNA synthesis and survival of mammalian cells irradiated with fast neutrons. *Magn Reson Med* 1987;5:307–317.

37. Osbakken M, Griffith J, Taczanowsky P. A gross morphologic, histologic, hematologic, and blood chemistry study of adult and neonatal mice chronically exposed to high magnetic fields. *Magn Reson Med* 1986;3:502–517.

38. Ossenkopp KP, Kavaliers M, Prato FS, et al. Exposure to nuclear magnetic imaging procedure attenuates morphine-induced analgesia in mice. *Life Sci* 1985;37:1507–1514.

39. Ossenkopp KP, Innis NK, Prato FS, et al. Behavioral effects of exposure to nuclear magnetic resonance imaging: I. Open-field behavior and passive avoidance learning in rats. *Magn Reson Imaging* 1986;4:275–280.

40. Papatheofanis FJ, Papthefanis BJ. Short-term effect of exposure to intense magnetic fields on hematologic indices of bone metabolism. *Invest Radiol* 1989;24:221–223.

41. Peeling J, Lewis JS, Samoiloff MR, et al. Biological effects of magnetic fields on the nematode *Panagrellus redivivus*. *Magn Reson Imaging* 1988;6:655–660.

42. Prasad N, Kosnik LT, Taber KH, et al. Delayed tumor onset following MR imaging exposure. In: *Book of abstracts*. Berkeley, CA: Society of Magnetic Resonance in Medicine, 1990:275.

43. Prasad N, Prasad R, Bushong SC, et al. Effects of 4.5 T MRI exposure on mouse testes and epididymes. In: *Book of abstracts*. Berkeley, CA: Society of Magnetic Resonance in Medicine, 1990:606.

44. Prasad N, Bushong SC, Thornby JI, et al. Effect of nuclear resonance on chromosomes of mouse bone marrow cells. *Magn Reson Imaging* 1984;2:37–39.

45. Prasad N, Lotzova E, Thornby JI, et al. Effects of MR imaging on murine natural killer cell cytotoxicity. *AJR Am J Roentgenol* 1987; 148:415–417.

46. Prasad N, Lotzova E, Thornby JI, et al. The effect of 2.35-T MR imaging on natural killer cell cytotoxicity with and without interleukin-2. *Radiology* 1990;175:251–263.

47. Prasad N, Wright DA, Ford JJ, et al. Safety of 4-T MR imaging: a study of effects of developing frog embryos. *Radiology* 1990;174:251–253.

48. Prasad N, Wright DA, Forster JD. Effect of nuclear magnetic resonance on early stages of amphibian development. *Magn Reson Imaging* 1982;1:35–38.

49. Prato FS, Ossenkopp KP, Kavaliers M, et al. Attenuation of morphine-induced analgesia in mice by exposure to magnetic resonance imaging: separate effects of the static, radiofrequency and time-varying magnetic fields. *Magn Reson Imaging* 1987;5:9–14.

50. Redington RW, Dumoulin CL, Schenck JL, et al. MR imaging and bioeffects in a whole body 4.0 Tesla imaging system. In: *Book of abstracts*. Berkeley, CA: Society of Magnetic Resonance Imaging, 1988;1:20.

51. Reid A, Smith FW, Hutchison JMS. Nuclear magnetic resonance imaging and its safety implications: follow-up of 181 patients. *Br J Radiol* 1982;55:784–786.

52. Roschmann P. Human auditory system response to pulsed radiofrequency energy in RF coils for magnetic resonance at 2.4 to 170 MHz. *Magn Reson Med* 1991;21:197–215.

53. Sacks E, Worgul BV, Merriam GR, et al. The effects of nuclear magnetic resonance imaging on ocular tissues. *Arch Ophthalmol* 1986;104:890–893.

54. Schwartz JL, Crooks LE. NMR imaging produces no observable mutations or cytotoxicity in mammalian cells. *AJR Am J Roentgenol* 1982;139:583–585.

55. Shellock FG, Schaefer DJ, Gordon CJ. Effect of a 1.5 T static magnetic field on body temperature of man. *Magn Reson Med* 1986;3:644–647.

56. Shellock FG, Crues JV. Temperature, heart rate, and blood pressure changes associated with clinical MR imaging at 1.5 T. *Radiology* 1987;163:259–262.

57. Shellock FG, Schaefer DJ, Grundfest W, et al. Thermal effects of high-field (1.5 Tesla) magnetic resonance imaging of the spine: clinical experience above a specific absorption rate of 0.4 W/kg. *Acta Radiol Suppl* 1986;369:514–516.

58. Shellock FG, Gordon CJ, Schaefer DJ. Thermoregulatory responses to clinical magnetic resonance imaging of the head at 1.5 Tesla: lack of evidence for direct effects on the hypothalamus. *Acta Radiol Suppl* 1986;369:512–513.

59. Shellock FG, Crues JV. Corneal temperature changes associated with high-field MR imaging using a head coil. *Radiology* 1986;167:809–811.

60. Shellock FG, Crues JV. Temperature changes caused by clinical MR imaging of the brain at 1.5 Tesla using a head coil. *AJNR Am J Neuroradiol* 1988;9:287–291.

61. Shellock FG, Schaefer DJ, Crues JV. Effect of a 1.5 Tesla static magnetic field on body and skin temperatures of man. *Magn Reson Med* 1989;11:371–375.

62. Shellock FG, Schaefer DJ, Crues JV. Alterations in body and skin temperatures caused by MR imaging: is the recommended exposure for radiofrequency radiation too conservative? *Br J Radiol* 1989;62:904–909.

63. Shellock FG, Rothman B, Sarti D. Heating of the scrotum by high-field-strength MR imaging. *AJR Am J Roentgenol* 1990;154:1229–1232.

64. Shivers RR, Kavaliers M, Tesky CJ, et al. Magnetic resonance imaging temporarily alters blood–brain barrier permeability in the rat. *Neurosci Lett* 1987;76:25–31.

65. Shuman WP, Haynor DR, Guy AW, et al. Superficial and deep-tissue increases in anesthetized dogs during exposure to high specific absorption rates in a 1.5-T MR imager. *Radiology* 1988;167:551–554.

66. Sperber D, Oldenbourg R, Dransfeld K. Magnetic field induced temperature change in mice. *Naturwissenschaften* 1984;71:100–101.

67. Stick VC, Hinkelmann ZK, Eggert P, et al. Beeinflussen starke statische magnetfelder in der NMR-Tomographie die gewebedurchblutung? [Strong static magnetic fields of NMR: do they affect tissue perfusion?] *Fortschr Rontgenstr* 1991;154:326–331.

68. Stojan L, Sperber D, Dransfeld K. Magnetic-field-induced changes in the human auditory evoked potentials. *Naturwissenschaften* 1988;75:622–623.

69. Sweetland J, Kertesz A, Prato FS, et al. The effect of magnetic resonance imaging on human cognition. *Magn Reson Imaging* 1987;5:129–135.

70. Teskey GC, Prato FS, Ossenkopp KP, et al. Exposure to time varying magnetic fields associated with magnetic resonance imaging reduces fentanyl-induced analgesia in mice. *Bioelectromagnetics* 1988;9:167–174.

71. Tesky GC, Ossenkopp KP, Prato FS, et al. Survivability and long-term stress reactivity levels following repeated exposure to nuclear magnetic resonance imaging procedures in rats. *Physiol Chem Phys Med NMR* 1987;19:43–49.

72. Thomas A, Morris PG. The effects of NMR exposure on living organisms. I. A microbial assay. *Br J Radiol* 1981;54:615–621.

73. Tyndall DA, Sulik KK. Effects of magnetic resonance imaging on eye development in the C57BL/6J mouse. *Teratology* 1991;43:263–275.

74. Tyndall DA. MRI effects on the teratogenicity of X-irradiation in the C57BL/6J mouse. *Magn Reson Imaging* 1990;8:423–433.

75. Vogl T, Krimmel K, Fuchs A, et al. Influence of magnetic resonance imaging on human body core and intravascular temperature. *Med Phys* 1988;15:562–566.

76. Von Klitzing L. Do static magnetic fields of NMR influence biological signals? *Clin Phys Physiol Meas (Bristol)* 1986;7:157–160.

77. Von Klitzing L. Static magnetic fields increase the power intensity of EEG of man. *Brain Res* 1989;483:201–203.

78. Von Klitzing L. A new encephalomagnetic effect in human brain generated by static magnetic fields. *Brain Res* 1991;540:295–296.

79. Weiss J, Herrick RC, Taber KH, et al. Bio-effects of high magnetic fields: a study using a simple animal model. *Magn Reson Imaging* 1990;8:166.

80. Willis RJ, Brooks WM. Potential hazards of NMR imaging. No evidence of the possible effects of static and changing magnetic fields on cardiac function of the rat and guinea pig. *Magn Reson Imaging* 1984;2:89–95.

81. Withers HR, Mason KA, Davis CA. MR effect on murine spermatogenesis. *Radiology* 1985;156:741–742.

82. Wolff S, Crooks LE, Brown P, et al. Tests for DNA and chromosomal damage induced by nuclear magnetic resonance imaging. *Radiology* 1980;136:707–710.

83. Yamagata H, Kuhara S, Eso Y, et al. Evaluation of dB/dt thresholds for nerve stimulation elicited by trapezoidal and sinusoidal gradient fields in echo-planar imaging. In: *Book of abstracts*. Berkeley, CA: Society of Magnetic Resonance in Medicine, 1991:1277.

84. Vyalov AM. Magnetic fields as a factor in the industrial environment. *Vestn Akad Med Nauk* 1967;8:72–79.

85. Vyalov AM. Clinico-hygenic and experimental data on the effect of magnetic fields under industrial conditions. In: Kholodov Y, ed. *Influence of magnetic fields on biological objects*. Moscow, 1971. Joint Publications Research Service, translator. JPRS 1974;63-38:20–35.

86. Barnothy MF. *Biological effects of magnetic fields*. Vols. 1, 2. New York: Plenum Press, 1964:1969.

87. Persson BR, Stahlberg F. *Health and safety of clinical NMR examinations*. Boca Raton, FL: CRC Press, 1989.

88. Tenforde TS. *Magnetic field effects on biological systems*. New York: Plenum Press, 1979.

89. Michaelson SM, Lin JV. *Biological effects and health implications of radiofrequency radiation.* New York: Plenum Press, 1987.

90. Tenforde TS. Thermoregulation in rodents exposed to high-intensity stationary magnetic fields. *Bioelectromagnetics* 1986;7:341–346.

91. Beischer DE, Knepton J. Influence of strong magnetic fields on the electrocardiogram of squirrel monkey (*Saimiri sciureus*). *Aerospace Med* 1964;35:939–944.

92. Tenforde TS, Gaffey CT, Moyer BR, et al. Cardiovascular alterations in Macaca monkeys exposed to stationary magnetic fields. Experimental observations and theoretical analysis. *Bioelectromagnetics* 1983;4:1–9.

93. Dimick RM, Hedlund LW, Herfkens RJ, et al. Optimizing electrocardiographic electrode placement for cardiac-gated magnetic resonance imaging. *Invest Radiol* 1987;22:17–22.

94. Abdullakhozhaeva MS, Razykov SR. Structural changes in central nervous system under the influence of a permanent magnetic field. *Bull Exp Biol Med* 1986;102:1585–1587.

95. Hong CZ. Static magnetic field influence on human nerve function. *Arch Phys Med Rehabil* 1987;68:162–164.

96. Budinger TF. Nuclear magnetic resonance (NMR) *in vivo* studies: known thresholds for health effects. *J Comput Assist Tomogr* 1981;5:800–811.

97. Shellock FG, Crues JV. MRI: safety considerations in magnetic resonance imaging. *MRI Decisions* 1988;2:25–30.

98. Shellock FG. Biological effects and safety aspects of magnetic resonance imaging. *Magn Reson Q* 1989;5:243–261.

99. Kanal E, Talagala L, Shellock FG. Safety considerations in MR imaging. *Radiology* 1990;176:593–606.

100. Reilly JP. Peripheral nerve stimulation by induced electric currents: exposure to time-varying magnetic fields. *Med Biol Eng Comput* 1989;27:101–112.

101. Bernhardt J. The direct influence of electromagnetic fields on nerve and muscle and muscle cells of man within the frequency range of 1 Hz to 30 MHz. *Radiat Environ Phys* 1979;16:309–323.

102. National Council on Radiation Protection and Measurements. Biological effects and exposure criteria for radiofrequency electromagnetic fields. Bethesda, MD: National Council on Radiation Protection and Measurements, 1986: NCRP Report No. 86.

103. Erwin DN. Mechanisms of biological effects of radiofrequency electromagnetic fields: an overview. *Aviat Space Environ Med* 1988;59(Suppl 11):A21–A31.

104. Gordon CJ. Thermal physiology. In: *Biological effects of radiofrequency radiation.* Washington: Environmental Protection Agency; 1984. EPA-600/8-830-026A:4-1–4-28.

105. Gordon CJ. Normalizing the thermal effects of radiofrequency radiation: body mass versus total body surface area. *Bioelectromagnetics* 1987;8:111–118.

106. Gordon CJ. Effect of radiofrequency radiation exposure on thermoregulation. *ISI Atlas Sci Plants Anim* 1988;1:245–250.

107. Beers J. Biological effects of weak electromagnetic fields from 0 Hz to 200 MHz: a survey of the literature with special emphasis on possible magnetic resonance effects. *Magn Reson Imaging* 1989;7:309–331.

108. Coulter JS, Osbourne SL. Short wave diathermy in heating of human tissues. Arch Phys Ther 1936;17:679–687.

109. Bottomley PA, Edelstein WA. Power disposition in whole body NMR imaging. *Med Phys* 1981;8:510–512.

110. Bottomley PA, Redington RW, Edelstein WA, et al. Estimating radiofrequency power disposition in body NMR imaging. *Magn Reson Med* 1985;2:336–349.

111. Wickersheim KA, Sun MH. Fluoptic thermometry. *Med Electronics* 1987;(Feb):84–91.

112. Berman E. Reproductive effects. In: *Biological effects of radiofrequency radiation.* Washington: Environmental Protection Agency; 1984; 600/8-83-026A.

113. Michaelson SM, Lin JC. *Biological effects and health implications of radiofrequency radiation.* New York: Plenum Press, 1987.

114. U.S. Food and Drug Administration. Magnetic resonance diagnostic device; panel recommendation and report on petitions for MR reclassification. *Federal Register* 1988;53:7575–7579.

115. Shellock FG, Kanal E. Policies, guidelines, and recommendations for MR imaging safety and patient management. *J Magn Reson Imaging* 1991;1:97–101.

116. Goldman AM, Grossman WE, Friedlander PC. Reduction of sound levels with antinoise in MR imaging. *Radiology* 1989;173:549–550.

117. Hayes DL, Holmes DR, Gray JE. Effect of a 1.5 Tesla nuclear magnetic resonance imaging scanner on implanted permanent pacemakers. *J Am Coll Cardiol* 1987;10:782–786.

118. Gangarosa RE, Minnis JE, Nobbe J, et al. Operational safety issues in MRI. *Magn Reson Imaging* 1987;5:287–292.

119. Alagona P, Toole JC, Maniscalco BS, et al. Nuclear magnetic resonance imaging in a patient with a DDD pacemaker. *Pacing Clin Electrophysiol* 1989;12:619.

120. Edelman RR, Shellock FG, Ahladis J. Practical MRI for the technologist and imaging specialist. In: Edelman RR, Hesselink J, eds. *Clinical magnetic resonance imaging.* Philadelphia: Saunders, 1990.

121. A new MRI complication? *ECRI. health devices alert.* 1988;(May 27):1.

122. Dormer KJ, Richard GJ, Hough JVD, et al. The use of rare-earth magnet couplers in cochlear implants. *Laryngoscope* 1981;91:1812–1820.

123. Shellock FG. *Ex vivo* assessment of deflection forces and artifacts associated with high-field MRI of "mini-magnet" dental prostheses. *Magn Reson Imaging* 1989;7(Suppl 1):IT-03.

124. Liang MD, Narayanan K, Kanal E. Magnetic ports in tissue expanders: a caution for MRI. *Magn Reson Imaging* 1989;7:541–542.

125. Lund G, Nelson JD, Wirtschafter JD, et al. Tatooing of eyelids: magnetic imaging artifacts. *Ophthalmic Surg* 1986;17:550–553.

126. Sacco DA, Steiger DA, Bellon EM, et al. Artifacts caused by cosmetics in MR imaging of the head. *AJR Am J Roentgenol* 1987;148:1001–1004.

127. Jackson JG, Acker JD. Permanent eyeliner and MR imaging. *AJR Am J Roentgenol* 1987;149:1080.

128. Pusey E, Lufkin RB, Brown RKJ, et al. Magnetic resonance imaging artifacts: mechanism and clinical significance. *Radiographics* 1986;6:891–911.

129. Buchli R, Boesiger P, Meier D. Heating effects of metallic implants by MRI examinations. *Magn Reson Med* 1988;7:255–261.

130. Davis PL, Crooks L, Arakawa M, et al. Potential hazards in NMR imaging: heating effects of changing magnetic fields and RF fields on small metallic implants. *AJR Am J Roentgenol* 1981;137:857–860.

131. Shellock FG, Crues JV. High-field MR imaging of metallic biomedical implants: an *in vitro* evaluation of deflection forces and temperature changes induced in large prostheses. *Radiology* 1987;165:150.

132. Shellock FG, Crues JV. High-field MR imaging of metallic biomedical implants: an *ex vivo* evaluation of deflection forces. *AJR Am J Roentgenol* 1988;151:389–392.

133. Dujovny M, Kossovsky N, Kossowsky R, et al. Aneurysm clip motion during magnetic resonance imaging: *in vivo* experimental study with metallurgical factor analysis. *Neurosurgery* 1985;17:543–548.

134. Shellock FG, Schatz CJ, Shelton C, et al. *Ex vivo* evaluation of 9 different ocular and middle-ear implants exposed to a 1.5 Tesla MR scanner. *Radiology* 1990;177:271.

135. Shellock FG, Schatz CJ. High-field strength MRI and otologic implants. *AJNR Am J Neuroradiol* 1991;12:279–281.

136. Shellock FG, Meeks T. *Ex vivo* evaluation of ferromagnetism and artifacts for implantable vascular access ports exposed to a 1.5 T MR scanner. *J Magn Reson Imaging* 1991;1:243.

137. Teitelbaum GP, Yee CA, Van Horn DD, et al. Metallic ballistic fragments: MR imaging safety and artifacts. *Radiology* 1990;175:855–859.

138. Shellock FG. MR imaging of metallic implants and materials: a compilation of the literature. *AJR Am J Roentgenol* 1988;151:811–814.

139. Shellock FG, Curtis JS. MR imaging and biomedical implants, materials, and devices: an updated review. *Radiology* 1991;180:541–550.

140. Holtas S, Olsson M, Romner B, et al. Comparison of MR imaging and CT in patients with intracranial aneurysm clips. *AJNR Am J Neuroradiol* 1988;9:891–897.

141. Huttenbrink KB, Grobe-Nobis W. Experimentelle Untersuchungen und theoretische Betrachtungen uber das Verhalten von Stapes-Metall-Prothesen im Magnetfeld eines Kernspintomographen. [Experiments and theoretical considerations on behavior of metallic stapedectomy-protheses in nuclear magnetic resonance imaging.] *Laryngologicie Rhinologie Otologie* 1987;66:127–130.

142. Becker R, Norfray JF, Teitelbaum GP, et al. MR imaging in patients with intracranial aneurysm clips. *AJNR Am J Neuroradiol* 1988;9:885–889.

143. Randall PA, Kohman LJ, Scalzetti EM, et al. Magnetic resonance imaging of prosthetic cardiac valves *in vitro* and *in vivo.* *Am J Cardiol* 1988;62:973–976.

144. Romner B, Olsson M, Ljunggren B, et al. Magnetic resonance imaging and aneurysm clips. *J Neurosurg* 1989;70:426–431.

145. Augustiny N, von Schulthess GK, Meier D, et al. MR imaging of large nonferromagnetic metallic implants at 1.5 T. *J Comput Assist Tomogr* 1987;11:678–683.

146. Teitelbaum GP, Bradley WG, Klein BD. MR imaging artifacts ferromagnetism, and magnetic torque of intravascular filters, stents, and coils. *Radiology* 1988;166:657–664.
147. Yuh WTC, Hanigan MT, Nerad JA, et al. Extrusion of an eye socket magnetic implant after MR imaging examination: potential hazard to a patient with eye prosthesis. *J Magn Reson Imaging* 1991;1: 711–713.
148. Kelly WM, Pagle PG, Pearson A, et al. Ferromagnetism of intraocular foreign body causes unilateral blindness after MR study. *AJNR Am J Neuroradiol* 1986;7:243–245.
149. Williams S, Char DH, Dillon WP, et al. Ferrous intraocular foreign bodies and magnetic resonance imaging. *Am J Ophthalmol* 1988;105: 398–401.
150. Shellock FG. *Guide to MR procedures and metallic objects: update 1999*. Philadelphia: Lippincott Williams & Wilkins, 1999.
151. Adey WR. Tissue interactions with nonionizing electromagnetic fields. *Physiol Rev* 1981;61:435–514.
152. Phelps LA. MRI and claustrophobia. *Am Fam Physician* 1990;42:930.
153. Flaherty JA, Hoskinson K. Emotional distress during magnetic resonance imaging. *N Engl J Med* 1989;320:467–468.
154. Fishbain DA, Goldberg M, Labbe E, et al. Long-term claustrophobia following magnetic resonance imaging. *Am J Psychiatry* 1988;145: 1038–1039.
155. Quirk ME, Letendre AJ, Ciottone RA, et al. Anxiety in patients undergoing MR imaging. *Radiology* 1989;170:463–466.
156. Quirk ME, Letendre AJ, Ciottone RA, et al. Evaluation of three psychological interventions to reduce anxiety during MR imaging. *Radiology* 1989;173:759–762.
157. Hricak H, Amparo EG. Body MRI: alleviation of claustrophobia by prone positioning. *Radiology* 1984;152:819.
158. Weinreb JC, Maravilla KR, Peshock R, et al. Magnetic resonance imaging: improving patient tolerance and safety. *AJR Am J Roentgenol* 1984;143:1285–1287.
159. Klonoff EA, Janata JW, Kaufman B. The use of systematic desensitization to overcome resistance to magnetic resonance imaging (MRI) scanning. *J Behav Ther Exp Psychiatry* 1986;17:189–192.
160. Granet RB, Gelber LJ. Claustrophobia during MR imaging. *N J Med* 1990;87:479–482.
161. McGuinness TP. Hypnosis in the treatment of phobias: a review of the literature. *Am J Clin Hypn* 1984;26:261–272.
162. Peterfy CG, Roberts T, Genant HK. Dedicated extremity MR imaging: an emerging technology. *Radiol Clin North Am* 1997;35:1–20.
163. Franklin PD, Lemon RA, Barden HS. Accuracy of imaging the menisci on an in-office, dedicated, magnetic resonance imaging extremity system. *Am J Sports Med* 1998;25:382–388.
164. Masciocchi C, Barile A, Navarra F, et al. Clinical experience of osteoarticular MRI using a dedicated system. *MAGMA* 1994;2:545–550.
165. Shellock FG, Stone K, Crues JV. Development and clinical applications of kinematic MRI of the patellofemoral joint using an extremity MR system. *Med Sci Sports Exerc* 1999;31:788–791.
166. Shellock FG, O'Neil M, Ivans V, et al. Cardiac pacemakers and implantable cardiac defibrillators are unaffected by operation of an extremity MR system. *AJR Am J Roentgenol* 1999;172:165–172.
167. Shellock FG, Crues JV. Aneurysm clips: assessment of magnetic field interaction associated with a 0.2-T extremity MR system. *Radiology* 1998;208:407–409.

Open MRI,
edited by Peter A. Rothschild and Debra Reinking Rothschild.
Lippincott Williams & Wilkins. Philadelphia © 2000.

CHAPTER 5

Sedation for Open Magnetic Resonance Imaging

Debra Reinking Rothschild

Magnetic resonance imaging (MRI) has become the diagnostic test of choice for a variety of conditions; however, some patients are unable or unwilling to undergo MRI without the aid of sedation. Sedation for these patients in the MRI suite presents challenges not found in the operating room or anywhere else in the hospital or clinic setting. The purpose of this chapter is to familiarize the radiologist and technologist with issues regarding sedation, particularly within the open MRI suite.

It must be understood that anesthesia and sedation are part of the same continuum. When the term *sedation* is used, the patient may actually be *anesthetized*, with its associated risks.

SEDATION FOR MAGNETIC RESONANCE IMAGING

Patients Requiring Sedation

Performance of an MRI examination requires that the patient lie motionless for each sequence. Some patients are unable or unwilling to lie still for the time required. Young children, patients in severe pain, claustrophobic and anxious patients, and patients with movement disorders present special challenges and often require sedation to successfully complete their MRI studies.

Pediatric Patients

Children younger than 5 years of age may require sedation. Infants younger than 12 months may often be scanned without sedation, especially in open MRI, if the patient is secured and the scan is scheduled during a normal nap time. Sleep deprivation can be helpful in this age group.

Patients Experiencing Severe Pain

Patients in severe pain are often unable to remain motionless during scanning and may require large doses of analgesics. Patients with pain from a malignancy are often in this category. Patients with low back pain often find that their pain is influenced by position and can be exacerbated by the supine position. Additionally, the supine position can elicit painful muscle spasms, further hindering the patient's ability to remain motionless and often resulting in an incomplete or nondiagnostic study.

Claustrophobia and Anxiety

A significant segment of the population experiences claustrophobia. Others do not have a history of claustrophobia but develop severe anxiety when attempting to undergo MRI and require sedation to complete the scan.

Patients with Movement Disorders

Patients with movement disorders, such as Parkinson's disease or other tremors, may be unable to lie motionless. Patients with torticollis may not be able to be positioned correctly or may be unable to maintain the necessary position for completion of the scan. General anesthesia may be the only way to obtain a diagnostic study in these patients.

Levels of Sedation

It must be recognized that sedation and anesthesia are part of the same continuum and that dividing sedation/anesthesia into the terms *conscious sedation*, *deep sedation*, and *general anesthesia* is somewhat artificial. Nonetheless, the terms *conscious sedation*, *deep sedation*, and *general anesthesia* are commonly used, and their definitions should be understood.

D. Reinking Rothschild: Open MRI, Hayward, California; Summit Medical Center, Oakland, California

Conscious sedation is defined by the American Academy of Pediatrics Committee on Drugs (AAP-COD) as

a medically controlled state of depressed consciousness that:

1. allows protective reflexes to be maintained,
2. retains the patient's ability to maintain a patent airway independently and continuously,
3. permits appropriate response by the patient to physical stimulation or verbal command, e.g. "open your eyes." (1)

In other words, the gag reflex (part of the protective reflexes) is maintained, the airway is open, and the patient follows simple directions.

The AAP-COD defines *deep sedation* as

a medically controlled state of depressed consciousness from which the patient is not easily aroused. It may be accompanied by partial or complete loss of protective reflexes, and includes the inability to maintain a patent airway independently and respond purposefully to physical stimulation or verbal command. (1)

In other words, the gag reflex is partially or completely lost, the tongue may fall back into the oropharynx causing airway obstruction, and the patient is unable to follow simple directions.

General anesthesia is defined by the AAP-COD as

a medically controlled state of unconsciousness accompanied by a loss of protective reflexes, including the inability to maintain a patent airway and respond purposefully to physical stimulation or verbal command. (1)

In other words, these patients do not have a gag reflex; airway obstruction frequently occurs; and yet, they may still move when sufficiently stimulated.

Although the distinctions between the various states of sedation and general anesthesia may at first seem clear-cut, the sedated patient is in a dynamic state. Delayed drug absorption can be an important factor, especially when administering drugs via oral, rectal, or intramuscular routes. The patient's state of sedation often varies according to the stimulation received. When pain or stimulation stops, the sedated patient can rapidly drift from the state of conscious sedation to deep sedation or even to a state more closely resembling general anesthesia, with its attendant risks and complications. Thus, many safeguards associated with general anesthesia, such as *nil per os* (NPO) intervals and monitoring during the procedure and recovery periods, should be undertaken even when only conscious sedation is planned. This critical point is often overlooked in radiology departments and imaging centers, with unfortunate and tragic results.

For an example of conscious sedation rapidly becoming anesthesia, one need only look to the hospital's preoperative area or postanesthesia recovery room. In both of these departments, it is a common experience to see a medicated (i.e., consciously sedated) patient complaining to the nurse of severe anxiety (in the preoperative area) or of severe pain (in the recovery room). Yet, as any experienced preoperative or recovery room nurse knows, as soon as the nurse leaves the patient's bedside (i.e., the stimulation stops), these med-

icated patients frequently doze off, sometimes developing respiratory depression, airway obstruction, and apnea. If this change in the patient's condition is immediately recognized, it can often be very easily treated. Sometimes, all the patient needs is to be talked to or patted, perhaps shaken on the shoulder to awaken the patient enough to maintain an open airway and resume breathing. Other times, a jaw-thrust maneuver to open the airway or positive-pressure ventilation, via an Ambu bag (Linthicum, MD), is required. The stimulation caused by the jaw-thrust maneuver or by ventilating the patient often awakens the patient enough that he or she no longer requires these interventions. On the other hand, if the patient is not monitored and the respiratory depression, airway obstruction, or apnea is not recognized, what could have been a temporary, easy-to-correct problem can cascade into cardiac arrest resulting in permanent brain damage or death. This can easily happen in an MRI scanner, in which it is difficult to see and hear the patient, electronic monitors are cumbersome and sometimes hazardous to use, pressure to maintain patient through-put exists, and the person assigned to observe the patient is often saddled with multiple other simultaneous responsibilities.

Administration of Sedation

Much debate exists concerning who should administer sedation for radiologic procedures (1–9). Administrative, medical, regulatory, and financial concerns are involved. Some MRI departments have two-tiered programs, in which patients are prescreened. Patients without complicating medical problems may be sedated by a nurse under the direction of the radiologist, although an anesthesia consultation may be obtained regarding patients with complicated or unusual conditions.

It is beyond the scope of this chapter to enter into this particular debate; however, certain standards should be followed, regardless of who administers the sedation. The AAP-COD (1), the American Society of Anesthesiologists (ASA) (9), and the American College of Radiology (10) have developed standards for sedation. The MRI center or department routines should, at a minimum, include patient preparation, monitoring during the sedation, and management of the postsedation recovery period.

Patient Preparation

Patient screening can detect conditions that may complicate sedation. Once these difficult patients are identified, MRI departments can ensure that appropriate measures, such as involvement of the anesthesia department, are taken to sedate these difficult and risky patients. Important patient information (9) includes the following:

- Major organ system disease, such as diabetes, cardiac, pulmonary, or hepatic disease
- Experience with previous anesthesia and sedation

TABLE 5-1. *Classification of physical status*

P-1	A normal healthy patient
P-2	A patient with mild systemic disease
P-3	A patient with severe systemic disease
P-4	A patient with severe systemic disease that is a constant threat to life
P-5	A moribund patient who is not expected to survive without the operation
P-6	A declared brain-dead patient whose organs are being removed for donor purposes

Reprinted with permission of the American Society of Anesthesiologists, 520 N. Northwest Highway, Park Ridge, IL 60068-2573.

- Medications and allergies
- NPO status
- History of alcohol, substance, or tobacco use

The ASA physical status table can be used to stratify patients (Table 5-1). In addition to ASA physical status and the factors above, the following specific conditions can have an enormous impact on the safety of sedation:

In adult patients:

- Obesity, pregnancy—more prone to airway obstruction, regurgitation, and aspiration of gastric contents
- Hiatal hernia, diabetes, gastroesophageal reflux—more prone to regurgitation and aspiration of gastric contents
- Obstructive sleep apnea—prone to airway obstruction with sedation
- Snoring—indicative of airway obstruction, more prone to airway obstruction when sedated
- Congestive heart failure—may be unable to lie flat without experiencing shortness of breath; the ability to lie flat when sedated in a patient who before sedation could not do so may indicate that the patient is oversedated
- Elevated intracranial pressure—retained carbon dioxide (CO_2) during sedation can further elevate intracranial pressure, diminishing an already compromised cerebral blood flow
- Other medical conditions, such as asthma and chronic obstructive pulmonary disease—may worsen during sedation

In pediatric patients:

- Airway abnormalities (Pierre Robin syndrome, micrognathia, macroglossia, and tonsillar hypertrophy)—more likely to experience airway obstruction when sedated
- Asthma—may experience exacerbation during sedation
- Cyanotic congenital heart disease—owing to complicated hemodynamic variables these patients may develop further hemoglobin oxygen desaturation when sedated
- Mental retardation, developmental delays, hyperactivity—more likely to experience sedation failure
- Previous failed sedation attempts—more likely to require higher doses or combinations of drugs, with higher risk of complications

TABLE 5-2. *Summary of fasting recommendations to reduce the risk of pulmonary aspiration*

Ingested material	Minimum fasting period (h)
Clear liquids[a]	2
Breast milk	4
Infant formula	6
Nonhuman milk[b]	6
Light meal[c]	6

Notes: These recommendations apply to healthy patients undergoing elective procedures. They are not intended for women in labor. Following the guidelines dose not guarantee complete gastric emptying.

The fasting periods noted above apply to all ages.

[a]Examples of clear liquids include water, fruit juices without pulp, carbonated beverages, clear tea, and black coffee.

[b]Because nonhuman milk is similar to solids in gastric emptying time, the amount ingested must be considered when determining an appropriate fasting period.

[c]A light meal typically consists of toast and clear liquids. Meals that include fried or fatty foods or meat may prolong gastric emptying time. Both the amount and type of foods ingested must be considered when determining an appropriate fasting period.

Reprinted with permission of the American Society of Anesthesiologists, 520 N. Northwest Highway, Park Ridge, IL 60068-2573.

An NPO interval is necessary to minimize the possibility of aspiration, an important point that is often overlooked by outpatient imaging centers. The ASA "Practice Guidelines Regarding Preoperative Fasting" (11) recommend a minimum fast of 2 hours for clear liquids, 4 hours for breast milk, 6 hours for infant formula or nonhuman milk, and 6 hours for a "light meal" (Table 5-2).

This NPO period is critical because sedatives depress the patient's gag reflex. Elective surgery is cancelled for a patient who does not adhere to the NPO period, even though cancelled surgery is a financial and scheduling burden for all involved. Vomited material can easily enter the pharynx. If the patient is only lightly sedated and partial reflexes are present, the patient may experience laryngospasm, in which the vocal cords and glottis close tightly to protect the lungs. Patients with laryngospasm cannot breathe and require immediate treatment. The stimulus for glottic closure must be removed and an airway must be established, by intubation if necessary. If the patient is more deeply sedated, with complete loss of the gag reflex, gastric material can enter the trachea. The patient can die immediately from mechanical obstruction of the airway. Aspirated liquid material, especially if it contains gastric acid, can cause enormous damage to the lungs, leading to respiratory failure, adult respiratory distress syndrome, and death. This NPO interval is more important in pediatric sedation because chloral hydrate (CH) itself is a gastric irritant that can cause vomiting.

Instructions should be given to the patient in advance of the planned sedation (Figs. 5-1 and 5-2). These instructions must emphasize the NPO period and the requirement for a

---

Sedation Instructions—Adult

Most patients can complete a scan at Open MRI, but patients occasionally are unable to complete the scan. Oral medications, such as Valium, which your referring doctor can prescribe, can help many patients complete the scan. If the oral medication is not sufficient, your doctor may have suggested sedation for your scan. Generally, this involves starting an intravenous line in your arm and injecting sedation or painkiller until you are comfortable enough to complete the scan.

Instructions:
1. Nothing to eat or drink from midnight the night before the scan, except for sips of water to take medications.
2. Most medications, especially analgesics (painkillers), can be continued with sips of water. Ask the anesthesiologist about specific medications.
3. You must have a responsible adult to drive you home from the MRI center. No driving or operating machinery for a minimum of 24 hours after the completion of the scan.
4. Complete the enclosed sedation questionnaire and bring it with you to the MRI center on the date of your examination.
5. Bring your medications and a list of your allergies when you come for your examination.
6. Wear comfortable clothing that will be easy for you to remove.
7. If you have not been contacted by the anesthesiologist 2 days ahead of the scheduled sedation, call the MRI center and ask to talk to the anesthesiologist.

Arrive at _____a.m./p.m. on _____.

FIG. 5-1. Sedation instructions for adults.

Sedation Instructions—Child

Your doctor has referred your child for an MRI at Open MRI. Many children, especially those older than 4 years of age, who can cooperate and follow instructions, can be scanned without sedation. The scanner at Open MRI is quiet, and your child will not be disturbed by the loud banging that some other MRI scanners produce. Children younger than 9 months usually do not require any sedation and will sleep through the examination, as long as they are adequately sleep deprived.

Some parents prefer that their children not receive sedative drugs. We have successfully scanned many pediatric patients with sleep deprivation alone. Parents should keep the child awake until he or she is so tired that the child simply falls asleep for the duration of the examination. Many children between the ages of 9 months and 4 years are more easily scanned if they receive sedation.

1. If your child does need sedation, it is important that he or she has an empty stomach. Generally, this means 8 hours without food or milk and at least 3 hours without water. However, very small children may be unable to go without food and drink for this period. The anesthesiologist will give you an exact time to stop oral intake, after taking into consideration the patient's age and weight and the exact time of the MRI examination.
2. Dress the child in comfortable cotton clothes. Make sure there are no zippers, snaps, or other metal objects on the clothing that could interfere with the magnet. Avoid T-shirts with decals, as many decals have metal particles that can cause artifact in the MRI image.
3. Bring extra diapers and juice or formula for the child to drink after the examination.
4. Sleep deprivation is very helpful. Arriving at the MRI center with a sleepy child will allow the examination to be completed with a minimum of drugs. Do not let the child take his or her afternoon nap on the day before the examination. Keep the child up at least 2 hours past his or her usual bedtime the night before the examination and wake him or her up an hour early on the morning of the examination. **Do not let your child fall asleep on the drive to the MRI center.**

Arrive at _____ a.m./p.m. on _____.

FIG. 5-2. Sedation instructions for children.

driver to accompany the sedated patient after the procedure. Informed consent should be obtained and documented (1,9).

Before sedation, the head, neck, and mouth should be examined for clues to airway abnormalities. Airway abnormalities can increase the likelihood of airway obstruction and make it more difficult to deliver positive-pressure ventilation, which may be needed if respiratory compromise occurs (1,9). A large "bull neck," obesity, micrognathia, macroglossia, hypertrophied tonsils, and unusual facies are some indications of airway abnormalities that can lead to problems.

Monitoring in Magnetic Resonance Imaging

Whenever sedative or anesthetic drugs are used, it is imperative to have equipment and personnel immediately available to diagnose and treat complications that are reasonably anticipated (1,9). Early recognition and treatment of complications can prevent minor, transient problems from becoming life-threatening events. The ASA "Practice Guidelines for Sedation and Analgesia" (1,9) mandate that a person be present to monitor the patient and that the following monitoring be performed:

- Visual.
- Level of consciousness.
- Ventilatory status, via observation or listening to the breath sounds. If the practitioner is physically separated from the patient, apnea monitoring such as via exhaled CO_2 may be used.
- Oxygenation status, via pulse oximetry.
- Hemodynamics via blood pressures and via electrocardiography (ECG) if significant cardiovascular disease is present.
- An individual who can recognize the complications of sedation, such as hypoventilation and airway obstruction, as well as establish a patent airway for positive-pressure ventilation, should be present.

The AAP guidelines further mandate that when deep sedation is used, a person be present whose only responsibility is to monitor the patient (1).

Supplemental oxygen must be available, and a means to artificially ventilate the patient [i.e., Ambu bag (Ambu, Inc., Brødby, Denmark) and masks], suction equipment, and other emergency resuscitative equipment (e.g., laryngoscopes, endotracheal tubes, and a defibrillator) must also be present (Table 5-3). All equipment must be available for the entire age and size range of patients being treated. The MRI center's defibrillator should have pediatric capabilities, if these patients are sedated.

Documentation

Documentation should be kept that records the patient's vital signs; oxygen saturation; respiratory function; as well as name, dosage, and time of administration of all drugs administered (1,9). A time-based anesthesia-type record is ideal (Fig. 5-3).

TABLE 5-3. *Example of emergency equipment and drug list for sedation for magnetic resonance imaging (MRI)*

Oxygen: piped-in is ideal; if cylinders are used in the MRI suite, they must be aluminum, not iron, and have MRI-compatible regulators and carts
Stethoscope
Plastic precordial stethoscope
Gurney: should be large enough for the patients who will be sedated; should be able to be safely taken into the MRI suite (given the field strength of the magnet)
Patient transfer board to facilitate moving patient from gurney to MRI table; extra-large board helpful for open scanners
Blood pressure cuffs: large and extra-large cuffs ("thigh cuffs") needed in open MRI; pediatric cuffs if pediatric patients are sedated
Noninvasive blood pressure monitor, MRI compatible, with extra long tubes to locate base unit away from the scanner
Pulse oximeter with probes (MRI compatible); pediatric probes if pediatric patients sedated
Capnography: in the MRI suite, an aspirating system is preferable to an infrared system
Means to give high concentration oxygen by positive-pressure ventilation [Ambu bag (Ambu, Inc., Brødby, Denmark) and masks in assorted sizes]
Intravenous solutions, tubing sets, micro-drip tubing for pediatric use, intravenous catheters in assorted sizes
Tourniquet, alcohol swabs, assorted syringes, needles, and sharps containers
Oral airways and nasal airways in assorted adult and pediatric sizes
Endotracheal tubes (adult and pediatric sizes)
Suction
   Suction catheters: rigid Yankauer catheters, as well as flexible suction catheters
   Laryngoscope handles, assorted blades, pediatric blades if pediatric patients sedated
   Defibrillator: should have pediatric capabilities if pediatric patients are sedated
   Electrocardiogram (MRI compatible) with accessories
Drugs
   Lidocaine jelly (for use with nasal airways)
   Epinephrine 1:1,000 and 1:10,000
   Ephedrine
   Phenylephrine
   Lidocaine
   Aminophylline
   Dextrose
   Sodium bicarbonate
   Calcium chloride
   Nitroglycerin tablets
   Anticholinergics: atropine, glycopyrrolate
   Diphenhydramine
   Reversal agents
      Flumazenil: to reverse benzodiazepines
      Naloxone: to reverse narcotics
   EMLA cream
   Pentobarbital
   Chloral hydrate
   Diazepam: oral tablets and intravenous solution
   Midazolam: intravenous solution and oral syrup

EMLA, eutectic mixture of local anesthetics.
Notes: Individual MRI center's needs may vary.
Based upon the 1996 Practice Guidelines for Sedation and Analgesia by Non-Anesthesiologists of the American Society of Anesthesiologists (ASA). A copy of the full text can be obtained from ASA, 520 North Northwest Highway, Park Ridge, IL 60068-2573.
Banyan sells Stat Kits, prepackaged emergency kits for physicians in suitcase-like containers. These kits contain many of the emergency drugs and equipment needed in a convenient form. Kits are available for adult and for pediatric patients. [Banyan International Corporation, 2118 E. Interstate 20, Abilene, TX 70604, (800) 351-4530, www.statkit.com.]

SEDATION RECORD   Date:

Patient name:		age:	height:	weight:
Examination:	diagnosis:		ref. Doctor:	
Allergies:	Medications:			
Medical history:				

PE:

Informed consent:

TIME: :00 :15 :30 :45 :00 :15 :30 :45 :00 :15

oxygen

medications

fluids

ETCO^2

O^2 SAT

BLOOD PRESSURE in MM HG

SYS ▼

DIAS ▲

230 220 210 200 190 180 170 160 150 140 130 120 110 100 90 80 70 60 50 40 30 20

HEART RATE IN BEATS PER MIN ●

NOTES:

Start time

Stop time

Monitors: circle as appropriate

BPC   IV

NIBPM

PCS

Pulse oximeter capnography

Recovery Notes:

Circle as appropriate: awake alert oriented presedation mental status

ambulating without assistance versus within 20% of presedation value

Released to: Time:

Discharge instructions and emergency phone number given to:

FIG. 5-3. Sedation record. BPC, blood pressure cuff; DIAS, diastolic; NIBPM, non-invasive blood pressure monitor; PCS, precordial stethoscope; PE, physical examination; SYS, systolic.

Emergency Plan

An emergency plan should be in place addressing the specific activities and roles needed in the event of a medical emergency within the MRI suite or facility. Will the patient be moved from the MRI suite before cardiopulmonary resuscitation or defibrillation, or will the equipment be brought to the patient? Who will call for assistance, and how will they be reached? If in a hospital, will the code team know how to reach the MRI suite? Who will be "in charge" of the code? Who will be responsible for maintaining the patient's airway and ventilation? Who will administer the drugs? Who will be responsible for recording of the drugs and activities? If in a freestanding facility, who will be called for assistance? Does the freestanding facility have a transfer agreement in place with an acute care hospital to care for any patient requiring such care? These may seem to be tedious and unnecessary details, but emergencies are never planned, and it is much better to have a plan in place and never need it than to risk having confusion add to the demands of caring for a "crashing" patient.

Magnetic Resonance Imaging Environment

The MRI suite presents unique challenges not found elsewhere in the hospital or clinic. Access to the patient, although rarely an issue in the operating or procedure room, is frequently difficult, even with open MRI. In standard tube-type MRI, the patient is enclosed in a tube and is inaccessible. Auditory noise levels in the high-field MRI suite can reach 65 to 85 dB or higher (12). Ear protection may be necessary, and auditory signals and alarms from the monitoring equipment can be obscured. Much "routine" monitoring is auditory; in many pulse oximeters, the tone of the beep is indicative of the oxygen saturation level.

Much has been written about anesthesia and sedation in the MRI suite (13–39).

The presence of a powerful magnet and radiofrequency pulses are variables not present in any other location in the hospital. The ferromagnetic attraction of the magnet can turn monitoring equipment into projectiles, and care must be taken to exclude ferromagnetic materials from the MRI suite. Oxygen must be available in areas in which patients are sedated. If piped-in oxygen is not available and cylinders are used, aluminum, not iron, oxygen cylinders and carts must be used.

The static magnetic field can also distort the electron beams within the monitors themselves, leading to unusual looking tracings and artifacts that can mimic pathology such as T-wave changes in the ECG (5,13,16,28,31,40). Additionally, the electronic monitors may introduce artifacts into the MRI images (5,13,14,31).

Standard anesthesia machines have been converted into MRI-compatible anesthesia machines by anesthesiologists (41,42). Other anesthesiologists have managed the issue by either using very long anesthesia circuits attached to an anesthesia machine that has been located as far as practical

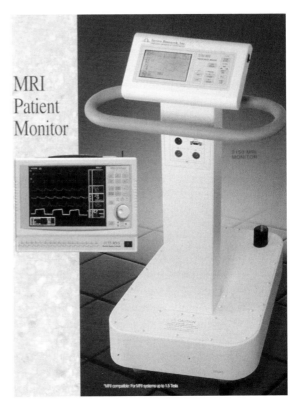

FIG. 5-4. Example of magnetic resonance imaging–compatible monitoring equipment. Photograph courtesy of Invivo Research, Inc., 12601 Research Parkway, Orlando, FL 32826.

from the bore of the magnet or by ventilating the patient with a manual anesthesia circuit, thereby completely avoiding the use of an anesthesia machine (13,15,43).

Burns from Wires

Several cases have been reported of patients who received burns, usually from ECG or pulse oximetry wires, while undergoing MRI (44–50), because the wire can act as an antenna and collect radiofrequency energy that is transmitted during the MRI scan. To minimize the risk of burns, the following guidelines should be followed (5,15):

- Electrically conductive materials not required for the study should be removed from the bore of the magnet and the vicinity of the patient.
- Electrically conductive material that must remain in the bore of the magnet should be kept from forming large loops.
- Electrically conductive material in the bore of the magnet should not be in direct contact with the patient.

Some authors recommend braiding any wires to prevent the formation of loops (15).

To remedy problems encountered in the MRI suite, several manufacturers have introduced MRI-compatible monitoring and anesthesia equipment (Fig. 5-4). MRI-compatible pulse oximeters use nonconducting fiber-optic cables instead of the ferromagnetic cabling used in traditional monitors. Some monitors have a second display unit that can sit outside the scan room, allowing observers both inside and outside the MRI room to have full access to the monitor output. MRI-compatible monitors and anesthesia equipment are available for use with MRI from 0.15 to 2.00 T. Even when MRI-compatible monitoring equipment is used, the practitioner must follow each manufacturer's instructions regarding use of leads and placement of the monitor itself. Ideally, equipment should be tested, before use, on the specific MRI with which it will be used (5).

Pulse Oximetry

Pulse oximetry displays the patient's pulse rate and hemoglobin saturation level in real time, allowing the detection of hypoxemia before cyanosis occurs. Pulse oximetry became rapidly accepted after its introduction in the early 1980s, and it has been credited with significant improvements in the safety of patients undergoing general anesthesia (51–53). Optimal use of pulse oximetry requires knowledge of its limitations (54). Oxygenation may remain normal in the presence of apnea if supplemental oxygen is given (55,56). Motion, hypotension, and vasoconstriction can cause the pulse oximeter to fail, either giving erroneously low readings or no reading at all. At oxygen saturations below 70%, significant variation between different manufacturers' pulse oximeters has been reported (57–59). CO_2 retention may occur and cannot be detected unless capnography is also used (55,56,60). Nonetheless, even with its limitations, pulse oximetry is an invaluable tool. When used in the MRI suite, the pulse oximeter probe should be placed as far away as possible from the body part being scanned.

Capnography

Capnography is valuable to assess the adequacy of ventilation of sedated patients. Pulse oximetry alone is not sufficient, especially when patients are receiving supplemental oxygen, because the saturation can remain high despite hypoventilation and elevated levels of CO_2 (55,56). Elevated levels of CO_2 can lead to tachycardia, arrhythmias, hypertension, and increases in intracranial pressure. Although these effects might be tolerated by healthy patients, they are not well tolerated by patients with preexisting diseases, such as hypertension, cardiac disease, or intracranial pathology. Freeman (60) reported that use of supplemental oxygen masked the presence of apnea. The resultant CO_2 retention was heralded by multifocal premature ventricular contractions in two of 64 patients. For the MRI suite, capnography using an aspirating system is preferable to an infrared system. The aspirating system requires only the presence of the plastic aspirating tube within the MRI scanner. A nasal cannula with a built-in channel for CO_2 monitoring is available. The practitioner

monitoring the patient must also be aware that hypoventilation can lead to either a high end-tidal CO_2 ($ETCO_2$), reflecting the high blood CO_2 levels, or a deceptively low $ETCO_2$. If hypoventilation is severe enough or if apnea occurs, the $ETCO_2$ will not accurately reflect the blood levels. The CO_2 cannot effectively be carried out by exhaled breaths if the patient is not breathing or if the breaths are too shallow. This issue is often overlooked.

Suction

Suction must also be available in any area in which sedation or anesthesia is administered (1,61). Emesis or secretions must be quickly removed from the oropharynx of the sedated patient to prevent laryngospasm or aspiration. Wall suction is preferable; portable suction machines are also available.

Postsedation Recovery

Once the scan is complete, the job of caring for the sedated patient is not over. One must ensure that predetermined recovery criteria are met before releasing the sedated patient to nonmedical personnel (1,9). This is especially true of pediatric patients, in whom the most commonly used drugs, CH and pentobarbital, have long half-lives (12,62) and in whom drugs are often administered via nonintravenous routes. Another complication is delayed drug absorption leading to late resedation, which can occur after oral, rectal, or intramuscular administration of drugs. If the postsedation observation period is too short, and drugs were administered via nonintravenous routes, the patient could absorb additional drug later than expected, perhaps even after release from the MRI center.

Before release from the facility, the following criteria should be met:

- The patient should be alert and oriented or returned to baseline mental status.
- Vital signs should be stable.
- If any reversal agents were given, such as flumazenil or naloxone, adequate time should have passed so that the patient does not become resedated once the reversal agent wears off.
- A responsible adult should accompany the patient home.
- Written instructions including an emergency telephone number should be given (1,9).

Coté collected a series of severe complications that occurred after sedation for diagnostic and therapeutic procedures (63). He reported 52 deaths, six permanent neurologic injuries, and 15 prolonged hospitalizations. Three children either died or suffered "neurologic devastation" on their way home from the hospital or clinic. These catastrophes were thought to be from airway obstruction when the children fell asleep and their heads fell forward. With the effects of residual sedatives, these children did not have the head and neck strength to unobstruct their airways (2).

DIFFERENCES BETWEEN TRADITIONAL AND OPEN MAGNETIC RESONANCE IMAGING WITH REGARD TO SEDATION

Patients Requiring Sedation

Some significant differences exist between sedation for open versus closed MRI. The most significant difference is that a much smaller percentage of patients require sedation for an open MRI than for a closed tube-type MRI. Conversely, depending on referral patterns in the local community and the open MRI center's marketing efforts, open MRI centers often attract an atypical patient population. Patients who present to open MRI centers are more likely to be severely anxious, claustrophobic, or large and unable to fit into a traditional closed scanner. Many of these patients have refused to be scheduled for a closed MRI and only consented to an MRI when offered an open MRI. Some of these patients were unable to complete a closed MRI examination even after they were given intravenous sedation. Nonetheless, many patients who were unable or unwilling to complete a closed tube-type MRI are able to complete an open MRI without incident. The experience and demeanor of the MRI staff and general comfort measures, such as soothing music, can have a tremendous and positive impact on these patients.

Pediatric Patients

As with adults, many children who would have required sedation for a closed scanner can undergo scanning in an open scanner without sedation. Although many closed MRI centers routinely sedate all children under the age of 8 years, most children over the age of 4 years can undergo scanning in an open scanner without sedation. When sedation is required, children can be scanned in the quieter open scanners with a lighter level of sedation than would be required in a noisier scanner. Allowing the parent to stay in the room with the child also decreases anxiety and helps the child tolerate the procedure.

Patient Size and Weight

Closed tube-type scanners usually are limited to patients who weigh less than 325 lb, owing to the table limit and gantry size. Even patients who weigh less than 325 lb may not fit into a tube-type scanner. Open scanners can usually scan patients up to 425 to 450 lb. The openness of the scanner allows even a very obese patient to fit comfortably within the scanner. However, obese patients can present a host of problems if they require sedation. The added adipose tissue, especially in the head and neck area, confers a much higher risk of airway obstruction in these patients when sedated. Obese patients are also at higher risk of regurgitation and aspiration of gastric contents. Sedated or anesthetized obese patients often do not have adequate spontaneous ventilation and may need to be ventilated. Owing to the added weight of the chest wall, they require higher ventilating pressures.

Scan Time

Another difference between open and traditional scanners is the open scanner's longer scan time. Some patients who could have tolerated a 2-minute sequence may find themselves unable to tolerate the same position for a 5- to 7-minute sequence. Patients undergoing conscious sedation may tolerate only the first 10 minutes of scanning and then begin to protest. It is imperative to complete the most important scans first and to use sequences with short scan times when caring for extremely anxious patients or patients in severe pain.

Benefits of Lower Field Strength Magnets

The lower field strength currently used in most open MRI scanners has definite clinical benefits. The risk of projectiles is much lower than with higher field strength tube-type scanners. The open architecture makes physical observation of the patient easier than with a closed MRI and allows a greater degree of direct access to the patient. The quieter operation can decrease the patient's anxiety level and can allow auditory contact with the patient during scanning. Auditory monitors can be heard over the operation of the lower field strength scanners. To the best of the author's knowledge, burns from wires or probes have not been reported with lower field strength scanners. Nonetheless, MRI-compatible equipment is widely available, and only MRI-compatible monitors are recommended.

Because magnetic field strength is the primary determinant of the fringe fields, lower strength magnets allow much more latitude with regard to use and placement of equipment. Most equipment, such as the pulse oximeter, blood pressure monitor, and infusion pumps, should be placed outside the 30-G line (28). With lower field strength magnets, placement outside the 30-G line is usually quite easy to accomplish, and monitors may be used much closer to a lower field strength magnet than a higher field strength magnet. Although the lower field strength present in currently available open scanners allows equipment to be brought closer to the magnet and patient, the gauss line plots from the magnet's manufacturer should be referred to before placement and use of equipment.

Sedation Techniques

Sleep Deprivation

Sleep deprivation is an old and safe technique for sedation. The infant's or child's scan is scheduled for a normal nap or sleep time. Parents are instructed to keep the child awake 2 to 3 hours later than his or her normal bedtime on the night before the examination and to awaken the patient an hour earlier than usual on the morning of the examination. The parents must not allow the child to fall asleep in the car on the way to the MRI center. Once at the MRI center and when the scanner is ready, parents and child are placed in a darkened, quiet room to rock the child to sleep. The child is then placed on the table and secured with foam, towels, and tape to prevent patient motion and to prevent the child from falling off the table. Although this technique is not always successful, it minimizes risk and often allows scanning of children whose parents prefer to avoid sedation. Sleep deprivation is particularly useful for infants under the age of 12 months, the age group that has the highest risk for complications of sedation and anesthesia, such as hypoxemia, apnea, airway obstruction, and hypotension (4).

Sleep deprivation also aids the success of sedation in all age groups. The success of sleep deprivation as a sole means of sedation depends on the noise level generated by the scanner. The quieter magnets allow greater levels of success with this technique. Open, low-field magnets are quieter than high-field, tube-type magnets. However, not all open models are quiet enough to successfully use sleep deprivation alone as a sedation technique.

Use of Pharmacologic Agents

The ideal sedative drug has a rapid, predictable onset; is easily and painlessly administered; does not cause any respiratory or cardiac depression; renders patients perfectly motionless for the exact duration of the examination; and allows them to awaken completely at the conclusion of scanning. No such drug exists. Therefore, numerous sedation techniques have been described (21–26,29,62,64). Important concepts to consider when administering sedation are as follows:

1. Many sedative drugs, when combined with others, act synergistically and cause a much greater effect than expected from simply adding the effects of each drug. For example, narcotics alone do not usually produce a significant hypnotic effect, but they do have a significant hypnotic effect when combined with a benzodiazepine such as diazepam. A small dose of narcotic plus a small dose of diazepam can cause a pronounced effect.
2. Administration of drugs via oral, rectal, or intramuscular routes can lead to erratic or delayed drug absorption. The clinician, believing that the patient requires a larger dose (instead of a longer induction time) may give additional drug. Both doses of medication may reach high blood levels simultaneously, leading to an excessively sedated patient. Although some have the impression that rectally and orally administered sedatives are safer than intravenous drugs, this is not necessarily the case. Owing to the possibility of erratic and delayed drug absorption, rectally administered drugs may be more dangerous than intravenous drugs. Once an intravenous drug has been given, the maximum effect is seen rapidly. When drugs are given orally or rectally, the practitioner does not always know when the drug has reached its peak effect. It is possible that the patient may absorb additional drug and become more sedated later than anticipated, sometimes even after release from the MRI facility.
3. After administration of sedative drugs, verification of a patent airway is essential, especially after positioning of the patient. Flexion of the head and neck should be avoided, as it may lead to airway obstruction.
4. The level of sedation varies according to the stimulation received. Once the stimulation of positioning and monitor placement are over, the patient may drift into a much deeper state of sedation or even anesthesia.

A cursory review of some common sedation drugs follows. Although every attempt is made to ensure accuracy at the time of publication, the practitioner should review package inserts before administration of any medications.

Because children are often sedated by the administration of oral, rectal, or intramuscular drugs, debate exists as to whether intravenous access is necessary for all sedated children. At a minimum, the equipment for and personnel capable of starting intravenous access should be immediately available (1,9).

Chloral Hydrate

CH has a long history of success as a sedative for pediatric patients. CH is generally given orally or rectally as a 25- to 100-mg per kg dose, up to a maximum of 100 mg per kg, or 2 g, whichever is less (62,64–69) (Table 5-4). After the initial dose, the child should be moved to a darkened, quiet room and allowed to fall asleep. The initial dose may take up to 30 to 60 minutes or longer to cause sleep. If a low dose (i.e., <100 mg/kg) was given initially, a second dose may be given, with the total dose not to exceed the maximum of 100 mg per kg, or 2 g. Once the child has fallen asleep, he or she should be gently placed on and secured to the MRI table and appropriate monitors applied. The head should not be flexed, as this may lead to airway obstruction. Personnel must ensure that the positioning does not cause any airway obstruction. The sedated child is unable to overcome obstruction, unlike an awake child. It is ideal to have the MRI suite waiting for the child, or valuable sleep time may be wasted. The author has had good success with CH in children younger than 18 months of age. The child usually awakens readily at the conclusion of the procedure when the monitors are removed and the child is moved off the table.

Advantages of CH include its ease of administration (oral or rectal), long history of use, and relatively low incidence of complications. Several different sedation schemes have been reported (see Table 5-4). Vade (70) reported the following dosing regimen:

• Children younger than 1 year—CH at a dose of 50 mg per kg, repeat dose of 50 mg per kg if the child is not sedated after 30 to 40 minutes.
• Children 1 to 2 years—75 mg per kg CH, plus hydroxyzine 0.8 mg per kg, with a repeat dose of 25 mg per kg CH, if needed.
• Children 2 to 4 years—75 mg per kg CH, plus hydroxyzine 0.8 mg per kg, with a repeat dose of 25 mg per kg CH, if needed. For this age group, Vade also added meperidine, 2 mg per kg, if needed.

TABLE 5-4. *Commonly administered drugs and doses*

Reference	Initial dose	Repeat dose	Maximum dosage	Complications	Comments
Coté (62)	Chloral hydrate (CH), 20–75 mg/kg p.o. or p.r.	—	CH, 100 mg/kg or 2 g, whichever is less	—	Peak effect may take 60 min or longer to accomplish
Greenberg (71)	CH, 100 mg/kg p.o.	NA	CH, 2.5 g	Hyperactivity 6%; vomiting 4%; mild respiratory depression 4%.	Higher failure rate in older children and with lengthy examination times
Vade (70)	≤1 yr: CH, 50 mg/kg p.o. or p.r.	CH, 50 mg/kg	CH, 100 mg/kg or 2 g	Prolonged sedation 3%; mild hypoxia 9%; moderate to severe hypoxia 0.5%; emesis 4%.	—
	1–2 yrs: CH, 75 mg/kg, plus hydroxyzine, 0.8 mg/kg p.o.	CH, 25 mg/kg	CH, 100 mg/kg or 2 g	Prolonged sedation 17%; mild hypoxia 5%; moderate to severe hypoxia 0.5%.	—
	2–4 yrs: CH, 75 mg/kg, plus hydroxyzine, 0.8 mg/kg	CH, 25 mg/kg	CH, 100 mg/kg or 2 g; meperidine, 2 mg/kg i.m. added if needed	—	—
Greenberg (65)	CH, 80–100 mg/kg	NA	—	Emesis 4%; hyperactivity 1.5%; respiratory compromise 1.2%.	Average age: 1.9 yr
Greenberg (69)	CH, 50–100 mg/kg; thioridizine, 2–4 mg/kg, max. 100 mg, 2 h before MRI	—	—	Emesis 5%; decreased oxygen saturation 6%; hyperactivity 2%.	Average age: 5 yr; 89% successfully scanned; all were patients with a history of failed sedation or were mentally retarded
Strain (68)	Pentobarbital, 2–6 mg/kg i.v.	Pentobarbital, 1–3 mg/kg i.v.	Pentobarbital, 100 mg	1- to 2-min induction time	0.5% sedation failures
Coté (62); Feld (90); Wilton (89)	Midazolam for pediatric premedication	0.3–0.5 mg/kg p.o. (62); 0.50–0.75 mg/kg p.o. (90); 0.2 mg/kg nasally (89)	NA	Note: if used as premedication, subsequent dosages of other drugs, especially narcotics, should be reduced. Onset of sedation 20–30 mins after p.o. administration (62).	In children, beta half-life of 106 min vs. 18 h for diazepam (62)
Physicians' Desk Reference (96)	Flumazenil	0.2 mg initial dose in adult	0.2 mg repeat dose as often as every minute, up to 1.0 mg	Reverses sedation from benzodiazepines within a few minutes.	May be associated with seizures in patients habituated to benzodiazepines; resedation may occur after effects of flumazenil dissipate
Physicians' Desk Reference (95)	Naloxone (Narcan)	0.1–0.2 mg q2–3min	May repeat q2–3min	Reverses respiratory effects of narcotics.	Titrate to desired effect, because rapidreversal of narcotics can lead to tachycardia, hypertension, nausea, and vomiting; resedation can occur

NA, not available.

In all age groups, all CH dosages were to a maximum of 100 mg per kg or 2 g, whichever was less. Vade reported a 100% success rate for children ages 1 to 4 years. Vade also reported that, although children under the age of 1 year who were given only CH had a 4% incidence of emesis, none of the children ages 1 to 4 who were also given hydroxyzine, 0.8 mg per kg, experienced emesis.

Greenberg (65,71) reported effective sedation using CH, 80 to 100 mg per kg, up to a maximum of 2.5 g. He reported successful sedation in 91% of children, and sedation failures were associated with increasing patient age and examination length. Greenberg reported an 89% success rate for sedation of children who either had failed previous sedation attempts or were mentally retarded (69) when thioridazine, 2 to 4 mg per kg, was added to CH.

Disadvantages of CH include its long and unpredictable induction time [up to 105 minutes (68)], its relatively high failure rate when used alone [up to 13% (68)], its higher failure rate in older children, its long half-life [9.67 hours in toddlers (2)], and serious complications including death. CH can cause hyperactivity and is a gastric irritant than can cause emesis in 4% of patients (65). Additionally, CH can cause airway compromise and depressed respiration leading to hypoxia (62,63,65,70). CH frequently requires redosing or supplementation with other sedative drugs. CH has been associated with death in a healthy young woman (72) and respiratory compromise in children with tonsillar hypertrophy (73). CH has been associated with respiratory insufficiency in children with subacute necrotizing encephalomyelopathy (74) and with respiratory failure in children with bronchiolitis (75). Neonates and those with liver disease have difficulty metabolizing CH and its metabolites and may experience a prolonged effect. Despite CH's popularity, some have completely abandoned its use owing to concerns with potential toxicity and mutagenicity (76,77). CH is a metabolite of trichloroethylene, which was banned in foods, drugs, and cosmetics after it was discovered that chronic high-dose exposure to trichloroethylene can induce malignancies in rodents (78). Trichloroacetic acid, a metabolite of trichloroethylene and CH, induces liver tumors in mice. However, chronic high doses in mice with CH may not be comparable to a one-time dose in humans. To avoid CH, other drugs with their own side effects would have to be substituted.

Barbiturates

Intravenous pentobarbital (Nembutal) is frequently used to sedate children (62,64,66,68,79,80). It is commonly administered at an initial dose of 2 to 6 mg per kg, titrated in increments, with additional doses of 1 to 3 mg per kg slowly administered up to a maximum dose of 100 mg. Strain (68) published a retrospective study of 749 children, over a 3-year period, who required sedation for computed tomography. The sedatives used included CH (35 to 75 mg/kg, with additional doses up to 100 mg/kg maximum), intramuscular pentobarbital (5 to 6 mg/kg initially, with sup-

plemental doses of 1 to 3 mg/kg), and intravenous pentobarbital. Strain reported that, by the end of the 3-year period, intravenous pentobarbital was used for 95% of the pediatric sedations. He reported an initial dose of 2 to 6 mg per kg intravenous pentobarbital, with additional doses of 1 to 3 mg per kg, up to a maximum of 100 mg. Induction time for intravenous pentobarbital was 1 to 2 minutes, compared to 30 to 45 minutes for intramuscular pentobarbital and 30 to 105 minutes for CH. A total of 419 patients underwent sedation with intravenous pentobarbital. Fifteen of these patients (4%) required a repeat dose, and two patients (0.5%) were considered sedation failures. In comparison, CH patients had a 13% failure rate, and 16% required repeat doses. Intramuscular pentobarbital patients had a 3% failure rate, and 14% required repeat doses.

Advantages of intravenous pentobarbital are its ability to be titrated to effect; low failure rate [0.5% (68)]; rapid onset of sedative effect; low, dose-dependent risk of respiratory depression; and reliability. Although pentobarbital may be administered intramuscularly, only the intravenous route allows personnel to effectively titrate the dose to the required level of sedation. The main disadvantages of intravenous pentobarbital are the necessity for intravenous access before proceeding with sedation and the prolonged duration of sedation after commonly administered doses.

Methohexital is a barbiturate commonly used rectally, intramuscularly, or intravenously (62,64,81–83). Rectally, the dose is 20 to 30 mg per kg as a 10% solution, with a maximum dose of 500 mg (62). Intramuscular use with 10 mg per kg (81) has provided successful sedation but is associated with painful injection owing to the high pH. Methohexital has been associated with seizures in epileptic patients (62) and has been associated with airway obstruction (62), apnea (83), and defecation when administered rectally (82).

Thiopental is a rapid-acting barbiturate that has been used for sedation and the induction of anesthesia (62,84). It has been given intravenously and rectally. Its high pH may be associated with tissue damage if extravasation occurs.

Propofol

Propofol (Diprivan), an intravenous sedative-hypnotic, has gained popularity for induction and maintenance of anesthesia since its introduction in the late 1980s. It has a rapid clearance, very rapid recovery characteristics, and a low incidence of nausea and vomiting. Propofol has been described for the sedation and anesthesia of patients undergoing MRI (24,30,62,64,85,86). Propofol self-administration via a patient-controlled analgesia pump for conscious sedation has been described (87). Propofol, however, can rapidly cause general anesthesia (62) and has been associated with respiratory depression and apnea, as well as with significant decreases in blood pressure (30). The *Physicians' Desk Reference* warnings section for propofol states that it should be administered "only by persons trained in the administration of general anesthesia and not involved in the conduct of the surgical/diagnostic procedure" (88).

Benzodiazepines

Benzodiazepines are useful for premedication and treatment of anxiety. Midazolam (Versed) is a water-soluble benzodiazepine that can be administered orally, intramuscularly, intravenously, or intranasally (89,90). For pediatric premedication, a dose of 0.3 to 0.5 mg per kg orally or 0.2 mg per kg nasally is given. Midazolam is available in a fruit-flavored solution for oral administration. Sedation occurs within 10 to 15 minutes after nasal administration and within 20 to 30 minutes after oral administration (62). Midazolam is particularly useful for brief periods of sedation, owing to its short half-life [beta elimination half-life of 106 + 29 minutes, versus 18 hours for diazepam in children (62)]. Although a premedication dose of midazolam may cause many children to fall asleep, the duration of sleep may not be sufficient to allow completion of an MRI examination but should be long enough to allow a stress-free intravenous start, particularly if the patient was pretreated with EMLA (eutectic mixture of local anesthetics) cream. In adults, intravenous midazolam in doses of 1.0 to 2.5 mg is effective for sedation (91).

Diazepam (Valium) is commonly given orally, intramuscularly, or intravenously and reaches its peak concentration approximately 1 hour after oral administration in adults (92). A typical adult dose is 2 to 10 mg orally, intramuscularly, or intravenously (93). Intravenous and intramuscular use are associated with pain on injection, because diazepam is insoluble in water and is dissolved in organic solvents, such as propylene glycol. The elimination half-life is long, 21 to 37 hours; can be dramatically increased with cirrhosis of the liver; and increases progressively with age (92). Desmethyldiazepam, the major metabolite of diazepam, is only slightly less potent than diazepam. Desmethyldiazepam has an elimination half-life of 48 to 96 hours and contributes to the prolonged drowsiness associated with diazepam (92).

The combination of benzodiazepines (midazolam or diazepam) and narcotics is synergistic and has been associated with numerous deaths (94).

EMLA Cream

EMLA cream, a relatively new topical anesthetic cream of lidocaine and prilocaine, provides topical anesthesia of the skin and is extremely helpful when starting intravenous lines in children. It must be applied at least 30 to 60 minutes before the needlestick. After application, it must be covered with an occlusive dressing (Fig. 5-5). Care must be taken to avoid contact of the EMLA cream with ocular or mucosal surfaces to avoid ocular anesthesia or ingestion (62). EMLA cream has the potential to cause methemoglobinemia if an excessively large amount of cream is applied for longer than necessary (62).

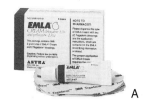
A

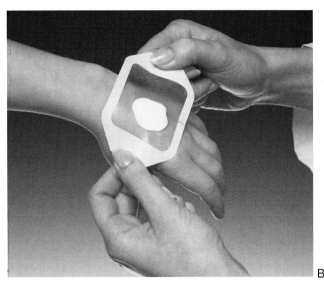
B

FIG. 5-5. EMLA (eutectic mixture of local anesthetics) cream **(A)** is a useful adjunct to the placement of intravenous lines. It must be covered with an occlusive dressing **(B)** and left in place at least 30 to 60 minutes. Photograph reproduced with permission of Astra Pharmaceuticals, L.P., 725 Chesterbrook Blvd., Wayne, PA 19087. EMLA is a registered trademark of Astra Pharmaceuticals.

Reversal Agents

Naloxone is an opioid antagonist that reverses the respiratory effects of narcotics. It should be available if narcotics are administered. For postprocedural respiratory depression in adults, the drug should be injected in 0.1- to 0.2-mg increments every 2 to 3 minutes and titrated to effect (95). Rapid reversal of opioids can result in nausea, vomiting, hypertension, and tachycardia. The duration of naloxone is less than that of many narcotics, and resedation is possible.

Flumazenil (Romazicon) is a specific benzodiazepine antagonist. It reverses the sedative effects of benzodiazepines within approximately 2 minutes. The initial dose (adult) is 0.2 mg intravenously over 15 seconds (96). This dose can be repeated at 60-second intervals, up to a maximum of 1 mg. The duration is shorter than that of most benzodiazepines, and the patient must be observed after administration of this drug because resedation may occur.

General Anesthesia

If general anesthesia is chosen for MRI, any technique that is appropriate for the particular patient can be selected.

Before the start of general anesthesia, the radiologic technologist should inform the anesthesiologist of the positioning and coils that are required and remind him or her of the effects of the magnetic field. Newer, very rapidly eliminated inhalational agents, such as desflurane or sevoflurane, allow the patient to awaken quickly at the conclusion of the examination. Total intravenous anesthesia may allow the administration of anesthesia without the necessity for an anesthesia machine. Nevertheless, a means of administering oxygen via positive-pressure ventilation and routine resuscitative equipment is still required.

CONCLUSION

Sedation for MRI is more challenging than sedation for other procedures. Identification of high-risk patients is valuable so that a more experienced individual can be present to administer the sedation and monitor these difficult patients. Sedation can rapidly become anesthesia, and a physician who can recognize and manage hypoventilation, airway obstruction, and other common problems is a necessity. Many of the safeguards required for general anesthesia, such as NPO intervals and an adult responsible for taking the patient home, are required for safe sedation in MRI. Monitoring during sedation is essential for safety, as is knowledge of pharmacologic principles. An MRI center whose sedation program does not meet AAP or ASA practice guidelines should carefully review its policies and procedures and make the changes necessary to ensure the safety of the patients they attempt to scan.

REFERENCES

1. American Academy of Pediatrics Committee on Drugs. Guidelines for monitoring and management of pediatric patients during and after sedation for diagnostic and therapeutic procedures. *Pediatrics* 1992;89:1110–1115.
2. Coté CJ. Monitoring guidelines: Do they make a difference? *AJR Am J Roentgenol* 1995;165:910–912.
3. Frush DP, Bisset GS. Sedation of children in radiology: time to wake up. *AJR Am J Roentgenol* 1995;165:913–914.
4. Malviya S, Voepel-Lewis T, Tait AR. Adverse events and risk factors associated with the sedation of children by non-anesthesiologists. *Anesth Analg* 1997;85:1207–1213.
5. Kanal E, Shellock FG. Patient monitoring during clinical MR imaging. *Radiology* 1992;185:623–629.
6. Cohen MD. Pediatric sedation. *Radiology* 1990;175:611–612.
7. Nelson MD. Guidelines for the monitoring and care of children during and after sedation for imaging studies. *AJR Am J Roentgenol* 1993;160:581–582.
8. Fisher DM. Sedation of pediatric patients: an anesthesiologist's perspective. *Radiology* 1990;175:613–615.
9. A Report by the ASA Task Force on Sedation and Analgesia by Non-Anesthesiologists. Practice guidelines for sedation and analgesia by non-anesthesiologists. *Anesthesiology* 1996;84:459–471.
10. American College of Radiology. ACR standard for use of intravenous conscious sedation, and ACR standard for pediatric sedation/analgesia. In: *1998 ACR standards*. Reston, VA: American College of Radiology, 1998:123–130.
11. ASA Task Force on Preoperative Fasting. Practice guidelines for preoperative fasting and the use of pharmacological agents to reduce the risk of pulmonary aspiration: application to healthy patients undergoing elective procedures. *Anesthesiology* 1999;90:896–905.
12. Kanal E, Shellock FG, Talagala L. Safety considerations in MR imaging. *Radiology* 1990;176:593–606.
13. Patteson SK, Chesney JT. Anesthetic management for magnetic resonance imaging: problems and solutions. *Anesth Analg* 1992;74:121–128.
14. Menon DK, Peden CJ, Hall AS, Sargentoni J, Whitwam JG. Magnetic resonance for the anesthetist. Part 1: physical principles, applications, safety aspects. *Anaesthesia* 1992;47:240–255.
15. Peden CJ, Menon DK, Hall AS, Sargentoni J, Whitwam JG. Magnetic resonance for the anesthetist. Part II: anesthesia and monitoring in MR units. *Anaesthesia* 1992;47:508–517.
16. Russell GB, Taekman JM, Cronin AJC. Anesthesia and magnetic resonance imaging. In: Russell GB, ed. *Alternate-site anesthesia: clinical practice outside the operating room*. Boston: Butterworth–Heinemann, 1997:69–81.
17. Gillies BS. Anesthesia outside the operating room. In: Barash PG, Cullen BF, Stoelting RK, eds. *Clinical anesthesia*, 2nd ed. Philadelphia: JB Lippincott, 1992:1470–1472.
18. Bendo AA, Hartung J, Kass IS, Cottrell JE. Neurophysiology and neuroanesthesia. In: Barash PG, Cullen BF, Stoelting RK, eds. *Clinical anesthesia*, 2nd ed. Philadelphia: JB Lippincott, 1992:888–889.
19. Smith DS, Askey P, Young ML, Kressel HY. Anesthetic management of acutely ill patients during magnetic resonance imaging. *Anesthesiology* 1986;65:710–711.
20. Roth JL, Nugent M, Gray JE, et al. Patient monitoring during magnetic resonance imaging. *Anesthesiology* 1985;62:80–83.
21. Avrahami E. Panic attacks during MR imaging: treatment with IV diazepam. *AJNR Am J Neuroradiol* 1990;11:833–835.
22. Shepherd JK, Hall-Craggs MA, Finn JP, Bingham RM. Sedation in children scanned with high field magnetic resonance: the experience at the Hospital for Sick Children, Great Ormond Street. *Br J Radiol* 1990;63:794–797.
23. Landrum A, Kittle D, Bildner C, et al. Propofol versus pentobarbital for autistic children and adolescents undergoing magnetic resonance imaging. *Anesth Analg* 1997;84:S440(abst).
24. Kain ZN, Gaal DJ, Kain TS, Jaeger DD, Rimar SR. A first-pass cost analysis of propofol versus barbiturates for children undergoing magnetic resonance imaging. *Anesth Analg* 1994;79:1102–1106.
25. Beebe DS, Tran P, Bragg M, Stillman A, Truwit C, Belani KG. Evaluation of a sedation protocol for MRI in pediatric patients. *Anesth Analg* 1997;84:S146.
26. Barkovich AJ. Techniques and methods in pediatric imaging. In: Barkovich AJ, ed. *Pediatric neuroimaging*, 2nd ed. Philadelphia: Lippincott–Raven Publishers, 1996:1–3.
27. Kovac A, Swanson B, Elliott C, Wetzel L. Effect of distance and infusion rate on operation of Medfusion 2010 Infusion Pump during magnetic resonance imaging (MRI). *Anesth Analg* 1999;88:S186(abst).
28. Polarz H, Browne AM, Martin E. Anesthetic management for intraoperative MRI. In: Lufkin RB, ed. *Interventional MRI*. St. Louis: Mosby, 1999:76–79.
29. Mize WA, Bisset GS. Pediatric orthopedics. In: Edelman RR, Hesslink JR, Zlatkin MB, eds. *Clinical magnetic resonance imaging*, 2nd ed. Philadelphia: WB Saunders, 1990:2114–2115.
30. Bloomfield EL, Masaryk TJ, Caplin A, et al. Intravenous sedation for MR imaging of the brain and spine in children: pentobarbital versus propofol. *Pediatr Radiol* 1993;186:93–97.
31. Messick JM Jr, Mackenzie RA, Nugent M. Anesthesia at remote locations. In: Miller RD, ed. *Anesthesia*, 3rd ed. New York: Churchill Livingstone, 1990:2069–2088.
32. Geiger RS, Cascorbi HF. Anesthesia in an NMR scanner. *Anesth Analg* 1984;63:619–625.
33. Dunn V, Coffman CE, McGowan JE, Ehrhardt JC. Mechanical ventilation during magnetic resonance imaging. *Magn Reson Imag* 1985;3:169–172.
34. Jorgensen NH, Messick JM, Gray J, Nugent M, Berquist TH. ASA monitoring standards and magnetic resonance imaging. *Anesth Analg* 1994;79:1141–1147.
35. Hollman GA, Elderbrook MK, VanDenLangenberg B. Results of a pediatric sedation program on head MRI scan success rates and procedural duration times. *Clin Pediatr* 1995;34:300.
36. Rao CC, Krishna G. Anaesthetic considerations for magnetic resonance imaging. *Ann Acad Med* 1994;23:531.
37. Fisher DM, Litt L, Coté CJ. Use of pulse oximetry during MR imaging of pediatric patients. *Radiology* 1991;178:891–892.
38. Malviya S, Voepel-Lewis T, Tait AR, Dipietro M, Prochaska G, Eldevik P. Sedation for MRI and CT procedures in children: recovery and adverse events. *Anesth Analg* 1999;88:S302(abst).

39. Voepel-Lewis T, Tait AR, Prochaska G, Malviya S. Sedation failures in children undergoing MRI and CT: Is temperament a factor? *Anesth Analg* 1999;88:S312(abst).

40. Shellock FG. Biological effects and safety aspects of magnetic resonance imaging. *Magn Reson Q* 1989;5:243–261.

41. Rao CC, Brandl R, Mashack JN. Modification of Ohmeda Excel 210 anesthesia machine for use during magnetic resonance imaging. *Anesthesiology* 1988;68:640.

42. Rao CC, McNiece WL, Emhardt J, Krishna G, Westcott R. Modification of an anesthesia machine for use during magnetic resonance imaging. *Anesthesiology* 1988;68:640–641.

43. Boutros A, Pavlicek W. Anesthesia for magnetic resonance imaging. *Anesth Analg* 1987;66:367.

44. Shellock FG, Slimp GL. Severe burn of the finger caused by using a pulse oximeter during MR imaging [Letter]. *AJR Am J Roentgenol* 1989;153:1105.

45. Kanal E, Shellock FG. Burns associated with clinical MR examinations. *Radiology* 1990;175:585.

46. Bashein G, Syrovy G. Burns associated with pulse oximetry during magnetic resonance imaging. *Anesthesiology* 1991;75:382–383.

47. Knopp MV, Essig M, Debus J, Zabel HJ, vanKaick G. Unusual burns of the lower extremities caused by a closed conducting loop in a patient at MR imaging. *Radiology* 1996;200:572–575.

48. Keens SJ, Laurence AS. Burns caused by ECG monitoring during MRI imaging [Letter]. *Anaesthesia* 1996;51:1188–1189.

49. Jones S, Jaffe W, Alvi R. Burns associated with electrocardiographic monitoring during magnetic resonance imaging. *Burns* 1996;22:420–421.

50. Brown TR, Goldstein B, Little J. Severe burns resulting from magnetic resonance imaging with cardiopulmonary monitoring. Risks and relevant safety precautions. *Am J Phys Med Rehabil* 1993;72:166–167.

51. Coté CJ, Goldstein EA, Coté MA, Hoaglin DC, Ryan JF. A single blind study of pulse oximetry in children. *Anesthesiology* 1988;68:184–188.

52. Coté CJ, Rolf N, Liu LMP, et al. A single blind study of combined pulse oximetry and capnography in children. *Anesthesiology* 1991;74:980–987.

53. Coté CJ. Pulse oximetry during conscious sedation [Letter]. *JAMA* 1994;271:429.

54. Council on Scientific Affairs, American Medical Association. The use of pulse oximetry during conscious sedation. *JAMA* 1993;270:1463–1468.

55. Chaney MA. Pulse oximetry during conscious sedation [Letter]. *JAMA* 1994;271:429.

56. Frumin MJ, Epstein RM, Cohen G. Apneic oxygenation in man. *Anesthesiology* 1959;20:789–798.

57. Barker SJ, Tremper KK. Pulse oximetry: applications and limitations. *Int Anesthesiol Clin* 1987;25:155–175.

58. Eichhorn JH, Cooper JB, Cullen DK, Maier WR, Philip JH, Seeman RG. Standards for patient monitoring during anesthesia at Harvard Medical School. *JAMA* 1986;256:1017–1020.

59. Severinghaus JW, Naifeh KH. Accuracy of response of pulse oximeters to profound hypoxia. *Anesthesiology* 1987;67:551–558.

60. Freeman ML, Hennessy JT, Cass OW. Carbon dioxide retention and oxygen desaturation during conscious sedation for ERCP, colonoscopy and upper GI endoscopy. *Gastrointest Endosc* 1991;37:233(abst).

61. ASA Guidelines for Nonoperating Room Anesthetizing Locations, Approved by the House of Delegates October 19, 1994, American Society of Anesthesiologists, Park Ridge, IL.

62. Coté CJ. Sedation for the pediatric patient. pediatric anesthesia. *Pediatr Clin North Am* 1994;41:31–58.

63. Coté CJ, Alderfer RJ, Notterman DA, Fanta KB. Sedation disasters: adverse drug reports in pediatrics—FDA, USP, and others. *Anesthesiology* 1995;83:A1183(abst).

64. Hopkins KL, Davis PC, Sanders CL, Churchill LH. Sedation for pediatric imaging studies. *Neuroimag Clin North Am* 1999;9(1):1–10.

65. Greenberg SB, Faerber EN, Aspinall CL. High dose chloral hydrate sedation for children undergoing CT. *J Comput Assist Tomogr* 1991;15:467–469.

66. Keeter S, Benator RM, Weinberg SM, Hartenberg MA. Sedation in pediatric CT: national survey of current practice. *Radiology* 1990;175:745–752.

67. Neuman GG, Kushins LG, Ferrante S. Sedation for children undergoing magnetic resonance imaging and computed tomography. *Anesth Analg* 1992;74:931–932.

68. Strain JD, Harvey LA, Foley LC, Campbell JB. Intravenously administered pentobarbital sodium for sedation in pediatric CT. *Radiology* 1986;161:105–108.

69. Greenberg SB, Faerber EN, Radke JL, Aspinall CL, Adams RC, Mercer-Wilson DD. Sedation of difficult to sedate children undergoing MR imaging: value of thioridazine as an adjunct to chloral hydrate. *AJR Am J Roentgenol* 1994;163:165–168.

70. Vade A, Sukhani R, Dolenga M, Habisohn-Schuck C. Chloral hydrate sedation of children undergoing CT and MR imaging: safety as judged by American Academy of Pediatrics guidelines. *AJR Am J Roentgenol* 1995;165:905–909.

71. Greenberg SB, Faerber EN, Aspinall AL, Adams RC. High-dose chloral hydrate sedation for children undergoing MR imaging: safety and efficacy in relation to age. *AJR Am J Roentgenol* 1993;161:639–641.

72. Jastak JT, Pallasch T. Death after chloral hydrate sedation: report of case. *JADA* 1988;116:345–348.

73. Biban P, Baraldi E, Pettenazzo A, Filippone M, Zacchello F. Adverse effect of chloral hydrate on two young children with obstructive sleep apnea. *Pediatrics* 1993;92:461–463.

74. Greenberg SB, Faerber EN. Respiratory insufficiency following chloral hydrate sedation in two children with Leigh disease (subacute necrotizing encephalomyelopathy). *Pediatr Radiol* 1990;20:287–288.

75. Mallol J, Sly PD. Effect of chloral hydrate on arterial oxygen saturation in wheezy infants. *Pediatric Pulmonol* 1988;5:96–99.

76. Fisher DM, Zwass MS. Chloral hydrate administration to children. *Anesth Analg* 1993;76:668–669.

77. Smith MT. Chloral hydrate warning. *Science* 1990;250:359.

78. Steinberg AD. Should chloral hydrate be banned? *Pediatrics* 1993;92:442–446.

79. Strain JD, Campbell JB, Harvey LA, Foley LC. IV Nembutal: safe sedation for children undergoing CT. *AJR Am J Roentgenol* 1988;151:975–979.

80. Kleinman PK, Spevak MR. Advanced pediatric joint imaging. *Radiol Clin North Am* 1990;28:1073–1074.

81. Varner PD, Ebert JP, McKay RD, Nail CS, Whitlock TM. Methohexital sedation of children undergoing CT scan. *Anesth Analg* 1985;64:643–645.

82. Liu LMP, Goudsouzian NG, Liu PL. Rectal methohexital premedication in children, a dose-comparison study. *Anesthesiology* 1980;53:343–345.

83. Yemen TA, Pullerits J, Stillman R, Hershey M. Rectal methohexital causing apnea in two patients with meningomyeloceles. *Anesth Analg* 1991;74:1139–1141.

84. Burckart GJ, White TJ III, Siegle RL, Jabbour JT, Ramey DR. Rectal thiopental versus an intramuscular cocktail for sedating children before computerized tomography. *Am J Hosp Pharm* 1980;37:222–224.

85. Frankville DD, Spear RM, Dyck JB. The dose of propofol required to prevent children from moving during magnetic resonance imaging. *Anesthesiology* 1993;79:953–958.

86. Cauldwell CB, Fisher DM. Sedating pediatric patients: Is propofol a panacea? [Editorial]. *Radiology* 1993;186:9–10.

87. Oei-Lim VLB, Kalkman CJ, Makkes PC, Ooms WG. Patient-controlled versus anesthesiologist-controlled conscious sedation with propofol for dental treatment in anxious patients. *Anesth Analg* 1998;86:967–972.

88. *Physician's desk reference*, 53rd ed. Montvale, NJ: Medical Economics, 1999:3414.

89. Wilton NCT, Leigh J, Rosen DR, Pandit UA. Preanesthetic sedation of preschool children using intranasal midazolam. *Anesthesiology* 1988;69:972–975.

90. Feld LH, Negus JB, White PF. Oral midazolam preanesthetic medication in pediatric outpatients. *Anesthesiology* 1990;73:831–834.

91. Stoelting RK. Benzodiazepines. In: Stoelting RK, ed. *Pharmacology and physiology in anesthetic practice*, 2nd ed. Philadelphia: JB Lippincott, 1991:128.

92. Stoelting RK. Benzodiazepines. In: Stoelting RK, ed. *Pharmacology and physiology in anesthetic practice*, 2nd ed. Philadelphia: JB Lippincott, 1991:120–121.

93. *Physicians' desk reference*, 53rd ed. Montvale, NJ: Medical Economics, 1999:2735.

94. Bailey PL, Pace NL, Ashburn MA, Moll JWB, East KA, Stanley TH. Frequent hypoxemia and apnea after sedation with midazolam and fentanyl. *Anesthesiology* 1990;73:826–830.

95. *Physicians' desk reference*, 53rd ed. Montvale, NJ: Medical Economics, 1999:981.

96. *Physicians' desk reference*, 53rd ed. Montvale, NJ: Medical Economics, 1999:2704.

SECTION II

Physics

Open MRI,
edited by Peter A. Rothschild and Debra Reinking Rothschild.
Lippincott Williams & Wilkins. Philadelphia © 2000.

CHAPTER 6

Open Magnetic Resonance Imaging Instrumentation

Louis Paladino

EVOLUTION OF OPEN MAGNETIC RESONANCE IMAGING SYSTEMS

Tremendous advances in open magnetic resonance imaging (MRI) technology have been made in the 1990s, but to understand where open MRI is headed, we must first consider the origin of MRI, or as it was popularly known before 1986, nuclear magnetic resonance imaging. It all began with Bloch and Purcell, who won the 1945 Nobel Prize for their efforts in the field of nuclear magnetic resonance. This was the genesis of many of the key aspects of MRI and of the new frontiers of open MRI that will cross into the new millennium. This chapter follows the evolution from the first medical image produced by Raymond Damadian in 1977 (Figs. 6-1 and 6-2), to the first commercially produced closed MRI systems in 1983, to one of its current descendants, the open system.

Consumers' demand for more open and comfortable MRI systems and the ever increasing industrial competition have precipitated an accelerated pace in the technological advances in open MRI systems. Open MRI encompasses a broad range of field strengths, from the early Toshiba (South San Francisco, CA) Access 0.064-T unit (Fig. 6-3) to the current Fonar (Melville, NY) Quad unit that operates at 0.6 T. Other manufacturers such as General Electric (Milwaukee, WI) and Siemens (Iselin, NJ) offer higher field (1.0- to 1.5-T) short-bore magnets. These magnets, although still designed with a cylindrical bore, use a bore that is much shorter than conventional longer bores. The short-bore magnets have proved superb for borderline claustrophobic patients, particularly when these patients are positioned feet first into the magnet. The open MRI industry seems to have settled on a range from 0.2 to 0.6 T. These systems are descendants of the earlier magnets introduced in the 1980s. The vertical field 0.3-T Fonar Beta 3000, introduced in 1983, provided 4 ft of space

on each side of the patient and an anterior-to-posterior dimension of 35 cm. The four-post 0.064-T Toshiba Access (see Fig. 6-3), introduced in 1987, was the first magnet to offer openings on all four sides, with an anterior-to-posterior dimension of 42 cm. It must also be remembered that although these systems were able to accommodate obese and claustrophobic patients, the signal-to-noise ratio suffered dramatically, and in turn image quality on these very low-field systems was often poor. The Image Enhancement System (Image Enhancement System, Inc., Hayward, CA), introduced by Peter Rothschild in 1992, improved image quality from low-field open systems while other improvements were developed. Image enhancement systems were so effective at noise reduction that they now appear on units with field strengths as high as 1.5 T.

Currently, no fewer than six major manufacturers offer truly open MRI scanners with such features as fluid attenuated inversion recovery (FLAIR), diffusion imaging, magnetic resonance cholangiopancreatography (MRCP), magnetic resonance angiography, and kinematics.

FIELD STABILITY, HOMOGENEITY, AND SHIMMING

The most important step in installation of an open MRI scanner is the shimming process. The shimming process can consist of passive shimming, in which the homogeneity of the magnetic field is accomplished by adding small ferromagnetic pieces to the iron bore; active shimming, in which an external power supply drives the shim coils; or a combination of the two. Although both methods are effective, passive shimming seems to be more reliable, because it requires less maintenance. *Homogeneity* is the measurement of the maximum field variation over a specific volume of interest at the magnet's center. This value is measured in parts per million (ppm) and is one of the most important measurements to ensure excellent image quality.

Careful monitoring of the shimming process has three very critical by-products:

L. Paladino: InSight Health Services Corporation, Myrtle Beach, South Carolina

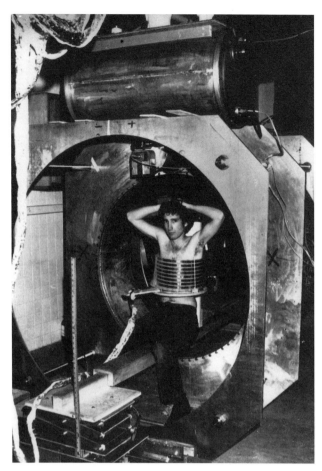

FIG. 6-1. The first image-producing magnet. This magnet is now displayed in the Smithsonian Institute. Photograph courtesy of Fonar, Inc., Melville, NY.

1. By far the most important is optimal image quality. It stands to reason that the more homogeneous a magnet is, the more accurate the spatial location of information is.
2. Image degradation occurs if the homogeneity of the magnetic field is suboptimal.

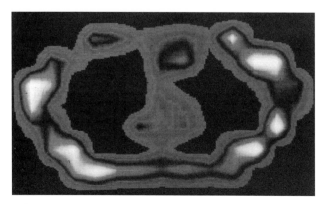

FIG. 6-2. The first magnetic resonance image ever produced, by Raymond Damadian in 1971. Photograph courtesy of Fonar, Inc., Melville, NY.

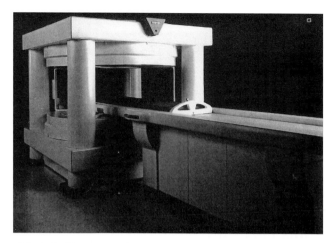

FIG. 6-3. The 0.064-T Toshiba Access introduced in 1987. Photograph courtesy of Toshiba America MRI, Inc., South San Francisco, CA.

3. A poor attempt at shimming could result in the need for a future reshimming of the magnet. This leads to downtime, which in a highly competitive imaging market may severely compromise a center's reputation.

Magnetic field uniformity (ppm) is calculated by using the following equation:

$$ppm = DH/Ho \times 10^6$$

where Ho equals the strength of the magnetic field in gauss and DH equals the minimum to maximum variation of magnetic field strength in gauss.

In MRI, a gradient magnetic field is applied on top of the static magnetic field to obtain positional information. Thus, if the static magnetic field is not uniform before the gradient magnetic field is applied, the positional information will deviate, resulting in image distortion. The magnetic flux density, symbolized by B (X, Y, Z), can be analyzed in the terms of [Zn, ZnX, ZnY, $Zn(X2 - Y2)$, $(XY)n$ ($n = 1, 2, 3$, etc.)]. Of these terms, the adjustable variables are, depending on the manufacturer, X, Y, YZ, Y1, Y2, Y3, Y4, Y5, Y6 or X, Y, ZY, Z1, Z2, Z3, Z4, Z5, Z6. The optimization of all these variables and the optimization of the peak-to-peak value is critical to homogeneity. These values should be monitored carefully when overseeing a new installation.

MAGNET TYPES

Over the years, many different magnet types have been used in MRI. Not all of the following magnet types are being used in today's open MRI market.

Air-Core Resistive Magnets

In a resistive magnet, current flows through a good conducting material, typically copper or aluminum, shaped in a circular coil to create a uniform magnetic field at the coil center. As the conductor is near room temperature, a resistance to the flow of current exists. In accordance with the rules of physics, to keep electrical costs down, careful attention must be paid to certain parameters—gap size and field strength—which must maintain specific proportional values. Proper proportions allow efficient water cooling.

The resistive magnet is subject to some distinct disadvantages. The dependence on an uninterrupted power supply, and in some cases the additional expense of a power conditioner, is a concern. An undependable power supply results in fluctuating ranges of image quality. When dealing with an air-core resistive magnet, a rather large fringe field is involved. Another disadvantage, although not nearly as critical as the power supply, is siting. Resistive magnets are normally delivered already configured, forcing the buyer to provide a large wall entrance. Particularly in an urban setting, this can be quite difficult.

The advantages of an air-core resistive magnet are that because no inherent magnetic material is required, this type of magnet is less expensive to produce, and air-core resistive magnets are lighter in weight. Other advantages are that the field can be ramped down rapidly and that coil maintenance is relatively easy.

Iron-Core Resistive Magnets

The iron-core resistive magnet can be classified as a hybrid between the heavy permanent magnet and the lighter air-core resistive magnet. Iron is used for shaping the imaging magnetic field and providing a return path. This iron yoke also provides inherent shielding.

The disadvantages of the iron-core resistive magnet are high power consumption; the necessity for a cooling system; and most important, the dependence on a precise temperature environment. An unstable environment causes severe image quality degradation. The most common design for this type of magnetic is the H- or C-shaped magnet.

Advantages of the iron-core resistive magnet include relatively low cost, a small fringe field due to the iron core, and a resistive magnet's ability to be ramped down quickly.

Permanent Magnets

Permanent magnets that are used for open MRI have field strength only as high as 0.3 T. These magnets are constructed of ferromagnetic ceramic blocks, and their poles are constructed of iron to help shape the magnetic field. Shimming screws are also added to manually shape the field as precisely as possible. Using neodymium iron boron (NdFeB) produces the most efficient and effective permanent magnet. The neodymium iron boron magnet has a magnetic energy 11 times greater than that of its predecessor, ferrite, and is also lighter in weight. The most common designs for this type of magnet are the H-shape and the C-shape.

Advantages of the permanent magnet include extremely low operating costs; low purchase costs; and because of the iron yoke, an extremely well-contained fringe field.

Disadvantages include the inability to ramp down the magnet in an emergency, a possible siting issue because of the magnet's weight, and the limit of field strength.

Superconducting Magnets

All high-field systems use superconducting magnets, which are constructed of materials that lose all resistance to current flow when kept at a controlled low temperature. The superconducting magnet is configured using multiple loops of wires. These wires are made of niobiumtitanium, which has zero current resistance at a temperature of 9.5 K and below, which is less than 10°C above absolute zero. Liquid helium has been found to be the most efficient way to maintain a proper environment for the superconducting magnet. Early superconducting MRI magnets also used liquid nitrogen, which boils at 77 K, to maintain the helium. However, the liquid nitrogen method adds to operating costs and complexity. Currently, electric-powered shield coolers (cryocoolers), or power heads, have replaced liquid nitrogen. A power supply is used to slowly build up current in the superconducting coil and consequentially the magnetic field. Once the magnetic field has reached full potential, the power supply is turned off and the current can, in theory, continue infinitely.

Advantages of the superconducting magnet are the capability for higher field strength, excellent field homogeneity, high signal-to-noise ratio, fast scanning, and low power consumption.

Disadvantages include high purchase costs; high cryogen costs; confining settings; noise; and because this is the most technically complex of all magnet structures, the possibility of longer down times.

MANUFACTURERS

Table 6-1 compares the seven manufacturers recognized by the open MRI industry. One of these manufacturers, Millennium, based in Canada, received FDA approval in the United States in late 1999.

CONCLUSION

It has been less than 30 years since the original MR image was produced in 1971. MRI has had an amazingly quick evolution in open MRI as well as in the industry of medical imaging as a whole. In the late 1980s, the first four-post open magnets were introduced, and in the early 1990s, higher field strength C- and H-shaped open magnets followed. MRI centers have taken the concept one step further by successfully combining psychology with the open technology to accommodate claustrophobic patients. They use new techniques for decreasing claustrophobic anxiety from

TABLE 6-1. *Currently manufactured open magnetic resonance imaging units*

Unit	Field strength	Minimum space required	5-G line	Magnet type	Weight (kg)	Vertical gap size (cm)	Power Requirements	Gradient strength	Rise time	Slew rate	Shimming	Required cooling
Toshiba (South Francisco, CA) OPART	0.35 T	388 sq. ft	9.5 ft	Superconductor	11,300	55	15 kVA (not including chiller)	10 mT/m	0.5 ms	SR 20	Passive	Cryogenless refrigerator
Fonar (Melville, NY) Quad 12000	0.6 T	900 sq. ft	7.5 ft	Resistive	63,000	49	100 kVA	12 mT/m	0.6 ms	SR 20	Active/passive	Water
Picker (Cleveland, OH) Proview	0.23 T	439 sq. ft	6.9 ft	Resistive	12,400	46	75 kVA	16 mT/m	0.6 ms	SR 25	Passive/active	Yes
Hitachi (Twinsberg, OH) Airis	0.3 T	365 sq. ft	6.6 ft[a]; 8.2 ft[b]	Permanent	15,734	43	3 kVA[c]	8 mT/m	0.7 ms	SR 11	Mechanical passive/active	No
Hitachi Airis II	0.3 T	380 sq. ft	6.6 ft[a]; 8.2 ft[b]	Permanent	15,734	43	3 kVA[c]	15 mT/m	0.5 ms	SR 20	Mechanical passive/active	No
Siemens (Iselin, NJ) Viva	0.2 T	307 sq. ft	8.5 ft	Permanent	10,999.6	41	15 kVA	15 mT/m	0.9 ms	SR 17	Passive/active	Small integrated chiller for gradients only
General Electric (Milwaukee, WI) Profile	0.2 T	247 sq. ft	5.6 ft	Permanent	10,000	44	3–4 kVA	15 mT/m	0.6 ms	SR 25	Mechanical-passive	No
Millennium (Vancouver, British Columbia, Canada) Virgo	0.35 T	241 sq. ft magnet room only	9.5 ft	Permanent	16,000	43	3–4 kVA	15 mT/m	0.6 ms	SR 25	Passive	No

[a]Lateral (specification provided by manufacturer).

[b]Vertical and longitudinal (specification provided by manufacturer).

[c]Average consumption for Hitachi Airis and Airis II. Capacity of service is 8 kVA for Airis, 10 kVA for Airis II (specifications provided by manufacturer).

aromatherapy to virtual reality glasses. Additionally, magnet rooms have evolved from antiseptic-feeling boxes in the 1980s to beautiful suites complete with skylights, windows, plush furnishings, and even waterfalls.

The rapid evolution of open MRI technology has seen expansion into hospital settings, which was almost unheard of as recently as 1995. This hospital expansion encompasses conventional open MRI in addition to interventional open MRI. Interventional open MRI now combines radiology with surgery. Although this is a relatively new technology, it is rapidly gaining acceptance and will be used for such procedures as diagnostic biopsies, MRI-guided drainage, MRI-guided nerve root management, vascular intervention, and direct delivery of drugs and chemotherapy.

The future of open MRI will show continual improvement in image quality and a trend to higher field strength magnets with images that are comparable with any closed MRI system.

Open MRI,
edited by Peter A. Rothschild and Debra Reinking Rothschild.
Lippincott Williams & Wilkins. Philadelphia © 2000.

CHAPTER 7

Physics of Open Magnetic Resonance Imaging

Leon Kaufman and Lawrence E. Crooks

Magnetic resonance imaging (MRI) is a medical diagnostic modality. As such, it is of value only if it is available to the people who can benefit from its use. Because MRI use is not limited by risk versus benefit considerations for most subjects, cost versus benefit is becoming the major determinant of use. In such cases, as the cost of a study decreases, the use (and presumably the benefit) increases. Decreasing the costs of MRI requires careful attention to the physics and engineering of the discipline. The major determinant of cost is field strength. By reducing the field strength, it becomes possible to use different approaches to magnet design, approaches that carry lower acquisition costs. Low-field systems can be sited in smaller rooms, which further reduces initial and ongoing costs. Other components that can lead to significant savings include radiofrequency (RF) transmitters and, in some cases, gradient coils.

Because of practical considerations, high-field systems are limited to cylindric configurations. These limitations are mainly concerned with cost and fringe fields and become less onerous as field strength decreases. Once the cylindrical magnet configuration can be avoided, alternatives in low-field magnets include some that are open. The era of open MRI started in 1988, with the commercial introduction of the Toshiba Access system (1). Not only was this system quickly accepted for dealing with difficult or ill patients, it also found application in interventional studies (2). Since then, Access has spawned a host of systems, creating a market for open MRI as a segment of its own, and has moved high-field systems to shorter bore configurations. For all practical purposes, the U.S. market consists of two segments: open low- and midfield MRI and high-field (1.5-T) short-bore systems, with the intermediate 1-T range shrinking to small portion of the total. Outside the United States,

patient preferences are less of a concern, and open MRI systems sell well because of their lower costs. Nevertheless, because the United States tends to lead the world in health care, it is to be expected that open MRI will become important on its own as patient preferences become a factor. As for the interventional market, predictions range from larger than the imaging market to just a niche.

PHYSICS OF LOW-FIELD STRENGTH OPERATION

As field strength decreases, so does the strength of the NMR signal emitted by the body. Nevertheless, imaging is a complex process that involves many factors. With decreasing field strength, noise from the body also decreases. Chemical shift and susceptibility artifacts decrease, permitting narrower bandwidths and consequent reductions in noise. T1 shortens (3,4) and T2 lengthens (4) this increasing signal level during imaging. Motion artifacts decrease, so that the fraction of study time spent on motion reduction can be used for data acquisition, and RF power deposition decreases dramatically. RF pulses can be tailored to improve section profiles and, more important, the hazard from RF heating is all but eliminated. At lower field, absolute magnetic field inhomogeneities get smaller (for imaging, a magnet with a 30 ppm homogeneity specification at 500 G is equivalent to one with a 1 ppm specification at 1.5 T). This fact and decreased susceptibility effects permit the use of gradient-echo techniques in which spin echoes may need to be used at higher fields (5). The shortened T1 values favor the use of three-dimensional (3D) fourier transform (TF) techniques, which can be designed to provide a wide range of contrast capabilities with good signal-to-noise ratios (SNRs) (6,7). Furthermore, for water-elevating lesions, for the same sequence, typically contrast is higher at the lower field. This is due to two factors: The shortened T1 of tissues permits contrast from T2 and hydrogen density [N(H)] changes to become visible at shorter repetition times (TRs) (8), and the change in T1 and T2 with water content

L. Kaufman: Radiologic Imaging Laboratory, Toshiba America MRI, Inc., South San Francisco, California

L. E. Crooks: Radiologic Imaging Laboratory, Toshiba America MRI, Inc., South San Francisco, California

is larger the lower the field (3,4). The impact of these effects depends on the type of study being performed, but, in general, for the same volume resolution and coverage and for equivalent contrast, there will be an SNR difference of 2 to 3 over a range of a factor of 25 in field strength.

MAGNETS FOR OPEN MAGNETIC RESONANCE IMAGING

High-field systems are still limited to cylindric configurations. The reasons for this fact are practical, not fundamental: With the technology as we understand it, the weight, fringe field, and cost characteristics of a high-field open unit are prohibitive for wide use. When the field strength is reduced to the mid to low range, various choices of magnet configurations become available. Resistive magnets were the early choices, but with the advent of practical permanent and superconducting magnet designs, the latter have been incorporated into the more recent commercially available products.

When considering magnet technology, the focus is on two basic components: the driver and the core of the magnet. The driver provides the motive force that establishes the magnetic field. Three kinds of driving technologies are available in the marketplace: (a) resistive, (b) permanent, and (c) superconducting. The Earth's magnetic field is a fourth source that has been discussed in the literature but has not become commercially available. The core is the medium on which the driver acts. Because a patient has to be able to be located in the magnet (a prerequisite for reimbursement), all magnets have at least a portion of their field in air. Air-core magnets feature a core that consists of air. These may have a return path (the region outside the core in which the magnetic field lines close) that is either air or iron. Iron-core magnets have, except for the patient volume, iron paths as return paths and for the drivers to act on. The relative merits of these approaches to magnet design are discussed in the following sections.

Resistive Drivers

In a resistive driver, a current is established on a good conducting material, typically copper or aluminum. (During the Manhattan Project, silver from the U.S. reserves was used for huge magnets for uranium separation, because copper and aluminum were needed for armaments.) The conductor is at or near room temperature, so it offers resistance to the flow of current. This resistance has two effects: Power has to be used to maintain the current flow and attendant magnetic field, and heat is generated in the conductor through resistive losses, so that water needs to be used to extract this heat. In addition, the stability of the field depends on power supply stability, a stability that comes at a price.

Given the conductor materials available, it is necessary to increase conductor cross-section to reduce resistance (and consequent power consumption). Doing so increases magnet cost, weight, and size. The task of the designer is to find some acceptable compromise among field strength and the three parameters mentioned above. An approximate measure is that iron-core resistive magnets consume approximately 125 kW per T.

The advantages of this approach are that the technology is well known and understood and entry is easy because a great deal of expertise exists or is easily acquired. The disadvantages are high power consumption, large cooling demand, a large conductor mass, and its consequent weight. When an iron core is used, the larger conductor mass forces an increase in the physical size of the core, which then results in further weight increases.

Permanent Drivers

In a permanent magnet, the field originates in blocks of permanently magnetized material. Currently available are ferrite magnets for low-field operation and Neomax (a rare earth alloy) for higher fields. The attractive aspect of permanent magnet drivers is that they are totally passive, requiring no added services such as electricity, cryogens, or cooling. The disadvantages are that the cost and field curve are very steep, especially when rare earth materials are needed for higher fields, and the weight of the permanent magnet material adds to the weight of an iron core.

A potential problem for the higher field units is that the magnet cannot be discharged in an emergency.

Superconducting Drivers

Some materials, generically known as *superconductors*, if kept at a sufficiently low temperature, lose all resistance to current flow. In typical magnets for MRI, this temperature has to be well below 10 K—that is, less than 10°C above absolute zero. A convenient way to achieve this is by the use of liquid helium, which has a temperature near 4 K. The liquid boils away owing to heat leaking into the magnet from room temperature. Because of cost, it is desirable to minimize the boil-off of the helium. One method used in the early years of commercial MRI is to use a surrounding container with liquid nitrogen, which has a temperature of 77 K, intermediate between helium and room temperatures. This, of course, adds liquid nitrogen consumption to the services needed for magnet operation. Later, electrical shield coolers were added to magnets to replace the liquid nitrogen shield; these coolers usually reached temperatures well below 77 K, thus improving the shielding effect. Recirculating coolers, which reliquefy vented helium gas, were also added to some magnets, even though this was not usually economical in the United States, owing to the relatively low cost of liquid helium.

More recently, electrical coolers that reach 4 K have become commercially available, opening the way to cryogenless superconducting magnets with low power consumption. It is worth noting that the high temperature superconducting (HTc) materials that were touted a few years ago as permitting magnets

TABLE 7-1. *Magnet tradeoffs*

Increased	Field	Homogeneity	Gap	Weight	Fringe field	Size	Cost
Field		−	−	+	+	+	+
Homogeneity	−		+	+	O	+	+
Gap	−	+		+	+	+	+
Weight	+	+	+		−	+	+
Fringe field	+	O	+	−		−	−
Size	+	+	+	+	−		+
Cost	+	+	+	+	−	+	

O, no change; +, increase; −, decrease.

cooled by liquid nitrogen have yet to provide the performance required by MRI magnets, but they have found use as superconducting leads, which bring current from the outside to the main windings during magnet charging and discharging.

Magnet designs will not change drastically when HTc materials become available, unless the operating temperature is near room temperature. The reason is as follows: When a liquid helium cryostat is used for cooling the superconductor and an intermediate temperature shield is added, being able to operate the superconductor at 40 to 77 K allows the cryostat to be eliminated. Then, magnet cost, size, and weight are reduced. On the other hand, if refrigerators are used to cool the superconductor, the liquid helium cryostat is already eliminated and only the intermediate shield remains, negating the advantage of higher temperature operation. Of course, a refrigerator that need not operate below 40 K will be of lower cost than one that needs to reach 4 K, but the magnet itself will not be significantly different. Today a vacuum vessel for a midfield superconducting magnet cooled by refrigeration is on the order of 15 cm^2; operation at 77 K would minimally reduce this cross-section.

The advantage of superconductors for MRI is relatively higher fields compared to the other technologies, with low weight and modest power consumption. The disadvantage is the need for cryogens (or, more recently, cryocoolers that can replace cryogens) and the technical complexity of these systems compared to other drivers, thus making entry more difficult. Superconductors become cheaper than other drivers at a certain field strength crossover point. Once the midfield range is reached, they have definite advantages in this respect.

Magnet Core

The driver can be shaped to obtain the desired imaging field and field return path without the aid of significant amounts of iron; these magnets are called *air-core magnets*. Iron can be used for shaping the imaging field and providing a return path; these magnets are called *iron-core magnets*. Some air-core magnets have an iron return path or shield.

The advantage of air-core magnets is their low weight. The disadvantages are inefficient conductor use, demands on the conductor configuration and manufacturing toler-

ances (because the homogeneity depends on conductor location), and large fringe fields requiring active or passive shielding. All of this, of course, results in increased costs.

Iron-core magnets make more efficient use of the driver, because the iron provides a medium that offers less resistance to the flow of the magnetic field lines. In iron-core magnets, fringe fields are relatively small and homogeneity is determined by the shape of the iron. The advantages of the iron core place fewer demands on the driver's configuration and tolerances. The main unavoidable disadvantage of these cores is weight.

Other nuances concerning the different drivers and cores need to be taken into account when designing an MRI system, but the characteristics described above are of a reasonably general nature and not amenable to significant manipulation. Commercially, the following driver-core combinations have become available at one time or another in the 15 years of clinical MRI: (a) resistive, superconducting, and permanent driver air-core, the first two sometimes with iron shielding, and (b) resistive, permanent, and superconducting driver iron-core. The number of posts in available iron-core designs can be one, two, or four. Magnet assembly technology results in elimination of eddy currents without the need for active gradient coil shielding. The design of these magnets involves tradeoffs among cost, size, weight, gap, homogeneity, fringe field, and field strength. Typically, larger gaps, higher homogeneities, smaller fringe fields, and higher field strengths require larger, heavier magnets of higher cost.

Designing a Magnet

Although all magnet designers are confronted by the same physics, the available technology and perceived merits of different characteristics generate occasionally disparate designs. The reason, of course, is that judgments are made as to the relative merits of different magnet performance parameters, so that the results look very different. Table 7-1 shows some of the tradeoffs made by magnet designers. For instance, a higher field strength can be realized by accepting a lower homogeneity, smaller gap, bigger fringe field, or higher weight, the last necessitating physically bigger magnets and higher costs. Cost increases with increased field strength, homogeneity, aperture, weight, and size and decreases with increased fringe field.

TABLE 7-2. *Single-variable comparison*

Magnet type	Weight (cost/B_0)	Homogeneity	Fringe field	Mechanical stability	Openness
Four-post	Lightest	Best	Smallest	Best	Intermediate
Two-post	Intermediate	Intermediate	Intermediate	Intermediate	Worst
One-post (C-type)	Heaviest	Worst	Largest	Worst	Best

In open iron-core magnets, another design choice is the number of posts used to separate the pole pieces. The magnets are typically supported by four posts, one at each corner; two posts, positioned either exactly at 180 degrees from each other or at a somewhat smaller angle; or one post that occupies essentially all of one side of the magnet (these are also known as *C-magnets*). If all performance specifications are the same, for any one kind of driver technology, the four-post magnets offer the lowest weight (and cost per unit field strength) at a given level of mechanical stability. If field strength, patient space, and weight are held fixed, four-post magnets also offer the best homogeneity, or smallest fringe field, and the highest mechanical stability. The one-post designs offer the least desirable results, and two-post designs offer results that fall somewhere between the other two designs (Table 7-2). Although C-magnets are attractive in that they have three unencumbered open sides, their efficiency is lower and they tend to have smaller gaps, a disadvantage for imaging of large subjects or for access during interventional procedures.

RADIOFREQUENCY COILS FOR OPEN MAGNETIC RESONANCE IMAGING

RF coil designs for open MRI contend with two generally applicable factors: The commercially available systems are vertical field configurations and the field of view (FOV) tends to be smaller than that found in conventional superconducting magnets (even though the increasingly popular short-bore high-field units are facing similar or more severe FOV limitations).

The vertical field configuration is particularly advantageous for head, neck, body, wrist, and knee imaging, in which a solenoid surrounding the anatomy of interest is particularly efficient. For quadrature detection (QD) configurations, a saddle can be added. For spine and breast imaging, the vertical field configuration is less advantageous. In spine imaging, rather than an efficient loop (essentially a one-turn solenoid), a figure-8 coil is needed, a design that is inherently less efficient. Combining the figure-8 coil with a solenoid around the body considerably increases SNR at depth, but at the price of having the whole body cross-section in the FOV. For imaging a prone woman's breast (the prone position increases patient comfort and stability), a solenoid surrounding the breast is ideal, because it generates a fringe field that extends into the chest wall. Such a coil cannot be used in a vertical field magnet, because its axis would have to be aligned with the field. Therefore, we use a QD configuration consisting of two saddle coils. These coils have small fringe fields and consequently relatively poorer penetration into the chest wall. As with every aspect of MRI, every choice of operating parameters affords advantages and disadvantages.

It is illustrative to show one set of choices we have made for coils (Fig. 7-1) for body parts in a vertical field open magnet:

- Head: Solenoid with horizontal axis along the subject and saddle with orthogonal and horizontal axis, combined in QD or array mode.
- Neck: Solenoid with horizontal axis along the subject, shaped to extend FOV (Fig. 7-2).
- Shoulder: Thin solenoid with horizontal axis, also appropriate for knee motion studies (9) (Fig. 7-3).

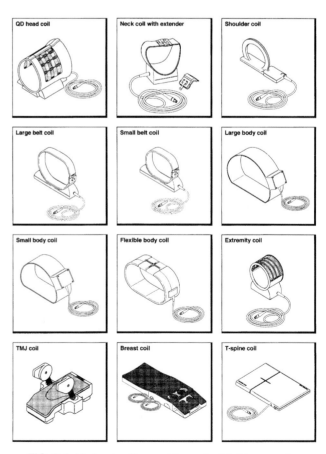

FIG. 7-1. Various coils used in vertical field magnets.

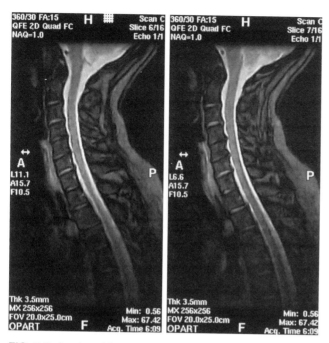

FIG. 7-2. A solenoid closely wrapped around the neck allows for an extended field of view. A, anterior; FA, flip angle; FOV, field of view; MX, matrix size; NAQ, number of acquisitions; P, posterior; QFE, quadrature field echo; Thk, thickness.

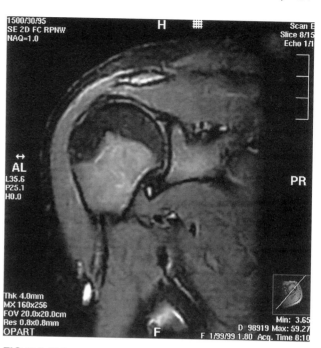

FIG. 7-3. Fat-suppressed image obtained with a shoulder coil. AL, anterior left; D, maximum density; F, foot; FC, flow compensated; FOV, field of view; MX, matrix size; NAQ, number of acquisitions; PR, posterior right; Res, resolution; RPNW, read and phase no wrap; SE, spin echo; Thk, thickness.

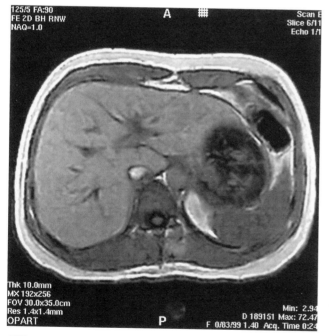

FIG. 7-4. Image obtained with a solenoidal coil surrounding the body. A, anterior; BH, breath hold; D, maximum density; F, foot; FA, flip angle; FE, field echo; FOV, field of view; MX, matrix size; NAQ, number of acquisitions; P, posterior; Res, resolution; RNW, readout no wrap; Thk, thickness.

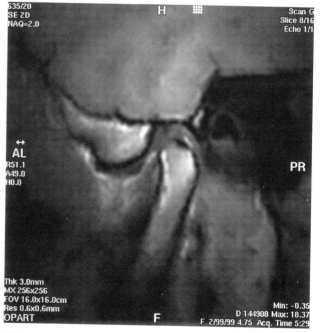

FIG. 7-5. Image of the temporomandibular joint obtained with a flat solenoidal coil. AL, anterior left; D, maximum density; F, foot; FOV, field of view; H, head; MX, matrix size; NAQ, number of acquisitions; PR, posterior right; Res, resolution; SE, spin echo; Thk, thickness.

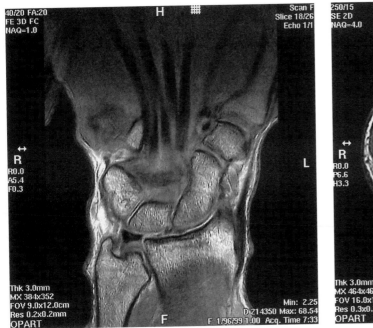
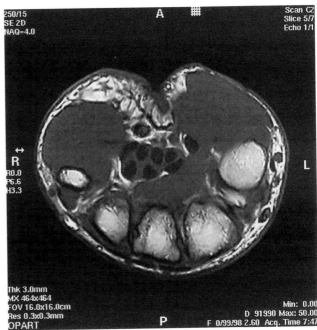

FIG. 7-6. Images of the wrist obtained with a flexible wrap-around coil. A, anterior; D, maximum density; F, foot; FA, flip angle; FC, flow compensated; FE, field echo; FOV, field of view; H, head; L, left; MX, matrix size; NAQ, number of acquisitions; P, posterior; R, right; Res, resolution; SE, spin echo; Thk, thickness.

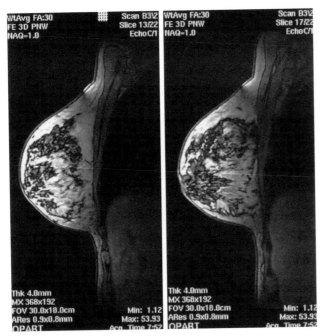

FIG. 7-7. Breast coil images obtained in a supine subject. ARes, acquisition resolution; FE, field echo; FOV, field of view; MX, matrix size; NAQ, number of acquisitions; PNW, phase no wrap; Thk, thickness.

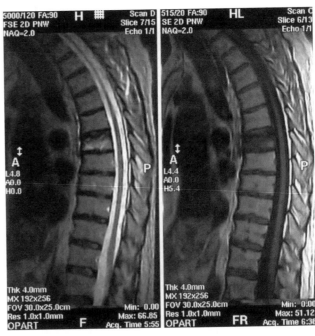

FIG. 7-8. Image obtained with a T-spine figure-8 coil. A, anterior; F, foot; FA, flip angle; FOV, field of view; FR, foot right; FSE, fast spin echo; H, head; HL, head left; MX, matrix size; NAQ, number of acquisitions; P, posterior; PNW, phase no wrap; Res, resolution; SE, spin echo; Thk, thickness.

- Body: Belt (or thin) or wide solenoid with horizontal axis along the subject, combined in QD or array mode with flat figure-8 coil, the latter used by itself for T-spine imaging. These can also be in a flexible wrap-around configuration (Fig. 7-4).
- Knee: Head-type configuration of smaller size.
- Small parts: Temporomandibular joint coil, flat solenoid with horizontal axis (Fig. 7-5), or wrist coil, wrap-around solenoid with horizontal axis (Fig. 7-6).

The common theme is to take as much advantage as possible of the solenoidal configuration and reduce coil size as much as possible to increase efficiency. When solenoids are not usable, we are forced to use alternate configurations:

- Breast: Two saddles with horizontal, orthogonal axis, combined in QD or array mode (Fig. 7-7).
- T-spine: A figure-8 coil. Penetration is limited, which is advantageous for a shallow feature such as the T-spine (Fig. 7-8).

SEQUENCING FOR OPEN IMAGING

Sequence development for open-magnet imaging needs to take into account and take advantage of the short T1 value of solid tissues at the field strengths at which these magnets operate. Also of importance are reduced chemical shift and susceptibility artifacts. One example involves strategies for the detection of lesions in areas in which water content is increased. This is a typical effect seen in tumors, edema, and infarcts. Considering the case in which there is no blood, for these lesions N(H), T1 and T2 are all elevated (8). In a spin-echo sequence, the elevation of N(H) and T2 increases signal, whereas the elevation of T1 decreases signal. Thus, N(H) and T2 effects are diluted by T1 effects. To obtain a lesion that is brighter than background, it is necessary to increase TR to the point at which T1 effects become unimportant, resulting in what is misnamed a *T2-weighted* image. In fact, a more accurate phrase would be *not T1-weighted*. To reliably achieve this condition, it is necessary to operate with a TR of at least 2 T1, preferably 2.5 to 3.0 T1. Because T1 increases with field strength, it is necessary to operate with a longer TR at the higher field. For instance, for brain tissue, the increase between 0.064 and 1.500 T is approximately a factor of 4, from 250 ms to approximately 1 second for white matter and from 300 ms to 1.2 seconds for gray matter. Thus, for a spin-echo sequence, the desired lesion contrast is easier to achieve and is more reliably achieved at the lower field. This has significant consequences in terms of SNR, because shorter TR values can lead to a larger number of data averages for fixed imaging time.

For watery lesions, the ability to use short TR values opens an avenue for imaging with three-dimensional (3D) FT sequences. The TR that can be achieved in 3D FT imaging is limited by practical time considerations, because this time increases linearly with the number of slices obtained. If

gradient-echo instead of spin-echo imaging is used, an angle smaller than 90 degrees results in a decrease of T1 effects. Lowering the angle at fixed TR has the same effect as lengthening TR for a 90-degree angle. This process cannot be carried to extremes, but it is more effective the larger the TR to T1 ratio. Thus, from a practical point of view, it is only achievable for short T1 values, for which it is highly effective. Furthermore, to obtain the desired contrast level, it is desirable to operate with a relatively long echo time (TE) to take advantage of T2 effects.

A significant benefit is derived in low-field operation from the fact that although solid tissues have shorter T1 values at low field, cerebrospinal fluid (CSF) has a T1 that is constant with field. Consequently, at the short TR at which lesion contrast is achieved, the signal from CSF is small. At high field, because TR has to be long, CSF signal is large, obscuring lesions that may be contiguous with CSF spaces. To summarize, low-field strengths offer many advantages for the detection of water-elevating lesions, including increased sensitivity to water changes, ability to operate with relatively short TR values, and the avoidance of confusing effects from bright CSF.

Clinical MRI started as a mid-field technique. Many of the sequences currently considered routine were originally developed at mid field (10,11), so contrast characteristics are more familiar. The contrast characteristics of midfield MRI are closer to low than high field. For instance, brain lesions

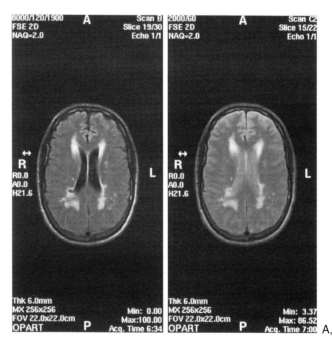

A, B

FIG. 7-9. A: Fast spin-echo fluid attenuation inversion recovery image in a multiple sclerosis patient (TR/TE/TI 8000/120/1900 at 0.35 T). **B:** Same sequence with TR/TE 2000/60. The first sequence produces one slice projection every 267 ms, whereas the second requires only 91 ms per slice projection. Cerebrospinal fluid is sufficiently hypointense not to mask lesions. A, anterior; FOV, field of view; FSE, fast spin echo; L, left; MX, matrix size; NAQ, number of acquisitions; P, posterior; R, right; TE, echo time; Thk, thickness; TR, repetition time.

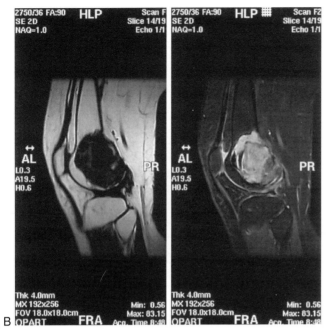

A, B

FIG. 7-10. Fat (A) and water (B) images of a knee with a large tumor, obtained with a single-shot, three-point Dixon technique. AL, anterior left; FOV, field of view; FRA, foot right anterior; HLP, head left posterior; MX, matrix size; NAQ, number of acquisitions; PR, posterior right; SE, spin echo; Thk, thickness.

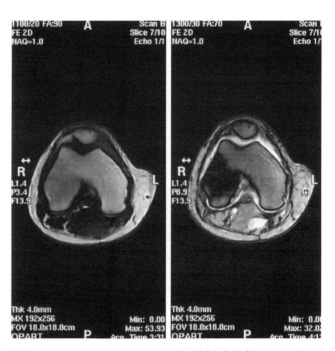

FIG. 7-11. Images in a patient with AVN. At left are gradient-echo images with water and fat in phase [echo time (TE) = 20 ms at 0.35 T] and at right out of phase (TE = 30 ms). A, anterior; FE, field echo; FOV, field of view; L, left; MX, matrix size; P, posterior; R, right; Thk, thickness.

are bright while CSF remains of lower intensity, so that fluid attenuation inversion recovery techniques are not needed to highlight periventricular lesions (Fig. 7-9). Fat signal gains in relative intensity compared to low field, but inversion recovery (see Fig. 7-3) and single-shot multipoint Dixon (12) techniques make it easier to suppress fat (Fig. 7-10). In gradient-echo imaging, water and fat are out of phase at a convenient TE of 10 or 30 ms and in phase at a TE of 20 ms. The former results in fast sequences for screening of bone marrow abnormalities (Fig. 7-11).

Another example of low-field sequencing involves MR angiography. In MR angiography, the clinically most successful techniques take advantage of wash-in effects (13). The blood entering the volume has not been excited previously and thus produces a great deal of signal after the first one or two excitations (14). Meanwhile, it is desirable to saturate the signal from stationary tissues by the same repeated excitations that produce signal from blood. This saturation is more effective the longer the T1, because recovery time is longer. Because high-field operation entails long T1 values, high contrast between blood and nonmoving tissues is easier to obtain, which permits more flexibility in trading vessel contrast for depth of penetration (FOV) than at low field, in which T1 values are short. For low-field systems, phase contrast angiography is an extremely attractive alternative. At midfield, the T1 of blood lengthens enough to make time-of-flight MR angiography techniques also attractive, so that both are usable (Figs. 7-12, 7-13, and 7-14). Similarly, CSF is easier to highlight at midfield (Figs. 7-15, 7-16, and 7-17; see Fig. 7-2).

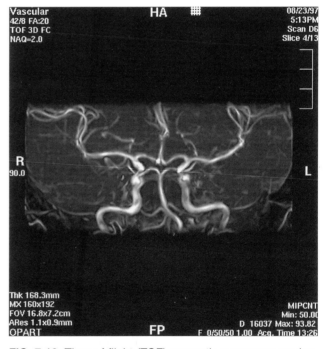

FIG. 7-12. Time of flight (TOF) magnetic resonance angiography on the head at 0.35 T. ARes, acquisition resolution; D, maximum density; F, foot; FA, flip angle; FOV, field of view; FP, foot posterior; HA, head anterior; L, left; MIPCNT, maximum intensity projection contrast; MX, matrix size; NAQ, number of acquisitions; R, right; Thk, thickness.

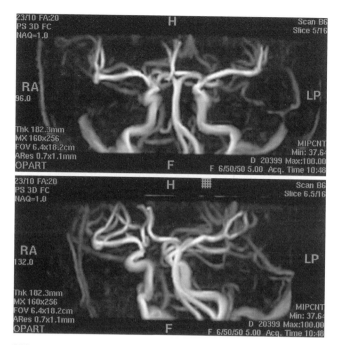

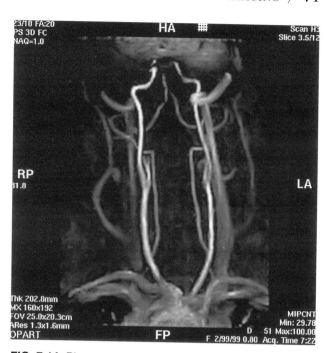

FIG. 7-13. Phase shift imaging of the head at 0.35 T. ARes, acquisition resolution; D, maximum density; F, foot; FC, flow compensated; FOV, field of view; H, head; LP, left posterior; MIPCNT, maximum intensity projection contrast; MX, matrix size; NAQ, number of acquisitions; PS, phase shift; RA, right anterior; Thk, thickness.

FIG. 7-14. Phase shift imaging of the neck at 0.35 T. ARes, acquisition resolution; D, maximum density; F, foot; FC, flow compensated; FOV, field of view; FP, foot posterior; HA, head anterior; LA, left anterior; MIPCNT, maximum intensity projection contrast; MX, matrix size; NAQ, number of acquisitions; PS, phase shift; RP, right posterior; Thk, thickness.

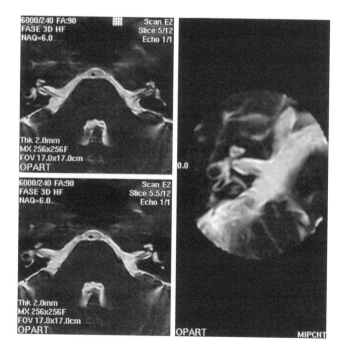

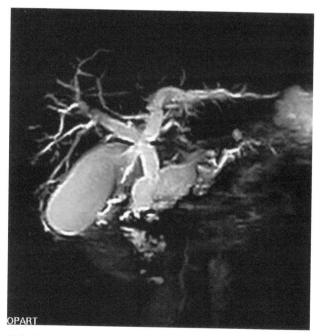

FIG. 7-15. Cranial nerves and auditory canal imaged with a long (128 echoes half Fourier) three-dimensional fast spin-echo technique. FA, flip angle; FASE, fast advanced spin-echo; FOV, field of view; HF, half Fourier; MIPCNT, maximum intensity projection contrast; MX, matrix size; NAQ, number of acquisitions; Thk, thickness.

FIG. 7-16. Biliary tract imaged with two-dimensional fast spin-echo technique (128 echos half Fourier).

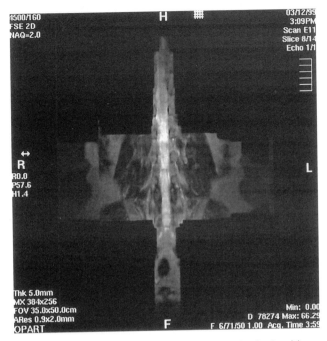

FIG. 7-17. Coronal image of the spinal canal, obtained by a double-curved reconstruction along the canal and foramina. ARes, acquisition resolution; D, maximum density; F, foot; FOV, field of view; FSE, fast spin echo; H, head; L, left; MX, matrix size; NAQ, number of acquisitions; R, right; Thk, thickness.

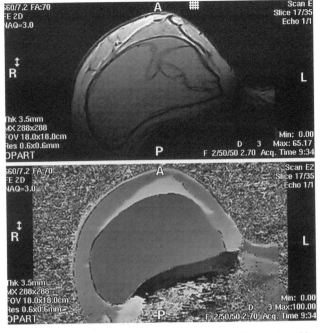

FIG. 7-18. Silicone, water, and fat are clearly differentiated in chemical shift images (*bottom*) in a subject with a collapsed implant. The chemical shift image is reconstructed from the same data set as the magnitude image (*top*) and has the same spatial resolution. A, anterior; D, maximum density; F, foot; FA, flip angle; FE, field echo; FOV, field of view; L, left; MX, matrix size; NAQ, number of acquisitions; P, posterior; R, right; Res, resolution; Thk, thickness.

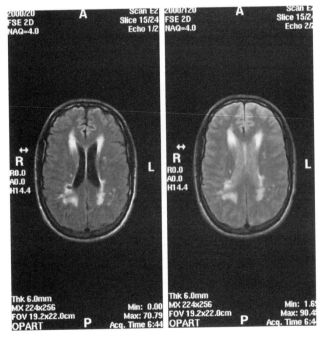

FIG. 7-19. Double-contrast fast spin-echo study in the head. Images have a repetition time of 2,000 ms and echo time (TE) of 20 and 120 ms and are obtained using half Fourier techniques to increase efficiency and keep the first echo to a short TE. The sequence requires 166 ms to acquire both echoes for one slice projection. A, anterior; FOV, field of view; FSE, fast spin echo; L, left; NAQ, number of acquisitions; MX, matrix size; P, posterior; R, right; Thk, thickness.

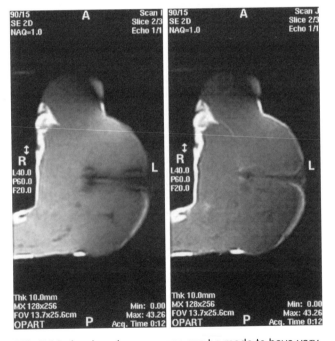

FIG. 7-20. A spin-echo sequence can be made to have varying sensitivity to magnetic susceptibility effects. This can be useful in interventional real-time imaging, in which an object such as a biopsy needle is being tracked. The image at right is a pure spin echo; the one at left is made susceptible to the needle's magnetic properties. A, anterior; FOV, field of view; L, left; MX, matrix size; NAQ, number of acquisitions; P, posterior; R, right; SE, spin echo; Thk, thickness.

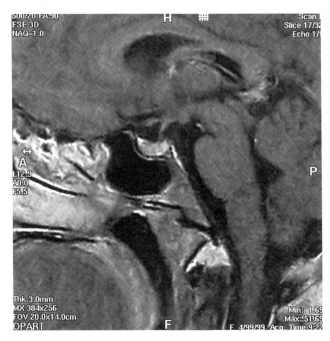

FIG. 7-21. Three-dimensional fast spin-echo image of the pituitary. A, anterior; F, foot; FOV, field of view; FSE, fast spin echo; H, head; MX, matrix size; NAQ, number of acquisitions; P, posterior; Thk, thickness.

Imaging of chemical shift is also accessible at low field for protons in water, fat, and silicone by reconstruction of phase images for 3D FT sequences. We have found this method particularly powerful in searching for extracapsular silicone in breast implant patients at fields as low as 0.065 T (15). The chemical shift images have the same resolution and SNR and do not require additional imaging time (Fig. 7-18).

Double-contrast fast spin-echo imaging adds to the flexibility with which contrast can be varied (Fig. 7-19). Asymmetric spin-echo sequences (16) can be used to highlight T2* effects (Fig. 7-20).

A crossover occurs between the efficacy of 2D versus 3D imaging (17), so either is effective. Particularly effective are 3D spin-echo techniques, which provide fine anatomic detail (Fig. 7-21).

SIGNAL TO NOISE RATIOS AND FIELD STRENGTH

A perception exists that SNR increases linearly with field strength. The physics of MRI show that signal increases as the square of the field and measurements and theoretical considerations (based on certain assumptions about the body) support a linear increase in noise with field, although this latter assumption should be considered with caution. Based on these two factors, "intrinsic" SNR should increase linearly with field. This simplistic view depends on disregarding all the factors that are important in imaging, resulting in a much smaller increase than presumed.

In addition to the intrinsic factor, SNR depends on the imaging conditions. Of interest is SNR per unit time for fixed voxel dimensions and imaged volume, as well as constant number of slices. For a 90-degree flip angle, the relative SNR is proportional to

$$\left[e^{-TE/T2}(1 - e^{-TE/T2})\sqrt{(\text{window length} \times \text{slices} / TR)} \right]$$

for 2D FT imaging. The reasons for the slices term are that if sequence A yields 10 slices and sequence B yields 20 slices with one excitation, then, to cover the same volume sequence A has to be run twice, whereas sequence B in the same time could be run once with two excitations and gain $\sqrt{2}$ in SNR. Similarly, the TR term comes in because if two sequences provide the same coverage for one excitation, then the sequence with the shorter TR can be run with more excitations and increase SNR accordingly. For 3D FT, there is an additional slices term. For a discussion of the relative merits of 2D versus 3D FT imaging, the reader is directed to reference 18. Based on imaging considerations, we can analyze how SNR will behave.

T1

As field strength increases, so does T1 (3,4). A longer T1 means smaller signals. For discussion purposes, consider T1 varying as the square root of field strength. For a short TR sequence, signal decreases linearly with T1, or as square root of field. For a long TR sequence, signal does not change much. For a fixed TR, the contrast is lower, or for fixed contrast, TR is longer (longer imaging time). In this case, the equivalent loss of SNR is smaller, approximately as the fourth root of field strength. Thus, for longer TR values, T1 effects result in a loss in signal that increases as the fourth root to square root of field.

T2

Clear evidence exists that T2 drops with field strength (4). Between 0.063 and 3.000 T, the T2 of brain drops from approximately 80 to 58 ms, for muscle from 37 to 30 ms, and for liver from 49 to 25 ms. For a TE of 30 ms, this results in signal drops from 16% to 50%, corresponding to a 1/20 to 1/8 power of field for the loss of SNR due to T2. The loss is smaller for shorter TE and bigger for longer TE values.

Window Length

Chemical shift, susceptibility, and inhomogeneity limit window lengths. As discussed, the artifacts depend linearly on field strength and window length. A shorter window reduces the artifacts but also decreases SNR as the square root of window length. The effect is that, at constant artifactual level, a square root of field strength term is available in the SNR, favoring low-field operation. In some sequences, this term is not usable—for example, when TE is very short—and in others it is not fully usable, but in general it provides relative advantages of factors of 2 to 3 in SNR for low-field operation.

Radiofrequency Power

As discussed, high-field systems compromise slice profile in the interest of savings in peak and average RF power. At mid and low fields these conditions are not important, and square profiles can be obtained (19). For a system in which a gap of 50% is needed to avoid interslice crosstalk, SNR loss for the slice itself may amount to 20%, and the gap can be considered an unused potential source of 50% more signal (20). Thus, the full SNR is not being achieved if the slice profile is poor. The loss in 2D FT imaging is sequence dependent. For 3D FT imaging, no difference exists.

Artifact Reduction

As discussed, artifact reduction schemes take time away from data collection, either by reducing the echo window length or number of sections or by lengthening TE, and may result in penalties in SNR per unit time. This loss depends on the particular sequence and can be as small as zero when artifact reduction is not needed and as big as 50% in some extreme cases, such as presaturation in multi-slice imaging.

Net Signal to Noise Ratio Change

From the aforementioned considerations it can be seen that SNR changes with field in a complex manner, which depends on the clinical purpose of the sequence, the type of sequence used, tissue imaged, coverage (including gaps), and artifacts. For a sequence such as MR angiography, a major part of the theoretical SNR available from increasing field strength can be obtained. For other sequences, the gain is small. An approximate rule is that, in many situations, the SNR increases as the third to fourth root of field strength, so that for a 25-fold increase in field, SNR doubles or triples.

Clinical Tests

Few studies have rigorously compared diagnostic efficacy at different field strengths. One, by the Australian government, was a broad-based evaluation of five units at 0.3, 1.0, and 1.5 T (21). Another was limited to head imaging, comparing 0.064-T and 1.500-T units (22), and a receiver operator characteristic study of multiple sclerosis and knee imaging was published more recently, in 1996 (23). The earliest such study compared field strengths of 0.5, 1.0, and 1.5 T (24). None has shown a statistically significant difference in efficacy. As of this writing, in the United States, approximately one-half of the market is for open (low-field and midfield) MRI systems, which may be the best indicator of the efficacy of these systems.

THE FUTURE

The public's discomfort with MRI "in a tube" has been somewhat of a surprise to those of us involved with the technology since its early stages. To a certain extent, this remains a U.S. phenomenon, where, as a society, we are much more attuned to individual comfort and patient choice than elsewhere. Nevertheless, it is safe to guess that the United States' propensity to export its culture (and other countries' propensity to import it) will make patient comfort an issue elsewhere. Furthermore, lower costs have an appeal outside the United States that is less dominant here. Thus, insofar as open MRI comes with a lower cost, its appeal is global. Furthermore, undertaking interventional procedures in an open system is far more appealing to surgeons than is doing so by remote control. It is safe to say that open MRI will be standard for interventional MRI.

There is no new physics in either open or closed-tube MRI. The major changes that make it possible have been in materials science (permanent magnets and rare earth refrigerators) and design philosophy. Physical factors are not limiting in obtaining even more open designs, but economic and siting considerations are. It is possible to build a one-sided magnet on which the patient lies. (In the most simple-minded scheme, consider a circular loop large enough that the central region has adequate homogeneity.) Any such magnet would have to contend with large fringe fields. All of this is manageable from a design point of view, but costs and siting may dictate against such a development. It is worth reminding the reader that anyone can build a one-of-a-kind unit. The challenge is to make (and sell, install, service, and upgrade) hundreds of them.

REFERENCES

1. Kaufman L, Arakawa M, Hale JC, et al. Accessible MRI. *Magn Reson Q* 1990;5:283.
2. Gronemeyer DHW, Seibel RMM, Busch M, Rothschild PA, Kaufman L. Interventionelle Kernspintomographie. In: Gronemeyer DHW, Seibel RMM, eds. *Interventionelle Computer-Tomographie, Ueberreuter Wissenschaft.* Berlin: Kapitel, 1989:24.
3. Koenig SH, Brown RD, Adams D, Emerson D, Harrison CG. Magnetic field dependence of 1/T1 in tissue. *Invest Radiol* 1984;19:76.
4. Chen J–H, Avram H, Crooks LE, Arakawa M, Kaufman L, Brito AC. *In vivo* relaxation times and hydrogen density at 0.063–4.8T in rats with implanted mammary adenocarcinomas. *Radiology* 1992;184:1.
5. Kramer DM, Li A, Kaufman L, Hake K. Two–gradient echo 2-DFT multi-section imaging: comparison with spin echo imaging. *J Neuroimag* 1992;2:195.
6. Rothschild PA, Schulz M, Kramer DM, Kaufman L. Magnetic resonance imaging characteristics of multiple sclerosis plaques imaged with two-dimensional and three-dimensional Fourier transform techniques at low and mid field strengths. *J Neuroimag* 1991;1:79.
7. Kramer DM, Guzman RJ, Carlson JW, Crooks LE, Kaufman L. Physics of thin-section MR imaging at low field strength. *Radiology* 1989;173:541.
8. Ortendahl DA, Hylton NM, Kaufman L, et al. Analytical tools for MRI. *Radiology* 1984;153:479.
9. Carlson JW, Gyori M, Kaufman L. A technique for MR imaging of the knee under large flexing angles. *Magn Reson Imag* 1990;8:407.
10. Crooks LE, Arakawa M, Hoenninger JC, et al. NMR whole body imager operating at 3.5 KGauss. *Radiology* 1982;143:169.
11. Brant-Zawadzki M, Norman D, Newton TH, et al. Magnetic resonance of the brain: the optimal screening technique. *Radiology* 1984;152:71.
12. Zhang W, Goldhaber DM, Kramer DM. Separation of water and fat MR images in a single scan at .35 T using "sandwich" echoes. *J Magn Reson Imag* 1996;6:909.

13. Blatter DD, Parker DL, Ahn SS, et al. Cerebral MR angiography with multiple overlapping thin slab acquisition. *Radiology* 1992;183:379.

14. Kaufman L, Crooks LE, Sheldon PE, Rowan W, Miller T. Evaluation of NMR imaging for detection and quantification of obstructions in vessels. *Invest Radiol* 1982;17:554.

15. Derby KA, Frankel SD, Kaufman L, et al. Differentiation of silicone gel from water and fat in MRI phase imaging of protons at 0.064T. *Radiology* 1993;189:617–620.

16. WT Dixon. Simple proton spectroscopic imaging. *Radiology* 1984;153:189–194.

17. Kramer DM, Kaufman L, Rothschild P, Hale J, Wummer J, Hake KK. Low-field 3-DFT MRI: conceptual, analytical and experimental aspects. *IEEE Transl Med Imag* 1991;10:382.

18. Carlson JC, Crooks LE, Ortendahl DA, Kramer DM, Kaufman L. Signal-to-noise ratio and section thickness in two-dimensional versus three-dimensional Fourier transform MR imaging. *Radiology* 1988;166:266.

19. Feinberg DA, Crooks LE, Hoenninger JC, et al. Contiguous thin multi-section MR imaging by two-dimensional Fourier transform techniques. *Radiology* 1986;158:811.

20. Kneeland JB, Shimakawa A, Wehrli F. Effect of intersection spacing on MR image contrast and study time. *Radiology* 1986;158:819.

21. MRI Technical Committee of the National Health Technology Advisory Panel. MRI Assessment Program final report. Canberra, Australia: Australian Institute of Health, August 1990.

22. Orrison WW, Stimac GK, Stevens EA, et al. Comparison of CT, low-field-strength MR imaging, and high-field-strength MR imaging. *Radiology* 1991;181:121–127.

23. Rutt BK, Lee DH. The impact of field strength on image quality in MRI. *J Magn Reson Imag* 1996;6:57–62.

24. Summary of safety and effectiveness data, premarket approval application No. P830074. Submitted to the U.S. Food and Drug Administration by the General Electric Company, 1989:11.

Open MRI,
edited by Peter A. Rothschild and Debra Reinking Rothschild.
Lippincott Williams & Wilkins. Philadelphia © 2000.

CHAPTER 8

Understanding Fast Scanning: Traversing K-Space

Mark L. Winkler

The purpose of this chapter is to provide the magnetic resonance imaging (MRI) practitioner with a simple, unified approach to fast scanning. This chapter presents a practical conceptual framework to understand the enhancement of data-acquisition speed used in conventional and fast imaging techniques.

K-SPACE

K-space is the raw data acquired during the MRI examination. It is also known as the *time domain* or *raw data file*. The k-space is mathematically processed with a Fourier transformation to produce the actual MR image (Fig. 8-1).

K-space is acquired as a series of lines with individual points defined along each line. Each line of K-space is defined by the phase-encoding gradient. Each point along the lines of k-space is defined by the frequency-encoding gradient (Fig. 8-2).

The data of k-space points is different from that of the points within the displayed images, as the points of k-space possess spatial and signal strength information for the entire image. The spatial and signal strength information contained within each data point is weighted differently by the Fourier transform depending on its location in k-space. The central portions of k-space contain predominantly signal strength information and therefore contribute principally to the signal-to-noise ratio (SNR) and contrast resolution of the image (Fig. 8-3). The peripheral portions of k-space contain predominantly spatial information and therefore contribute principally to the spatial resolution of the image (Fig. 8-4).

An additional property of k-space is its symmetry. This allows the MR image to be created with only a portion of the k-space being acquired (Fig. 8-5).

M. L. Winkler: Department of Health Sciences, University of Nevada, Las Vegas, Las Vegas, Nevada; Steinberg Diagnostic Medical Imaging, Las Vegas, Nevada

The speed with which the k-space is traversed determines the scan time. This chapter explores the various methods of speeding up this travel through k-space. These are described as walking, striding, skipping, running, sprinting, or oscillating through the k-space, depending on the individual imaging techniques used. No one fast imaging technique fits all applications. The clinician must tailor the sequence choice to match the clinical needs. The availability of fast scanning techniques has increased the number of tools available to most efficiently obtain the clinical diagnosis.

SPIN-ECHO IMAGING

Spin-echo imaging (1) may be thought of as walking through the k-space. With conventional spin-echo imaging, scan time is proportional to the repetition time (TR) of the examination, the number of phase-encoding steps, and the number of excitations. The limitation of conventional imaging is that as any of the three variables are reduced, image quality suffers.

If the TR is reduced, image quality suffers from a reduction in SNR as well as a limitation in contrast. For proton- or T2-weighted images, this limitation in contrast may be unacceptable, forcing the use of relatively long TR values, resulting in long scan times.

If the number of phase-encoding steps is decreased, image quality suffers either a decrease in SNR or a limitation in resolution. For high-resolution neurologic or musculoskeletal work, this resolution limitation may be unacceptable.

If the number of excitations is decreased, image quality again suffers a decrease in SNR. In addition, the improvement in scan time is eventually limited to one excitation. For a T2-weighted examination with a TR of 3000, 192 phase-encoding steps, and only one acquisition, scan time is still 9 minutes, which is not acceptable in the fast scan era.

Thus, it is clear that other methods of traversing through k-space are necessary to improve scan time.

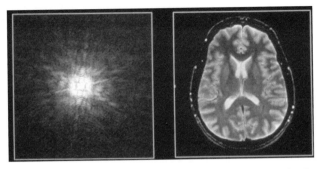

FIG. 8-1. The k-space or raw data (left) are mathematically processed with a Fourier transformer to produce the actual MR image (right).

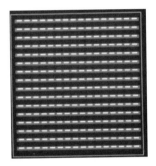

FIG. 8-2. K-space is acquired as a series of lines with individual points defined along each line. Each line of k-space is defined by the phase-encoding gradient. Each point along the lines of k-space is defined by the frequency-encoding gradient.

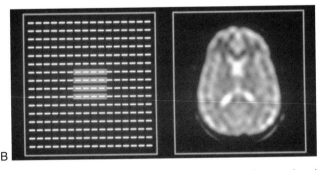

A, B

FIG. 8-3. The center of the k-space **(A)** contributes signal information to the magnetic resonance image providing SNR and contrast **(B)**.

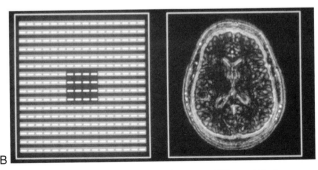

A, B

FIG. 8-4. The periphery of the k-space **(A)** contributes spatial information to the magnetic resonance image providing resolution **(B)**.

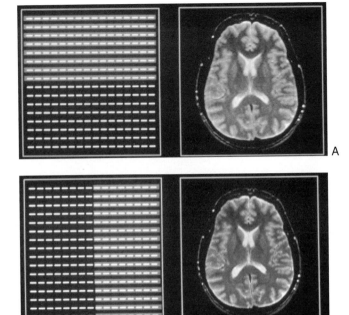

A

B

FIG. 8-5. K-space symmetry. **A:** Symmetry of the k-space allows the magnetic resonance image to be created with only slightly more than half of the phase-encoding lines. **B:** Symmetry of the k-space allows the magnetic resonance image to be created with only slightly more than half of the frequency-encoding points.

PARTIAL FLIP IMAGING

With partial flip imaging (2,3), one strides through k-space through the use of a shorter TR than would conventionally be necessary for the desired contrast. The reduction in flip angle used with partial flip imaging allows a reduction in TR while preserving contrast.

The advantage of partial flip imaging is the effective increase in TR, which allows a reduction in scan time. The disadvantage of partial flip imaging is that it generally uses gradient-recalled echoes, which bring with them their own limitations. The use of gradient-recalled echoes leads to increased sensitivity to magnetic susceptibility, phase cancellation effects, and a limitation in the length of echo time (TE) such that true T2-weighted images cannot be obtained. Partial flip imaging with gradient-recalled echoes is also known as *field-echo imaging*.

So-called T2*-weighted images are merely proton density–weighted images performed with partial flip imaging with gradient-recalled echoes. The reduction in flip angle produces a very long effective TR so that fluid becomes bright. T2* images differs from true T2 spin-echo images because TE is limited, magnetic susceptibility effects are increased, and phase cancellation effects may be present.

A primary clinical use of partial flip imaging is to produce images with bright fluid to create myelographic and

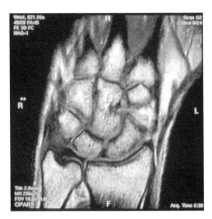

FIG. 8-6. Partial flip imaging performed on an open 0.35-T system allows for the very short repetition times needed for three-dimensional volume imaging. T1-weighted coronal image of the wrist (2 mm × 0.39 mm × 0.39 mm voxel).

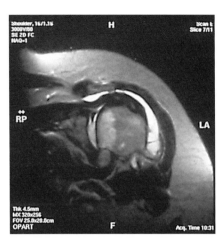

FIG. 8-7. Variable repetition time (TR) imaging performed on an open 0.35-T system produces the contrast of a long TR examination in the scan time of a medium TR examination. T2-weighted coronal image of the shoulder (4.5 mm × 0.78 mm × 0.78 mm voxel).

arthrographic effects. Partial flip imaging may also be used with very short TRs for three-dimensional (3D) volume imaging, which is particularly useful for acquiring multiple thin-slice T1- or T2*-weighted images (Fig. 8-6).

VARIABLE REPETITION TIME IMAGING

With variable TR (4) imaging, k-space is traversed by using a shorter TR than would conventionally be needed for the desired contrast. The central lines of k-space, which contribute predominantly to the signal strength of the image, are acquired with a longer TR, whereas the more peripheral lines of k-space, which contribute predominantly to resolution, are acquired with a shorter TR, allowing a time savings. Thus, an effective increase in TR, with its benefits for contrast and SNR, occurs without the increase in scan time that would be necessary with a conventional procedure, in which all portions of the k-space are traversed with equal TR. Alternatively, one can decrease scan time with respect to a conventional study without sacrificing contrast or SNR.

The advantages of variable TR include the option of reducing scan time by 20% to 40% for a given image contrast, or alternatively, increasing the effective TR to improve contrast and SNR without increasing scan time.

The disadvantages of variable TR include a decrease in the number of slices available with respect to a conventional sequence, because the number of slices is limited by the shortest TR used in the peripheral lines of k-space. An additional disadvantage of variable TR is that blurring in phase-encoding direction can be prominent if the technique is used too aggressively.

The primary clinical use of variable TR is to produce bright fluid to create myelographic and arthrographic images without suffering the gradient-echo limitation of increased magnetic susceptibility effects, phase cancellation

effects, or limitation in TE. This technique has been largely supplanted by fast spin-echo (FSE) imaging techniques with the exception of shoulder imaging, for which true T2 spin-echo contrast is preferable (Fig. 8-7).

HALF FOURIER IMAGING

With half Fourier imaging (5), one skips through the k-space to improve scan time. This is done by relying on the symmetry of the k-space and acquiring only one-half of the total number of phase-encoding steps that are routinely acquired.

The advantages of half Fourier imaging include the ability to break the one acquisition time barrier with scan time savings of up to 50% and the ability to maintain the contrast and resolution of conventional spin-echo images. The disadvantage of half Fourier imaging is the loss of SNR with respect to conventional spin-echo imaging, which has longer image acquisition times.

The primary clinical uses of half Fourier imaging are to acquire true proton- and T2-weighted brain images without the contrast or resolution compromises found in other fast imaging techniques and to provide breath-holding images of the abdomen of realistic duration. Half Fourier imaging may be implemented with conventional spin-echo techniques, partial flip imaging techniques, or other fast imaging techniques.

MATCHED BANDWIDTH IMAGING

With matched bandwidth imaging (6), one skips through k-space by again relying on the symmetry of the k-space data. With this imaging technique, only slightly more than one-half of the total number of frequency-encoded data

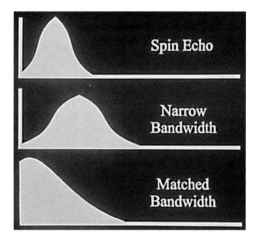

FIG. 8-8. Matched bandwidth imaging. **A:** Conventional echo: Apex of echo is the echo time (TE). Area under the curve is proportional to the square root of the signal-to-noise ratio (SNR). **B:** Narrow bandwidth echo has a lengthened data collection time to improve SNR but suffers from a lengthened TE. **C.** Matched bandwidth echo allows a reduction in TE to enhance contrast and a simultaneous lengthening of the data collections time to enhance the SNR. This is made possible by the symmetry of the k-space, which allows many frequency-encoding points not to be acquired (see Fig. 8-5).

points are acquired, which allows a reduction in TE to enhance contrast and a simultaneous reduction in bandwidth to enhance SNR (Fig. 8-8).

The advantages of matched bandwidth imaging are a reduction in echo time, an improvement in SNR, and an improvement in the number of slices for given TR. Disadvantages of matched bandwidth imaging include altered motion and flow sensitivity and slightly diminished resolution in the frequency-encoding direction.

Matched bandwidth imaging finds tremendous clinical utility at midfield, in which it is used to improve contrast

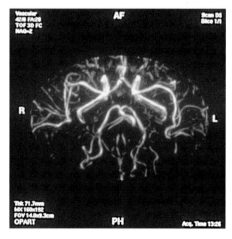

FIG. 8-9. Matched bandwidth imaging performed on an open 0.35-T system allows a reduction in echo time to improve magnetic resonance angiography.

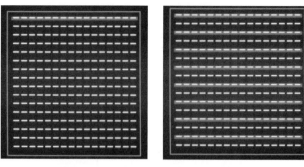
A, B

FIG. 8-10. Spin echo versus fast spin echo. **A:** Conventional spin-echo examinations acquire one place-encoding line per repetition time (TR). **B:** Fast spin-echo examinations acquire multiple phase-encoding lines per TR.

(shortened echo times for T1-weighted images), increase SNR, and increase the number of slices per TR. At mid and high field, matched bandwidth techniques allow reduction in echo times to improve MR angiography (Fig. 8-9).

FAST SPIN-ECHO IMAGING

With FSE imaging (7), k-space is traversed by acquiring multiple phase-encoding lines per TR—that is, a multi-echo sequence is acquired with all of the echoes being combined into a single image (Fig. 8-10).

The advantages of fast SE include a dramatic time savings (typically by a factor of 2 to 4) and minimization of magnetic susceptibility effects due to the use of repeated 180-degree radiofrequency (RF) pulses between echoes.

The disadvantages of FSE imaging include the possibility for image blurring if the sequence is not properly optimized and a limitation in the number of slices acquired per TR because the echo train is so long. The former limitation can be minimized by reducing the spacing between echoes or by increasing the resolution in the phase-encoding direction. The latter limitation can be overcome by increasing the TR beyond that which is conventionally used. The repeated 180-degree RF pulses produce bright fat on T2-weighted images and diminished sensitivity to intracranial hemorrhage owing to the reduction of magnetic susceptibility effects.

The primary clinical role of FSE imaging is to acquire T2-weighted scans at significant time savings or, alternatively, to acquire T2-weighted scans with moderate time savings and significant improvements in resolution (Fig. 8-11). The FSE technique is being successfully used in the brain, spine, and musculoskeletal system and is being increasingly used for body imaging.

FSE imaging may be implemented using both spin and field echoes. The field echoes are acquired before and after the spin echoes, allowing the echo train to be more closely packed. The spin echoes are used for the center of k-space and thus determine contrast. The field echoes are used for the periphery of k-space and thus determine resolution. The pres-

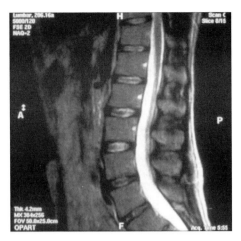

FIG. 8-11. Fast spin-echo imaging performed on an open 0.35-T system produces fast, high-resolution T2-weighted images. T2-weighted sagittal image of the lumbar spine (4.2 mm × 1.3 mm × 0.97 mm voxel).

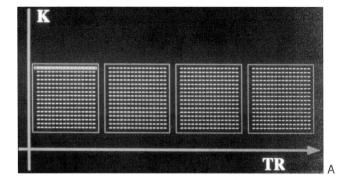

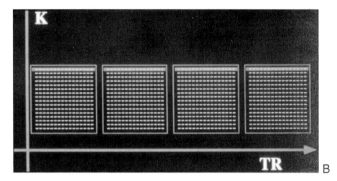

FIG. 8-12. Spin echo versus QuadScan. **A:** Conventional spin-echo examinations acquire one place-encoding line per repetition time (TR). **B:** QuadScan examinations acquire multiple phase-encoding lines per TR and build multiple images simultaneously.

ence of the field echoes decreases the fat intensity, increases the magnetic susceptibility, and decreases the RF power deposition of the FSE sequence. They allow the sequence to be acquired more quickly and with imaging characteristics more similar to a conventional spin-echo sequence.

FSE imaging may also be implemented with half Fourier imaging. Half Fourier imaging is used to effectively increase the echo train length. This may be done to increase the number of slices or reduce the minimum TR of the FSE acquisition. The price paid for using half Fourier imaging is a reduction in SNR. The echo train length may be effectively lengthened to allow for single-shot T2-weighted images. Contrast remains similar to a conventional FSE sequence with bright fat and low magnetic susceptibility effects.

QUADSCAN IMAGING

With QuadScan imaging (8), k-space is traversed by acquiring phase-encoding lines with data for multiple images. In contrast to FSE imaging, in which the multiple phase-encoding lines per TR contribute to building one image, with QuadScan imaging, each phase-encoding line per TR contributes to building multiple images simultaneously (Fig. 8-12). Thus, QuadScan is for short TR imaging (T1-weighted spin-echo imaging and T2*-weighted field-echo imaging) what FSE imaging is for long TR imaging (T2-weighted spin-echo imaging).

A main advantage of QuadScan is the ability to acquire fast T1-weighted images with true spin-echo contrast. The time savings is typically by a factor of 2 to 4. Because the number of slices per TR is increased two-, four-, or sixfold, very short TRs may be used to improve contrast over a conventional spin-echo examination while simultaneously improving coverage. QuadScan is also useful for T2*-

weighted field-echo imaging to dramatically increase the number of slices per TR to enhance coverage. SNR per unit of acquisition time is also improved over a conventional spin-echo or field-echo sequence (Fig. 8-13).

The main disadvantage of QuadScan imaging is that phase-encoding artifacts from one image are displayed across all images acquired simultaneously. Another disadvantage is that

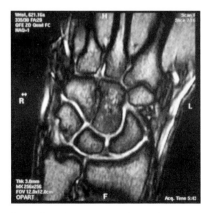

FIG. 8-13. QuadScan imaging performed on an open 0.35-T system dramatically increases the coverage and signal-to-noise ratio of a conventional field-echo examination. T2*-weighted coronal image of the wrist (3 mm × 0.47 mm × 0.47 mm voxel).

the number of images contributed by a single place-encoding line is equal to the number of repetitions. Thus, the increasing number of repetitions may partially offset the time savings.

The primary clinical uses of QuadScan are to improve the speed, contrast, and coverage of conventional Tl-weighted spin-echo examinations or to improve the coverage of field-echo examinations.

FAST FIELD-ECHO IMAGING

With fast field-echo (FFE) imaging (9), one sprints through the k-space using a gradient-recalled echo image with the shortest possible TR and TE the system will allow.

The advantage of FFE imaging is a tremendous increase in imaging speed, potentially down to the subsecond range. The disadvantage of snapshot imaging is that the ultrashort TR and TE combination that is used has poor contrast. This loss of contrast with snapshot imaging is compensated for by a variety of techniques, including the use of preparation pulses, segmentation of the k-space (10), and reordering of the k-space (11).

The use of a preparatory 180-degree inversion pulse enables FFE imaging to acquire very high-contrast Tl-weighted images, similar to inversion recovery. Other contrast weighting may be obtained by using more complex preparatory pulse schemes.

K-space segmentation may be used to increase the contrast control by limiting the data acquisition to a small segment on the inversion recovery curve. With k-space segmentation, only a segment of k-space is acquired for each preparatory pulse. Over the course of several preparatory pulses, the entire k-space is filled. The advantages of space segmentation are a significant improvement in contrast control and the potential for improved temporal resolution with gated studies. The only disadvantage of k-space segmentation is that scan time is increased by the number of segments used.

K-space reordering alters the order in which the central k-space lines are acquired to maximize contrast and SNR control. This technique may be used not only in FFE imaging but also with FSE imaging to obtain short echo times and with MR angiography to obtain improved background suppression.

The primary clinical roles of FFE imaging are to produce fast thin-slice images and to improve the temporal resolution of MRI. The snapshot technique is the fastest method to produce multiple thin-slice T1-weighted neurologic and musculoskeletal examinations. This is typically done with 3D volume imaging. The high speed of FFE imaging also allows for very high temporal resolution, which is useful for perfusion, cine cardiac, and breath-holding abdominal studies.

ECHO PLANAR IMAGING

With echo planar imaging (EPI) (12), one rapidly oscillates through k-space allowing for ultrafast acquisition of the raw data. With EPI, a weak constant phase-encoding gradient is used in combination with a rapidly switching or oscillating frequency-encoding gradient to scan the k-space.

EPI may be done in spin-echo or gradient-echo versions. Spin-echo versions use preparatory pulses to create images with predominantly T1-, proton density–, or T2-weighted contrast and have less artifacts from magnetic field inhomogeneities than do pure gradient-echo versions. In addition to preparatory pulses, contrast control with EPI may be enhanced with k-space segmentation or reordering. Gradient-echo versions of EPI are exceptionally fast and are best used for cine cardiac imaging, when an entire study of the heart can be completed in a single heartbeat, which renders the method insensitive to arrhythmias.

Although EPI's sheer speed is advantageous, the technique is technically demanding and requires substantial hardware modification. Strong fast gradients, rapid data-handling capabilities, high magnet homogeneity, and autoshimming are necessary to successfully implement EPI. Image quality provided by EPI is generally inferior to more conventional MRI techniques. Therefore, EPI is normally used for specialized examinations rather than for routine clinical imaging.

The clinical role for EPI is not yet defined. The technique could be used to rapidly scan even the sickest or most uncooperative patient in a matter of seconds. Examination times would be limited only by patient setup, coil tuning, sequence downloading, and image reconstruction and review. Body imaging without breath-holding may render body imaging more patient- and operator-friendly. Cardiac imaging requiring neither breath-holding nor electrocardiography gating is also possible.

REFERENCES

1. Crooks LE, Ortendahl DA, Kaufman L. Clinical efficiency of nuclear magnetic resonance. *Radiology* 1983;146:123–128.
2. Haase A, Frahm J, Matthaei D, et al. FLASH imaging: rapid NMR imaging using low flip-angle pulses. *J Magn Reson Imag* 1986;67:258.
3. Winkler ML, Ortendahl DA, Mills TC, et al. Characteristics of partial flip angle and gradient reversal MR imaging. *Radiology* 1988;166:17–26.
4. Mattinger LD, Shen LL, Mattinger GW, et al. Performance optimization of mixed TR sequences. *Proc Soc Magn Reson Med* 1992;2:625.
5. Feinberg DA, Hale JD, Watts JC, et al. Halving MR imaging time by conjugation: demonstration at 3.5 kGauss. *Radiology* 1986;161:527–531.
6. Kaufman L, Winkler ML. Matched bandwidth technology: cost implications. *Admin Radiol* 1987;6:32–38.
7. Hennig J, Nauerth A, Friedburg H. RARE imaging: a fast imaging method for clinical MR. *Magn Reson Med* 1986;3:823–833.
8. Yon C, Shen L, Wuj, Kritzer M. Parallel multi-slice imaging with limited peak RF power. *Proc Soc Magn Reson Med* 1993;1:427.
9. Haase A. Snapshot FLASH MRI: applications to T1, T2, and chemical shift imaging. *Magn Reson Med* 1990;13:77–89.
10. Edelman RR, Waliner B, Singer A, et al. Segmented turboFLASH: a method for breath-hold magnetic resonance imaging of the liver with flexible contrast. *Radiology* 1990;177:515–521.
11. Holsinger AE, Riederer SJ. The importance of centric phase encoding order in snapshot imaging. *Proc Soc Magn Reson Med* 1990;1:11–14.
12. Stehling MK, Turner R, Mansfield P. Echo-planar imaging magnetic resonance imaging in a fraction of a second. *Science* 1991;254:43–50.

Open MRI,
edited by Peter A. Rothschild and Debra Reinking Rothschild.
Lippincott Williams & Wilkins. Philadelphia © 2000.

CHAPTER 9

Fast Spin-Echo Imaging

Karen Procknow

What do *FSE, TSE, turbo-SE, FAST-SE*, and *RARE* have in common? They are all acronyms for fast spin-echo (FSE) imaging sequences. Whatever the name for these fast imaging sequences, the primary benefit is *speed*. Before the introduction of FSE sequences, we relied on gradient-echo sequences to reduce acquisition times. The quest for speed has led to FSE sequences, which provide scan times routinely two to 32 times faster than conventional SE sequences. The FSE sequence is not a gradient-echo sequence in which a gradient is used to refocus the echo and the echo time (TE) and flip angle primarily determine contrast for the acquisition. In FSE, multiple 180-degree refocusing radiofrequency (RF) pulses are used to generate the echoes used in the sequence. The contrast seen in FSE images is T2 decay, similar to conventional SE information, not T2* as is seen in gradient-echo images.

The time saved by FSE sequences can be used in magnetic resonance imaging (MRI) in several ways to

1. Increase through-put through reduced scan times
2. Use longer repetition times (TRs), which increase signal-to-noise ratio (SNR) and improve T2 contrast
3. Select higher matrices for increased resolution

How are FSE sequences acquired? What do *echo train length* (ETL) and *echo spacing* (ESP) mean? This chapter answers these questions.

First, let us discuss data collection for a conventional SE sequence in which scan time equals TR multiplied by the number of phase-encoding steps (phase matrix) multiplied by the number of excitations (NEX).

The application of a 90-degree RF excitation pulse followed by a 180-degree refocusing RF pulse generates an echo. The timing from the application of the initial 90-degree excitation pulse to next 90-degree excitation pulse is called *TR*. The size of the phase-encoding matrix (or number of phase-encoding steps) determines the number times that the TR must be repeated to complete an acquisition. For example, with a 128 phase-encoding matrix, the TR must be repeated 128 times. The number of times the TR is repeated at each phase-encoding step is determined by the NEX selected (Fig. 9-1). The result of this MRI experiment after application of a Fourier transform is one image at a prescribed TE.

FSE sequences differ from conventional SE sequences in several ways:

1. An FSE sequence has multiple 180-degree RF refocusing pulses per 90-degree RF excitation pulse. In a conventional SE, multiple echoes—usually 1 to 4 (Fig. 9-2)—can be generated; in FSE sequences, however, a larger number of echoes—generally 8 to 14 (Fig. 9-3)—are generated.
2. In an FSE sequence, a phase-encoding step is collected for every 180-degree RF refocusing pulse, whereas in a conventional SE sequence, only one phase-encoding step is collected.
3. In a conventional SE sequence, an image is created for each of the echoes generated in the TR period. However, in an FSE sequence, only one or two images are created regardless of the number of echoes generated in each TR period.

In an FSE sequence, after the application of the 90-degree RF excitation pulse, a series of 180-degree refocusing RF pulses are generated. These multiple 180-degree RF pulses are known as the *echo train* and the number of echoes in the train as the *ETL*. The name or acronym used for this series of echoes depends on the manufacturer of the system used. For each of the 180-degree refocusing pulses, a phase-encoded echo is created by the application of a different amplitude phase-encoding gradient for each of the echoes.

In an FSE sequence with an 8-echo train for each TR period, eight phase-encoding steps are acquired. The collection of multiple phase-encoding steps per TR changes the formula for calculating scan time. Scan time for FSE sequences is calculated as follows:

$$\text{Scan time} = \text{TR} \times (\text{phase matrix/ETL}) \times \text{NEX}$$

K. Procknow: Mid-Field and Open Products, General Electric Medical Systems, Milwaukee, Wisconsin

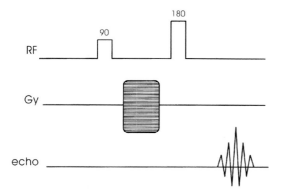

FIG. 9-1. Basic spin-echo sequence in which Gy represents the phase-encoding steps needed for the acquisition. RF, radiofrequency.

Following is a comparison of scan times for an SE sequence with a TR of 2,000 ms, 128 phase-encoding steps, and 2 NEX versus an FSE sequence with the same parameters and an ETL of 8:

SE $(2,000 \times 128 \times 2)/60,000 = 8$ minutes, 31 seconds

FSE $[2,000 \times (128/8) \times 2]/60,000 = 1$ minute, 2 seconds

The FSE sequence completes the 128 phase-encoding steps eight times faster than the conventional sequence. The time saved is directly related to the ETL. The greater the number of echoes, the greater the time saved.

This time savings is a significant benefit, but as we all know, there is no "free lunch" in MRI. One parameter that is affected in an FSE sequence is the number of slices that can be obtained in an acquisition. Another major hurdle in FSE imaging is controlling the image contrast. In conventional SE imaging, contrast is primarily dependent on the TR and TE selected. These parameters remain constant throughout the acquisition for an SE sequence. In FSE imaging, the TR is constant, but the multiple TEs contribute to the contrast for the image. The number of different TEs used is determined by the ETL selected.

Two factors determine how the contrast is seen in an FSE image when the multiple echoes are combined into one

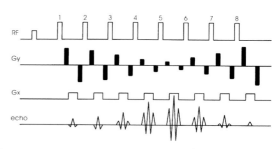

FIG. 9-3. Diagram for a fast spin-echo pulse sequence with 8 echoes. Gx, frequency encoding; Gy, phase-encoding steps for the acquisition; RF, radiofrequency.

composite image. The first factor, which cannot be controlled, is the natural T2 decay (Fig. 9-4) that occurs in the echo train over the TR period.

The ETL and ESP contribute to the amount of T2 decay included in the acquisition. The longer the ETL and the greater the ESP, the greater the T2 decay over the TR period (Fig. 9-5). This T2 decay over the ETL contributes to the edge blurring seen in FSE images as compared to conventional SE images. The greater the signal difference due to T2 decay over the acquisition, the greater the edge blurring in the image. Increasing the phase resolution of the acquisition can help decrease this edge blurring. Decreasing the ESP also helps decrease edge blurring.

The introduction of FSE blurring cancellation methods reduces edge blurring in FSE images. FSE blurring cancellation options use modified k-space–filling techniques to reduce the contrast difference from one portion of k-space to the next, which results in a reduction of blurring in the image.

If collected sequentially, the first echo in the echo train contributes the most signal, because the smallest amount of T2 dephasing has occurred. Each successive echo contributes a smaller amount of signal to the image. The last echo has very little signal left to contribute to the composite image. This means that if nothing is done to alter the way information is collected for an FSE acquisition, the early echoes have greater influence than the later echoes in determining image contrast.

The second factor that contributes to image contrast is the relationship between the strength, or amplitude, of the

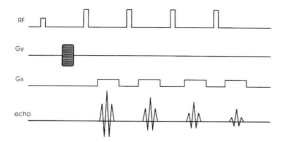

FIG. 9-2. Diagram for a conventional spin-echo pulse sequence with 4 echoes. Gx, frequency encoding; Gy, phase-encoding steps for the acquisition; RF, radiofrequency.

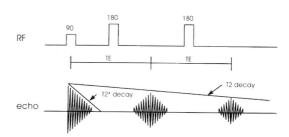

FIG. 9-4. The strength of an echo decreases as the echo time (*TE*) becomes longer, owing to T2 decay. RF, radiofrequency.

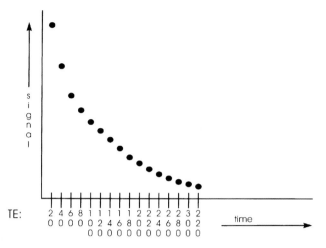

FIG. 9-5. Change in signal intensity for a train of 16 echoes with a 20-ms echo spacing due to T2 decay. Note the larger signal differences in the echoes at the beginning of the train of echoes compared to those at the end of the echo train. Large signal differences from echo to echo increase the edge blurring seen in the image. TE, echo time.

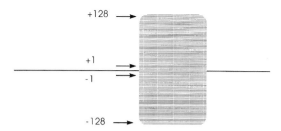

FIG. 9-7. Data must be collected for each phase-encoding step before an acquisition is complete.

phase-encoding gradient applied and the amount, or strength, of the signal for the echo generated (Fig. 9-6). The amount of signal in the echo controls contrast information. The stronger or higher the amplitude of the phase-encoding gradient, the smaller the signal of the echo generated. The weaker or lower the amplitude of the phase-encoding gradient, the stronger or larger the signal of the echo created.

This MRI mechanism of gradient amplitude offers a means to control the size of the signal. Control over signal resulting from echoes collected at multiple TEs in an FSE sequence influences contrast of the image.

In a conventional SE sequence, the application of the phase-encoding gradient is done in a sequential fashion. In the acquisition of a 256-phase matrix, 128 different amplitudes are applied in the positive and negative direction (Fig. 9-7).

The strongest negative phase-encoding gradient is applied first; each successive phase encoding is slightly stronger

until all 128 negative phase encodings have been done. At this point, one-half of the acquisition has been completed. Data acquisition proceeds with the positive 128 phase encodings until the strongest positive phase encoding has been done. Once the last positive phase encoding has been collected, the data for one excitation or NEX have been completed (Fig. 9-8).

When all the signal collected from the individual echoes for each phase-encoding step is combined (sent through a Fourier transform), it is estimated that as much as 90% of the contrast information is contributed by the 16 lowest gradient amplitudes (phase encodings +8 . . . → . . . −8), which means that approximately 90% of the signal is coming from only 16 phase-encoding steps (Fig. 9-9).

What do the rest of the phase-encoding steps contribute to the image? The higher amplitude gradient phase encodings provide the spatial information (i.e., edge detail) for the image (Fig. 9-10).

What we have described is the collection of the raw data for the formation of an MRI. This collection of the MRI data is first stored in a format known as *k-space*. Another way to think of k-space is as the amount of information or data that must be collected so that it may be mathematically manipulated by a Fourier transform to form an image.

As shown in Figures 9-11 and 9-12, k-space contains both phase- and frequency-encoded information, which, after reconstruction, becomes the MRI.

Thus far, we have determined that the amplitude of the phase-encoding gradient affects the size of the echo to be

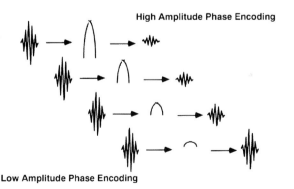

FIG. 9-6. The signal strength of the first echo is greatly reduced by the application of a strong or high-amplitude gradient, whereas the fourth echo is dephased only slightly by the application of a weak or low-amplitude gradient.

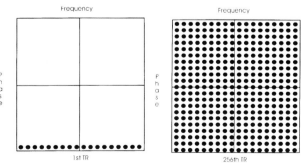

FIG. 9-8. A: Data collection for the first phase encoding for a 256-phase matrix. B: Completion of the collection of all phase-encoding steps for the acquisition. TR, repetition time.

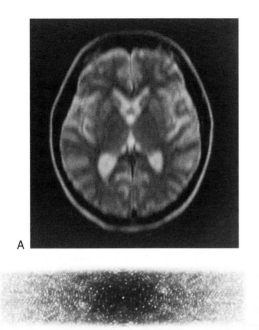

A

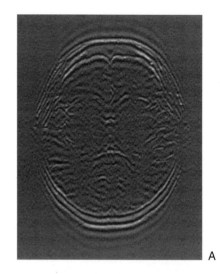

B

FIG. 9-9. A: This image was created from the central phase-encoding steps. **B:** Raw data in k-space for the central or lowest phase-encoding steps used to create **(A)**.

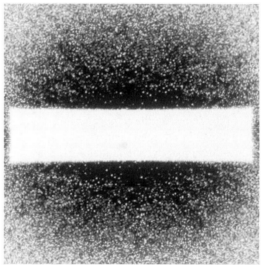

A

B

FIG. 9-10. A: This image was created from the high-amplitude gradient phase-encoding steps. **B:** Raw data in k-space for the outer or highest phase-encoding steps used to create **(A)**.

sampled in the frequency-encoding dimension. We have also determined that lower amplitude gradients have the most effect on contrast of the image. These two facts are depicted in Figures 9-13 and 9-14.

Image contrast in FSE sequences is manipulated by changing the order in which the phase-encoding steps are acquired during the acquisition of the MRI data. In an FSE sequence, the TE selected defines how the phase-encoding steps are collected. Remember that the TE selected is a target, or effective, TE because all the echoes in the echo train contribute to the final image contrast. The MRI system acquires the data so the lowest amplitude phase-encoding steps or central views of k-space are applied at the time of the desired TE (contrast) for the acquisition (Fig. 9-15). The lowest amplitude gradients contribute up to 90% of signal and determine the contrast of the image.

The order in which the phase-encoding gradients are applied results in the maximum amount of signal (contrast information) for the composite image being generated from the echoes collected at the desired TE. Signal from the undesired TEs is suppressed by placing the highest amplitude phase-encoding gradients at these TEs. The higher amplitude gradients dephase almost all of the signal that would have been generated by these echoes, so they contribute little to the contrast of the image. When comparing the amount of signal generated by different echoes, the amplitude of the gradient is generally more important to image contrast than is the amount of T2 decay. In very late echoes (roughly, TEs >150 ms), there is very little signal to be refocused, no matter what the gradient amplitude.

The terms *effective TE* or *target TE*, instead of *TE*, are used in FSE imaging because the contrast seen in FSE images is created by combining multiple different TEs—not just one TE, as in conventional SE images (Fig. 9-16).

The contrast in an FSE image is similar to that seen in a conventional SE image. How similar depends on the ETL. The shorter the ETL, the more closely the FSE image contrast resembles the conventional SE image with a similar TE. In an FSE acquisition in which the full-echo train contributes to the contrast for only one effective TE, the resulting contrast and image quality may differ slightly from a conventional SE (Fig. 9-17) owing to the large number of echoes contributing different amounts of signal over a long period of T2 decay.

However, in an FSE sequence, in which the echo train is split to provide two contrasts (proton density and T2), the

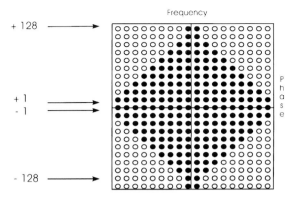

FIG. 9-11. The outer portion of k-space contains phase and frequency information that contributes to the detail of the image, whereas the central portion contains phase and frequency information that determines the contrast of the image.

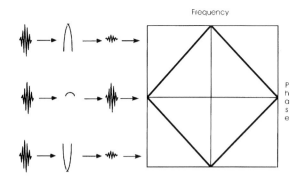

FIG. 9-13. The different gradient amplitudes applied to acquire data for an image are shown along with the signal generated from the echoes sampled at these phase-encoding steps. The data acquired fill k-space, creating a pattern with large signal in the center and decreasing signal intensity from the echoes at the edges.

contrast and image quality more closely resemble that of a conventional variable echo sequence (Fig. 9-18).

Additionally, in a full-echo train the effective TE is selectable, whereas in a split-echo train the effective TE for the second contrast is determined by the ETL and ESP. Furthermore, twice the number of TR periods are needed to complete a split-echo train with two effective TEs with the same ETL and phase-encoding matrix as compared to a full-echo train with one effective TE, owing to the echo train's being split between the two effective TEs. Therefore, scan time for an SE train is twice that of a full-echo train with identical parameters. Increasing the ETL is one way to decrease scan for SE train acquisitions; however, the effective TE for the second image increases. Another way to decrease the scan time for an SE train is to share data for the two effective TEs. For example, in an 8-ETL acquisition, if the first 5 echoes were used to create the image for the first effective TE and the data from the fifth echo also were used to create the image for the second effective TE, the acquisition time would be the same as if a 10-ETL was used. When compared to images from a 10-ETL, the images from an 8-ETL with one shared echo have less T2 effects, because the T2

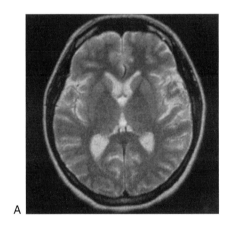

A

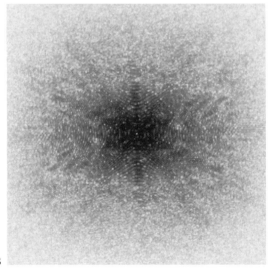

B

FIG. 9-12. This image **(A)** is created from the raw data stored in k-space **(B)**.

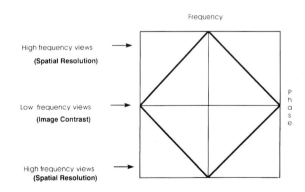

FIG. 9-14. The outer edges of k-space contribute information to define the detail or resolution in an image, whereas the central portion determines the contrast for the image. The signal from the echoes at the edge of k-space contribute little to the contrast of the image because it is small; however, frequency information in these echoes provides spatial resolution for the image.

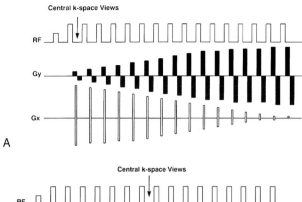

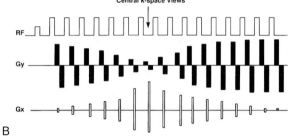

FIG. 9-15. The top lines of these diagrams depict a 90-degree radiofrequency (*RF*) pulse with multiple 180-degree refocusing RF pulses. The middle lines (*Gy*) depict the positive and negative phase-encoding gradient amplitudes applied for each echo in the echo train. The bottom lines (*Gx*) depict the amount of signal generated for each echo for the gradient strength applied. **A:** The contrast of the acquisition in this example is weighted toward the first echo time because the lower phase-encoding gradients are applied at the beginning of the echo train. **B:** The contrast in this example is weighted toward the echo time at the middle of the echo train because the lower amplitude phase-encoding steps are applied to the middle echoes.

decay over the ETL is less. As with everything in MRI, trade-offs exist. As the number of shared echoes increases, edge blurring may increase.

When using FSE sequences, several parameters affect the number of slices that can be acquired in a given TR. The first is the ETL. The longer the echo train becomes, the fewer the number of slices that may be acquired in the TR period. Increasing the ETL is comparable to increasing the TE in

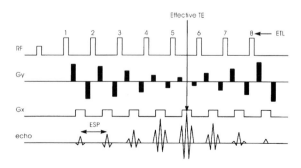

FIG. 9-16. The effective echo time (*TE*) for this 8–echo train length (*ETL*) fast spin-echo acquisition is echo 5 in the echo train. Gx, frequency encoding; Gy, phase encoding; RF, radiofrequency.

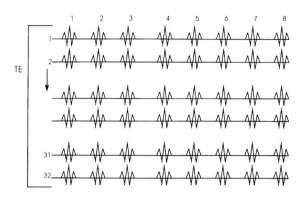

FIG. 9-17. All of the echoes in the echo train for this full-echo train fast spin-echo sequence with an 8–echo train length contribute to the contrast of the image created from this acquisition with one effective echo time (*TE*). With an echo train length of 8 and a phase matrix of 256, 32 repetition time periods are needed to complete the acquisition.

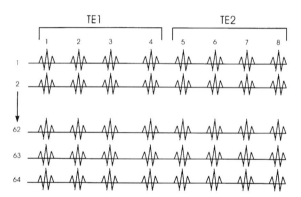

FIG. 9-18. In the case of a split-echo train, the first half of the echo train contributes to the contrast of the first image and the second half of the echo train is used to create a second image for a fast spin-echo sequence with two effective echo times (*TE1* and *TE2*). With an echo train length of 8 and a phase matrix of 256, 64 repetition time periods are needed to complete the acquisition. The number of repetition time periods in a split-echo train is twice that of a full-echo train, owing to the splitting of the echo train between the two effective TEs.

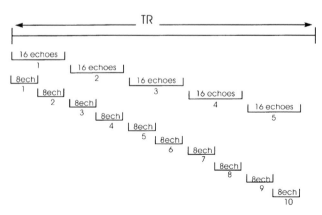

FIG. 9-19. This diagram demonstrates the influence of the echo train length on the number of slices that can be collected in a single repetition time (*TR*) period. ech, echoes.

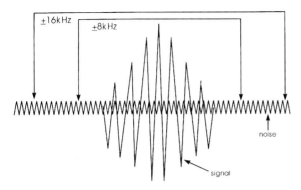

FIG. 9-20. As the receiver bandwidth decreases, the amount of noise acquired with the echo decreases, improving the signal to noise ratio.

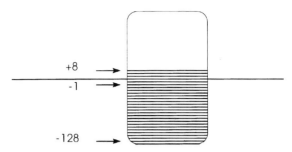

FIG. 9-22. Phase-encoding scheme for a half Fourier acquisition.

conventional SE sequence, given its impact on the number of slices that can be collected during a single TR. The longer the prescribed TE is, the longer it takes to acquire the information for that echo, and the fewer slices can be acquired in that TR. The same is true when increasing the ETL. The greater the number of echoes, the longer it takes to collect all the information for a single slice location (Fig. 9-19).

To maximize the number of slices per TR in FSE sequences, the echoes are acquired as fast or as close together as possible. The time between the echoes is known as *ESP*. The ESP is generally set to the minimum possible timing. On some MRI systems, it may be done automatically, or some limited control may be available. The minimum ESP is affected by all the parameters that affect selection of a minimum TE, such as the receiver bandwidth, field of view, matrix, and slice thickness. On some systems, the effective TE is a multiple of the ESP; on others, the ESP is determined by the effective TE selected. The receiver bandwidth has a large impact on ESP. As the receiver bandwidth is decreased, the SNR increases (Fig. 9-20).

The narrower the bandwidth, the larger the ESP, owing to the increased sampling time required to frequency encode the data (Fig. 9-21).

Consideration must be given to the trade-offs of selecting the narrowest bandwidth acceptable versus the effect of large ESP. Although a narrow receiver bandwidth improves SNR of the acquisition, a large ESP induces more edge blurring. However, by decreasing the frequency-encoding matrix, it may be possible to select a narrower receiver bandwidth without inducing more edge blurring, owing to the ESP's not being increased because of the reduced sampling time for a bandwidth. Reducing the frequency-encoding matrix decreases pixel resolution in the frequency direction, but it also increases SNR.

Another consideration in FSE imaging is the selection of effective TE for long ETLs and the effect the ETL has on image blurring. The longer the ETL, the more T2 effects seen in the image. Imaging blurring may be increased depending on the effective TE selected. Increasing the effective TE for long ETLs can decrease blurring, because the T2 decay changes are less from echo to echo as the effective TE increases.

Single-shot FSE (SS-FSE) is a variation of the FSE sequence. In SS-FSE, all the phase-encoding steps are acquired in a single TR period. The acquisition times for SS-FSE sequences are very short, making it possible to produce motion-resistant images or to acquire images during a breath-hold period. For an SS-FSE acquisition, a half Fourier technique is used—in which only one-half the phase-encoding steps are collected (Fig. 9-22).

In a half Fourier acquisition, all the central views of k-space along with one-half of the phase-encoding steps are acquired. Due to the conjugate symmetry of the data in k-

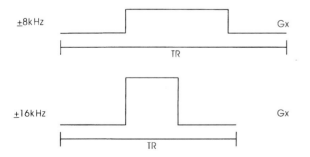

FIG. 9-21. As the receiver bandwidth decreases or narrows, the time to acquire same amount of frequency-encoded data increases. The Nyquist theorem states that any signal must be sampled at least twice per cycle to be represented, or reproduced, accurately. Gx, frequency encoding; TR, repetition time.

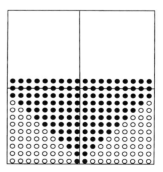

FIG. 9-23. The bottom portion of k-space represents the data collected for a half Fourier acquisition, and the top half is the portion that is mathematically constructed.

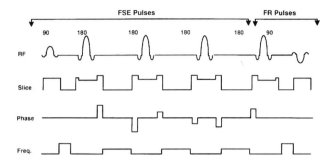

FIG. 9-24. Pulse sequence diagram for a fast recovery (*FR*) fast spin-echo (*FSE*) sequence. Freq., frequency; RF, radio-frequency.

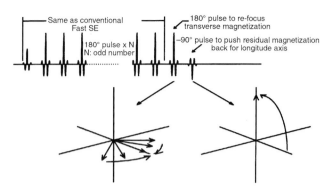

FIG. 9-25. In a fast recovery fast spin-echo (*SE*) sequence, recovery pulses are added at the end of the echo train to refocus the remaining horizontal magnetization and then push it back to the vertical plane.

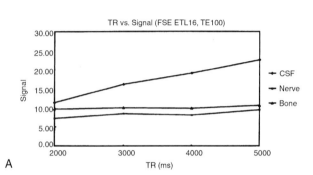

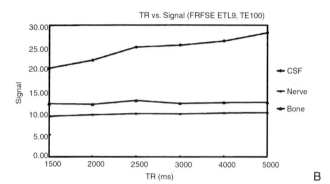

FIG. 9-26. Comparison of signal from a fast spin-echo (*FSE*) sequence **(A)** and a fast recovery FSE (*FR-FSE*) sequence **(B)**. Note how signal from cerebrospinal fluid (*CSF*) has increased in signal intensity in the FR-FSE sequence as compared to the FSE sequence relative to the repetition time (*TR*). ETL, echo train length; TE, echo time.

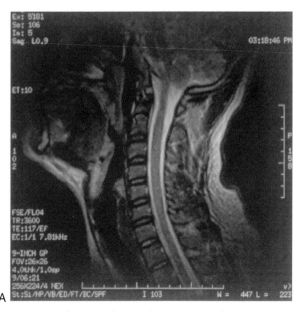

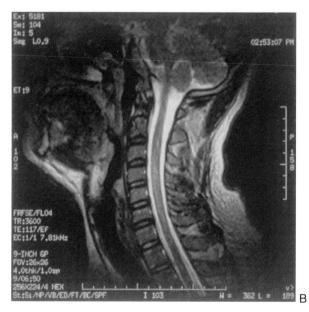

FIG. 9-27. Comparison images of the cervical spine from a fast spin-echo (FSE) sequence **(A)** and a fast recovery FSE (*FR-FSE*) sequence **(B)**. Note the increased signal from cerebrospinal fluid in FR-FSE compared to FSE.

space, the remainder of the phase-encoding data is mathematically constructed (Fig. 9-23), which reduces the acquisition time for the sequence. However, the SNR is also reduced by the square root of 2, owing to acquisition of only a portion of the phase-encoding steps.

In SS-FSE, the ETL is determined by the phase-encoding matrix. For a 256-phase matrix, 128 phase-encoding steps plus eight additional steps to complete the central views of k-space are required to create an image using a half Fourier technique. The echo train for an SS-FSE acquisition with a 256-phase matrix is 136 echoes. SS-FSE images are heavily T2 weighted—owing to the large amount of T2 decay over the ETL—making them ideal for MR cholangiography.

Another variation of the FSE sequence is to add recover pulses at the end of the echo train to push the remaining transverse magnetization back to the longitudinal plane (Figs. 9-24 and 9-25).

The 180-degree refocusing RF pulse and the negative 90-degree RF pulse recovery pulses in a fast recovery FSE reduce the time needed to wait for recovery of the transverse magnetization to the longitudinal plane. Thus, shorter TRs can be used, resulting in a reduced acquisition time yet maintaining a bright signal from fluid such as cerebrospinal fluid (Figs. 9-26 and 9-27). In fact, in a fast recovery FSE sequence, fluid is bright whether the contrast for the acquisitions is T1 weighted, T2 weighted, or proton density weighted.

Open MRI,
edited by Peter A. Rothschild and Debra Reinking Rothschild.
Lippincott Williams & Wilkins. Philadelphia © 2000.

CHAPTER 10

Protocol Development Strategy for Open Magnetic Resonance Imaging

William H. Faulkner, Jr.

The lower field strength of currently available open scanners begs a detailed discussion of lower field strength magnetic resonance imaging (MRI). Lower field MRI systems have been in use for many years. In fact, most of the early clinical systems were 0.6 T or less. High-field systems then became more popular, mostly owing to their improved signal-to-noise ratio (SNR) over lower field systems. A major benefit of the high-field MRI systems is reduced scan times. Proponents of lower field systems, however, continued to tout the benefits of imaging below 1.0 T. Those benefits included

1. Reduced chemical shift artifact
2. Reduced magnetic susceptibility–related artifacts
3. Greater T1 contrast in body imaging owing to the shorter T1 times at lower field strength
4. Reduced pulsation or flow artifacts

Even as these benefits remain, additional improvements in magnet design, radiofrequency (RF), gradient coil design, and newer pulse sequences have given lower field systems the ability to produce MR images that rival those produced on high-field systems and in reasonable scan times.

Although these improvements have been a tremendous benefit for those imaging with lower field systems, a comprehensive understanding of basic MRI principles and protocols is essential for both radiologists and technologists if consistently high-quality MR images are expected. The major hurdle to overcome when imaging at lower magnetic field strengths is the inherently low SNR. MRI noise is analogous to the static heard on the radio when the receiver is too far away from the transmitter or is not optimally tuned to the transmitter. The very small MRI signal comes from the hydrogen nuclei in tissues. By selecting protocol parameters with an emphasis on either increasing signal or reducing noise, adequate SNR images can be produced.

W. H. Faulkner, Jr.: William Faulkner & Associates, LLC, Chattanooga, Tennessee

For the sake of accuracy, it is important to note the human eye does not perceive SNR; rather it perceives the contrast-to-noise ratio (CNR). Contrast is the difference in MRI signal intensity between tissue A and tissue B. CNR is simply the ratio of the SNR of tissue A to the SNR of tissue B. The higher the contrast between two tissues, the lower the SNR required for the eye to perceive the difference. Conversely, the closer two tissues are in signal intensity (i.e., the lower the contrast), the greater the SNR required to perceive them as separate tissues. SNR is the limiting factor in the ability to detect low contrast.

MAGNETIC RESONANCE IMAGE QUALITY

An MR image can be thought of as consisting of three major elements: (a) SNR, (b) image contrast, and (c) spatial resolution. In general, emphasizing either SNR or spatial resolution causes a reduction in the other. For example, if spatial resolution is increased by reducing the field of view (FOV), a gain in spatial resolution is at the cost of SNR. In this example, the SNR must be sufficient to compensate for the gain in spatial resolution; otherwise, the result may be an image with increased spatial resolution but inadequate SNR to allow a diagnosis.

The previous example illustrates the interdependence of imaging parameters. This chapter evaluates the major imaging parameters and their interrelationships. Also, the objective of developing protocols that exploit the advantages of imaging at low magnetic field strengths, in particular below 0.5 T, is discussed. Because the major hurdle to overcome is reduced SNR, we first look at the parameters that influence SNR.

SIGNAL-TO-NOISE RATIO

Pulse Sequence Parameters

In a spin-echo sequence, the repetition time (TR) and echo time (TE) are used primarily to control image contrast. They

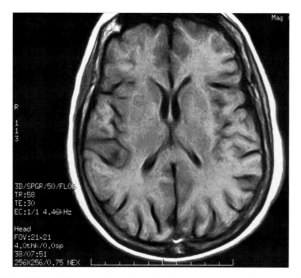

FIG. 10-1. T1-weighted (gradient echo) three-dimensional Fourier transform. Repetition time, 58 ms; echo time, 30 ms; bandwidth, 4.46 kHz; flip angle, 50 degrees.

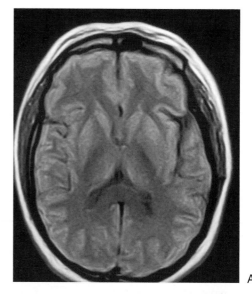

A

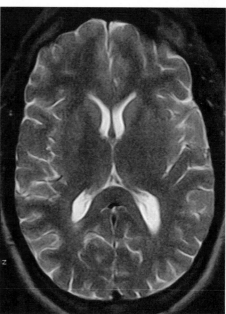

B

FIG. 10-2. A: Proton density–weighted, fast spin-echo sequence. Repetition time, 2,500 ms; echo time, 21; bandwidth, 10.4 kHz. **B:** Fast spin-echo, T2-weighted sequence. Repetition time, 6,800 ms; echo time, 90; bandwidth, 10.4 kHz.

also affect the inherent SNR of an MR image. Lower TR selections allow only those tissues with short T1 times, such as fat, to recover longitudinal magnetization between repetitions of the sequence, producing high signal in the resultant image. Tissues with long T1 times, such as water, are relatively saturated and produce little signal. Other tissues produce some signal; however, the signal from all tissues is much greater if a longer TR is used to allow greater longitudinal recovery. Although the selection of a longer TR produces images in which proton density (PD) contrasts predominate, it should be remembered that images acquired with a short TR have inherently lower SNRs compared to those acquired with a longer TR, assuming all other factors remain unchanged (Fig. 10-1).

The TE affects image contrast as well as SNR. Long TEs are selected when T2-weighted images are desired. Increasing the TE causes tissues with a short T2 time (e.g., fat) to produce little signal when compared to those with longer T2 times (e.g., water), owing to the dephasing of the spins that occurs after the excitation pulse. The longer the TE, the greater the dephasing; therefore, less MRI signal is induced in the receiver coil. As with TR, increasing the TE alters the image contrast (i.e., greater T2 weighting); however, the longer the TE, the lower the SNR (Fig. 10-2).

In gradient-echo (GRE) sequences, T2-like contrasts (i.e., bright signal from fluids) can be obtained with short TRs by using flip angles of less than 90 degrees. As a general rule of thumb, reducing the flip angle has the same effect on image contrast as increasing the TR, in that they both reduce saturation. Reducing the flip angle produces an image with less T1 weighting and more PD weighting (assuming a short TE). Generally, to sufficiently reduce T1 weighting, flip angles of 30 degrees or less are chosen. Lower flip angles, however, produce a smaller amount of transverse magnetization. Because the amplitude of the MRI signal is related to the magnitude of the transverse magnetization vector, lower flip angles inherently produce low SNR.

The available SNR is further reduced if a longer TE is chosen to produce T2*-weighted images (Fig. 10-3).

Pulse sequence and timing parameter selections are made based on the desired contrast (T1, T2, T2*, or PD), but they also have an impact on the available SNR. GRE sequences generally have less inherent SNR, particularly when a low flip angle and increased TE are selected.

Voxel Volume

When developing MRI protocols, voxel volume is usually considered the factor that determines spatial resolution.

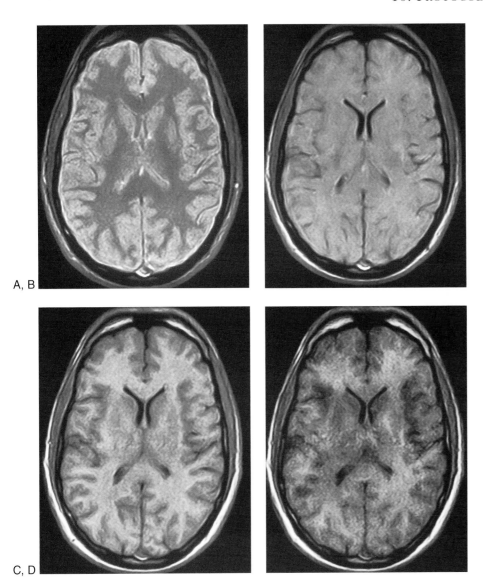

A, B

C, D

FIG. 10-3. Gradient reversal images with various flip angles. Note the change in gray/white signal intensity. Three-dimensional Fourier transform. Repetition time, 58 ms; echo time, 30. **A:** Flip angle, 10 degrees. **B:** Flip angle, 30 degrees. **C:** Flip angle, 60 degrees. **D:** Flip angle, 90 degrees.

Although this is true, it is important to remember the voxel volume has a tremendous impact on SNR, in that SNR is directly proportional to voxel volume. If voxel volume is doubled, SNR is doubled. Conversely, if voxel volume is halved, SNR is halved. When developing MRI protocols, the biggest compromise with which one must contend is that between spatial resolution and SNR.

Voxel volume is determined by three operator-selected parameters: (a) acquisition matrix, (b) slice thickness, and (c) FOV. The acquisition matrix is determined by the number of steps of the phase-encoding gradient and the number of samples taken during the application of the frequency-encoding gradient (also known as the *readout gradient*). Because of the way MRI data are acquired and encoded, the number of frequency samples does not affect scan time; the number phase-encoding steps, however, does. Thus, when one wants to increase spatial resolution without affecting the scan time, a greater number of frequency samples is the parameter to be altered. Regardless of whether the frequency matrix or the phase matrix is increased, the resulting

reduction in voxel volume reduces the SNR. Newer techniques such as zero interpolation increase the apparent spatial resolution without significantly reducing the SNR by increasing the number of "lines" in k-space but filling them with zeros. It should be noted that these techniques do not change voxel volume and therefore do not increase the actual spatial resolution. They can, however, produce images with slightly sharper edge definition (Fig. 10-4).

Small slice thicknesses, such as 3 mm, are required in many studies, such as cervical spine, internal auditory canal, pituitary, orbit, and extremities. Unfortunately, thinner slices also produce images with lower SNR when compared to those acquired with thicker slices. Although it is important to acquire certain images using thin slices, it is also important to remember that these images will exhibit inherently low SNRs. Several techniques, discussed later in this chapter, can be used to "buy back" the SNR lost owing to the use of thin slices.

Of all the parameters that control voxel volume, the greatest effect is seen with the FOV. The FOV affects the voxel volume in two directions. As a result, if the FOV is

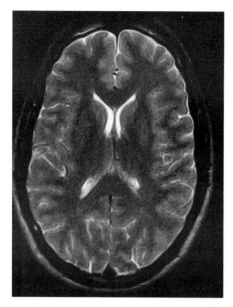

FIG. 10-4. Example of zero interpolation imaging of the brain. Image acquired at 256 × 256 and ZIPPED (zero interpolation processing) to 512 × 512.

reduced by only 20%, SNR is reduced by 40%. Conversely, increasing the FOV only 20% (e.g., increasing from 20 to 24 FOV) causes a 40% increase in SNR. One should be careful with the selection of the FOV. Because the FOV affects the size of the image seen on the screen and consequently the film, some operators may tend to select an FOV that fills the screen as much as possible. Such an approach can have disastrous consequences for the SNR, particularly at low field. Even though the image may be the size desired, inadequate SNR can result in nondiagnostic images. Acquiring the data with a large FOV and then applying a magnification, or zoom, factor so the image fills the screen do not increase spatial resolution. Magnifying an image is a photographic process that magnifies the pixel. Images with a large magnification factor fill the screen but can appear quite blurry. Because of the substantial affect on the SNR by the FOV, operators should ensure that adequate SNR is available for the desired FOV. When correcting image quality issues related to inadequate SNR, increasing the FOV may be a good first step.

Sampling Time

SNR is also related to the time spent sampling, or "listening to," the MRI signal. Two major parameters are related to sampling time: (a) receiver bandwidth and (b) the number of signal averages (NSA), or number of excitations (NEX).

Number of Signal Averages

Of the two parameters just mentioned, NSA is the most used. However, of all the parameters affecting SNR, it is also the most inefficient. NSA is the number of times each line of k-space is filled. It is analogous to coats of paint. If two signal averages are selected, the image data are acquired twice and the signals from each data point are averaged. Doubling the NSA doubles the scan time but not the SNR. Every time the MRI signal is sampled, noise is also acquired. Noise is random and, therefore, the SNR is proportional to the square root of the NSA. For example, if the NSA of a given sequence is increased from two to four (i.e., by a factor of 2), the scan time is doubled, but the increase in SNR is equal to only the square root of 2. It is interesting to note that doubling the NSA produces the same SNR gain as increasing the FOV by 20%. Increasing the FOV does reduce the spatial resolution, but it does not increase the scan time. To double the SNR by increasing the NSA, NSA would have to increase by a factor of 4 (because the square root of 4 is 2). However, a fourfold increase in scan time would also result. Because the NSA has such a small effect on SNR but a significant effect on scan time, it is best to select other parameters with SNR in mind so that one is not dependent on the NSA selection to produce an image with high SNR.

Receiver Bandwidth

Receiver bandwidth also affects sampling time and therefore SNR. Manufacturers that design systems to allow users direct control over receiver bandwidth provide a real "power tool" parameter for low-field imaging. Receiver bandwidth determines the range of frequencies the analog-to-digital converter can accurately detect. According to the Nyquist theorem, accurate sampling of a group of waveforms requires that they be sampled at twice the rate of the highest frequency. Most alternating/direct current converters acquire 256 samples (dictated by selecting a 256-frequency matrix) in 8 ms. As shown in the first equation below, this would allow for an absolute receiver bandwidth of 32 kHz (±16 kHz).

$$256/8 = 32 \ (\pm16)$$

$$256/16 = 16 \ (\pm8)$$

$$256/32 = 8 \ (\pm4)$$

Narrowing receiver bandwidth as shown in these equations increases the sampling time. The result is an increase in SNR: SNR is equal to 1 divided by the square root of the receiver bandwidth. For example, reducing receiver bandwidth by a factor of 2 increases the SNR by the square root of 2, or 1.41 (41%). By reducing receiver bandwidth, we are, in effect, reducing the amount of noise sampled relative to signal. Reducing receiver bandwidth does not cause an increase in scan time. As with most of MRI, some trade-offs exist.

Using a lower receiver bandwidth increases the sampling, or readout, time (previous equations). Increasing the readout time causes the minimum TE that can be obtained to increase. The result of this increase in minimum TE is increased T2 contrast (although slight) and an increase in flow-related artifacts. Flow-related artifacts are less prominent at low field when compared to the same bandwidth at high field (Fig. 10-5). A trade-off encountered at both low

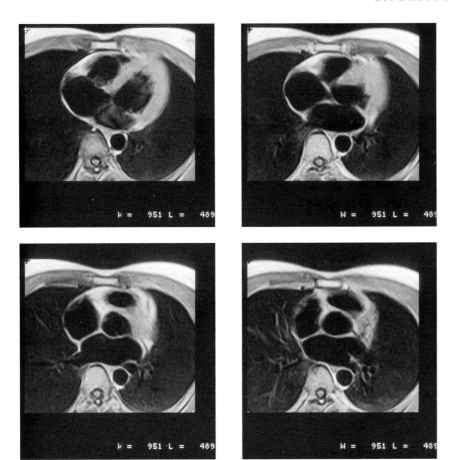

FIG. 10-5. Cardiac images using cardiac gating show lack of flow-related artifacts. Courtesy of General Electric Medical Systems, Milwaukee, WI.

and high field, however, is the reduction in the number of slices allowed in a two-dimensional (2D) multi-slice sequence as receiver bandwidth is reduced.

Many manufacturers have overcome some of the TE issues using a technique known by some as *partial echo* or *fractional echo*. Partial echo essentially uses the symmetric properties of k-space in the frequency direction. As shown in Figure 10-6, if we read the back two-thirds of the echo, the front one-third can be interpolated from the sampled data. Doing so can reduce the minimum TE and allow more time within the TR to excite other slices.

At high field, the major drawback of using reduced bandwidth techniques is the increase in the chemical shift artifact. Chemical shift artifact is seen as a black line along a fat and water interface. This shift is a result of the difference in precessional frequency between fat and water. Chemical shift is field strength–dependent and is 3.5 ppm. At 1.5 T, the Larmor frequency is approximately 64 MHz. Multiplying 3.5 by 64 yields 224. Therefore, at 1.5 T, water will precess 224 Hz faster than fat. With a receiver bandwidth of 32 kHz (±16 kHz), each pixel would represent 125 Hz (32,000/256). In this example, with a value of 125 Hz per pixel, the chemical shift would be 224 Hz/125 Hz per pixel, or 1.8 pixels. This would be seen on the image as a black line along one side of a fat/water interface and a bright line on the other side 1.8 pixels wide. If receiver bandwidth were reduced to 4 kHz (±2 kHz) at high field, each pixel would represent 15.6 Hz. The amount of chemical shift would

then be 224 Hz/15.6 Hz per pixel, or 14.3 pixels. This would produce a more noticeable chemical shift artifact.

At lower field strengths, however, lower bandwidths can be used without paying the penalty of chemical shift artifact. For example, consider a 0.2-T field strength with the same FOV and frequency matrix as in the previous example. At 0.2 T, the Larmor frequency is 8.52 MHz, producing a chemical shift of 29.8 Hz (3.5 × 8.52). Using a (4±2)–kHz bandwidth at 0.2 T,

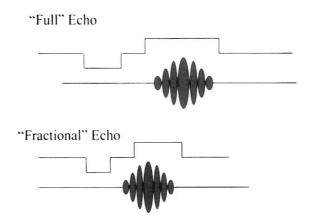

FIG. 10-6. Partial echo. These images illustrate the shifting of the echo in the readout window, which allows for a shorter echo time. The frequency data for the "front" of the echo are interpolated from the "back" of the echo.

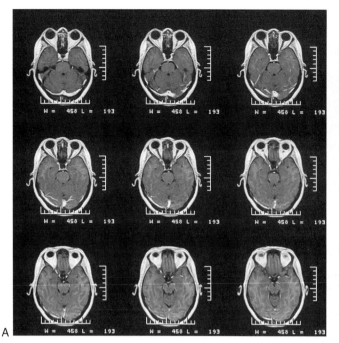
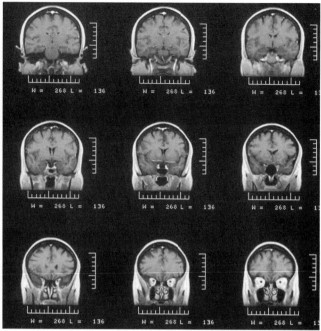

FIG. 10-7. A: Axial images obtained from a three-dimensional volume set. **B:** Reformatted coronal images from the axial data set in **A**.

the resultant pixel shift would be 1.9 pixels, essentially the same amount of pixel shift seen at 1.5 T with a ±16-kHz bandwidth. Because chemical shift and flow artifacts are not as prominent at low field, reducing receiver bandwidth should be attempted when increased SNR is needed.

Even at lower field strength, however, reducing receiver bandwidth is not without certain penalties. As receiver bandwidth is reduced, the time spent sampling the echo (also known as the *readout period*) is increased. Increasing the readout period causes the minimum TE to increase. With standard spin-echo or GRE sequences, increasing the readout period can easily reduce the number of slices allowed for a given TR. Due to the use of lower bandwidths with lower field systems, it is not uncommon to find that a given TR allows fewer slices than are seen at higher field with the same TR.

Fast spin-echo (FSE) sequences present additional issues related to receiver bandwidth. As receiver bandwidth is reduced and the readout period is increased, the spacing (or time) between the echoes increases. Increasing the echo spacing (ESP) can increase image blurring as well as pulsation or flow artifacts. FSE sequences tend to have higher SNRs, however, than do conventional spin-echo sequences. Thus, somewhat higher receiver bandwidths can be used with FSE sequences. As a general rule of thumb, receiver bandwidth for FSE sequences should be kept to approximately 6 or 7 kHz.

Three-Dimensional Acquisitions

Using conventional 2D acquisitions has certain limitations related to SNR and CNR. As thinner slices are used to improve spatial resolution, the SNR drops accordingly. With 2D acquisitions, we have to prescribe a certain amount of gap between slices to minimize "cross-talk" between slices. Cross-talk causes a reduction in CNR due to the tissue saturation. If one wishes to increase the number of slices for coverage, an increase in TR can be entered—increasing scan time and changing tissue contrast.

A three-dimensional (3D) acquisition excites a slab of tissue and uses phase encodings in the slice (z) direction to "partition" the slab into slice locations. As a result, the SNR in a 3D acquisition is proportional to the square root of the number of slices. Furthermore, because the slices (or partitions) are produced by gradient-encoding steps, the slices are truly contiguous without cross-talk. If data is acquired with isotropic voxels, the data set can be retrospectively reformatted into any plane, depending on the system's postprocessing capabilities (Fig. 10-7).

Increasing the number of slices in a 3D acquisition increases SNR but also increases the acquisition time. Although any pulse sequence could be used in a 3D acquisition, GRE sequences are generally used because of the ability to use a low TR and thus keep scan time to a minimum. With high-field systems, GRE sequences demonstrate a good bit of signal loss, distortion, or both at air/tissue interfaces owing to magnetic susceptibility effects. Magnetic susceptibility is field strength–dependent and is therefore less at low field. Magnetic susceptibility is also proportional to TE and voxel volume. The inherently high SNR of a 3D acquisition allows the selection of smaller voxel volumes while maintaining SNR. The reduction in magnetic susceptibility effects at low field and the ability to acquire small voxel volumes make 3D techniques a valuable tool for open MRI (see Figs. 10-1 and 10-3).

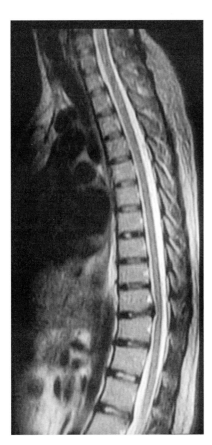

FIG. 10-8. Sagittal T2-weighted fast spin-echo images of the thoracic spine obtained using a phased-array coil. (Courtesy of General Electric Medical Systems, Milwaukee, WI.)

Surface Coils

An integral component of any MRI system is the RF subsystem, which includes the coils used to receive the MRI signal from the tissue. MRI coils are simply antennae. The better the design, the less the inherent noise and, therefore, the higher the SNR. With vertical field magnets, the receiver coils have a solenoid design. A solenoid coil is more efficient and therefore inherently has higher SNR than a flat-type coil used with horizontal field magnets. As a general rule of thumb, the smaller the coil and the closer it is to the patient, the better the SNR. The area of coverage is directly related to the diameter or the width of the solenoid coil. Increasing the coil size increases the area of coverage or allows imaging of larger patients. The penalty, however, is low SNR. Whenever possible, the operator should choose a coil that optimally matches the size of the patient and anatomy being imaged.

Advances in technology have led to improved designs even with solenoid coils. The term *quadrature* is used to describe coils designed to be circularly polarized. This type of design generally increases SNR up to 40% over conventional coils.

Imaging of the spine, particularly in the sagittal plane, presents a dilemma for many operators. To minimize scan time and cover a large area in head-foot direction, larger coils are required. As mentioned, larger coils have a negative impact on SNR. A solution has been found in the design and implementation of phased-array coils. A phased array consists of multiple small coils. Each coil has its own receiver. With this design, the electrical interaction between the individual coils in the array is minimized and thus the noise is reduced. The resulting image is a combination of coverage of the entire array. The SNR, however, is closer to that of each individual coil in the array (Fig. 10-8).

MAGNETIC RESONANCE IMAGE CONTRAST

Pulse Sequences and Parameters

The tissue contrast seen in an MR image is a function of intrinsic parameters that include T1 relaxation, T2 relaxation, proton (spin) density, flow/motion, magnetization transfer, perfusion, and diffusion. As a rule, the operator does not have control over these intrinsic parameters but rather controls the extrinsic parameters that include TR, TE, time of inversion (TI), and flip angle. Magnetic susceptibilities also play a role in determining the contrast seen in an MR image.

Two basic types of pulse sequences exist in MRI: spin echo and GRE. Spin-echo pulse sequences use a 180-degree refocusing pulse before the formation of the echo. The application of an RF refocusing pulse reduces the effects of magnetic susceptibility seen in an MR image. When imaging at lower magnetic fields, susceptibility effects are inherently reduced. Spin-echo sequences can be used to produce T1-weighted, T2-weighted, or PD-weighted images, depending on the selection of the timing parameters. One major drawback to conventional spin-echo sequences is the long TRs (typically >2,000 ms) required to produce images with minimal T1 contrast contribution.

Fast Spin Echo

Advances in pulse sequence design have led to the implementation of so-called RARE (*rapid acquisition relaxation enhanced*) or FSE sequences. FSE sequences use a train of echoes within a single TR period. Each echo is associated with a different phase-encoding gradient amplitude, and thus each echo fills a different line of k-space. Using an FSE sequence, scan times are reduced by a factor of the number of echoes in the train, a parameter known as the *echo train length* (ETL).

Because each image is made up of multiple echoes, each with a different amount of T2 weighting, the image contrast is affected by more than one echo. The higher the ETL, the more echoes with varying T2 weighting contributing to the image (Fig. 10-9). The result is a distinctive blurring of the image. The blurring is directly related to the ETL, both in relation to the number of echoes in the train and to the length of time it takes to play out the echo train. Another major factor affecting the length of the echo train is the ESP—the time between each echo in the train. Although ESP is not usually under the

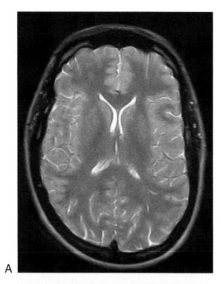

A

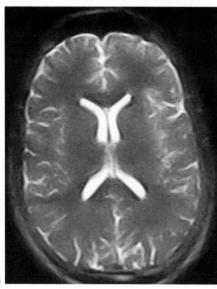

B

FIG. 10-9. Comparison of fast spin echo with an echo train of 15 **(A)** and a single-shot fast spin echo **(B)** with an echo train length of 160. The single shot **(B)** has an acquisition time of 33 seconds versus 9 minutes for **(A)**.

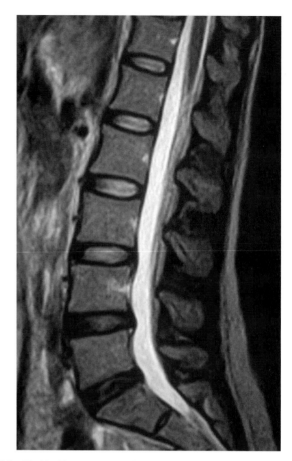

FIG. 10-10. Fast recovery fast spin-echo sequence. Repetition time, 3,700 ms; echo time, 108; bandwidth, 8.9 kHz; echo train length, 9. The fast recovery allows the use of shorter repetition time and echo time to obtain bright cerebrospinal fluid.

direct control of the operator, it can be controlled indirectly by the receiver bandwidth. As receiver bandwidth is reduced, the readout time of the frequency-encoding gradient increases and thus ESP increases. Reducing receiver bandwidth in an FSE sequence improves SNR, but it also increases image blurring.

One of the major benefits of FSE is the ability to acquire sequences with a long TR without a severe time penalty. Using a TR of at least 4,000 ms greatly minimizes saturation and therefore provides high SNR. Additionally, when the TE is increased for T2 weighting, tissues with high contrast are very easily distinguished even if the SNR is low.

An advance in pulse sequence design has led to the introduction of an imaging option known as *fast recovery*. Fast

recovery uses an additional RF pulse at the end of the echo train to drive residual transverse magnetization back to the longitudinal plane. The main benefit is the ability to use shorter TRs and TEs while retaining the high SNR and contrast of longer TRs (Fig. 10-10).

Gradient Echo

As discussed, GRE sequences do not use an RF refocusing pulse and thus do not correct for field inhomogeneities and chemical shift. GRE sequences also allow the use of lower flip angles. Using lower flip angles allows the user to acquire images with PD- or T2-like contrasts while using lower TRs.

Two basic types of GRE sequences exist: steady state and spoiled. A steady state exists whenever the TR is much less than the T2 and T1 of a given tissue. Because cerebrospinal fluid (CSF) has a long T1 and T2, use of a steady-state sequence can provide images with high signal from CSF. If a low flip angle is used in conjunction with a moderately long TE, images with T2* contrast are produced. At low field, the lower susceptibility causes the T2* decay to be longer compared to similar sequences acquired at high field. Thus,

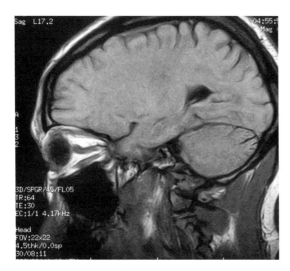

FIG. 10-11. Sagittal gradient reversal (gradient echo) three-dimensional Fourier transform image of the orbit. Repetition time, 58 ms; echo time, 30; flip angle, 50 degrees; bandwidth, 4.46 kHz. The optic nerve and extraocular muscles are well visualized. Note that the orbital fat does not become as bright as with higher field strength magnetic resonance images.

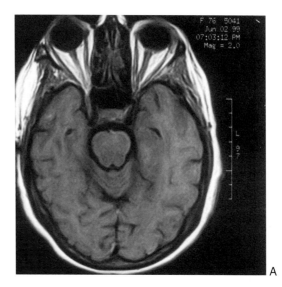

A

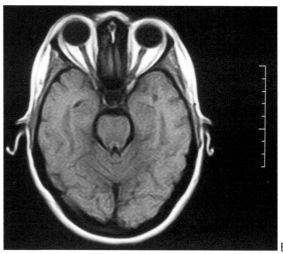

B

FIG. 10-12. Comparison of an axial three-dimensional Fourier transform (gradient echo) of the brain **(A)** with a spin-echo two-dimensional Fourier transform **(B)**. Three-dimensional Fourier transform sequences have higher signal to noise ratios; therefore higher resolution sequences and thinner slices can be used.

slightly longer TEs should be selected for T2*-weighted GRE sequences at low field. The example shown in Figure 10-11 is an axial 2D GRE acquired with a 52 TE. Use of the same parameters at high field would produce an image with severe magnetic susceptibility artifact.

For T1 weighting, an additional gradient magnetic field at the end of the pulse sequence or shifting the phase of the excitation pulse with each repetition of the pulse sequence can eliminate, or "spoil away," any residual transverse magnetization between repetitions. This spoiling removes high signal from fluid seen with steady-state sequences. Although it is possible to produce images with T2* contrast using spoiled GRE sequences (low flip angle and moderately high TE), their primary utility is to provide GRE images with heavy T1 weighting. For T1-weighted images, it is necessary to use as low a TE as possible to reduce the T2-contrast influence in the image. Because GRE sequences do not use a 180-degree refocusing RF pulse before the echo, shorter TEs are possible, particularly with lower receiver bandwidths. Figure 10-12 demonstrates the improved T1 contrast between gray and white matter seen with the GRE acquisition.

Inversion Recovery Sequences

In addition to the aforementioned benefit of allowing the selection of long TRs without a significant time penalty, FSE sequences offer the ability to efficiently perform inversion recovery sequences. Inversion sequences use a 180-degree pulse at the beginning of the pulse sequence,

followed by a period known as the *TI*. Choosing a TI that is 69% of a tissue's T1 nullifies the signal from that tissue (1).

Two types of inversion sequences are commonly used at both low and high field: short tau inversion recovery (STIR) and fluid attenuated inversion recovery (FLAIR). STIR uses a relatively short TI to null the signal from fat. At lower fields, STIR is one of two methods for suppressing fat signal. It is important to remember, however, that STIR suppresses the signal from fat based on its short T1 recovery time. Any tissue that has a short T1 time close to that of fat can also be suppressed; this may include hemorrhage and gadolinium enhancement (2). STIR sequences are very useful in imaging the musculoskeletal system (Fig. 10-13). Because they rely on the T1 recovery time of fat, they do not

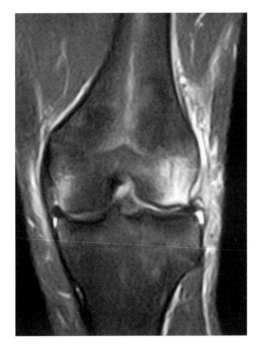

FIG. 10-13. Short inversion time inversion recovery (fast short tau inversion recovery) of the knee. This technique incorporates a 6-echo train. Repetition time, 3,750 ms; echo time, 37; bandwidth, 7.8 kHz; inversion time, 75. A bone contusion in the lateral femoral condyle is well seen with short tau inversion recovery imaging.

suffer from inhomogeneous fat suppression, which is seen with the spectral fat-saturation techniques used at high field.

FLAIR uses a long TR, TE, and TI to produce T2-weighted images. Using a relatively long TI, the signal from CSF can be nullified, making FLAIR especially useful in brain imaging.

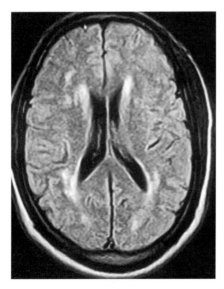

FIG. 10-14. Fluid-attenuated inversion recovery is a fast technique that uses an echo train of 6. Repetition time, 6,000 ms; echo time, 108; bandwidth, 8.93 kHz, inversion time, 1,400. Note that the periventricular high signal intensity ischemic lesions are nicely demonstrated against the dark cerebrospinal fluid.

Often, neuropathology is difficult to see at the gray/white matter interface in the deep white matter and around CSF spaces. FLAIR suppresses the signal from CSF and increases the contrast between the brain tissue and lesions such as stroke and white matter diseases (Fig. 10-14). Owing to FLAIR's high contrast sensitivity, many sites have replaced the conventional PD-weighted sequence in the brain with FLAIR (3).

DEVELOPING PROTOCOLS FOR LOW-FIELD IMAGING

Brain and Spine Imaging

When developing MRI protocols for low-field systems, one must keep in mind the inherent lower SNR. If short scan times are desired, due to the patient's inability to tolerate conventional scan times, trade-offs have to be made in either spatial resolution or SNR. As long as the tissue contrasts are high, shorter scan times can be gained by giving up SNR. Several previously discussed methods can be used to produce images with high contrast and thus lessen the dependence on SNR. For good T1 contrast between gray and white matter, a spoiled GRE can be used. If acquired as a 3D data set, high SNR and thin slices can be produced. Such an acquisition can be useful when imaging small structures such as the seventh and eighth intracranial nerves, orbits, and pituitary (Fig. 10-15). Acquiring the data set with relatively isotropic voxels can allow retrospective reformatting of the image data. Reducing receiver bandwidth can be an additional source of SNR, even with 3D sequences. However, increases in the minimum TE, due to reducing receiver bandwidth, may cause loss of contrast or introduction of chemical shift mismapping at the fat/water interfaces.

FSE sequences with TRs of 4,000 ms or higher can greatly reduce the T1 saturation and increase the SNR and tissue contrasts. Additional imaging options such as fast recovery can be of benefit by reducing scan time through the use of lower TRs without the SNR or contrast penalties. This increase in SNR can be used to reduce the scan time or, better yet, allow increased spatial resolution. Using FSE, it should be easy to obtain a 5-mm slice data set in the brain in approximately 5 minutes or less (Fig. 10-16).

Gadolinium Studies

Without the ability to spectrally suppress fat, it is often difficult to visualize gadolinium enhancement in certain areas, such as the orbit, at low field. Several approaches can be used to address this issue. Using a technique based on the Dixon technique of fat and water suppression, images can be acquired with various TEs to obtain both fat and water images (4). The water image is essentially fat suppressed. If this type of technique is not available, a GRE sequence can be acquired with a TE such that fat and water are 180 degrees out of phase. At 0.2 T, for example, a TE of 16.5 ms produces an image with fat and water out of phase (Fig. 10-

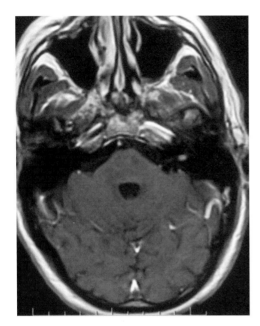

FIG. 10-15. Three-dimensional Fourier transform (gradient echo). Repetition time, 67 ms; echo time, 33; flip angle, 60 degrees; bandwidth, 4.81 kHz; slice thickness, 3.5 mm. This high-resolution T1 image of the internal auditory canals with contrast shows a small, approximately 3-mm, intracanalicular acoustic neuroma.

17). This technique holds great promise in postcontrast T1 studies of the knee and orbits with fat suppression. In the brain, magnetization transfer may also prove beneficial in improving contrast between gadolinium-enhancing lesions and brain tissue (5).

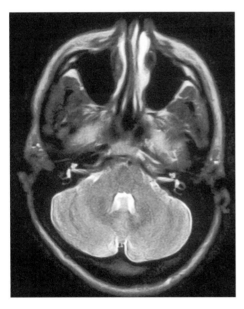

FIG. 10-16. Fast spin-echo sequence with extremely high resolution demonstrates the separation of the seventh and eight cranial nerves in the internal auditory canal. The semicircular canals are also well seen. This sequence was performed in a 0.2-T open magnet. Repetition time, 3,500 ms; echo time, 91; bandwidth, 7.8 kHz.

Body Imaging

The main problems encountered when using MRI to image the chest, abdomen, or pelvis are cardiac motion, respiratory motion, and flow. Fortunately, flow and respiratory artifacts, although still present, are much less severe at low field. SNR is generally not a real problem owing to the necessity for a larger FOV and generally thicker slices. Most, if not all, low-field systems require some type of receiver coil to be used. As always, SNR can be optimized by choosing the proper coil size for the patient. Reducing receiver bandwidth can also increase SNR; however, using too low a receiver bandwidth can result in increased flow and motion artifacts.

When imaging the liver for lesion detection, strong T1 contrasts are useful. With low-field systems, it is quite easy to obtain the proper contrast. The spleen can be used as a guide for parameter selection. Using the shortest TE possible, the TR should be selected so the resultant images show normal liver to be hyperintense relative to normal spleen. Many liver lesions follow the signal intensity of normal spleen. The higher the contrast between the liver and the spleen, the greater the probability of good contrast between normal and abnormal liver tissue.

Respiratory artifacts can be minimized using a respiratory compensation or triggering technique. The only problem may be the inability to control the TR, as it may be dependent on the respiratory cycle. As an alternative, 2D, spoiled GRE sequences can often be acquired in a breath-hold, eliminating any artifact due to respiratory motion. Additionally, GRE sequences can be acquired with specific TEs to image fat and water either in phase, or out of phase. This type of imaging, often known as *opposed phase imaging*, is useful for studies of the liver, pancreas, and adrenal glands (Fig. 10-18). At 0.2-T field strength, fat and water are out of phase at 16.5 ms. The difference in signal intensity is apparent in the left adrenal mass when the 17 TE is compared to the minimum TE.

FSE sequences can be used to provide high-quality T2-weighted images. Again, when selecting the receiver bandwidth, care should be taken not to exacerbate flow/motion artifacts. Additionally, FSE techniques are prone to image blurring. This blurring can be worsened by an increase in the ESP resulting from reduced receiver bandwidth. Keeping the ETL at 6 or less can also minimize blurring.

Musculoskeletal Imaging

Low-field systems offer several advantages when imaging the musculoskeletal system. The T1 times of tissues at lower field produce excellent contrast on T1-weighted images. Many open systems allow the patient to be offset in his or her position on the table or by side-to-side movement of the table, allowing the body part of interest to be imaged at, or very close to, magnet isocenter. Imaging at isocenter provides the most homogeneous magnetic field, thereby optimizing SNR. Patients presenting for certain examinations, such as of the wrist and elbow, can be imaged with their arm by their side, significantly increasing patient comfort and cooperation (Fig. 10-19).

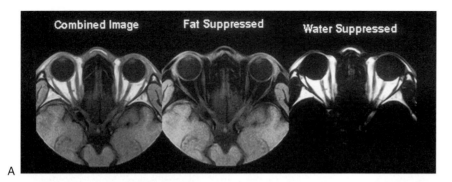

A

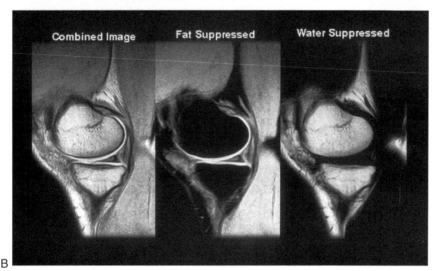

B

FIG. 10-17. A: Combined, fat-suppressed, and water-suppressed images of the orbit. Fat-suppressed images with gadolinium may, in the future, overcome the limitations of not being able to obtain fat saturation images on open magnetic resonance imaging. **B:** Combined, fat-suppressed, and water-suppressed images of a meniscal tear. (Courtesy of General Electric Medical Systems, Milwaukee, WI.)

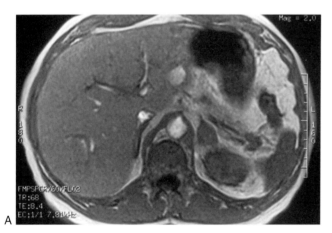

A

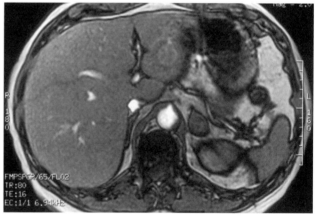

B

FIG. 10-18. In-phase **(A)** and out-of-phase **(B)** images of the left adrenal gland and kidney. **A:** Gradient echo, three-dimensional Fourier transform. Echo time, minimum; repetition time, 68 ms; echo time, 8.4; bandwidth, 7.81; flip angle, 60 degrees. **B:** Gradient echo. Echo time, 17 ms; repetition time, 80 ms; echo time, 16; bandwidth, 6.9 kHz; flip angle, 65 degrees. The echo time of 17 ms is such that fat and water are 180 degrees out of phase. This results in the black line around the adrenal gland, liver, spleen, and kidney. The exact echo time to produce an out-pf-phase image depends on field strength. In evaluation of adrenal adenomas, out-of-phase imaging can be very helpful to help confirm the diagnosis of an adenoma.

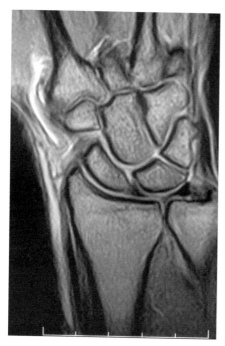

FIG. 10-19. High-resolution coronal gradient echo of the wrist. Repetition time, 750 ms; echo time, 25; flip angle, 30 degrees.

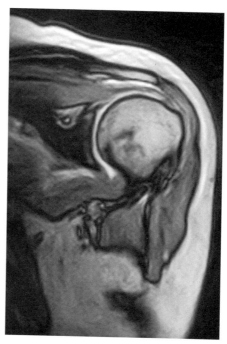

FIG. 10-20. Gadolinium arthrogram of the shoulder. Repetition time, 300 ms; echo time, 17; bandwidth, 3.47; flip angle, 90 degrees. Note that the echo time of 17 produces an out-of-phase image.

Musculoskeletal examinations often require thin slices at various oblique angles to demonstrate small structures such as the anterior cruciate ligament. Given these requirements, 3D acquisitions can be of considerable benefit in musculoskeletal protocols: They provide high SNR, thin contiguous slices, and the ability to reformat the data set assuming isotropic voxels are prescribed. Spoiled GRE sequences can be used if T1 weighting is desired; steady-state sequences can be used to provide T2* contrast to better visualize fluid. For optimum fluid sensitivity, STIR sequences are often used in musculoskeletal imaging. Although often low in SNR and therefore not well suited for high-resolution imaging, the sensitivity to fluid, particularly in marrow pathology, makes STIR a powerful component of any musculoskeletal protocol.

When gadolinium is required, the high signal from fat often blends with the signal from tissues whose T1 time has been altered by the gadolinium. Use of the aforementioned techniques for suppressing fat can be quite useful. The example shown in Figure 10-20 shows a shoulder joint injected with a gadolinium and saline mixture (2.0 cc gadolinium in 150 mL saline). The contrast above the rotator cuff is easily identified. This type of sequence can also be used in postcontrast studies of marrow abnormalities.

STIR should not be used after the injection of gadolinium because it can suppress the signal from the gadolinium-enhanced tissues as well as from fat.

FSE sequences, when used to produce PD-weighted images, are often subject to too much blurring to provide adequate visualization of some pathologies such as meniscal tears (6). This blurring is more pronounced as the ESP increases. Also, as receiver bandwidth is reduced for SNR gains, the readout time increases, increasing the ESP. Thus, conventional spin-echo sequences may be the better choice for T2 imaging of the meniscus.

CONCLUSION

MRI using lower field open scanners offers many advantages over high-field closed imaging. Patient comfort and acceptance are major advantages. As the patient population becomes more aware of choices, primarily through direct advertisement, they have begun to ask specifically for open MRI. Advances in hardware and software have and will continue to improve the overall image quality as well as shorten scan times. Software developments will also add to the capabilities of lower field open systems, allowing them access to today's newer applications, such as diffusion imaging, contrast-enhanced MR angiography (Fig. 10-21), and fat/water imaging (see Fig. 10-17).

Regardless of improvements, the primary drawback remains the inherently lower SNR when compared to high-field systems. Technologists with extensive knowledge of

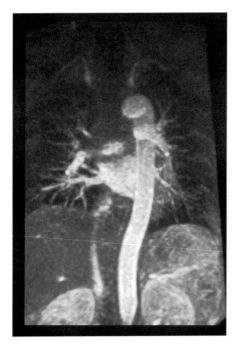 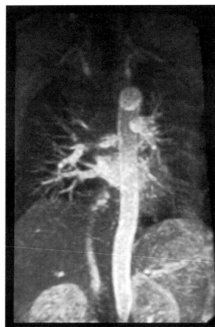

FIG. 10-21. Contrast-enhanced magnetic resonance angiography of the heart and thoracic aorta. (Courtesy of General Electric Medical Systems, Milwaukee, WI.)

basic MRI fundamentals are critical if a facility wishes to provide its referring physicians and, most important, its patients with the highest quality diagnostic MRI examinations.

REFERENCES

1. Woodward P, Friemarck RD. *MR for technologists.* New York: McGraw-Hill, 1995.
2. Krinsky G, Rofsky NM, Weinreb JC. Nonspecificity of short inversion time inversion recovery (STIR) as a technique of fat suppression: pitfalls in image interpretation. *AJR Am J Roentgenol* 1996;166(3):523–526.
3. Kates R, Atkinson D, Brant-Zawadzki M. Fluid-attenuated inversion recovery (FLAIR): clinical prospectus of current and future applications. *Top Magn Reson Imag* 1996;8(6):389–396.
4. Daniel BL, Butts K, Glover GH, Cooper C, Herfkens RJ. Breast cancer: gadolinium-enhanced MR imaging with a 0.5 T open imager and three-point Dixon technique. *Radiology* 1998;207(1):183–190.
5. Peretti-Viton P, Taieb D, Viton JM, et al. Contrast-enhanced magnetization transfer MRI in metastatic lesions of the brain. *Neuroradiology* 1998;40(12):783–787.
6. Anderson MW, Raghavan N, Seidenwurm DJ, Greenspan A, Drake C. Evaluation of meniscal tears: fast spin-echo versus conventional spin-echo magnetic resonance imaging. *Acad Radiol* 1995;2(3):209–214.

SECTION III

Clinical Imaging

Open MRI,
edited by Peter A. Rothschild and Debra Reinking Rothschild.
Lippincott Williams & Wilkins. Philadelphia © 2000.

CHAPTER 11

Open Magnetic Resonance Imaging of the Brain

R. Craig Platenberg

Magnetic resonance imaging (MRI) has rapidly become the imaging modality of choice for the evaluation of disease processes involving the central nervous system (CNS). The superior soft tissue contrast differentiation and the ability to scan in any arbitrary plane make MRI ideal for imaging the brain as well as virtually every other anatomic system. The brain, because of its location, size, and contour, is usually the first organ studied with any new imaging modality. MRI was no exception. In the early days of MRI, examinations were performed with very low field strengths. Optimum signal-to-noise ratios (SNRs) were somewhat difficult to obtain; as a result, an initial push for scanning at higher field strength occurred.

Improvements in gradient strength, coil design, and sequence performance have made imaging at lower field strengths a convincing reality. High-quality, high-resolution, and, more important, clinically diagnostic images of the brain, posterior fossa, skull base, pituitary, and internal auditory canals are routinely obtained on open MRI systems. With attention to the physical realities of scanning at lower field strengths, the MRI physician may perform imaging sequences that produce results of comparable quality to those obtained in high-field closed magnets. As interest in open scanning develops and as more research is focused at lower field strength, advanced imaging techniques originally thought to be restricted to high-field systems are becoming available at lower fields. Although differences between high and lower field open systems exist, "bad MRI" is "bad MRI" regardless of the field strength used. The objective of this chapter is to limit the factors contributing to poor MRI examinations, providing background information of the CNS at lower field strengths, and optimizing scan quality on open systems. In addition, imaging of commonly encountered disease processes of the brain on lower field open MRI systems is discussed.

FIELD STRENGTH AND OTHER TECHNICAL CONSIDERATIONS

When tissues are placed within an external static magnetic field, the hydrogen protons in that tissue occupy one of two energy states: Some protons align with and some protons align against the direction of the main magnetic field according to quantum mechanics beyond the scope of this text. A net magnetization vector is formed along the direction of the main magnetic field. This net magnetization vector is related to the size of the static field strength. Progressively higher field strengths yield a greater difference in the number of protons in the lower energy state and a larger net magnetization vector. The intensity of the signal obtained in MRI is proportional to the population difference of these protons (1). Higher field strength magnets generate greater signal intensity per given time than lower field strengths for the same time spent. The SNR has a relatively linear relationship to the field strength only if the receiver bandwidth is held constant and the repetition time (TR) is long compared to the T1 time of the tissue. If the receiver bandwidth is allowed to vary with field strength (which is commonly done in clinical imaging), the SNR scales as a square root of field strength (2). This physics parameter has important implications for practical scanning. One may increase scan time at lower field to obtain equivalent SNRs relative to high field; however, increasing scan times does not correlate to a linear increase in signal intensity. A better solution for improving SNR exists: One may increase the field of view (FOV) without a time penalty to gain more SNR. Only slight increases in the FOV may yield important improvements in the SNR. Changing the number of phase-encoding steps affects the spatial resolution and the scan time, as well as allows user flexibility in manipulating the SNR. Many critics of lower field strength open MRI systems object to operator-chosen matrices that favor time over spatial resolution. However, use of an asymmetric matrix and slightly larger FOV may balance competing factors of SNR and spatial resolution.

R. C. Platenberg: Wide Open MRI, Med-Ted International Corporation, McLean, Virginia

TABLE 11-1. *Routine brain, internal auditory canal (IAC), and pituitary (PIT) scan parameters*

TR/TE (ms)	Sequence	Field of view	Echo train length	Slice thickness (mm)	Matrix	Pixel dimension	Time	Number of averages
470/17	T1 SAG-Ax	211 × 250		5	215 × 256	0.98 × 0.98	6:46	2
6,300/100/ 2,200 IT	FLAIR Ax	250 × 250	8	5	256 × 256	0.98 × 0.98	6:40	2
4,300/126	FSE	250 × 250	16	5	256 × 256	0.98 × 0.98	4:35	2
3,700/120	HI RES FSE	250 × 250	12	5	300 × 360	0.83 × 0.69	6:25	2
30/10	PIT/IAC COR T1	180 × 180		3	216 × 256	0.83 × 0.70	6:22	1
420/18	PIT/IAC COR T1	220 × 220		3	256 × 256	0.86 × 0.86	7:10	4

Ax, axial; COR, coronal; FLAIR, fluid attenuated inversion recovery; FSE, fast spin echo; HI RES, high resolution; IT, inversion time; SAG, sagittal; TE, echo time; TR, repetition time.

The contrast-to-noise ratio (CNR) is the ratio of different signals from different types of tissues. The ability to detect a lesion from the surrounding background tissue is much more important than the measured value of SNR or of imaging film parameters that, at best, only contribute to film aesthetics. Relative CNRs for T1-weighted imaging reach a maximum in the range of 1.0 to 1.5 T and then decrease above this range (3). Ten patients were scanned by Rutt and Lee (3) at 1.5 and 0.5 T. Identical scan times and identical scan parameters—except bandwidth—were performed. The bandwidth was varied in proportion to the field strength. The calculated advantage in CNR for 1.5 T over 0.5 T is less than 20% for T1-weighted images with variable bandwidth. The CNR varies with sequences as well as with tissue types studied. In this same paper, for the evaluation of multiple sclerosis (MS) lesions using receiver operating characteristic analysis, more difference was found between the skill levels of the radiologists interpreting the MRI than was found between lesion detection at 0.5 or 1.5 T (3).

Image clarity is an elusive entity that is a subjective and personal observation. Spatial resolution relates to the ability to distinguish two points that are close together in a matrix as separate from one another. Spatial resolution relates to the slice thickness, the FOV, and the imaging matrix. These features determine the size of the picture element or pixel in two dimensions and the volume element or voxel in three dimensions. The smaller the pixel element, the higher the spatial resolution and, as a result, the higher potential background noise. In general, the smaller the pixel element, the lower the SNR and the greater the time required to produce adequate signal. A trade-off exists between signal, contrast, and resolution. Typical brain studies have voxel dimensions

TABLE 11-2. *Pixel dimensions*

FOV	Phase/frequency encode steps									
	256	224	220	208	196	192	180	176	172	160
150	0.5859	0.6696	0.6818	0.7212	0.7653	0.7813	0.8333	0.8523	0.8721	0.9375
160	0.625	0.7143	0.7272	0.7692	0.8163	0.8333	0.8888	0.9091	0.9302	1.0
180	0.7031	0.8036	0.8182	0.8654	0.9184	0.9375	1.0	1.023	1.047	1.125
200	0.7813	0.8929	0.9091	0.9615	1.020	1.042	1.111	1.136	1.163	1.25
210	0.8203	0.9375	0.9545	1.009	1.071	1.094	1.167	1.193	1.221	1.313
220	0.8594	0.9821	1.0	1.058	1.122	1.146	1.222	1.25	1.279	1.375
240	0.9375	1.071	1.091	1.154	1.224	1.25	1.333	1.364	1.395	1.5
250	0.9766	1.116	1.136	1.202	1.276	1.302	1.389	1.420	1.453	1.563
260	1.016	1.161	1.182	1.25	1.327	1.354	1.444	1.477	1.512	1.625
270	1.055	1.205	1.227	1.298	1.378	1.406	1.5	1.534	1.569	1.688
280	1.094	1.25	1.273	1.346	1.429	1.458	1.556	1.591	1.628	1.75
300	1.172	1.339	1.364	1.442	1.531	1.563	1.667	1.705	1.744	1.875
310	1.25	1.429	1.445	1.538	1.633	1.667	1.778	1.818	1.860	2.0

FOV, field of view.
Pixel dimensions must be calculated for existing scan protocols to ensure they fall within ACR guidelines using the following formulas:
FOV/frequency steps = In-plane frequency pixel dimension
FOV/frequency steps = In-plane phase pixel dimension
ACR pixel dimensions: Guidelines using FOV and plane pixel size. The minimum dimension for the brain is a ratio of less than or equal to 1.2.
From *ACR magnetic resonance image site accreditation guideline book.* Twinsburg, OH: Hitachi Medical Systems, 1999.

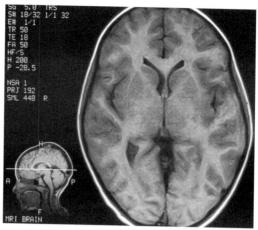

A

B

FIG. 11-1. Comparison of two-dimensional T1-weighted, spin-echo image versus a three-dimensional spoiled gradient-echo, heavily T1-weighted image. **A:** Two-dimensional T1-weighted, spin-echo image [repetition time (*TR*)/echo time (*TE*) 820/20]. The cerebrospinal fluid is dark (low signal). The subcutaneous fat is bright white (high signal intensity). The ability to differentiate gray matter from white matter is somewhat less apparent. **B:** Three-dimensional spoiled gradient-echo image that is very heavily T1 weighted. The cerebrospinal fluid is low signal intensity and fat is high signal intensity—similar to routine spin-echo T1 imaging. Note, however, that the difference between the gray matter and the white matter is more pronounced using this type of sequence (TR/TE 50/18). The flip angle of this study was 50 degrees versus the 91- and 180-degree flip angle parameters performed with routine spin echo.

of 0.9 mm × 0.9 mm × 5 mm or smaller in transverse, coronal, and sagittal imaging. Pituitary studies tend to be 0.7 mm × 0.8 mm × 3 mm as does high-resolution imaging of the internal auditory canals. Volumetric/three-dimensional (3D) scans can be performed with pixel sizes of 0.6 mm × 0.7 mm × 1 mm, similar to that obtained at high field (Table 11-1). The American College of Radiology site accreditation for

MRI systems recommends a maximum pixel dimension of no more than 1.2 mm and slice thickness on routine brain imaging of no more than 5 mm (Table 11-2). The pixel element and slice thickness of open systems are well within this recommendation (4). It is important to be able to differentiate one tissue from another. Protons react to radiofrequency (RF) pulses applied to them in a static field by being

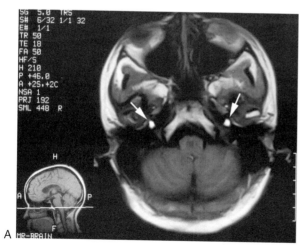

A

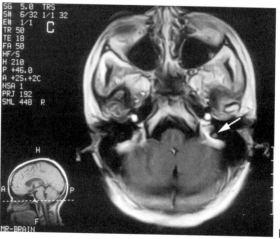

B

FIG. 11-2. Pre– and post–contrast enhancement characteristics of spoiled gradient-echo, heavily T1-weighted images. **A:** Three-dimensional spoiled gradient-echo T1 sequence obtained before the administration of contrast material. Note that in the carotid arteries in the skull base, the hyperintensity is consistent with entry slice phenomenon in-flow or hyperintensity from blood entering from outside the slice of interest (*arrows*). This feature may be seen in routine spin-echo imaging as well but is somewhat more pronounced with the spoiled gradient-echo techniques. **B:** Three-dimensional spoiled gradient-echo image obtained after contrast administration. Enhancement in the sigmoid sinus and jugular vein is also apparent. These findings must not be confused for abnormalities.

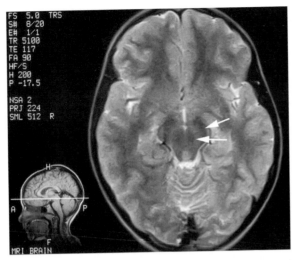

FIG. 11-3. A fast spin-echo image obtained through the mid-brain with a repetition time/echo time of 5,100/117. The echo train length is 8. A series of these images were obtained in 7 minutes and 20 seconds. Note the thin rim of hyperintensity in the subcutaneous fat in this very thin individual. In addition, the low signal intensity in the substantia nigra and the red nucleus (*arrows*) is somewhat less conspicuous than that which would be seen on a conventional T2-weighted spin-echo image.

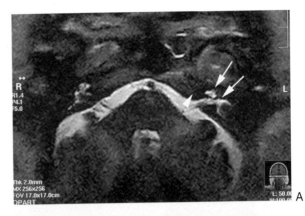

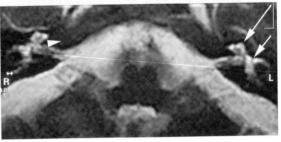

FIG. 11-4. Three-dimensional fast spin-echo sequence. **A:** Source image with 2-mm slice thickness obtained with a repetition time/echo time of 6,000/240. This study was acquired in 7 minutes and 18 seconds. **B:** A maximum-intensity projection composite image of the 15 slices of the source image compressed. Demonstration of the vestibule (*arrow*), cochlea (*long arrow*), vestibulocochlear nerve (*arrowhead*), and cerebellar pontine angle is noted.

displaced from the main field direction. The width and voltage of the RF pulse applied to the protons determine the extent to which the protons will tip relative to the magnetic field. When the RF pulse is turned off, the spins realign in an oscillatory fashion with the main field. The record of the net magnetization vector occurs as a result of the T1 and T2 properties of the tissue stimulated. Different tissues have different T1 and T2 relaxation times. The ability to differentiate one tissue from another is related to the different T1 and T2 values of the tissues at different field strengths. The T1 values for gray and white matter are similar at very low field strengths. As a result, the ability to differentiate gray matter from white matter may be more difficult. The use of T1-weighted gradient-echo or spoiled gradient-echo techniques allows the MR user to evaluate the difference between gray and white matter and overcome this seeming limitation (Fig. 11-1).

Gadolinium-containing contrast material decreases the T1 relaxation time of tissues. This correlates with increased signal intensity on T1 spin-echo images and brain areas, in which disruption of the normal blood–brain barrier becomes bright on T1 images. Diagnostic concerns exist regarding T1 relation of spoiled gradient-echo techniques and, as a result, some authors recommend that postgadolinium images be obtained using T1-weighted spin-echo techniques (5,6). However, not all open MRI radiologists agree. With spoiled gradient-echo images, inflow effects may be seen in the posterior fossa and circle of Willis (Fig. 11-2). Blood flow in the vertebral arteries and carotid arteries at the skull base because of inflow effects may appear as hyperintensities.

These should not be confused with lesions in skull base vasculature. A combination of T1 spin-echo and spoiled gradient-echo images for postcontrast imaging allows for obtaining the strengths of both of these separate sequences. The recommended dose of ionic contrast materials is 0.1 mmol per kg. This dose may not be sufficient for optimizing lesion detection for contrast-enhancing lesions at lower field strengths. Routinely, 20 cc nonionic gadolinium compounds are administered to patients scanned on open systems. The use of nonionic contrast material may make the administration of higher concentrations of contrast material more feasible. Contrast agents optimized for lower field strength systems are under investigation.

Fast spin-echo (FSE) techniques have significantly decreased the time needed to obtain high-quality T2-weighted images. In routine spin-echo imaging, one line of imaging data is acquired per repetition and placed into a matrix called *k-space*. The number of phase-encoding steps determines the number of TRs needed to obtain an image. This k-space filling method resulted in T2 imaging times of 13 to 15 minutes were common. FSE techniques using multiple echo trains have allowed a significant decrease in scan time relative to routine T2-weighted spin-echo images. With

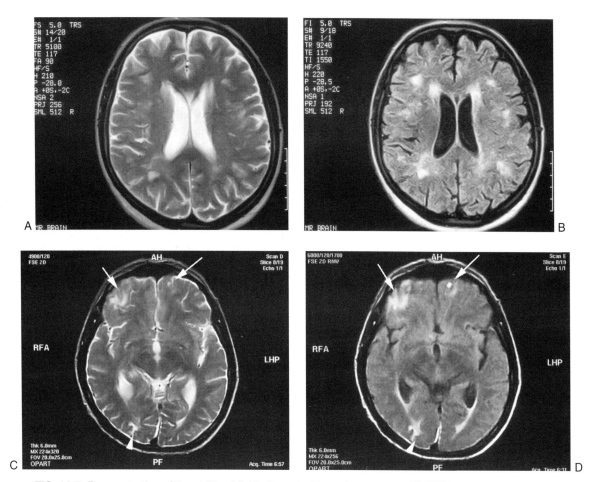

FIG. 11-5. Demonstration of the ability of fluid attenuated inversion recovery (FLAIR) imaging to accentuate the difference between lesions and background. **A:** A T2-weighted axial image obtained in a 55-year-old woman with a history of multiple sclerosis (MS). Repetition time (*TR*)/echo time (*TE*) is 5,101/17 on this routine fast spin-echo image. Multiple lesions are seen in the subcortical and periventricular white matter. **B:** A FLAIR image at the same slice location with a TR/TE of 92,040/117 and an inversion pulse of 1,550. Note the improved lesion to background contrast-to-noise ratio on the FLAIR images, making the areas of MS demyelination much more conspicuous. **C:** A heavily T2-weighted image using a fast spin-echo technique with TR/TE of 4,900/120 in a patient who sustained closed-head injury and cerebral contusions. Abnormal signal intensity is seen in the right frontal lobe (*arrow*) and the left inferior frontal region (*long arrow*) and is somewhat less conspicuous in the right occipital area (*arrowhead*). **D:** A FLAIR image obtained through this same slice in the same patient with TR/TE/inversion pulse of 6,000/120/1,700. The right frontal cortical lesion is much more conspicuous (*arrow*). The left frontal and right occipital lesions are readily apparent (*arrowhead*). Abnormal signal intensity in the occipital white matter and the periventricular area is also more easily identified on this FLAIR image.

an echo train length (ETL) of 8, scan times in theory may be lowered to one-eighth of the time required for routine spin echo. Very heavily T2-weighted images can now be obtained in as little as 5 to 6 minutes. FSE imaging produces a range of contrast over the TR. Fat signal intensity is higher in FSE images than in conventional spin-echo images (Fig. 11-3). Susceptibility to iron is reduced with FSE techniques. These features must be kept in mind when performing FSE sequences. 3D FSE studies can be performed on some open systems (Fig. 11-4). This 3D FSE has many potential uses and allows for the volumetric evaluation of the internal auditory canals.

Proton density imaging is the result of sequences obtained relying on the difference in tissue proton concentration rather than on T1 and T2 relaxation effects. Proton density imaging usually displays the signal intensity of cerebrospinal fluid (CSF) as isointense with brain. Lesions of the surrounding periventricular tissues become more conspicuous on proton density images because the signal from CSF is not bright, whereas lesions from vascular insults, tumors, and infections are of higher signal intensity. Many radiology residents are trained to evaluate proton density images of the brain as the first sequence of interest, correlating the T1 and T2 images with the findings seen on pro-

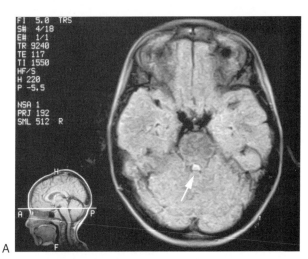
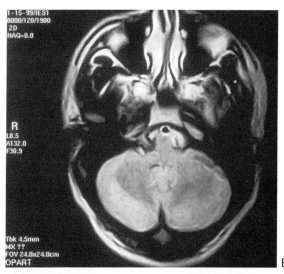

FIG. 11-6. Fluid attenuated inversion recovery (FLAIR) images with pulsation artifact. **A:** A FLAIR axial image through the fourth ventricle demonstrating abnormal hyperintensity (*arrow*) within the fourth ventricle secondary to pulsation of cerebrospinal fluid. The repetition time (*TR*)/echo time (*TE*) and inversion time are 9,240/117/1,550. **B:** FLAIR axial image demonstrates the increased signal intensity in the prepontine space around the basilar artery that may be seen on some FLAIR images. The parameters on this FLAIR sequence at a different field strength were TR/TE/inversion pulse of 8,000/120/1,900.

ton density images. Fluid attenuated inversion recovery (FLAIR) has rapidly become the sequence of choice over proton density images, especially when evaluating cortical abnormalities. FLAIR imaging allows greater lesion-to-background contrast (Fig. 11-5). Marked improvement in lesion detection may result especially in the supratentorial region. T2 and FLAIR imaging, however, complement one another in the posterior fossa. FLAIR imaging is especially susceptible to patient motion. In addition, pulsation of the CSF may be seen as high signal intensity on these images. Attention to the foramen magnum, skull base, and prepontine cisterns, as well as the aqueduct of Sylvius and foramen

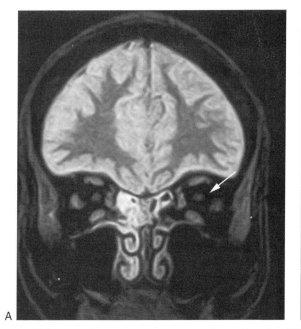
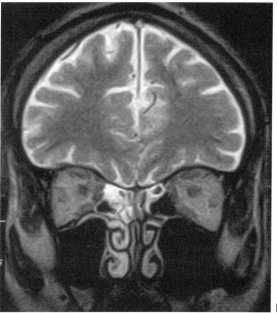

FIG. 11-7. Fat suppression versus fast spin-echo (FSE) techniques at lower field. **A:** A short tau inversion recovery (STIR) coronal image with a repetition time (TR)/echo time (TE) of 2,000/25 and inversion time of 100. Note that the normally bright signal intensity in the orbits is low signal intensity on this study (*arrow*). The subcutaneous fat is also lower signal intensity on this study. **B:** An FSE T2 coronal image (TR/TE 3,600/117) at the same level. The high signal intensity in the orbital fat and subcutaneous fat is demonstrated in contrast to the signal from these same areas on STIR imaging.

of Monro, is important. Hyperintensities on FLAIR images in these regions may be secondary to CSF flow and should not be confused with lesions (Fig. 11-6).

Fat-suppressed imaging is usually performed using inversion recovery sequences. Short tau inversion recovery is a sequence obtained after a preparatory 180-degree pulse is applied at the proper time before the routine spin-echo 90-degree and 180-degree refocusing pulse. With the proper time of inversion, one can obtain nullification of signal intensity from fat. This form of fat suppression is somewhat nonselective and unfortunately cannot effectively be used after contrast administration (Fig. 11-7). Comparison of T1 images pre- and postcontrast material is, as a result, the method of analysis at lower field strength. Subtraction techniques are possible on separate workstations but are not routinely performed by clinical radiologists. RF fat-suppression techniques are not yet possible with open MRI because of the very short separation of the fat and water excitation peaks at lower field strengths. The difference between the fat and the water peaks is related to the main field strength of the system. Very heavily T2-weighted images with very long TRs, on the order of 8,000 to 9,000 ms, and long TE are another way of obtaining very heavily T2-weighted images with less signal intensity from fat. These offer a type of fat-suppressed image. Fat and water separation imaging may play a role in the future.

One must optimize image quality by applying the principles and techniques discussed in this book. Knowing the underlying variables that influence the competing features of SNR, CNR, and spatial resolution will assist in designing sequences for brain imaging. Taking the time to understand and apply these techniques with open MRI will result in image quality that is optimal and diagnostic and in a study performed in a more patient-friendly environment.

BRAIN ANATOMY

Most MRI studies of the brain begin with a T1-weighted sagittal sequence, which allows excellent visualization of midline anatomic structures, such as the corpus callosum, pituitary gland, infundibulum, pineal gland, third ventricle, aqueduct of Sylvius, pons, quadrigeminal plate, fourth ventricles, and the cerebellar vermis, to name a few important structures (Fig. 11-8). Sagittal views off midline allow inspection of the temporal lobes, Sylvian fissures, and anatomic divisions between the frontal and parietal cortex and identification of the sensory motor strip. Sagittal FLAIR or T2-weighted images are helpful for the evaluation of signal changes in the corpus callosum that are present in patients with MS (7,8) (Fig. 11-9). Transverse (axial) T1-weighted, FLAIR, and T2-weighted images complete the routine evaluation of the brain. Very heavily T1-weighted images demonstrate cortical anatomy well. The spoiled gradient-echo sequences described earlier are very helpful in evaluation for cortical detail and developmental abnormalities and are routinely performed on all

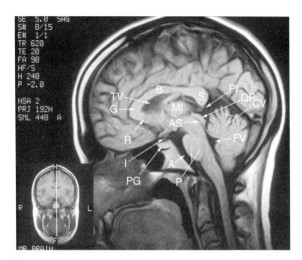

FIG. 11-8. A T1-weighted sagittal image demonstrating midline sagittal anatomy. The various portions of the corpus callosum shown include the rostrum (*R*), genu (*G*), body (*B*) and splenium (*S*), pituitary gland (*PG*), infundibulum (*I*), pineal gland (*PI*), third ventricle (*TV*), aqueduct of Sylvius (*AS*), pons (*P*), quadrigeminal plate (*QP*), fourth ventricle (*FV*), cerebellar vermis (*CV*), aqueduct of Sylvius prepontine space (*A*), and craniocervical junction.

brain studies in the author's open MRI practice. The ability to localize specific areas of the frontal, parietal, temporal, and occipital cortex assist in determining lesion location. The deep gray matter structures are also well demonstrated on heavily T1-weighted images. The contrast difference between gray and white matter can be shown at the level of the centrum semiovale, periventricular corona radiata, forceps major, and forceps minor. In addition, the anterior and posterior limbs of the internal capsule are identified. The caudate nucleus, to include the head and body, the globus pallidus, and putamen, is an easily recognizable structure (Fig. 11-10).

T2-weighted images depict fluid as high signal intensity, which allows evaluation of the ventricular system and CSF spaces. T2-weighted images also may demonstrate white matter fasciculi, which represent specialized white matter bundles in the brain (Fig. 11-11).

Midbrain images with T1 and T2 techniques demonstrate the midbrain cisterns (interpeduncular, crural, and ambient wing of the parimesencephalic cisterns), suprasellar cistern, and supracerebellar cisterns. T2 images show substantia nigra and red nucleus; however, because the effects of visualization of iron are field dependent, these structures are less conspicuous at lower field strength (Fig. 11-12). Cortical spinal tracts and the medial lemniscus can be seen in the posterior fossa, as can the inferior olive pyramid and inferior cerebellar peduncle. The middle cerebellar peduncles, cerebellar pontine angle cistern, internal auditory canal, cochlea, vestibule, cerebellar hemispheres, and superior cerebellar peduncles are also demonstrated with T2

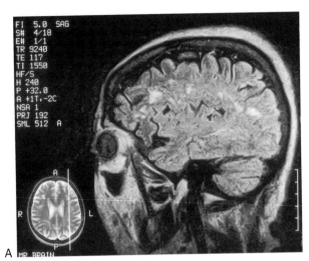
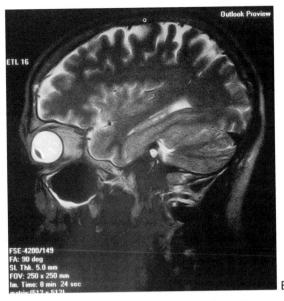

FIG. 11-9. Sagittal fluid attenuated inversion recovery (FLAIR) and T2-weighted images. **A:** A FLAIR image obtained off midline in a patient with multiple sclerosis demonstrating multiple subcortical and deep white matter areas of abnormal signal intensity. **B:** A high-resolution heavily T2-weighted FSE image with a 512 matrix, from a different patient, off midline obtained through the orbit and temporal lobe. Demonstration of portions of the inner ear structures are noted on this study as well.

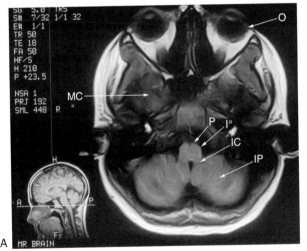
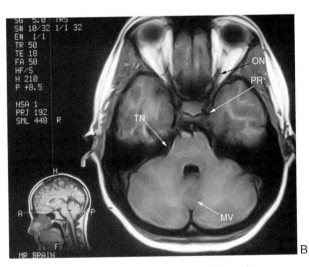

FIG. 11-10. T2 axial anatomy with a heavily T1-weighted spoiled gradient-echo sequence. **A:** Through the inferior medulla, one may see the pyramid (*P*), inferior olive (*I*^{O}), inferior cerebellar peduncles (*IC*), inferior portion of the cerebellum (*IP*), floor of the middle cranial (*MC*) fossa, and portions of the skull base and inferior orbits (*O*). **B:** The optic nerve (*ON*), pericavernous region (*PR*), trigeminal nerve (*TN*), portions of the temporal bone, middle cerebellar peduncles, and midline vermis (*MV*). *Continued.*

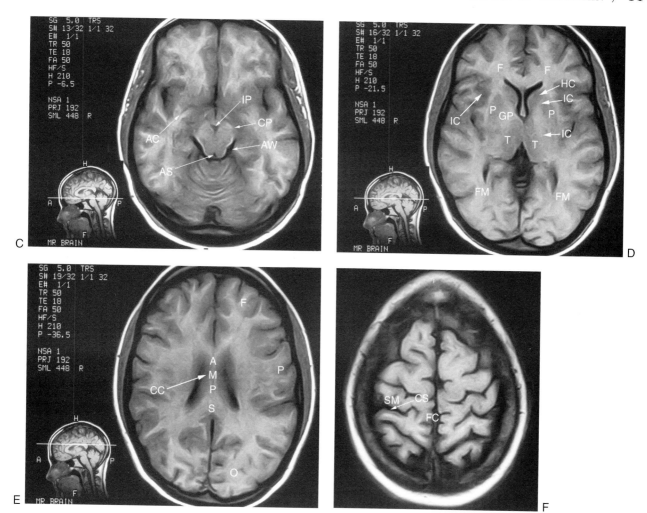

FIG. 11-10. *Continued.* **C:** An image obtained through the midbrain demonstrates portions of the anterior commissures (*AC*). The midbrain cisterns, the interpeduncular cistern (*IP*), crural portion (*CP*) of the perimesencephalic cistern, and the ambient wing (*AW*) of the perimesencephalic cistern are seen. The aqueduct of Sylvius (*AS*) is also demonstrated. **D:** An image obtained at the level of the third ventricles. The thalami (*T*), anterior and posterior limbs of the internal capsule (*IC; short arrow*), globus pallidus (*GP*), and putamen (*P*) are demonstrated. The head of the caudate (*HC*) is also noted. The forceps major (*FM*) and forceps minor (*F*) are seen. The insular cortex is demonstrated (*IC; long arrow*). **E:** Obtained at the level of the corpus callosum (*CC*). The anterior (*A*), mid (*M*), and posterior (*P*) bodies as well as the splenium (*S*) of the corpus callosum are well seen. The superior portion of the body of the lateral ventricles is noted. Portions of the frontal (*F*), parietal (*P*), and superior occipital (*O*) cortex are demonstrated. **F:** Obtained through the high parietal convexity. The sensory motor strip (*SM*), the central sulcus (*CS*), and the falx cerebri (*FC*) are noted.

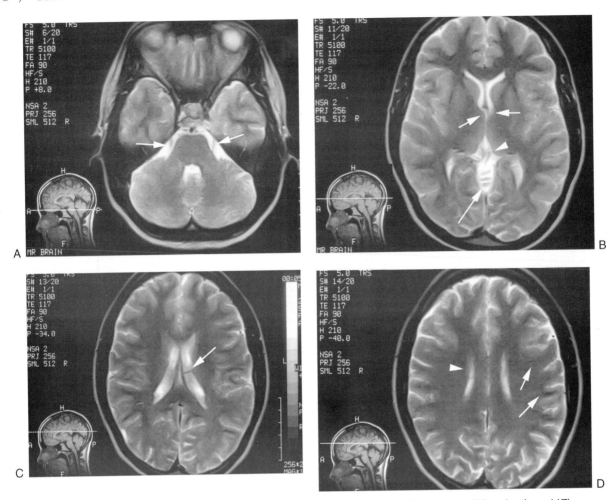

FIG. 11-11. T2-weighted anatomy on a fast spin-echo axial series (repetition time, 5,100; echo time, 117). **A:** Hyperintensity in the cerebrospinal fluid space in the prepontine region. The trigeminal nerve stands out in relief as it courses through the cerebrospinal fluid (*arrows*). The fourth ventricle is also demonstrated. **B:** Frontal horns of the lateral ventricles and the foramen of Monro (*arrows*): A small third ventricle is seen in this patient and normal trigones of the lateral ventricle. Internal cerebral veins are seen in the superior cerebellar cistern (*arrowhead*). The very tip of the vermis is also demonstrated on this study (*long arrow*). **C:** The superior body of the lateral ventricles. The thalamostriate vein traveling to meet the internal cerebral vein is seen on the left (*arrow*). The splenium of the corpus callosum is a prominent structure on this image. **D:** Through the superior portion of the corona radiata and inferior portion of the centrum semiovale: Differences in signal intensity in the subcortical white matter in the midparietal area are consistent with the superior longitudinal fasciculus (*arrows*). The superior orbital frontal fasciculus is a subtle structure on the right representing a more subtle linear area of lower signal intensity (*arrowhead*).

FIG. 11-14. ▸ Images through the orbits and periorbital area. **A:** A heavily T2-weighted coronal image demonstrating the optic nerve surrounded by cerebrospinal fluid (*arrows*). The intraconal fat is lower signal intensity because of how heavily T2 weighted this image is. The extraocular muscles are demonstrated. The subfrontal region and paranasal sinuses are seen as well. The olfactory sulcus is a prominent structure. **B:** A transverse T1-weighted image through the orbits in a patient who had had head trauma and a contusion along the medial temporal region. The patient also has a tentorial parafalcine subdural hematoma. The orbits, however, are well demonstrated. The extraocular muscles taper normally. The optic nerves are well seen. The suprasellar cistern is identified as well. **C:** A precontrast coronal image through the pituitary fossa in a patient with a large macroadenoma: The macroadenoma extends to the suprasellar cistern and compresses the optic chiasm. There is also abutment of the internal carotid arteries and the cavernous sinus bilaterally. **D:** A postcontrast image demonstrating the mass effect on the floor of the third ventricle and hypothalamus as well as the contour and extent of the lesion within the sella turcica and suprasellar region.

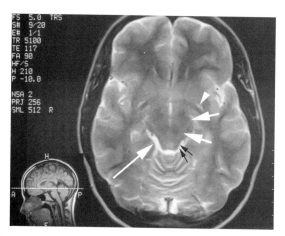

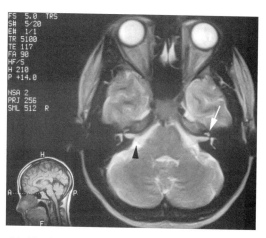

FIG. 11-12. T2 fast spin-echo axial image demonstrates very subtle low signal intensity in the red nuclei and substantia nigra (*arrows*). This illustrates the relative insensitivity to iron of lower field strength systems using spin-echo and fast spin-echo images. Gradient-echo imaging using T2* technique may increase the conspicuity of iron. Anatomic structures of interest on this image include the anterior commissures (*arrowhead*), the ambient wings of the perimesencephalic cistern (*long arrow*), the aqueduct of Sylvius, and the peri-aqueductal gray matter (*black arrows*).

FIG. 11-13. Fast spin-echo T2-weighted axial images through the temporal bone. The cochlear portions of the vestibule (*arrow*) and internal auditory canals are well visualized on this routine magnetic resonance image of the brain. The vestibulocochlear nerve (*arrowhead*) and cerebellopontine angle cisterns are seen as well.

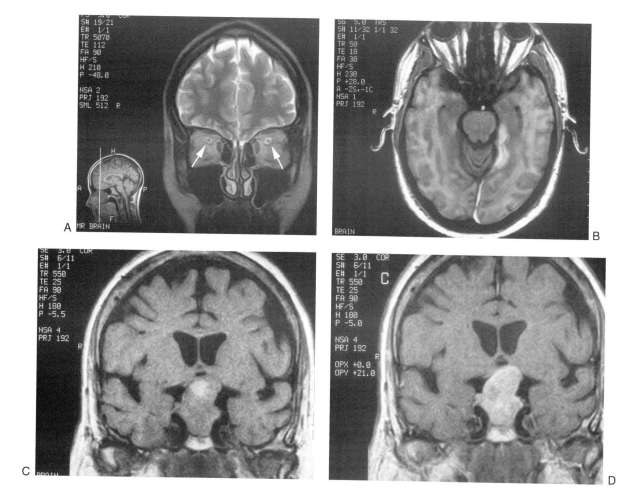

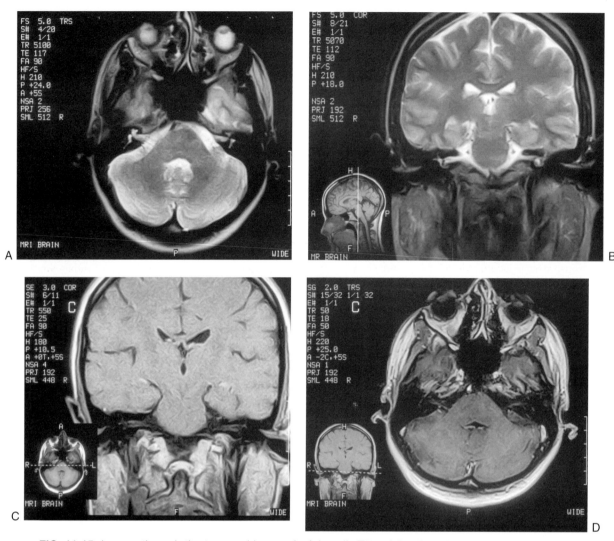

FIG. 11-15. Images through the temporal bones. **A:** A heavily T2-weighted routine image of the brain depicts the internal auditory canals, vestibulocochlear nerve, cochlea, and vestibule. This study was performed with a repetition time (*TR*)/echo time (*TE*) of 51,000/117 with 210 phase-encoding steps and 256 readout steps. **B:** A heavily T2-weighted routine brain coronal image showing the cerebellopontine angles, internal auditory canals, and semicircular canals. **C:** A 3-mm postgadolinium coronal image of the internal auditory canals. The vestibulocochlear nerves enhance slightly bilaterally, which is normal. A spin-echo technique with a TR/TE of 5,500/25 with a 3-mm slice. **D:** A transverse image through this same region using a thin-slice spoiled gradient-echo T1 technique. Performed with a TR/TE of 50/18 and a 50-degree flip angle. A volumetric study with a 2-mm slice.

techniques (Fig. 11-13). 3D FSE imaging of the internal auditory canals may demonstrate the vestibulocochlear nerves, cochlea, and vestibule to a great degree.

Imaging of the orbits, optic nerves, cavernous sinus, suprasellar cistern, hypothalamus, and third ventricle may be performed with coronal techniques (Fig. 11-14). High-resolution pre- and postcontrast images through the orbit and pituitary, as well as internal auditory canals, are performed routinely to evaluate patients with symptoms referable to these anatomic structures (Fig. 11-15).

BRAIN TUMORS

Approximately 1.1 million cancers are diagnosed in the United States each year. Of these cancer patients, more than 34,000 have tumors of the brain (9). Approximately one-half of these lesions originate within the brain tissue or its coverings, and the other half originate outside the brain and metastasize to the CNS (10). The tumors that originate within the brain are called *primary*, or *intrinsic*, brain tumors. Tumors that originate elsewhere and metastasize to

TABLE 11-3. *Brain tumors*

Intraaxial
    Metastasis
    Gliomas
        Astrocytomas—low grade
        Anaplastic
        Glioblastoma multiforme
        Oligodendroglioma
        Ependymoma
        Choroid plexus tumors—extraaxial versus intraaxial
    Ganglioglioma
    Desmoplastic infantile ganglioglioma
    Dysplastic gangliocytoma
    Central neurocytoma
    Neural ectodermal tumors
        Embryonal cell
        Medulloblastoma
    Pineal tumors
    Central nervous system lymphoma
    Hemangioblastoma
    Neuroblastoma
Extraaxial tumors
    Metastasis—dural
    Subarachnoid space
        Meningioma
        Schwannoma
        Epidermoid tumors
Dermoid tumors
Teratomas
Lipoma

This is a histologic classification of tumors broken down into those arising within the brain parenchyma and those arising in the brain coverings or outside the brain parenchyma.
From ref. 9, with permission.

the brain are termed *secondary*, or *metastatic*, tumors. Differentiating whether a tumor stems from brain parenchyma cells or from the cells of the brain coverings is difficult at times. However, imaging procedures may help determine the location of the origin of these tumors. If the tumor is located within cells of the brain tissue, the tumor is termed *intraaxial*. If the tumor arises from the brain coverings, the tumor is termed *extraaxial*. Tumors may also be classified according to whether they are above the tentorial membrane, in which case they are termed *supratentorial*, or below the tentorial membrane, in which case they are termed *infratentorial*. Tumors may also be classified by their histology or pathologic features (Table 11-3).

The goal of imaging is to determine the tumor size, shape, contour, signal characteristics, presence of hemorrhage, site of origin, and location in the brain. It is important to determine whether the tumor is supratentorial or infratentorial, intraaxial or extraaxial, and primary or metastatic to the brain. The ultimate goal is to predict the underlying histology of the lesion, which can only be confirmed on pathologic analysis. Digital imaging allows precise measurements of tumor dimension and volume. The border the tumor shares with adjacent brain has implications for its behavior. Supratentorial tumors are easily differentiated from those

that are infratentorial when imaging is obtained in all three planes. Determining whether a tumor is intraaxial or extraaxial may be difficult, and some features attributed to one category may overlap the other.

Tumors within the brain parenchyma (intraaxial) have the center of the tumor (sometimes termed the *epicenter*; however, this is a geologic term probably better suited to earthquakes) located within the brain tissue. These tumors distort the junction between the gray and white matter. The sulci of the brain are compressed. The brain and brain tissues infiltrated by intraaxial tumor are displaced outward, toward the skull.

Tumors that are located within the coverings of the brain or occur outside of the parenchyma (extraaxial) are centered outside the brain parenchyma, have a broad base relative to the skull or dura, push the gray/white junction toward the midline of the brain, and displace the cortex away from the mass. An interface forms between the tumor and the brain that may be associated with sulcal widening at the edges of extraaxial tumors. Extraaxial tumors may exhibit enhancement of the surrounding dura. These extraaxial tumors may also have cortical vessels situated between the mass and the adjacent brain (Fig. 11-16).

Histologic prediction based on imaging features is critical in helping to provide information needed for patient management. Extraaxial tumors tend to fall into three categories: (a) meningiomas, (b) metastasis, and (c) schwannoma. The schwannoma is discussed later, under Temporal Bone. Meningiomas are the most common extraaxial tumor and represent 15% of all intracranial neoplasms. Although many different histologic types of meningiomas exist, these tumors are usually benign, and the patient's prognosis is usually quite good after surgical resection (11). Meningiomas are dura-based lesions arising from the inner dural layer and may occur over the convexities, in the parafalcine region, sphenoid wings, cerebellopontine angle (CPA) cistern, subfrontal area, olfactory groove, and tentorium. Meningiomas may even occur within the ventricular system (12). Meningiomas tend to be isointense to gray matter on T1 and T2 pulse sequences. They have a sharply marginated border and a broad-based attachment to the dura (Fig. 11-17). These tumors enhance briskly after contrast material. Angiographically, this contrast enhancement pattern has earned these tumors the nickname of the "mother-in-law" or "unwanted guest" lesion, in which enhancement comes early and stays late. The enhancement is brisk, and, on postgadolinium images, even small meningiomas tend to be bright. Meningiomas frequently contain calcium, which is readily apparent on computed tomography (CT) but rarely seen on MR images. Calcification may be seen in 20% to 30% of meningiomas. Meningiomas may also have hemorrhage in approximately 5% of patients. Necrosis, however, is not common. Adjacent brain edema may vary from minimal to significant. Adjacent mass effect may vary as well (Fig. 11-18). Thickening of the adjacent skull is better demonstrated on CT. An en plaque, or thin flat variety, meningioma is occasionally seen. A "dural tail" is a common

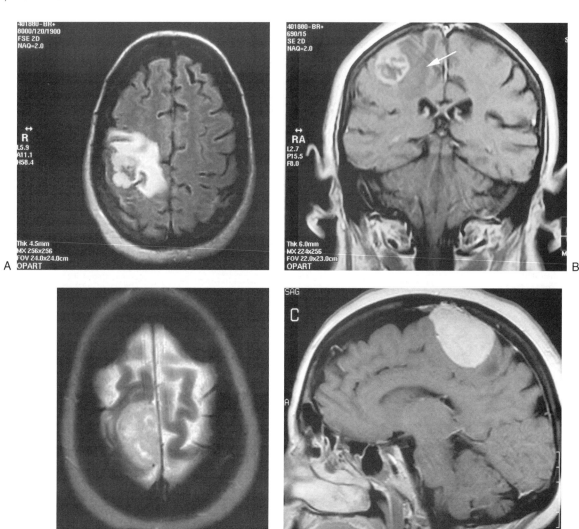

FIG. 11-16. Intraaxial versus extraaxial masses. **A:** A fluid attenuated inversion recovery axial image in a 56-year-old woman with renal cell cancer with metastatic disease demonstrates a mass centered at the gray/white junction characterized by the darker signal intensity surrounded by the hyperintensity of tumor edema. The gray/white junction is obliterated where the mass is located. The adjacent cortical sulci are somewhat compressed, and tumor infiltrates the surrounding brain tissue. **B:** A post–contrast-enhanced T1 coronal image demonstrates the center of the mass at the level of the gray white junction. The mass is large and abuts the brain cortex but does not have its attachment outside the brain substance. The edema on this image is low signal intensity, medial to the mass (*arrow*). **C:** A T2 axial image of an extraaxial mass: This mass is a parafalcine meningioma in a 58-year-old woman. The mass has a broad-based attachment to the falx. The mass pushes the brain cortex away and a small vessel characterized as a very dark punctate low signal region in the posterior medial aspect of the tumor is also pushed away from the interface between the tumor and the brain. **D:** An enhanced T1 sagittal image clearly demonstrates a meningioma, the interface between the tumor and the brain, and widening of the subarachnoid space anterior and posterior to the mass.

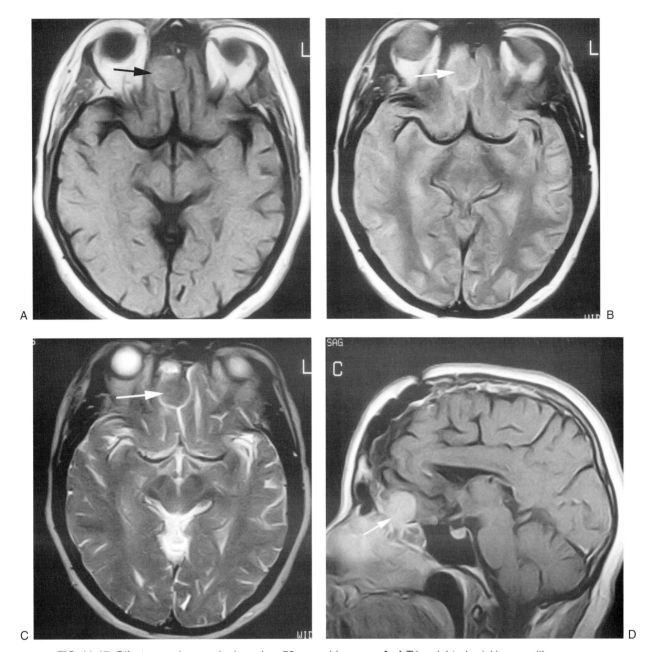

FIG. 11-17. Olfactory region meningioma in a 58-year-old woman. **A:** A T1-weighted axial image with a repetition time (TR)/echo time (TE) of 740/20. **B:** A proton density axial image with TR/TE 4,590/26. **C:** A T2-weighted axial image with TR/TE 4,590/120. The sharply marginated, rounded extraaxial mass is isointense to gray matter on all of these three sequences (*arrows*). **D:** A sagittal T1 image with TR/TE 620/20 demonstrates brisk enhancement of this subfrontal meningioma (*arrow*).

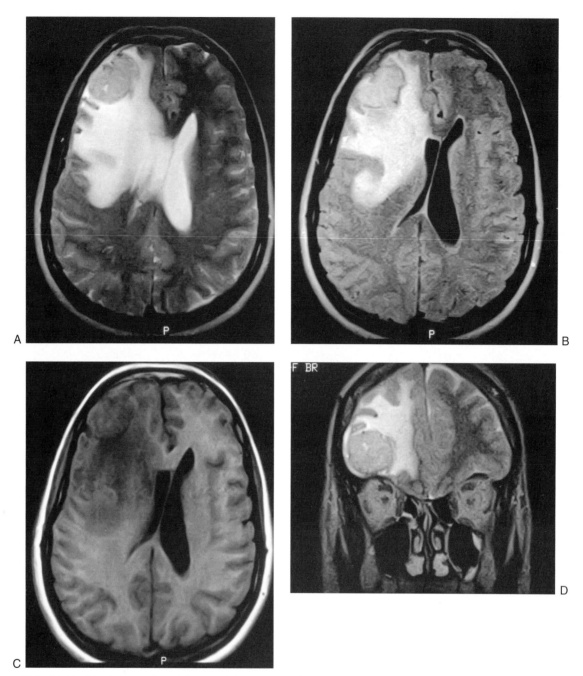

FIG. 11-18. Meningioma in a 52-year-old woman in the inferior frontal region of the anterior frontal fossa. **A:** A T2-weighted axial image, with a repetition time (TR)/echo time (TE) of 5,100/117, demonstrates the isointense extraaxial mass with significant adjacent edema and mass effect. **B:** A fluid attenuated inversion recovery axial image with TR/TE 9,500/117 and an inversion time of 1,550. The vasogenic edema surrounding the mass is more easily demarcated from the lateral ventricular surface. Left to right subfalcine shift is present. The septum pellucidum of the ventricle is markedly shifted off the midline. **C:** A T1 axial image using a spoiled gradient-echo technique with TR/TE 50/18 and a flip angle of 50 degrees. Edema is characterized by lower signal intensity that is not quite as low as cerebrospinal fluid. **D:** A coronal T2-weighted image with TR/TE 4,100/117 shows the extraaxial mass cortical vessels medially are deviated and superiorly displaced, demonstrating an interface between the tumor and adjacent brain. Vasogenic edema is hyperintense signal seen at this level.

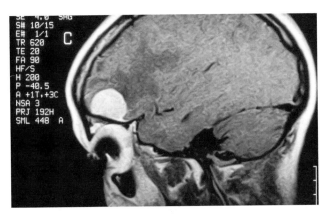

FIG. 11-19. T1 sagittal postgadolinium image demonstrates a frontal meningioma with a dural tail as a thin wisp of dural enhancement in the posteroinferior aspect of the tumor. This finding, initially thought to be a reliable indicator of meningioma, may be seen with a variety of extraaxial masses, such as metastatic disease, or even intraaxial masses that abut the inner table.

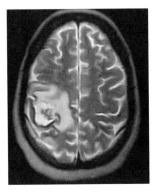

FIG. 11-20. The patient in this figure had renal cell metastasis (see Fig. 11-16). This T2-weighted image, however, has very low signal intensity along the brain cortex consistent with hemosiderin deposition. Hemosiderin can be seen on open magnetic resonance images and should be in the differential diagnosis for a low signal intensity band.

observation in meningiomas; however, other lesions of the dura may have a dural tail, and this finding is not specific for meningioma (Fig. 11-19). Some lesions that may be difficult to differentiate from meningiomas include cortical glioma, dural metastasis, or an intraaxial mass that abuts the inner table with a broad interface (13).

Extraaxial metastasis may originate in the dura or spread to the dura from a metastatic focus in the adjacent bone. Virtually any malignant tumor may metastasize to the skull and have an extraaxial component; however, the more common tumors to produce metastasis include lung, breast, and prostate cancer and melanoma (14). Breast and lung cancer are the two most common lesions to be associated with metastasis isolated to the dura. In young children, leukemia and neuroblastoma are the most common conditions to involve the dura. Metastases have a varying appearance on T1 and T2 images; however, usually these lesions are hypointense on T1 and hyperintense on T2 images. This difference in T2 contrast may help differentiate metastasis from meningioma. Contrast enhancement is usually brisk in extraaxial lesions.

Other extraaxial lesions include arachnoid cysts, epidermoids, dermoids, teratomas, and lipomas. Arachnoid cysts are benign lesions that form secondary to failure of fusion of the arachnoid membranes. These tumors account for 1% of all intracranial mass lesions and are usually asymptomatic observations by MRI. Frequent locations include the middle cranial fossa, parasellar cistern, Sylvian fissure, CPA, vermian area, and over the convexities. Arachnoid cysts are isointense to CSF on T1 and T2 images.

Epidermoids are congenital lesions that result from cellular rests of ectodermal elements becoming encapsulated during neural tube closure *in utero*. These lesions tend to insinuate themselves in the CSF spaces, predominantly in

the CPA cistern. They tend to be isointense with CSF on T1 and T2 images; however, hyperintensity occasionally is seen on T1 images, depending on the mucoproteinaceous component of the tumor. Dermoid tumors have a more complex histology than epidermoid tumors. Although similar in origin, the dermoid contains not only stratified squamous epithelium like the epidermoid tumors, but also hair, hair follicles, and sebaceous glands. Dermoids tend to have signal characteristics like lipid, which is hyperintense on T1 and less intense on T2 images. Fluid levels may also be seen. Teratomas may have fat, bone, teeth, and hair within the mass. The presence of these substances contributes to the signal characteristics observed by MRI.

Lipomas are congenital lesions usually found in the midline and are frequently associated with other congenital or developmental abnormalities. Lipomas are isointense to fat and therefore are hyperintense on T1 and exhibit lower signal intensity on T2 images. FSE, T2-weighted imaging may demonstrate a lower fat signal intensity, and, as a result, care must be exercised in interpreting FSE images of the lipid-containing lesions.

Intraaxial Neoplasms

Metastasis to the CNS represents spread of malignant cells outside the primary place of origin into the bloodstream with subsequent tumor emboli into the brain. Parenchymal metastatic tumors are frequently centered at the gray-white junction. Common tumors that metastasize to the brain are lung, breast, and renal cancer; melanoma; and tumors of the head and neck soft tissues. Hemorrhagic metastasis tends to be secondary to renal cell, anaplastic thyroid melanoma, and choriocarcinoma (Fig. 11-20). Solitary metastasis may be seen in 30% to 40% of cases; however, most metastasis usually presents in multiple locations (Fig. 11-21). In an adult, a solitary lesion in the posterior fossa is

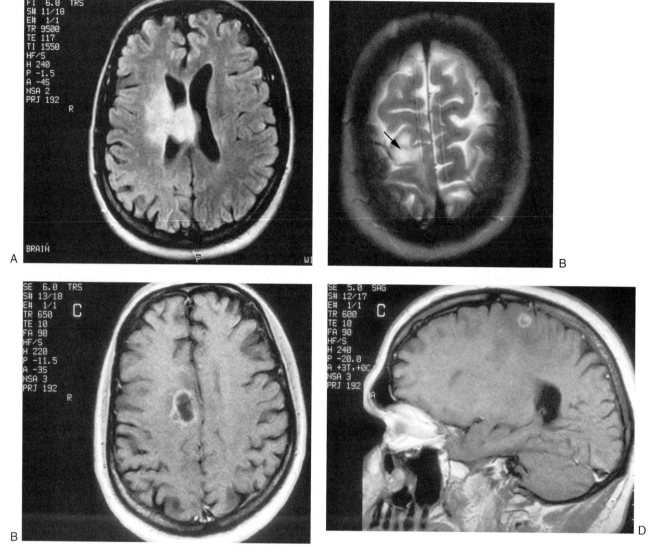

FIG. 11-21. Metastatic disease in a 50-year-old man with tonsillar carcinoma metastatic to the brain. **A:** A fluid attenuated inversion recovery axial image demonstrates abnormal signal intensity adjacent to the body of the right lateral ventricle. **B:** A T2-weighted axial image high over the convexity with subtle abnormality seen in the high frontal parietal cortex (*arrow*). **C:** A post–contrast enhancement T1-weighted axial image demonstrates a ring-enhancing abnormality at the level of the corpus callosum. **D:** T1-weighted coronal postgadolinium image shows a second lesion in the high parietal convexities—another a nodular ring-enhancing mass. Use of contrast material improves lesion conspicuity and detection.

most commonly secondary to metastasis. The most common tumor types to metastasize to the posterior fossa in an adult are lung and breast (Fig. 11-22) carcinoma.

Contrast enhancement improves lesion detection. MRI studies with the use of contrast material are superior to other modalities for detecting metastatic disease (15). Enhancement may be peripheral or diffuse, ringlike or nodular. The border may be thick, thin, nodular, or irregular. Enhancement may change depending on the type of treatment.

Primary brain tumors arise from cells found within the brain parenchyma. Gliomas of the brain are the most com-

mon and include astrocytomas, glioblastoma multiforme (GBM), oligodendroglioma, ependymoma, medulloblastoma, neuroblastoma, gangliocytoma, and ganglioglioma. Astrocytomas of the brain make up 25% to 30% of all gliomas. Glioblastomas account for 55% of all brain tumors, ependymomas and medulloblastomas for 6%, and oligodendrogliomas for 5%. The other histologic tumor types represent 2% or less of intracranial neoplasms. Certain tumors have a propensity for either supratentorial or infratentorial locations in the brain. In addition, the percentage of tumor types is different in children compared with adults. In chil-

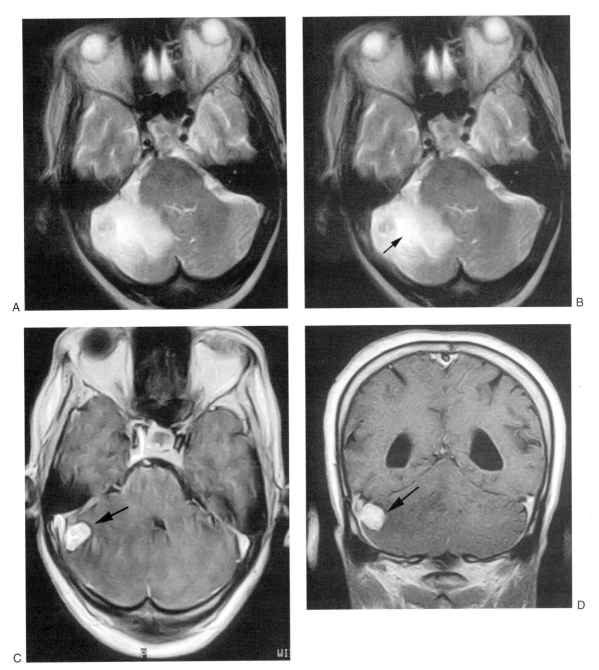

FIG. 11-22. A solitary metastasis in the posterior fossa of a 72-year-old woman with non–small cell lung carcinoma with metastasis to the brain. **A:** T2-weighted axial image. **B:** Fluid attenuated inversion recovery axial image demonstrates hyperintensity in the posterior fossa consistent with vasogenic edema. On the T2 image a subtle distinction exists between the tumor and the surrounding edema (*arrow*). After contrast administration, T1 axial **(C)** and coronal **(D)** images demonstrate a briskly enhancing intraaxial soft tissue mass that extends to the cortical edge (*arrows*).

dren, 60% to 70% of tumors occur infratentorially. In adults, the majority of tumors occur supratentorially.

The World Health Organization classification for brain tumors divides astrocytomas into low-grade astrocytoma, which appears as a low-signal abnormality on T1 images

and hyperintense on T2 images without necrosis, hemorrhage, or contrast enhancement (Fig. 11-23); anaplastic astrocytoma, which is low signal on T1, high signal on T2 images, and tends to enhance in a diffuse heterogeneous manner; and GBM. The GBM is the most aggressive and

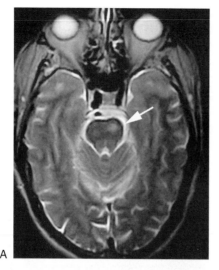

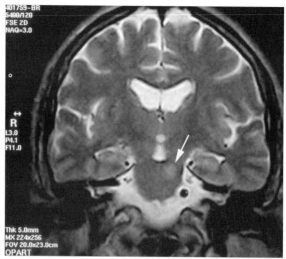

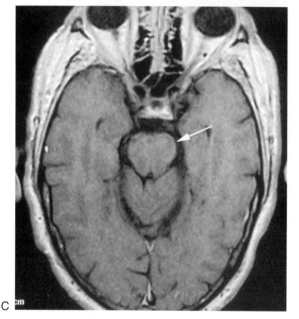

FIG. 11-23. A 55-year-old man with pupillary dilatation. **A:** T2-weighted axial image demonstrates abnormal signal intensity in the left upper pons in the pontomesencephalic junction (*arrow*). **B:** A heavily T2-weighted coronal image shows a subtle hyperintensity in this region (*arrow*). **C:** An axial image after the injection of intravenous contrast material. Note the mild mass effect in the upper pons (*arrow*) and no contrast enhancement in this region. The patient has no history of hypertension or diabetes. The absence of abnormality in the periventricular white matter eliminates suspicion of microvascular disease. This is the typical appearance of a pontine astrocytoma.

ominous of all gliomas: The mean 2-year survival rate for GBM is 10% to 15%. Russel and Rubenstein state that more than 50% of astrocytomas dedifferentiate into GBM (11). In fact, some maintain that the majority of GBMs may have begun as low-grade astrocytomas. GBMs have local mass effect, irregular borders, enhancing margins, and central necrosis (Fig. 11-24). The enhancement pattern varies from the nodular to ringlike or diffuse. Grading tumors based on these imaging features is not precisely accurate. Glioblastomas may cross the corpus callosum and have a butterfly-like appearance on imaging (Fig. 11-25). When these butterfly lesions are seen, the differential diagnosis is between lymphoma of the CNS and glioma. GBM may metastasize within the CNS, and multicentric GBM may be noted on MRI.

Oligodendrogliomas make up 4% to 5% of all gliomas. These tumors exhibit calcification in up to 50% of the cases. Calcification may be difficult to detect by MRI. These tumors are hyper- to isointense on T1 and hyperintense on T2-weighted images. Half of these tumors enhance with contrast material. Frontal and temporal lobe locations are the most frequent (Fig. 11-26), and the 5-year survival rate is 50% to 65%.

Ependymomas account for 1% to 3% of all primary brain tumors. They represent the third most common tumors in children, with astrocytoma and medulloblastoma first and second, respectively. Ependymomas arise from ependymal cells lining the ventricular system. Extraventricular rests of ependymal cells may be responsible for the parenchymal location of some ependymomas. These tumors are iso- to hypointense on

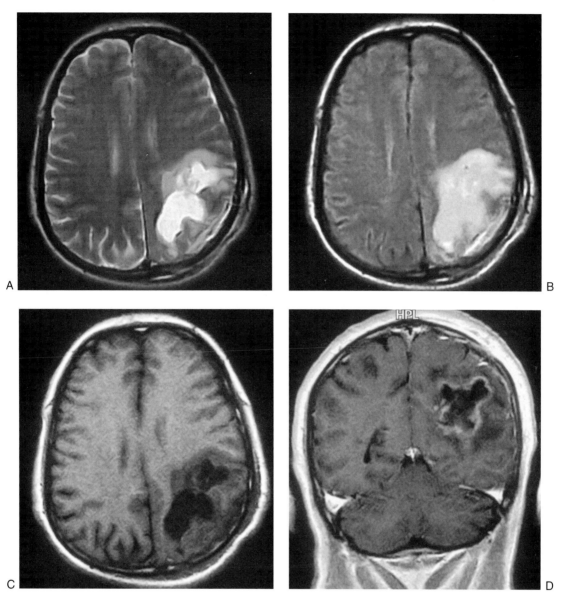

FIG. 11-24. Glioblastoma multiforme. **A:** A T2-weighted axial image demonstrates a heterogeneous lobulated mass with solid and cystic components. **B:** A fluid attenuated inversion recovery axial image shows vasogenic edema and mass effect on the posterior aspect of the left lateral ventricle. **C:** A T1-weighted axial image without contrast administration shows the heterogeneous nature of this cystic and solid mass. **D:** A coronal T1-weighted image after contrast administration shows the necrotic mass.

T1 and hyperintense on T2 images, and they usually enhance after contrast administration. Ependymomas metastasize in the CSF in 5% to 13% of cases. The 5-year survival rate in patients with ependymomas ranges from 37% to 64%.

Gangliogliomas are rare tumors, representing 0.3% to 1.3% of primary brain tumors. These tumors most frequently involve the cerebral hemispheres. They have cystic changes in 30% to 50% of cases, 30% may calcify, and the MRI appearance varies because of these factors.

Medulloblastomas account for 12% to 25% of infratentorial tumors in childhood. A more precise term for these tumors is *primitive neural ectodermal tumors*. In adults, this tumor accounts for 6% to 8% of all primary tumors. In children, the tumor usually presents as a posterior fossa mass involving the vermis and fourth ventricle. In adults, the tumors may appear in the cerebellum, somewhat lateral to the midline. Medulloblastomas appear hypo- to isointense on T1 and hyperintense on T2-weighted images. Calcifica-

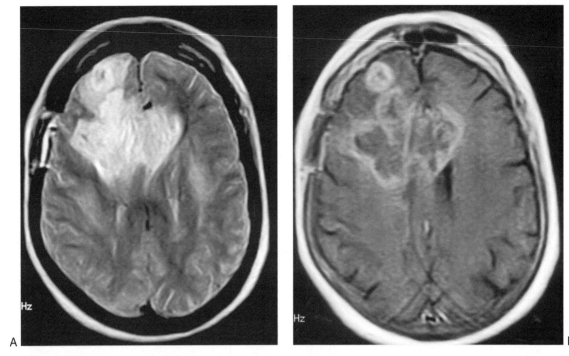

FIG. 11-25. A: An axial proton density image in a 71-year-old man with a butterfly glioma of the corpus callosum. **B:** A post–gadolinium-enhanced axial T1 image demonstrates involvement of the right and left portions of the corpus callosum. The differential diagnosis in this case would include lymphoma.

tion may be present, and these masses enhance to a variable degree. Up to 7% of medulloblastomas metastasize outside the CNS to the bone, lymphatic, peritoneum, liver, and lungs (9). In some groups of patients with medulloblastoma, a survival rate of up to 95% may be obtained.

An incomplete list of pineal region tumors includes primary parenchymal tumor, such as pineocytoma or pineoblastoma; germ cell tumors; teratomas; choriocarcinomas; and dermoid, epidermoid, and pineal cysts. Germ cell tumors are the most common pineal region tumors in Japan, accounting for 5% to 15% of all childhood intracranial tumors there. This tumor, however, accounts for only 0.4% to 3.4% of all intracranial tumors in the west. Pineocytomas are the least aggressive primary pineal tumor. Pineoblastomas are included in the category of embryonal cell tumors and represent aggressive tumors that may metastasize.

Lymphoma may involve the brain as a primary lesion or as metastatic disease. Primary CNS lymphoma represents 0.3% to 2.0% of all primary intracranial tumors. These tumors are hypercellular and may appear mildly hyperintense on T1 images. These lesions appear hyperintense on T2 images as well, and marked contrast enhancement occurs in the majority of cases.

Hemangioblastomas are found in the cerebellum in the majority of tumors; however, these tumors represent only 1% of all intracranial tumors. The MRI appearance is iso- to hypointense on T1 images and hyperintense on T2 images, with a nodule or ring-enhancing pattern noted after contrast administration. Hemangioblastomas may be seen in patients

with von Hippel–Lindau (VHL) disease. Forty-five percent to 60% of patients with VHL may have hemangioblastomas. However, not all patients with hemangioblastomas have VHL. Twenty percent to 30% of patients with hemangioblastomas are found to have VHL.

Congenital or Developmental Lesions of the Brain

A detailed discussion of congenital or developmental lesions of the brain is outside the scope of this text. The reader is referred to basic neuroradiology texts for detailed descriptions of these lesions (16–19). Cortical malformations may occur secondary to abnormalities in brain development during the stages of cellular proliferation, cellular migration to the developing cortex, and cortical organization. See Table 11-4 for a list of congenital abnormalities based on disorders of various stages of development. Cellular proliferation abnormality may result in hemimegalocephaly, focal cortical dysplasia, tuberous sclerosis, hamartomas, and gangliogliomas (20). Disorders of cortical migration include band heterotopias, lissencephaly, marginal glioneuronal heterotopia, and nodular cortical dysplasia (20). Cortical organization disorders include polymicrogyrii, schizencephaly, and cortical dysplasia with band lesions.

The anatomic appearance of congenital malformation of the CNS can be well imaged on open MRI systems. However, patients with abnormalities referable to congenital or developmental lesions are usually imaged in the hospital set-

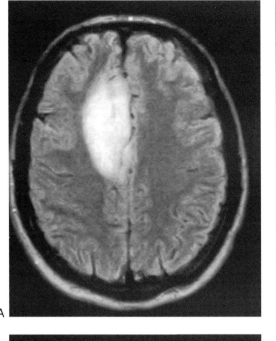

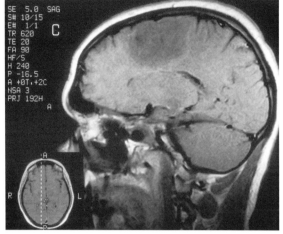

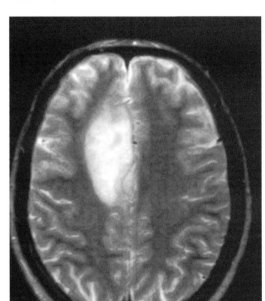

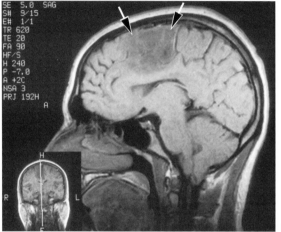

FIG. 11-26. A: A hyperintensity in the right posterior frontal region in this 45-year-old man on a fluid attenuated inversion recovery axial image. **B:** A sagittal T1 image without contrast demonstrates the low signal intensity in the posterior frontal region. **C:** A T2-weighted (axial) image shows mild heterogeneity within the tumor, which abuts the midline. This mass is located intraaxially. **D:** After contrast administration, no abnormal contrast enhancement of this oligodendroglioma (*arrows*) is seen. A computed tomographic scan (not shown) of this area demonstrated no calcifications.

ting. As more and more open MRI units are found within the hospital setting, more case material on patients with congenital abnormalities may be seen. In outpatient clinical practice, congenital malformations tend to comprise the minority of referrals for scanning. Patients are scanned in high-field university-based MR systems initially. Follow-up imaging may be performed at an open MRI facility. No technical or clinical limitations exist to performing imaging studies of the pediatric brain in open systems. Representative examples of CNS malformation are provided to illustrate the capabilities of open systems in the evaluation of CNS malformations (20) (Figs. 11-27 through 11-30).

Hydrocephalus

Hydrocephalus is manifested by ventricular dilatation; it represents an obstruction at some level to the normal flow of CSF from its site of origin in the choroid plexus in the lateral third and fourth ventricles through the ventricular system into the subarachnoid space with subsequent absorption through the arachnoid granulations over the convexities. Obstruction may occur at the foraminal outlets of the lateral ventricle, foramen of Monro, the aqueduct of Sylvius, the outlet of the atria of the lateral ventricle, the outlets of the fourth ventricular system (foramen of Luschka or the foram-

TABLE 11-4. *van der Knaap and Valk classification of congenital cerebral, cerebellar, and spinal malformations*

Disorder type	Gestational time of onset
Disorders of dorsal induction	
Primary neurulation	3–4 wk
Cranioschisis (anencephaly, cephalocele)	
Rachischisis (myelocele, myelo-meningocele, Chiari malformation, hydromyelia)	
Secondary neurulation	4 wk to postnatal
Myelocystocele	
Diastematomyelia	
Diplomyelia	
Meningocele	
Lipomeningocele	
Lipoma	
Dermal sinus	
Tight filum terminale	
Neurenteric anomalies	
Caudal regression syndrome	
Disorders of ventral induction	5–10 wk
Holoprosencephaly	
Septooptic dysplasia	
Agenesis of septum pellucidum	
Cerebral hemiatrophy/hemihypoplasia	
Hypoplasia/aplasia of cerebellar hemispheres	
Hypoplasia/aplasia of cerebellar vermis	
Dandy-Walker syndrome	
Craniosynostosis	
Diencephalic cyst	
Disorders of neuronal proliferation, differentiation, and histogenesis	2–6 wk
Micrencephaly	
Megalencephaly	
Unilateral megalencephaly	
Aqueductal anomalies	
Colpocephaly	
Porencephaly	
Multicystic encephalopathy	
Hydranencephaly	
Disorders of histogenesis	
Neurocutaneous syndromes	
Tuberous sclerosis	
Sturge-Weber syndrome	
von Hippel–Lindau disease	
Neurofibromatoses	
Vascular malformations	
Malformative tumors	
Disorders of sulcation and migration	2–5 wk
Agyria/pachygyria	
Lissencephaly	
Polymicrogyria	
Schizencephaly	
Neuronal heterotopias	
Hypoplasia/aplasia of corpus callosum	
Myelination disorders	7 mo to 2 yr
Hypomyelination, retarded myelination	
Secondarily acquired injury of normally formed structures	
Encephaloclastic hydranencephaly	
Encephaloclastic porencephaly	
Encephaloclastic schizencephaly	
Encephaloclastic multicystic encephalopathy	
Hydrocephalus secondary to aqueductal stenosis	
Hemorrhage and infarction	
Unclassified	
Arachnoid cysts	

Adapted and modified from van der Knapp MS, Valk J. Classification of congenital abnormalities of the CNS. *AJNR Am J Neuroradiol* 1988;9:315; and ref. 19.

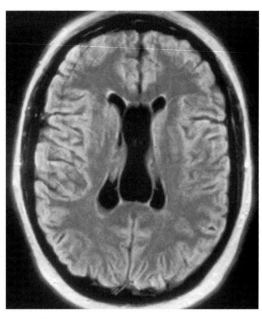

FIG. 11-27. This T1 axial image demonstrates a cavum septum pellucidum and cavum vergae in a 29-year-old woman. This asymptomatic observation represents lack of fusion of the arachnoid of the septum pellucidum. This is a normal anatomic variant.

ina of Magendie), along the subarachnoid space, or at the arachnoid granulations. *Communicating* hydrocephalus refers to conditions in which CSF is able to egress the ventricular system but cannot escape the subarachnoid space. *Noncommunicating* hydrocephalus describes conditions in which CSF cannot egress the ventricular system.

Communicating Hydrocephalus

Communicating hydrocephalus usually results from obstruction at the level of the arachnoid granulations over the superior meninges. Dilatation of the lateral ventricle temporal horns, rounding or dilatation of the anterior third ventricle, and fourth ventricular dilatation are present in the face of normal or compressed cortical sulci. Abnormal signal intensity on FLAIR and T2-weighted images around the lateral ventricles may be seen with communicating or noncommunicating hydrocephalus and reflects impaired absorption of the CSF in the ventricular system or "transependymal resorption" of CSF. Balanced or well-compensated hydrocephalus may have no abnormal signal intensity around the ventricular system despite marked ventricular dilatation (Fig. 11-31). The pressure within the ventricular system cannot be objectively ascertained by MRI. Measurement of the CSF opening pressure after lumbar or direct ventricular puncture is the only truly objective way to confirm increased intraventricular pressure. However, MRI of hydrocephalus can assist in measuring the ventricular size, shape, and contour as well as

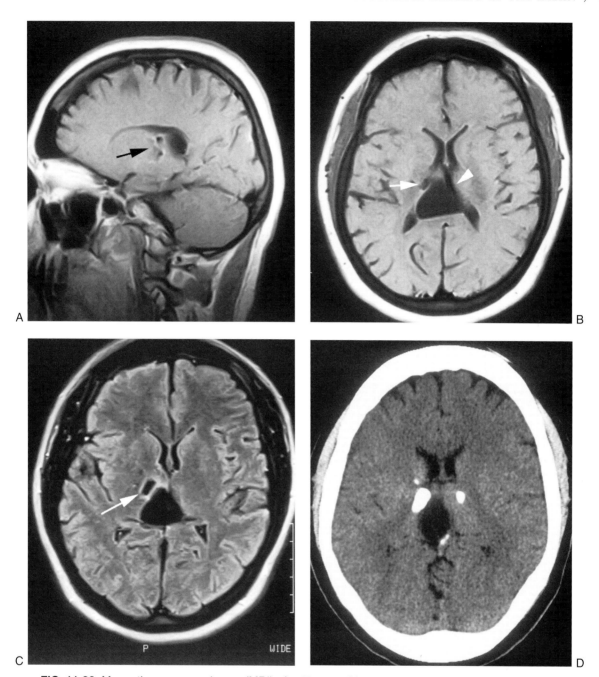

FIG. 11-28. Magnetic resonance image (MRI) of a 43-year-old woman who was born 2 months prematurely. The patient had germinal matrix hemorrhages that have resolved. The patient had this MRI for headaches. **A:** A slightly off-midline T1 sagittal image demonstrates focal abnormalities in the thalamus (*arrow*) and a cerebrospinal fluid signal intensity above the internal cerebral veins representing a cavum velum interpositum. **B:** A T1-weighted axial image shows low signal intensity in the right thalamus (*arrow*) and the internal cerebral veins being displaced somewhat inferiorly and to the left (*arrowhead*). **C:** A fluid attenuated inversion recovery axial image demonstrates low signal intensity in the medial aspect of the right thalamus (*arrow*). **D:** A computed tomographic (CT) image shows calcifications in the regions of the thalamus and terminal matrix. This illustrates the difficulty in detecting calcification by MRI. Low signal is seen on the right on the MR images; however, no signal change on the left is identified by MRI. The calcifications are easily identified by CT on the left and right sides. The calcifications are the sequelae of hemorrhage and ischemia in the perinatal period.

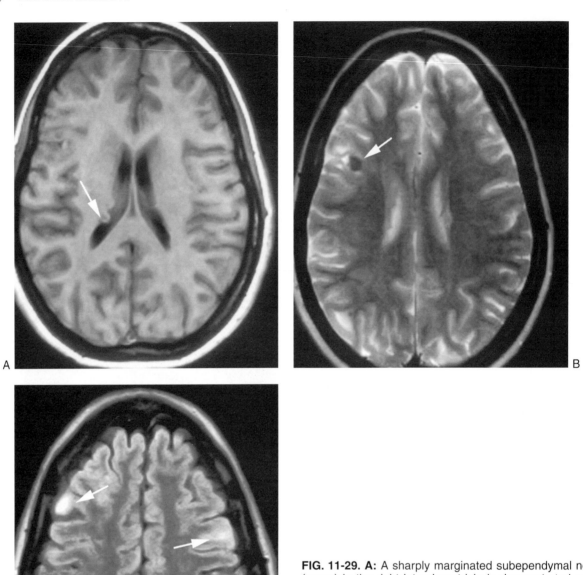

A

B

C

FIG. 11-29. A: A sharply marginated subependymal nodule (*arrow*) in the right lateral ventricle is demonstrated on this T1-weighted axial image. **B:** An axial T2-weighted image exhibits a low signal intensity hamartomatous lesion in the right frontal subcortical area (*arrow*). **C:** Fluid attenuated inversion recovery imaging demonstrates multiple focal hyperintensities in the cortical and subcortical areas consistent with band hypertropias (*arrows*) in this patient with tuberous sclerosis (TS). TS is a familial phacomatosis with multisystem involvement. This patient had seizures and adenoma sebaceum and was intellectually challenged—consistent with the classical clinical triad for TS.

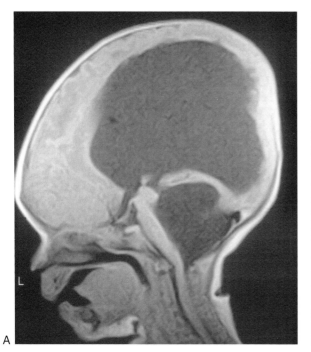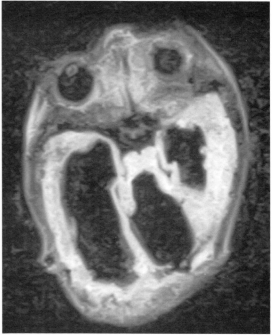

A

B

FIG. 11-30. A 1-week-old infant with abnormal head size. **A:** A sagittal T1-weighted image in the midline demonstrates a markedly dilated fourth ventricle, agenesis of the inferior vermis, and massive hydrocephalus, which are features seen in the Dandy-Walker malformation. The best concept explaining the etiology of this malformation is that of impaired permeability of the fourth ventricle with subsequent vermian dysgenesis. This is a disorder of ventral induction that occurs between 5 and 10 weeks' gestation. **B:** A T1-weighted axial image demonstrates the markedly dilated fourth ventricle as well as the massive dilation of the temporal horns of the lateral ventricles.

allow visualization of the anatomy of the ventricles and CSF spaces.

Noncommunicating Hydrocephalus

Aqueduct stenosis is the most common form of noncommunicating hydrocephalus and may be developmental or acquired (Fig. 11-32). Developmental hydrocephalus may be diagnosed *in utero* by ultrasound evaluations. Early shunting of the ventricular system allows optimum brain development without the pressure effects of the expanded ventricular system on the adjacent brain. Acquired aqueduct stenosis may result from previous subarachnoid hemorrhage from meningitis. Other forms of noncommunicating hydrocephalus may result from tumors, abscesses, or hemorrhagic lesions that compress the outlets of the ventricular system.

WHITE MATTER DISEASE

Lesions and abnormalities of the white matter stem from many diverse etiologies. MRI is a very sensitive but nonspecific tool, especially when it comes to evaluating diseases of the white matter. Some features of white matter disease tend to narrow the differential diagnosis. The discussion of each

entity is beyond the scope of this text, and the interested reader is referred to basic neuroradiology and neurology texts for further investigation. An organized approach or a systematic classification, however, is absolutely necessary when discussing the diverse categories of white matter disease. Classification of disease based on the underlying metabolic disorder may be helpful (Table 11-5) (21). This approach, however, includes diseases of white matter, gray matter, and those that affect both structures. Classification according to patient age provides some order in analyzing MR images. A simplified discussion of white matter disease based on whether myelin forms normally and is subsequently destroyed (demyelinating disease) versus abnormal formation of myelin (dysmyelination) is popular and follows.

Demyelinating Diseases

Demyelinating diseases are those entities in which myelin is formed normally and then destroyed by a variety of causes. This set of diseases may be subdivided into primary demyelinating disease, in which no etiology is yet known, and secondary demyelinating disease, in which the cause of demyelination is relatively certain (Table 11-6).

MS is by far the most common demyelinating disease imaged in open MRI. The diagnosis of MS is based on clinical signs and symptoms and neurologic deficits separated in

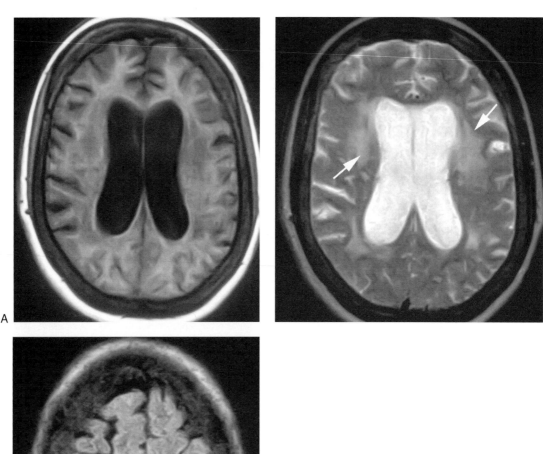

A

B

C

FIG. 11-31. Balanced or well-compensated normal-pressure hydrocephalus in 66-year-old woman with confusion, gait disturbance, and incontinence. These symptoms are the classic clinical triad for normal-pressure hydrocephalus. **A:** An axial T1-weighted image demonstrates the appearance of the dilated lateral ventricles. **B:** An axial T2-weighted image demonstrates no ring of hyperintensity around the ventricular surface, which is inconsistent with transependymal flow of cerebrospinal fluid. Severe small vessel white matter disease lesions are seen in the deep and subcortical white matter (*arrows*). **C:** Axial fluid attenuated inversion recovery imaging through the right parietal convexity demonstrates no sulcal widening. This mismatch between the ventricular size and sulcal size is not consistent with global atrophy.

time and space. MRI, however, plays a critical role in the evaluation of patients thought to have MS and in patients with known disease. The MRI finding of three or more lesions in the periventricular white matter represents a typical imaging presentation (Fig. 11-33). This disease occurs in patients of virtually any age, but it is most common in patients 20 to 50 years old. However, more than 10% of patients presenting with MS may be older than 55 years. MS lesions may involve any region of the brain, but are most common in the periventricular white matter, especially in the white matter of the atrium and occipital horns; corpus callosum; optic nerves; apparatus; chiasm; and posterior fossa. MS may also involve the spinal cord, with the cervical spine most commonly affected (Fig. 11-34). MS lesions are generally hypointense on T1 and hyperintense on proton density,

FLAIR, and T2-weighted images. Pathognomonic ovoid lesions occurring in the periventricular region represent demyelinating plaques following periventricular radial veins and are termed *Dawson's fingers* (Fig. 11-35). Chronic lesions tend to have low signal on T1 images similar to CSF and have the appearance of microcystic encephalomalacia. Contrast enhancement illustrates lesions associated with breaks in the blood–brain barrier. Correlation of enhancement with disease activity has been suggested; however, this has not been confirmed, and many enhancing lesions do not have associated neurologic symptoms. Enhancement is usually nodular or ringlike in nature. Involvement of the corpus callosum is extremely helpful in differentiating MS from periventricular microvascular disease, which is commonly seen in the older population. The corpus callosum may

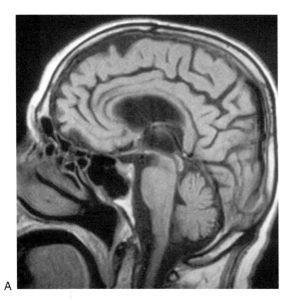

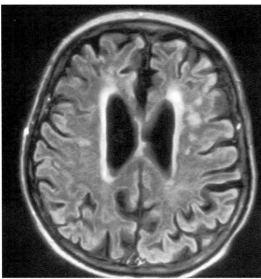

FIG. 11-32. Obstructive hydrocephalus. **A:** This sagittal T1-weighted image demonstrates an enlarged third ventricle with bowing of the corpus callosum. However, the fourth ventricle is of normal size. **B:** An axial fluid attenuated inversion recovery image demonstrates enlarged lateral ventricles with a ring of hyperintensity along the ventricle surface consistent with transependymal flow of cerebrospinal fluid.

TABLE 11-5. *Common causes of white matter disease*

Peroxisomal disorders
  X-linked adrenoleukodystrophy
  Neonatal adrenoleukodystrophy
  Zellweger's syndrome
Lysosomal disorders
  Lipidosis
    Krabbe's disease (globoid cell leukodystrophy)
    Metachromatic leukodystrophy
    Fabry's disease
    Tay-Sachs disease
    Niemann-Pick disease
    Gaucher's disease
  Mucopolysaccharidoses
    Type I Hurler's
    Type II Hunter's
    Type III San Filippo
    Type IV Morquio
    Type VI Maroteaux-Lamy
Mitochondrial disorders
  Leigh disease (subacute necrotizing leukoencephalopathy)
  Kearns-Sayre syndrome
  Mitochondrial myopathy encephalopathy lactic acidosis strokes
  Myoclonic epilepsy with ragged red cell fibers
  Wilson's disease (?)
Aminoacidopathies/aminoacidurias
  Aminoacidopathies
    Phenylketonuria (enzyme defect)
    Tyrosinemia
    Maple syrup urine disease
    Homocystinuria
    Methylmalonic acidemia
    Glutaric acidemia type I
  Aminoaciduria
    Oculocerebrorenal (Lowe's) syndrome (transport defect)
Primary white matter disorders
  Alexander's disease
  Canavan's disease
  Pelizaeus-Merzbacher disease
  Cockayne disease
Differential diagnosis
  Hypoxia-ischemia—periventricular leukomalacia
  Acute disseminated encephalomyelopathy
  Demyelination
  Progressive multifocal leukoencephalopathy
  Infection—acquired immunodeficiency syndrome
  Therapy—radiation, methotrexate
  Carbon monoxide poisoning

From ref. 21, with permission.

become atrophic in a focal or diffuse manner. The abnormal hyperintensities seen in the corpus callosum in MS are unusual in patients with small vessel disease. As a result of this observation, especially in older patients suspected of having MS, sagittal T2-weighted or FLAIR imaging is necessary. Additionally, lesions tend to be smaller than 1 cm; however, a tumefactive variety of MS may have large lesions that mimic neoplasia.

The cervical spinal cord is the most common cord segment involved with MS. Two percent to 20% of patients with cervical lesions due to MS may have normal MRI stud-

ies of the brain. Follow-up MRI allows documentation of the ebb and flow of this disease process, which is multiphasic and can remit and relapse or be relentlessly progressive. Other conditions in the differential diagnosis of MS include sarcoid, small vessel disease, Lyme disease, and migraine-related white matter disease.

Establishing the diagnosis of the secondary demyelinating diseases may rest on the patient's clinical context. The lesions associated with these entities tend to be hypointense on T1 imaging and hyperintense on proton density, FLAIR, and T2-weighted images. Clinical history and lesion loca-

TABLE 11-6. *Categories of demyelinating disease*

Primary demyelinating disease
    Multiple sclerosis
Secondary demyelinating disease
    Acute disseminated encephalomyelitis
    Progressive multifocal leukoencephalopathy
    Subacute sclerosing panencephalitis
    Acquired immunodeficiency syndrome
    Disseminated necrotizing leukoencephalopathy
    Subcortical atherosclerotic encephalopathy
    Binswanger's disease
    Central pontine myelinolysis
    Radiation changes
    Drugs, alcohol, and toxins

tion may help to focus the radiographic interpretation. Acute disseminated encephalomyelitis is a postviral monophasic cell-mediated response to a primary viral infection. It has been seen in association with measles, varicella, and other viruses, and it represents immune complex deposition in the white matter. These lesions may improve or completely regress with time.

Progressive multifocal leukoencephalopathy is a demyelinating disease caused by the human JC SV40 papovavirus. Up to 65% of the population is exposed to this virus by adolescence. This entity is manifest in the immunocompromised state seen in acquired immunodeficiency syndrome, immunosuppressant therapy for transplant treatment, lymphoma, or end-stage renal disease. Lesions may be focal or diffuse, and they frequently have a cotton-wool appearance. Lesions also tend to be peripheral in the white matter and more posteriorly located.

The differential diagnosis for vascular white matter disease includes a spectrum of entities including dilated Virchow-Robin spaces, small vessel ischemic-gliotic change, lacunar infarctions, and subcortical atherosclerotic encephalopathy. Binswanger's disease is a progressive dementia affecting older men and women associated with hypertension, lacunar infarctions, and predominant white matter involvement with gray matter sparing.

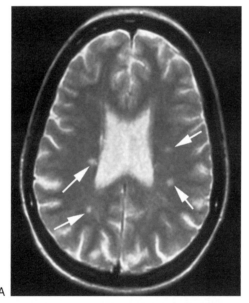

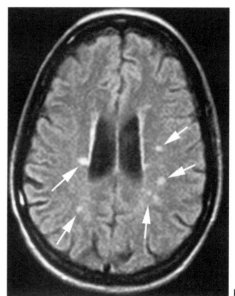

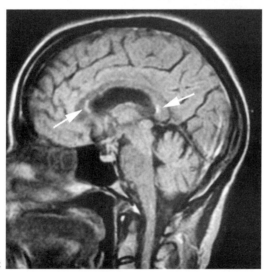

FIG. 11-33. A: Periventricular punctate areas of abnormal increased signal intensity (*arrows*) are seen on this T2-weighted axial image in this patient with a known diagnosis of multiple sclerosis. **B:** An axial fluid attenuated inversion recovery (FLAIR) image demonstrates focal hyperintensities (*arrows*) in the periventricular and supraventricular regions, some of which are punctate. **C:** A sagittal FLAIR image shows abnormal increased signal intensity in genu and splenium of the corpus callosum (*arrows*). These findings in the corpus callosum are characteristic of demyelinating disease and are not found in microvascular disease.

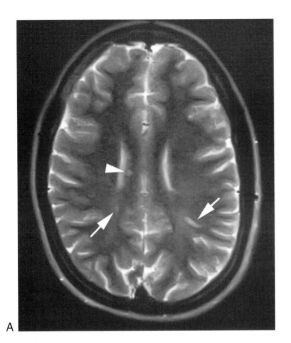

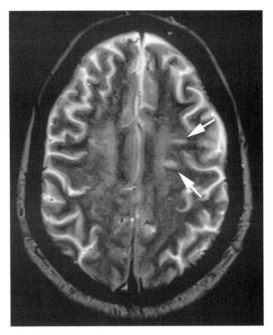

FIG. 11-35. This axial T2-weighted image in a patient with multiple sclerosis demonstrates periventricular linear and ovoid lesions consistent with the appearance of Dawson's fingers (*arrows*).

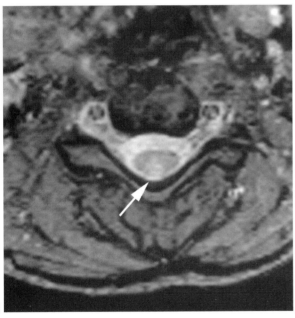

FIG. 11-34. Multiple sclerosis (MS) in a 32-year-old woman. **A:** The T2-weighted axial image demonstrates a lesion in the corpus callosum (*arrowhead*) and a subtle lesion in the right and left occipital white matter (*arrows*). **B:** A transverse image obtained through the cervical spinal cord at the C3 level. Posteriorly located low signal intensity is identified and is consistent with an MS plaque involving the cervical spinal cord (*arrow*).

wedge-shaped appearance of the demyelinating area in the midpons presents as hyperintensity on T2-weighted images.

Drugs such as cocaine and heroin, chemotherapy such as methotrexate and cyclosporine, and toxins such as lead and hexachlorophene are an incomplete list of agents associated with white matter lesions. The history of exposure helps establish the proper diagnosis. Trauma- and radiation-induced white matter disease should be in the differential diagnosis in the proper clinical setting.

Disseminated necrotizing leukoencephalopathy may result from radiation treatment and intrathecal methotrexate administration. This was first demonstrated in children being treated for leukemia; however, this disease entity may be seen with other forms of chemotherapy and radiation treatment regimes in children or adults. The features tend to represent hyperintensity in the periventricular white matter on proton density, FLAIR, and T2-weighted images as patchy diffuse matter.

Dysmyelinating Diseases

Dysmyelinating diseases are conditions associated with the abnormal formation of myelin. Individuals tend to present in childhood, and an MRI diagnosis is rarely made without the proper history and laboratory documentation of the underlying pathologic enzymatic defect. Some features of these entities, however, may be detected by MRI.

Metachromatic leukodystrophy is the most common dysmyelinating disease that has multifocal nonenhancing

Central pontine myelinolysis, or osmotic demyelination syndrome, is seen in patients who have had rapid correction of hyponatremia, severe alcoholism, or severe debilitation. White matter involvement in the pons with central pontine myelinolysis is typical, but thalamic and deep gray matter–basal ganglia involvement has also been reported. A characteristic

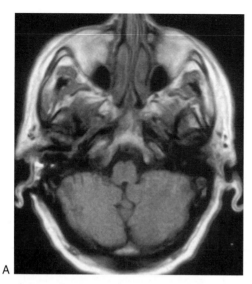 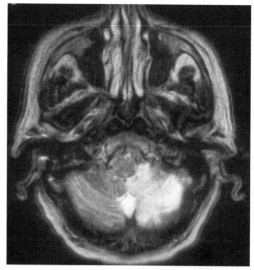

FIG. 11-36. Acute and chronic large vessel infarction. **A:** An axial T1-weighted image in the region of the posterior fossa in a 71-year-old woman with stroke symptoms demonstrates mass effect with no significant signal abnormality. **B:** A T2-weighted axial image through the same region demonstrates abnormal increased signal intensity in the brain parenchyma. These findings are consistent with an acute to subacute large vessel infarction. *Continued.*

lesions, with a predilection for the frontal lobes. Alexander's disease is a nonneoplastic primary white matter disorder associated with an enlarged head in the neonatal form. Lesions tend to start in the frontal region and progress posteriorly. Involvement of the basal ganglia has been reported. Canavan's disease is a spongiform degeneration of white matter that is also associated with an enlarged head size. Symmetric involvement of the white matter is noted.

Adrenoleukodystrophy is caused by an impairment in the oxidation of very-long-chain fatty acids. These fatty acids accumulate in the white matter and adrenal glands. This disorder affects young boys and is manifested as extensive demyelination starting in the posterior-occipital regions and traveling anteriorly. Adrenoleukodystrophy has features of both a dysmyelinating and demyelinating disease. Enhancement with gadolinium tends to occur around the advancing edge of this disorder.

Krabbe's disease is associated with basal ganglia and thalamic involvement. Calcifications in these areas may be seen on CT and are less apparent on MRI. Pelizaeus-Merzbacher is a form of sudanophilic leukodystrophy, which is a class of demyelinating disease characterized by an affinity for staining with Sudan Red on histologic slides. Symmetric, diffuse white matter disease is noted on MRI, with low signal in the deep gray matter thalamus and substantia nigra that is thought to be secondary to iron deposition.

The diagnosis of MS and the evaluation of disease progression are frequently made using open MRI. Many of the conditions are imaged in hospital settings, and many are performed on high-field systems. As open MRI becomes more prevalent, the neuroimaging literature should contain repre-

sentative examples of these more uncommon dysmyelinating disorders.

VASCULAR DISEASE

Cerebrovascular disease is a significant cause of neurologic deficits in the United States. It has been estimated that approximately 150,000 people have cerebrovascular accidents each year in the United States (22). Decreased blood flow to the brain frequently results in dramatic neurologic changes. Reversible ischemia and completed infarctions in the acute phase may be clinically indistinguishable. Brain imaging is performed to detect the size and extent of infarctions, exclude underlying lesions such as tumors or infections, and evaluate for the presence of hemorrhage. Acute cerebral ischemia may involve the large vessels, which include the carotid arteries, vertebral arteries, and arteries of the circle of Willis, or small vessels, which are penetrating arterioles in the base of the brain and periventricular region. The appearance on MRI of stroke and ischemic changes in these vessels has been described in basic neurology and neuroradiology texts. The following sections review large vessel disease, small vessel disease, and vascular malformations.

Large Vessel Disease

Three different ischemic models of large vessel disease have been described by Yuh et al. (23,24). These models include infarction or complete ischemia, incomplete ischemia, and watershed infarctions. Complete ischemia, or infarction, may

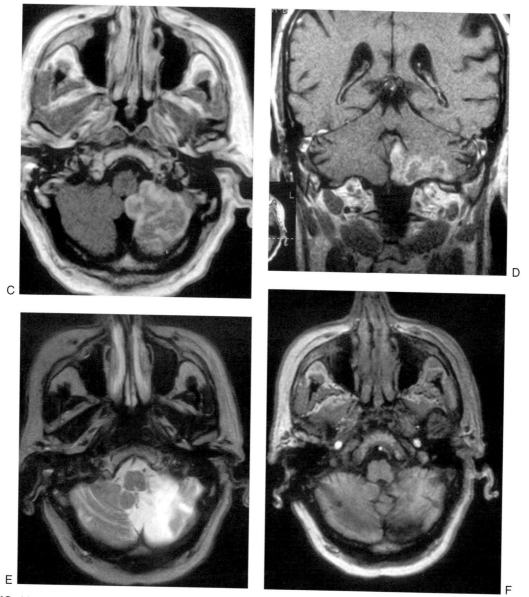

FIG. 11-36. *Continued.* **C:** An axial image using T1 technique after the administration of contrast material with enhancement in a curvilinear gyriform pattern. **D:** A T1-weighted coronal image obtained through the posterior fossa demonstrates abnormal contrast enhancement. **E:** This image was obtained 2 years and 5 months after the preceding images. This T2-weighted axial image through the posterior fossa exhibits marked volume loss in the site of the previous infarction. **F:** A transverse heavily T1-weighted axial image through this area shows volume loss and encephalomalacia.

result from thromboembolic occlusions of the carotids, vertebral arteries, or proximal larger vessels of the circle of Willis. Vascular flow alterations, alteration of arterial flow void, and arterial enhancement are noted. The finding of arterial enhancement correlates with clinical severity of ischemic lesions better than the presence of arterial occlusion on angiography (25).

Mass effect is subtle in acute stroke and may occur before signal changes in the parenchyma. Signal changes may be absent on routine MRI in the first 4 to 8 hours. Diffusion imaging depicts early ischemic changes before FLAIR and T2 imaging. Edema and brain swelling peak within the first 3 days, and parenchymal signal changes on T2 images follow. In acute stroke, parenchymal enhancement is usually absent, reflecting a lack of contrast agent delivery to the infarcted tissue.

Subacute strokes are those of more than 1 week's duration. Absence of signal flow void in arteries and brain swelling may persist, and parenchymal enhancement may still be seen. Chronic strokes are usually those detected more than 3 weeks after the stroke occurred. Volume loss, or encephalomalacia; prominence of the subarachnoid space; and local ventricular dilatation are noted. Additionally, some parenchymal enhancement may still be seen (Fig. 11-36).

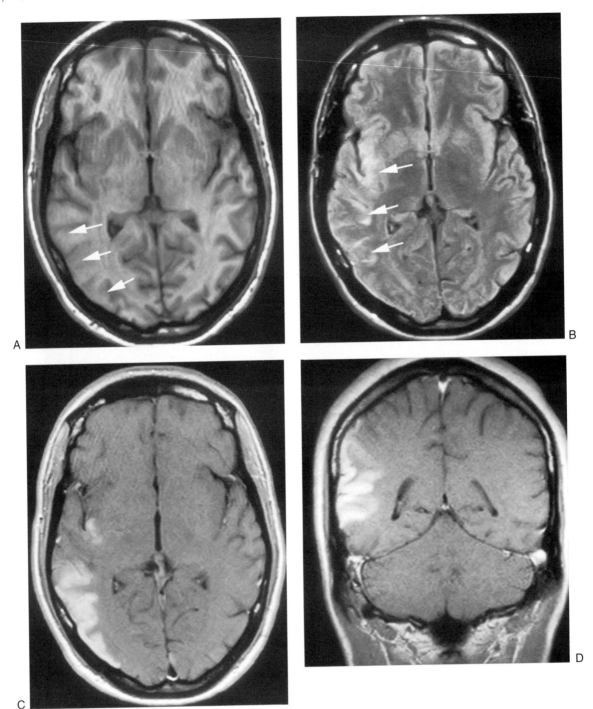

FIG. 11-37. A 37-year-old man with diplopia, headaches, and memory loss. **A:** A T1-weighted axial image at the level of the third ventricle demonstrates subtle effacement of the cortical sulci in the right parietal occipital temporal region (*arrows*). **B:** An axial fluid attenuated inversion recovery image through the same level demonstrates minimal hyperintensity on the right (*arrows*). **C:** A T1 axial image after contrast administration with brisk, thick enhancement of the cortex and underlying white matter. **D:** A coronal T1-weighted postcontrast image demonstrates thick contrast enhancement as well. The patient subsequently had complete resolution of neurologic symptoms, and follow-up imaging (not shown) demonstrated no large vessel infarction, which is consistent with reversible ischemic neurologic deficit. This event occurred near the region of the watershed between the parietal, occipital, and temporal cortices.

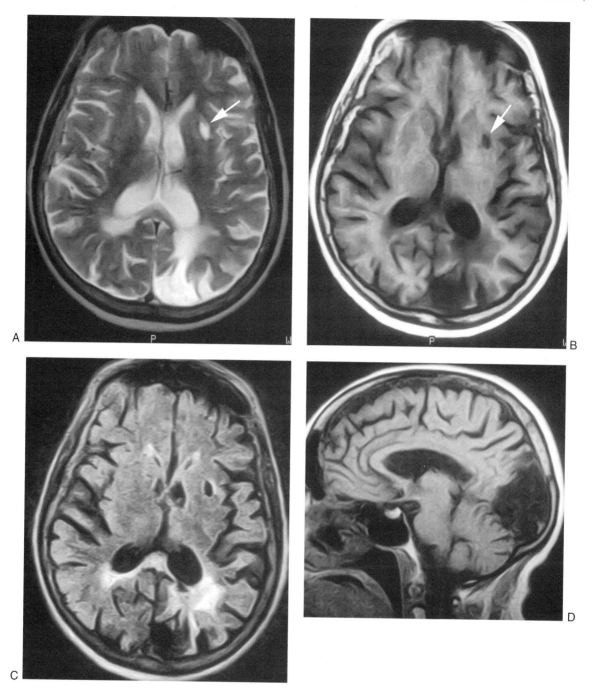

FIG. 11-38. Lacunar and large vessel infarction. **A:** A T2-weighted axial image demonstrates abnormal signal intensity in the left anterior putamen (*arrow*) and in the left occipital cortex. **B:** A heavily T1-weighted axial image demonstrates low signal intensity in the putamen (*arrow*) and left occipital region. **C:** An axial fluid attenuated inversion recovery (FLAIR) image demonstrates abnormal signal intensity in the occipital region in the left consistent with gliosis and on the right consistent with microvascular disease. Low signal intensity on this FLAIR image is consistent with focal encephalomalacia. **D:** This T1-weighted sagittal image demonstrates large vessel infarction in the occipital territory. This patient exhibits the typical imaging features of chronic large vessel infarction as well as a chronic small vessel lacunar infarction in the left putamen.

Incomplete ischemia has many forms, including transient ischemic attack, reversible ischemic neurologic deficits, and partial reversible ischemic neurologic deficit. Incomplete ischemia represents temporary interruption of blood flow to the brain that resolves before the formation of a completed infarction. In the acute phase, brain swelling may be seen, and arterial enhancement is usually absent. Extensive intense parenchymal enhancement involving both the gray and white matter may be seen early in incomplete ischemia (Fig. 11-37). Parenchymal signal changes are often subtle or absent on T2-weighted images. In the subacute and chronic phases, any signal change or mass effect usually has resolved, and parenchymal enhancement is absent. In cases of partially reversible ischemic neurologic deficits, the portions of the brain that are not reversibly affected follow the temporal sequences described for complete infarction.

Watershed infarctions represent decreased blood flow to areas of brain at the distal edges of the major vascular territories. A watershed exists between the anterior and middle cerebral arteries, middle cerebral arteries, and posterior cerebral arteries. These areas are vulnerable to decreased blood pressure or to vascular occlusions with intact collateral vessels. Brain swelling and abnormal signal intensity are characteristic in the watershed territory on T2-weighted images, and early parenchymal enhancement is noted.

Small Vessel Disease

Small vessel disease, or microvascular disease, occurs in the penetrating end arterioles that supply blood to the deep gray matter or anterior perforating substance. These penetrating end arterioles also provide blood to the periventricular and deep white matter. Atherosclerotic disease, vascular changes from hypertension, or diabetes mellitus may be responsible for the MRI changes seen. Microvascular disease is manifested by enlarged perivascular subarachnoid Virchow-Robin spaces, periventricular hyperintensities, or subcortical atherosclerotic disease. Vasculopathy, effects of migraine, and amyloid angiopathy are differential diagnosis considerations.

A large perivascular space in the region of the anterior commissure may be a normal finding in younger individuals. If prominent dilatation of these spaces, especially involving the supraventricular small vessels, is seen in an elderly individual, this finding may be considered secondary to small vessel ischemia. The signal intensity seen on all sequences is identical to CSF. Periventricular Virchow-Robin space dilatation may be as large as 1 cm.

Periventricular hyperintensities have been described as unidentified bright objects, microvascular ischemic-gliotic changes, and leukoareosis. The presence of periventricular hyperintensities in older individuals may have no correlation with the patient's neurologic status. Periventricular lesions appear to be less clinically significant than lesions detected within the subcortical white matter in distinguishing vascular dementia from Alzheimer's disease (26).

T2-weighted imaging in small vessel ischemic disease demonstrates increased signal intensity. FLAIR or proton density images may demonstrate increased signal intensity as well. T1 images generally show no abnormality. If low signal intensity is seen on T1-weighted images, an infarction of the small vessels termed a *lacunar infarction* is suspected (Fig. 11-38). Acute lacunar infarctions may not be low signal intensity on T1 images. Contrast enhancement may help establish the diagnosis of early lacunar infarction. Diffusion imaging is helpful in evaluating the presence of early lacunar infarctions. Additionally, subcortical signal abnormalities on T2-weighted images may be indicative of subcortical atherosclerotic encephalopathy or multiinfarct dementia.

VASCULAR MALFORMATIONS

Four types of vascular malformations exist: In a prospective autopsy study of 4,069 consecutive brain sections, McCormick demonstrated venous anomalies, or "venous angiomas," in 2.5% of specimens, capillary telangiectasia in 0.68%, arteriovenous malformations in 0.58%, and cavernous malformations in 0.39% (27).

Venous anomalies are veins that drain a larger portion of brain than normal. If the venous anomaly is large, signal flow void may be seen on T1- or T2-weighted images. Venous anomalies appear as branching structures joined to form one large venous draining trunk. Contrast enhancement may make these lesions more conspicuous. Occasionally, venous anomalies are associated with a cavernous malformation. Cavernous venous malformations may resemble a tumor on MRI. They present a sharply marginated, lobulated mulberry-like lesion that is seen with hemorrhage in various stages. These lesions tend to be hyperintense on T1 images and may have focal areas of low signal intensity secondary to hemosiderin. An increased incidence is seen in a familial form of cavernous malformation. Capillary telangiectasias are not detectable by MRI. These lesions are secondary to dilated capillary vessels found in the pons, cortex, and white matter. If hemorrhage is found in the pons of a younger individual, especially a young woman, this may be the only manifestation of a capillary telangiectasia. Arteriovenous malformations are abnormal, abrupt transitions from feeding arteries to abnormal draining veins. These lesions constitute a shunt of blood from the arterial supply to the draining veins with no intervening capillary bed (Figs. 11-39 and 11-40). Small arteriovenous malformations bleed 77% of the time. Large arteriovenous malformations bleed approximately 50% of the time but usually present as a neurologic deficit or seizure. Tubular flow void, hemosiderin formation, and solid clumps of vessels may be seen by MRI. When evaluating MRI of patients with arteriovenous malformation, it is important to discuss the nidus size, the location of the arte-

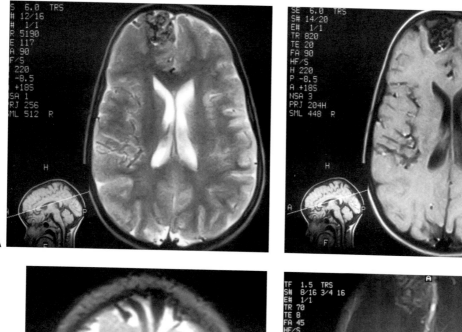

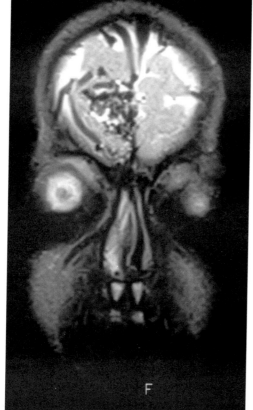

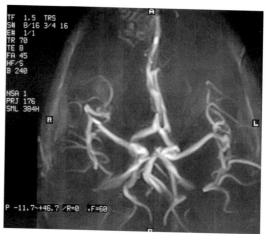

FIG. 11-39. Scans from a 6-year-old girl with a right frontal arteriovenous malformation (AVM). **A:** A T2-weighted image shows a tangled clump of vessels in the right frontal cortex. **B:** A T1-weighted image showing the signal flow void in the nidus of the AVM. **C:** A T2-weighted coronal image with prominent cortical veins noted as well as portions of the nidus. **D:** A magnetic resonance angiogram (MRA) maximum intensity projection image faintly shows the nidus at the upper edge of the field of view and prominent right anterior cerebral arteries. The feeding arterioles are not well identified in this MRA, thus demonstrating the limitations of MRA (regardless of field strength) for the evaluation of smaller vascular supply to AVMs.

riovenous malformation and eloquent or less eloquent brain cortex, the presence of deep venous drainage, and the feeding arteries as well as draining veins. These features determine the Spetzler classification, which in turn determines the type of neurosurgical or neurointerventional treatment. MR angiography frequently underestimates the feeding arteries to an arteriovenous malformation and is not a substitute for conventional angiography in the initial evaluation and treatment of patients with arteriovenous malformation.

With staged neurointerventional procedures, MRI is useful to follow the response to embolic therapy. MR angiography techniques are discussed in Chapter 24.

PITUITARY

Evaluation of the pituitary is routinely performed using MRI. Attention to the slice thickness and high-resolution

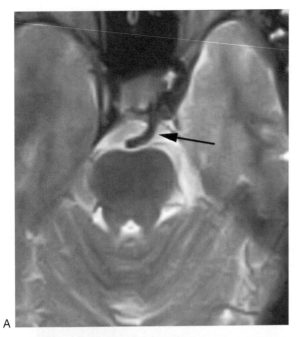

A

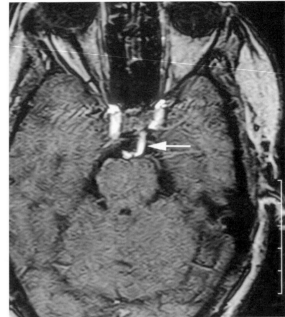

B

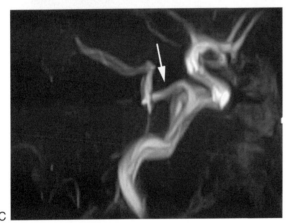

C

FIG. 11-40. A: A T2-weighted transverse image in a 31-year-old woman who complained of headaches. A prominent tubular structure in the prepontine space extends from the left juxtasellar internal carotid artery to the midbasilar artery (*arrow*). This finding is not to be confused with an arteriovenous malformation, which is illustrated in Fig. 11-39. **B:** A source image from a three-dimensional time of flight magnetic resonance angiogram of the circle of Willis. The carotid-basilar connection is seen as high signal intensity on this study (*arrow*). **C:** A maximum intensity projection image demonstrates the persistent trigeminal carotid-basilar anastomosis (*arrow*), a relatively rare congenital anomaly that represents persistence of fetal circulation. The trigeminal carotid-basilar anastomosis is the most frequent, with hypothalamic-otic and pro-atlanto-axial anastomoses being less frequent.

imaging is necessary for pituitary and parasellar scanning no matter the field of strength of the underlying magnet system. Open MRI machines are capable of pixel resolution similar to high field and, in this regard, no difference exists between MRI systems. The pituitary evaluation commonly involves the use of intravenous contrast material. Dynamic imaging of the pituitary after contrast administration provides the greatest difference between the normal gland and the nonenhancing pituitary tumors. This is especially important if surgery is contemplated and less critical if medical therapy is advocated. Dynamic MRI with lower field open MRI may be somewhat problematic. T1-weighted gradient-echo images may be performed during and shortly after contrast bolus administration. Starting conventional T1 spin-echo sequences before and during contrast administration is another way to achieve a pseudodynamic scan. Higher gradient strengths (usually encountered on higher field strength systems) allow greater ease in acquiring these types of images. As gradient strengths increase in open MRI, dynamic pituitary imaging may approach high-field techniques. Some individuals advocate nonenhanced pituitary

imaging for microadenoma detection and, in this situation, with high-resolution techniques, optimum imaging may be obtained without contrast or dynamic imaging.

The normal anatomy of the anterior and posterior pituitary is routinely imaged on sagittal MR images of the brain. With 3-mm coronal imaging and smaller pixel size, imaging of the pericavernous anatomy and anatomy of the sella turcica, suprasellar cistern, optic chiasm, and hypothalamus is available. Frequent indications for MRI of the sella include evaluation for microadenomas. Microadenomas are pituitary tumors smaller than 10 mm. Macroadenomas are pituitary tumors larger than 10 mm. Gland size in women is usually 9 mm or less, and in men 8 mm or less. In children, the gland size should be approximately 6 mm or less. In postpartum women, the gland may be as large as 12 mm and still be normal. The pituitary gland is homogeneous in signal intensity, the upper surface is smooth, and the pituitary stalk or infundibulum is midline. In microadenoma, focal heterogeneity or low signal intensity is seen on T1-weighted images (Fig. 11-41). The superior gland is convex upward, and the infundibulum may

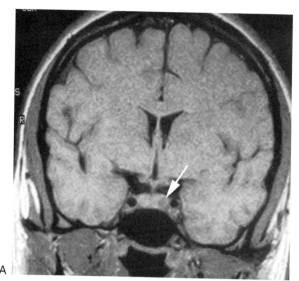

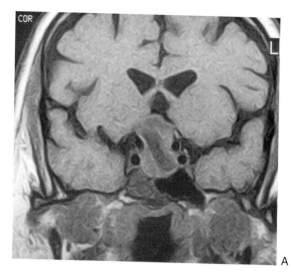

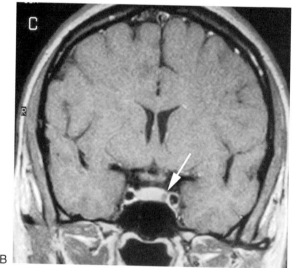

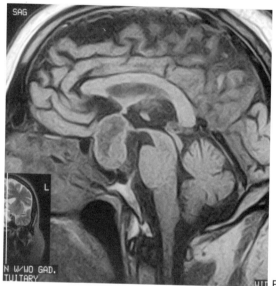

FIG. 11-41. T1-weighted pre- and postcontrast coronal images through the pituitary gland are shown in this 23-year-old woman with clinical suspicion of a microadenoma. **A:** The precontrast T1-weighted image (3-mm slice thickness) shows heterogeneity in the left mid to posterior position of the pituitary gland, which is consistent with a microadenoma (*arrow*). **B:** After the administration of contrast material, the gland enhances in a homogeneous manner. The microadenoma is not enhancing and stands out as a hypointense structure (*arrow*).

FIG. 11-42. Magnetic resonance imaging studies in the coronal and sagittal planes using T1 techniques on a 63-year-old man with blurred vision and a macroadenoma. **A:** Coronal T1-weighted image (3-mm slice thickness). The patient has had surgery and has a somewhat linear surgical defect extending from the left inferior portion of the gland to the right superior portion of the macroadenoma. The macroadenoma extends into the suprasellar cistern and abuts not only the optic chiasm but involves the hypothalamus and anterior portion of the third ventricle. **B:** Sagittal T1-weighted image (3-mm slice thickness).

deviate from the microadenoma. After contrast administration, the majority of microadenomas are hypointense to the briskly enhancing gland. Enhancement of microadenomas, however, may be seen on delayed images obtained 10 to 20 minutes or later after the administration of contrast material.

Macroadenomas are common tumors that may have mass effect on the cavernous sinus, suprasellar cistern, optic chiasm, or third ventricle. These masses tend to enhance in a heterogenous manner. Macroadenomas may also extend into the cavernous sinus and have mass effect on the chiasm (Fig. 11-42). When a macroadenoma involves the optic chiasm, it

is important for neurosurgical treatment purposes to determine whether the mass displaces the optic chiasm anteriorly (prefixed chiasm) or posteriorly (postfixed chiasm).

Metastatic disease, meningiomas, granulomatous disease, pituitary apoplexy, and abscess formation may all occur in the pituitary fossa. The empty sella syndrome may be secondary to dehiscence of the diaphragma sella, a dural membrane surrounding the superior portion of the pituitary. This may have the appearance of CSF signal intensity in the pituitary gland and may mimic an arachnoid cyst as well. Rathke cleft cyst may be seen in the anterior sella or in the suprasellar region

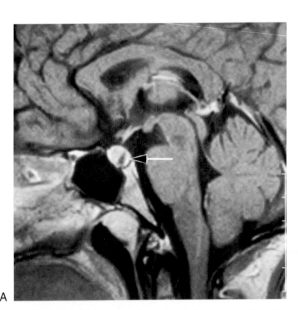

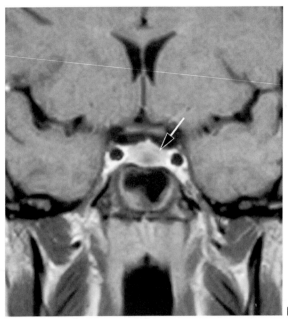

FIG. 11-43. Postcontrast T1-weighted sagittal **(A)** and coronal **(B)** images demonstrate a focal wedge-shaped elliptical area between the pituitary lobes that does not enhance (*arrows*). This is consistent with the appearance of a Rathke cleft cyst.

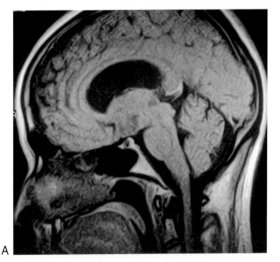

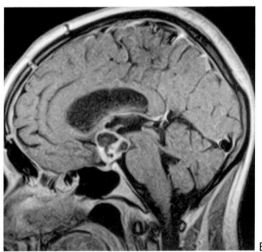

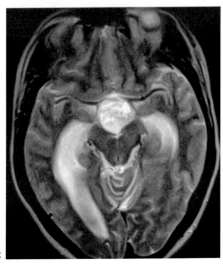

FIG. 11-44. A: A sagittal T1-weighted image before contrast administration is seen. A soft tissue mass is present in the suprasellar cistern and hypothalamus. Mass effect on the anterior third ventricle is present. **B:** After gadolinium administration, curvilinear contrast enhancement is seen in the region of the soft tissue mass on a sagittal T1-weighted image. **C:** An axial T2-weighted image demonstrates the hyperintensity and heterogeneous signal within this soft tissue mass, which extends into the interpeduncular cistern of the midbrain. Note that the temporal horns are markedly dilated in this patient who has hydrocephalus as a result of this craniopharyngioma.

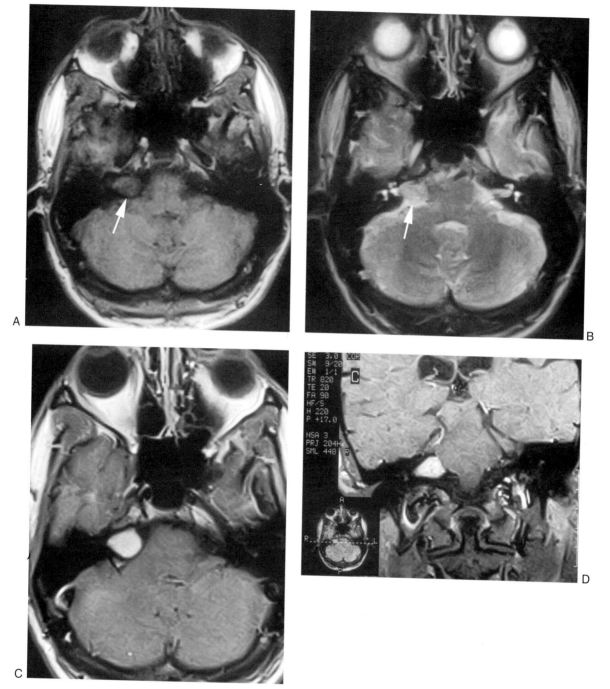

FIG. 11-45. Acoustic schwannoma. **A:** This axial T1-weighted precontrast image demonstrates abnormal soft tissue in the right cerebellopontine angle and internal auditory canal (*arrow*). **B:** An axial T2-weighted image through this same area demonstrates abnormal soft tissue in the right cerebellopontine angle cistern and extending into the internal auditory canal (*arrow*). Widening of the internal auditory canal is seen on this image. This feature helps differentiate an acoustic schwannoma, which widens the internal auditory meatus, from a meningioma, which usually does not have associated widening of the internal auditory canal. **C:** An axial T1-weighted postgadolinium image depicts the brisk contrast enhancement of an acoustic schwannoma, which in this case is predominately located in the cerebellopontine angle cistern. **D:** The coronal T1-weighted postgadolinium representation of this entity.

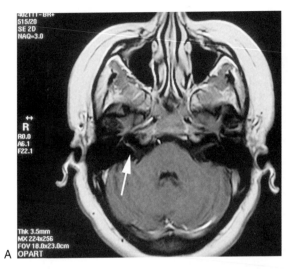

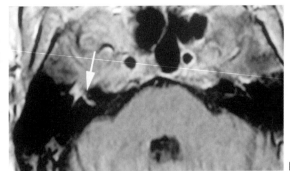

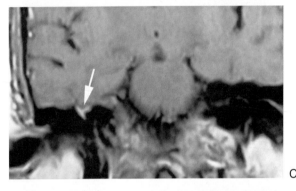

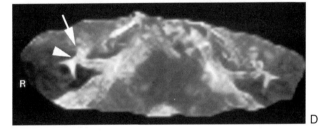

FIG. 11-46. A: An axial T1-weighted postgadolinium image (3.5-mm slice thickness) through the internal auditory canal in a patient with right Bell's palsy. Faint enhancement of the facial nerve in the intracanalicular segment is present (*arrow*). **B:** An axial T1-weighted postgadolinium image demonstrates enhancement in the facial nerve and at the level of the geniculate ganglion (*arrow*) in another patient with right Bell's palsy. Enlargement of the geniculate ganglion may be secondary to a facial nerve schwannoma; however, a facial neuritis is also in the differential diagnosis. **C:** A coronal T1-weighted axial postgadolinium representation of the abnormal enhancement in the region of the geniculate ganglion (*arrow*). **D:** A three-dimensional representation of a stack of 1.5-mm fast spin-echo images. This represents a compression or maximum intensity projection image through the internal auditory canals. Portions of the cochlea (*arrow*), vestibule (*arrowhead*), and the vestibulocochlear nerves are noted in this example.

(Fig. 11-43). Lipomas and epidermoids may be detected in the suprasellar region.

Craniopharyngiomas comprise 1.2% to 1.3% of all intracranial tumors. They are formed from metaplasia of squamous epithelium from the anterior pituitary or the anterior infundibulum. These tumors may be very large, may calcify in up to 80% of cases, and may exhibit cyst formation. Craniopharyngiomas tend to briskly enhance after contrast administration (Fig. 11-44). Mass effect on the chiasm is frequently noted. The differential diagnosis of masses in these regions includes chiasmatic glioma, hypothalamic hamartomas, hypothalamic glioma, and metastasis.

TEMPORAL BONE

High-resolution thin-section CT is an excellent modality for imaging the external, middle, and inner ear structures of the temporal bone. MRI plays a role in the evaluation of patients with suspected skull base tumors such as glomus jugulare, glomus tympanicum, chordoma, hemangiopericytoma, or chondrosarcoma. MRI is superior to CT in the evaluation of

patients with unilateral sensorineural hearing loss and facial palsy (Fig. 11-45). Thin-section MRI allows high-resolution images of the facial nerve (cranial nerve VII) and the vestibulocochlear nerve (cranial nerve VIII) (Fig. 11-46). Very thin (1.5-mm) images may be performed with 3D FSE techniques. Contrast enhancement is necessary not only to exclude acoustic schwannoma but also to evaluate for intracanalicular schwannoma, facial nerve schwannoma, hemangioma neuritis, metastasis, and meningiomas. Any of the aforementioned may involve the intracanalicular portion of the internal auditory canal or the CPA. Exquisite depiction of temporal bone anatomy is possible on open MRI with attention to the technical considerations discussed earlier.

ORBITS

The most common indication for orbital imaging is for the evaluation of Graves' thyroid eye disease, lymphoproliferative disease, lymphoma, or orbital pseudotumor (Fig. 11-47). These examinations may be performed using CT or MRI. Evaluation of the optic nerve, especially the intra-

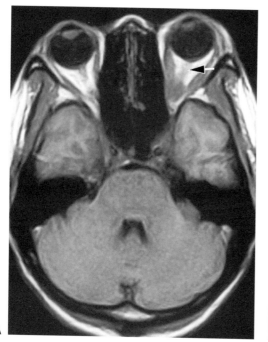
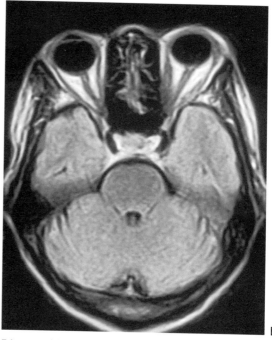

A

B

FIG. 11-47. A magnetic resonance image of a 54-year-old woman with left proptosis and visual changes. Imaging of the brain demonstrated enlargement of the medial rectus on the left. **A:** An axial T1-weighted image (3.5-mm slice thickness) of the orbits demonstrates the enlarged medial rectus without normal tapering (*arrow*), which is consistent with pseudotumor. **B:** Axial fluid attenuated inversion recovery images through the orbit also demonstrate this finding. Note the high signal intensity of the intraconal fat on both of these sequences. Short tau inversion recovery images (see Fig. 11-7) are helpful to evaluate the bright signal for fat.

canalicular portion and optic chiasm, is better performed using MRI. Coronal, heavily T2-weighted images aid in determining signal changes in the optic nerves that may be seen with optic neuritis or MS. High-resolution axial and coronal images are also performed. Oblique sagittal images aid in defining the course of the optic nerve as well. Gadolinium contrast material is mandatory in all cases of suspected mass or optic nerve compression. Open MRI systems are limited in this area in that fat saturation images performed after contrast administration, which can be critical in detecting subtle abnormalities, are currently unavailable. This fat saturation technique is easily performed at high-field strength using RF pulse saturation. But, at lower field strengths, this difference is smaller, making selective RF fat suppression difficult. Short tau inversion recovery imaging or very heavily T2-weighted imaging (described earlier in this chapter) can be performed with open MRI for fat saturation images. This is a nonselective form of fat saturation and cannot be performed after contrast administration. Despite this limitation, some advantages of lower field open MR merit consideration: Fat saturation tends to be more homogeneous at lower field strengths and, because of the lower static magnetic field, the chemical shift artifact between the water/fat interface at the posterior aspect of the orbit is decreased.

REFERENCES

1. Rajan SS. *MRI: a conceptional overview.* New York: Springer-Verlag, 1998.
2. Hoult DI, Chen CN, Sank VG. The field dependence of NMR imaging. *Magn Reson Med* 1986;3:722–746.
3. Rutt BK, Lee. DH. The impact of field strength on imaging in MRI. *J Magn Reson Imag* 1996;(6):57–62.
4. ACR Commission on Standards and Accreditation. *ACR MRI accreditation program description.* Reston, VA: ACI, August 1997.
5. Hauwe L, Parizel PM, Van Goethem JW, De Scheppera AM. Clinical usefulness of contrast-enhanced MPRAG of the brain. *J Neuroradiol* 1996;38:S14–S18.
6. Bourgoyne PM, Sarizin L, Duong HD, Roy D, Wolfson C, Vezina JL. Comparison of gadolinium enhanced T1-weighted SE and 3-D fast SPGR imaging in evaluation of intracranial lesions. *Radiology* 1994;193:295.
7. Bastianello S, Bozzao A, Paolillo A, et al. Fast spin echo and fast fluid-attenuated inversion-recovery versus conventional spin-echo sequences for MR quantification of multiple sclerosis lesions. *AJNR Am J Neuroradiol* 1997;18:699.
8. Wilms G, Marchal G, Kersschot E, et al. Axial vs. sagittal T2-weighted brain MR images in the evaluation of multiple sclerosis. *J Comput Assist Tomogr* 1991;15:359–364.
9. Feignbaum F, Manz H, Platenberg RC. *Principles of neuroscience.* Philadelphia: Lippincott Williams & Wilkins, 1999.
10. Preston-Martin S. Epidemiology of primary CNS neoplasms. *Neuro-epidemiology* 1996;14:273–290.
11. Russel DS, Rubenstein LJ. *Pathology of tumors of the nervous system,* 5th ed. Baltimore: Williams & Wilkins, 1989.
12. Jelinek J, Smirniotopulos JG, Parisi JE, et al. Lateral ventricular neoplasms of the brain: differential diagnosis based on clinical, CT and MR findings. *AJNR Am J Neuroradiol* 1990;11:567–574.

13. Leads NE. Brain tumors. In: *Neuroimaging clinics of North America*. Philadelphia: WB Saunders, 1993.

14. Grossman RI, Yosem DM. *Neuroradiology requisites*. St. Louis: Mosby–Year Book, 1994.

15. Sze G, Milanoc E, Johnson C, et al. Detection of brain metastasis: comparison of contrast enhanced MRI with unenhanced MRI and enhanced CT. *AJNR Am J Neuroradiol* 1990;11:785–791.

16. Atlas SW. *Magnetic resonance imaging of the brain and spine*. New York: Raven Crest, 1991.

17. Seugso H, Lee MD, Krinshna CVG, Rao MD. *Current computed tomography and MRI*. New York: McGraw-Hill, 1987.

18. Rosenberg RN, Heinz ER. *The clinical neurosciences—neuroradiology*. New York: Churchill-Livingstone, 1984.

19. Kluczknik RL, Wolpert SM, Anders ML. Congenital and developmental abnormalities of the brain. In: Wolpert S, Barnes PD, eds. *MRI in pediatric neuroradiology*. St. Louis: Mosby–Yearbook, 1992.

20. Edwards MK, Barnes P. Pediatric neuroimaging. In: *Neuroimaging clinics of North America*. Philadelphia: WB Saunders, 1999.

21. Lee BCP. Magnetic resonance imaging of metabolic and primary white matter disorders in children. *Neuroimag Clin North Am* 1993;3:276.

22. National Heart, Lung and Blood Institute. *The stroke belt initiative projects*. Baltimore: National Heart, Lung and Blood Institute, 1996.

23. Yuh WTC, Crain MR. Magnetic resonance imaging of acute cerebral ischemia. In: Drayer B, ed. *Neuroimaging clinics of North America*, Vol. 2. Philadelphia: WB Saunders, 1992.

24. Crain MR, Yuh WTC, Green GM, et al. Cerebral ischemia: evaluation with contrast-enhanced MRI imaging. *AJNR Am J Neuroradiol* 1991;12:631–639.

25. Mueller BP, Yuh WTC, Chandran KB, et al. MRI arterial enhancement and acute stroke: a correlation of angiographic findings and in vitro experience. Presented at the 29th Annual Meeting of the American Society of Neuroradiology. Washington, DC, 1991.

26. Bowen DC, Bancar WW, Loewenstein PA, et al. MRI signal abnormalities in memory disorder and dementia. *AJNR Am J Neuroradiol* 1990;11:283–290.

27. Newton TH, Potts DG. *Radiology of the skull and brain angiography*, Vol. 2, Book 4. Great Neck, NY: Medibooks, 1974.

Open MRI,
edited by Peter A. Rothschild and Debra Reinking Rothschild.
Lippincott Williams & Wilkins. Philadelphia © 2000.

CHAPTER 12

Open Magnetic Resonance Imaging of the Spine in Outpatient Practice

John L. Sherman, Peter A. Rothschild, and Elizabeth J. DuBose

The role of magnetic resonance imaging (MRI) in the spine has been well established, but this procedure has been unavailable to many very large or severely claustrophobic patients. This is where the use of open MRI has been so revolutionary. The areas of greatest proven value for open MRI of the spine include diseases related to the disc, degenerative processes, trauma, inflammation, neoplasm, and congenital malformations.

TECHNIQUE

MRI of the cervical spine for degenerative disease is probably the most difficult study to perform consistently, regardless of the field strength or scanner type. Patient movement, vascular pulsation, and swallowing can render the most exquisite sequence a waste of time. Some small discs and spurs are seen only on T1-weighted sequences (Fig. 12-1) and some only on T2-weighted sequences (Fig. 12-2). The thinner the sections, the better, as long as image quality can be maintained. Slice thicknesses of 3 to 4 mm and high in-plane resolution are optimal for diagnosis. Techniques using a three-dimensional Fourier transformation (3D FT) acquisition can achieve 2.5-mm slice thickness with good signal even at lower field strength. In some patients, it may be necessary to use 5-mm slice thickness to satisfy the need for adequate signal, especially in very large patients and when larger diameter coils are used. If spinal

cord disease (myelopathy) is the primary reason for the MRI study, thicker sections are acceptable and preferable. Very heavily T2-weighted fluid attenuated inversion recovery (FLAIR) sequences can be useful for evaluation of occult spinal cord disease. The FLAIR sequence is sensitive to motion artifact, but this is less of a problem at midfield and low field than at high field. The FLAIR sequence replaces standard spin-echo or fast spin-echo sequences. Short tau inversion recovery (STIR) and fast STIR are excellent techniques for evaluation of intramedullary disease, especially in the cervical spine. These images tend to have more noise and are less visually pleasing than fast spin-echo images, but they are also more sensitive to pathology.

Lumbar spine open MRI is considered a "bread and butter" technique and does not vary substantially among MRI scanners. Many open MRI centers find that imaging of the lumbar spine is their most frequently performed examination. Slice thickness is not as critical to imaging of the back as it is to imaging of the neck. The open scanner techniques make excellent use of T2-weighted fast spin-echo sequences to produce clear and detailed myelographic images of the lumbar spinal canal (Fig. 12-3). A four-sequence study is routine, but at most open MRI centers, one of the sequences can be eliminated in some patients if the examination is being monitored by a radiologist. For suspected intramedullary disease, we use at least four, and usually six to seven, sequences, including pre- and postcontrast (gadolinium chelate) T1-weighted sagittal and axial sequences and precontrast T2-weighted sagittal and axial sequences (Fig. 12-4). The T2-weighted axial sequence may use a gradient-echo (T2*-weighted) technique. A sagittal proton density–weighted sequence can also be obtained. STIR sequences can be helpful to evaluate for metastatic disease or trauma in the vertebral bodies (Fig. 12-5).

J. L. Sherman: Department of Radiology, University of Colorado School of Medicine, Denver, Colorado; Medical Director, Open MRI of Colorado, Colorado Springs, Colorado

P. A. Rothschild: Department of Radiology, University of California, San Francisco, San Francisco, California; Open MRI, Hayward, California; Open MRI, Louisville, Kentucky

E. J. DuBose: Open MRI, Hayward, California; Open MRI, Louisville, Kentucky

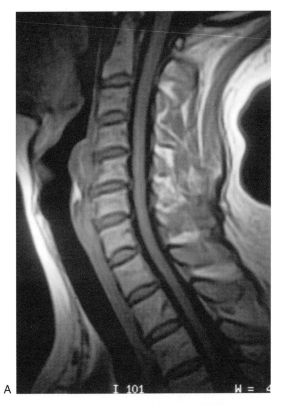

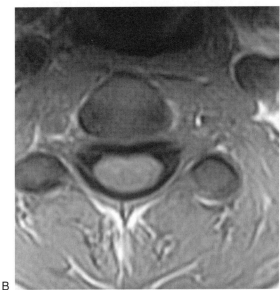

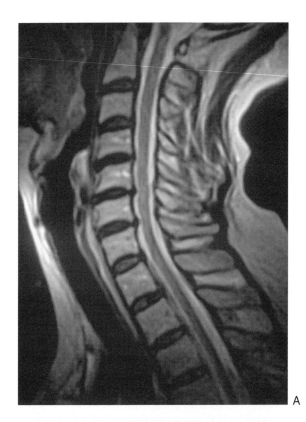

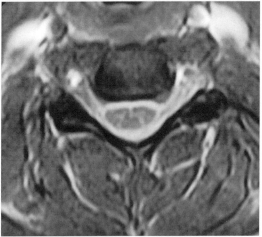

FIG. 12-1. Minimal disc bulges at multiple levels. **A:** The T1-weighted sagittal two-dimensional Fourier transform image of the cervical spine demonstrates small disc bulges at the C4-5, C5-6, and C6-7 levels. These bulges appear smaller than in Figure 12-2A, which is the corresponding T2-weighted sagittal image. T1-weighted sagittal and axial images of the cervical spine can be of great assistance in accurately judging the size of disc bulges and protrusions as well as spurring. **B:** High-resolution axial T1-weighted three-dimensional image. Note the anterior and posterior rami of the exiting nerve roots. High-resolution, 14 cm × 14 cm field of view of the cervical spine can be obtained with open magnetic resonance imaging.

FIG. 12-2. Minimal disc bulges at multiple levels. **A:** T2-weighted sagittal image of the cervical spine demonstrates small disc bulges at the C4-5, C5-6, and C6-7 levels. Disc bulges appear somewhat larger on the T2-weighted gradient reversal or fast spin-echo images than their true size, which is more accurately represented by the T1-weighted images (as demonstrated in Fig. 12-1A). **B:** Axial T2-weighted images of the cervical spine in the same patient demonstrate widely patent intervertebral foramina at this level.

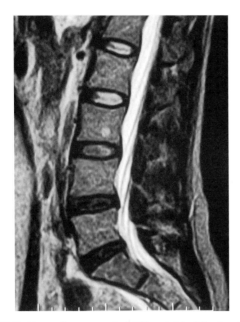

Spine protocols on an open MRI should allow routine evaluation of disc hydration, end plate/bone marrow reaction, facet joints, and disc margins. Tears of the annulus fibrosus are depicted as small focal areas of hyperintensity on sagittal T2-weighted images (Fig. 12-6) and on T1-weighted gadolinium-enhanced MRI.

Thoracic spine MRI uses the standard sequences indicated for the lumbar spine (Fig. 12-7). The challenge of thoracic MRI is complete visualization of the entire craniocaudal length of the spine with adequate resolution to detect small lesions. A cervical or lumbar "pilot" scan is always recommended to assist correct identification and numbering of the thoracic spinal levels. Neurosurgeons prefer a cervical spine pilot if they plan to operate in the thoracic spine. Axial images are necessary even when the sagittal scan appears negative. New phase-array coils on open MRI should be very beneficial in the thoracic spine

FIG. 12-3. Normal paracentral T2-weighted fast spin-echo sagittal image with a 9-echo train. The exiting nerve roots should be easily identified in the thecal sac on the parasagittal T2-weighted images with high resolution.

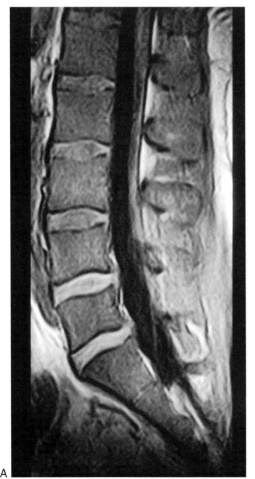

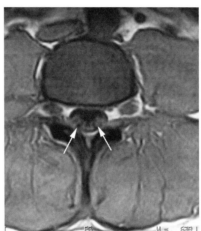

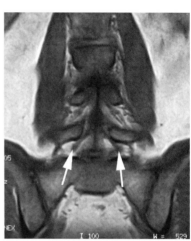

B, C

A

FIG. 12-4. Sagittal **(A)**, axial **(B)**, and coronal **(C)** T1-weighted three-dimensional Fourier transform (3D FT) images of the lumbar spine. 3D FT T1-weighted images are excellent in obtaining anatomic information in the lumbar spine. The fat signal intensity does not become as bright as with higher field strength magnets, and this is most helpful in identifying pathology. **B:** The nerve roots can be identified layering dependently in the thecal sac (*arrows*). **C:** The coronal images are also helpful in identifying far posterolateral disc herniations as well as giving an excellent view of the intervertebral foramina. Note the dorsal root ganglion in the intervertebral foramina (*arrows*).

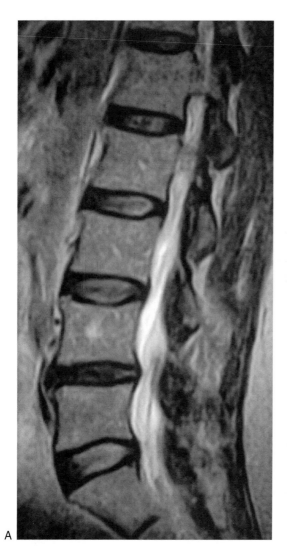
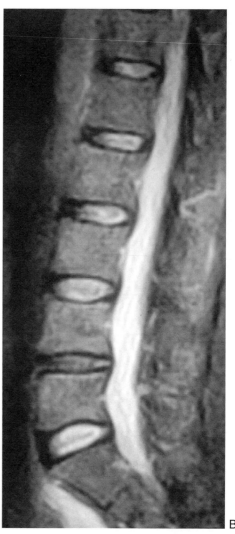

FIG. 12-5. Minimal 1-mm disc bulge at L4-5. Sagittal T2-weighted fast spin-echo **(A)** and corresponding short tau inversion recovery (STIR) **(B)** images demonstrate disc desiccation at the L4-5 disc with normal hydration of the remainder of the discs and normal marrow signal intensity. This is all best demonstrated on the STIR image. However, STIR images do not exhibit the same signal to noise ratio as fast spin-echo imaging; therefore, higher resolution images can be obtained with fast spin-echo techniques. Fast spin-echo T2-weighted images are used routinely in most open facilities where fast STIR images are used to evaluate for trauma or marrow-replacing disease processes. STIR images are also helpful in evaluating extension of tumor process or infection into the paraspinous fat.

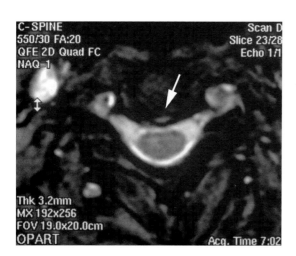

FIG. 12-6. Tear in the annulus fibrosis. T2-weighted axial gradient reversal images demonstrate a linear area of high signal intensity in the annulus fibrosis (*arrow*) consistent with an annular tear and a small protrusion of disc material. Axial T2-weighted images also nicely demonstrate the intervertebral foramina in the cervical spine; however, T2-weighted images can sometimes overestimate the narrowing of intervertebral foramina, and therefore, a T1-weighted axial image can be helpful in obtaining a more accurate picture of the exact narrowing to the intervertebral foramina.

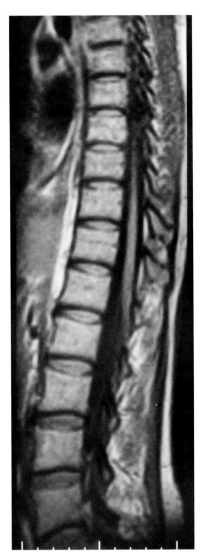

FIG. 12-7. Normal lower thoracic and upper lumbar spine. The patient was not well positioned in the scanner, and the study does not show the complete thoracic cord on one sagittal image. Proper positioning of the patient in the scanner can be assisted with the use of magnetic resonance fluoro techniques, which acquire an image approximately every 1 to 2 seconds and demonstrate the resulting reconstructed image almost immediately on the screen in the scan room. These fluoro techniques can also be helpful in an interventional procedure and in performing joint injections with gadolinium.

VERTEBRAE AND DISCS

Disc-space degeneration, herniation of the nucleus pulposus, or both result from a combination of chronic degenerative structural changes and mechanical stress. Initially, circumferential tears develop in the most centrally located lamellae. In addition, the progressive desiccation of the nucleus pulposus with age results in diffuse disc bulging, decreased disc-space height, and increased mobility of the vertebral elements.

Degenerative changes in the disc are often associated with changes in the vertebral end plate and bone marrow (Modic) changes. In some patients, disruption of the vertebral end plate permits fibrovascular tissue to invade the adjacent marrow space. This fibrous tissue is characterized by low signal on T1-weighted MR images and high signal on T2-weighted images (type I changes) (Fig. 12-8). Type I changes are thought to be indicative of an acute or subacute inflammatory disorder that may explain pain. In other patients, fatty marrow replaces the normal marrow adjacent to the disc and appears as high signal on T1-weighted images and low to intermediate signal on T2-weighted images (Modic type II changes) (see Fig. 12-8). In patients with severe degenerative disc disease and bony sclerosis, the sclerotic end plate and subcortical bone appears as low signal intensity on T1- and T2-weighted images (type III changes) (1).

Degenerative Disc and Facet Disease

Lumbar disc degeneration is the most common cause of back and leg pain. As disc degeneration progresses, disc protrusion and subsequent herniation occur secondary to the combined influences of degenerative changes and mechanical stress from forward flexion and axial rotation. Disc herniation requires a relatively gelatinous nucleus and usually is seen in younger patients. When it occurs, disc herniation is usually in the posterolateral region, in which the annulus is structurally weakest, and it can produce a radicular pain syndrome.

Types of Disc Herniations

Specialists in the treatment and diagnosis of spinal disc disease generally agree on the use of nomenclature, including the terms *annular bulge*, *disc protrusion*, and *extrusion* (2).

1. By definition, a herniated nucleus pulposus occurs when the gelatinous nucleus squeezes through a cleft or defect in the annulus fibrosus (Fig. 12-9). When the margin of the disc circumferentially extends beyond the vertebral end plate, the finding should be termed an *annular bulge*. An annular disc bulge is a common finding in the aging spine. An annular disc bulge may be associated with radial tears of the annulus.
2. If a focal area of extension of the nucleus is seen beyond the vertebral margin but remains beneath the outer annular/posterior longitudinal ligament complex, it should be termed a *disc protrusion* (Fig. 12-10).
3. The extension of nuclear material completely through the outer annulus into the epidural space is termed an *extrusion* (Fig. 12-11). When the extruded disc tissue has separated from the native disc, it can be called a *free fragment* or a *sequestration*.

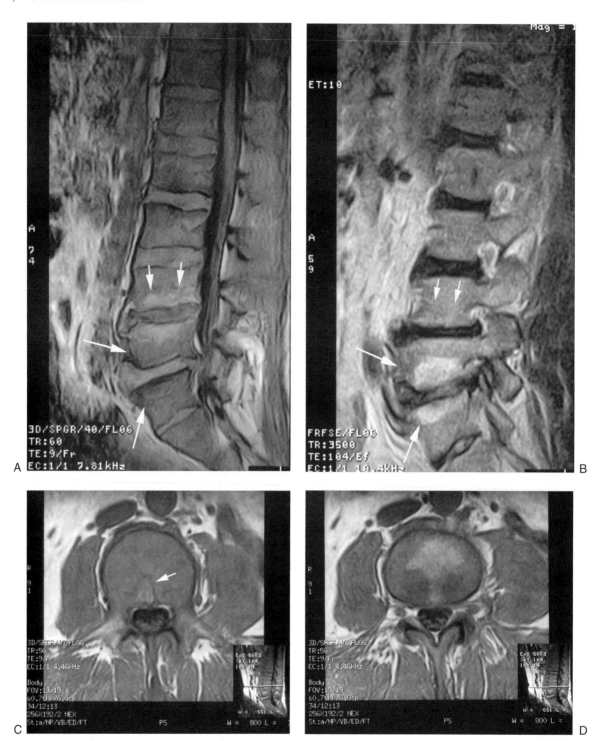

FIG. 12-8. Modic type I and II changes. T1-weighted three-dimensional Fourier transform (3D FT) **(A)** and fast spin-echo T2-weighted **(B)** sagittal images demonstrate Modic type II (*short arrows*) changes at the L4-5 level, which shows high signal intensity on the T1-weighted images secondary to fatty replacement of the normal marrow and appears similar in signal intensity to the surrounding marrow fat on the T2-weighted images. At the L5-S1 level, Modic type I (*long arrows*) changes are somewhat low in signal intensity on T1-weighted images and become bright on the T2-weighted images. **C:** The axial T1-weighted images at a different level in the same patient demonstrate the normal basivertebral venous plexus extending into the midportion of the vertebral bodies (*arrow*). This should not be mistaken for a cleft in the vertebral disc, because this is clearly not at the disc level. Reference images, which are common on open magnetic resonance imaging, can be very helpful in accurately identifying the correct level. **D:** Axial T1 3D FT image at the L4-5 disc level. Both exiting L4 nerve roots in the intervertebral foramina are surrounded by normal fat. In **A**, a small disc is seen at the S1-2 level. Accurately numbering lumbar vertebral bodies is crucial to ensure that surgery is performed at the correct level. If doubt remains as to the exact number of vertebrae, it can be helpful to call the last lumbar vertebra *L-6* instead of *S-1*. This ensures that proper attention is paid to numbering of the vertebral bodies by the referring physician before any procedure is performed.

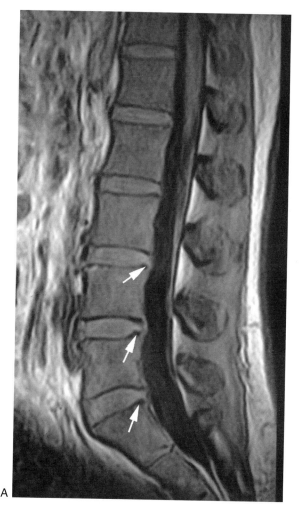

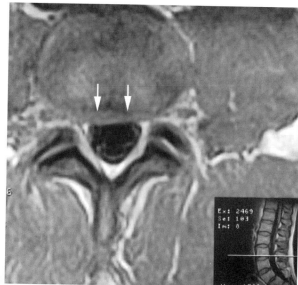

FIG. 12-12. Multiple small disc bulges. **A:** Sagittal T1-weighted three-dimensional Fourier transform (3D FT) image (*arrows*). **B:** Axial 3D FT T1-weighted image demonstrates 1- to 2-mm disc bulges that appear to minimally efface the thecal sac (*arrows*).

axial images a[...]
The lateral an[...]
axial images. A[...]
niques are rec[...]
lower, higher, o[...]
sac (Fig. 12-16[...]

The use of G[...]
ment even in t[...]
fibrosus elicits [...]
Granulation tis[...]
Inflamed nerve [...]
this observation[...]
active disease in[...]
bly in patients w[...]
Pre- and postco[...]
technique for s[...]
versus recurrent [...]
postoperatively [...]

Scanning shou[...]
tion, because so[...]
seen on delayed [...]
disc fragment, pr[...]
increasing the ap[...]
images (Fig. 12-[...]
be differentiated [...]
lunar appearance [...]

Degenerative Ce[...]

It is difficult t[...]
process of a disc [...]
Degenerative spir[...]
cially in men and [...]
incidence of symp[...]
because minor ce[...]
go unreported. Te[...]
head and neck MI[...]
with no subjective [...]
of degenerative spi[...]
67% occurrence ra[...]
older than 64 years[...]
for those aged 45 [...]
degenerative disc [...]
gle-level changes [...]
patients.

The vertebra can[...]
consisting of the int[...]
the inferior facet. Pr[...]
other joints. As the [...]
height, and the abili[...]
the force vectors on [...]
increased mobility, [...]
result from settling[...]
Increased mobility at[...]
mation of osteophyte[...]

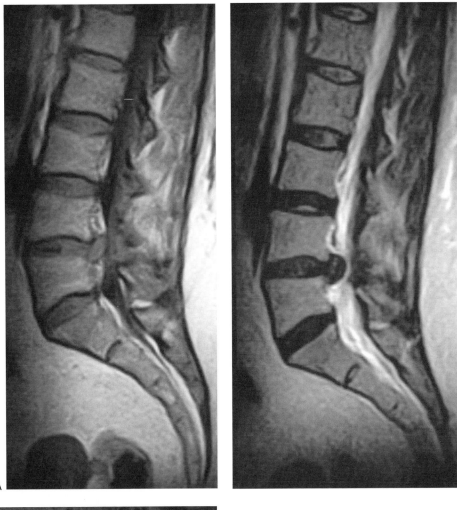

A

B

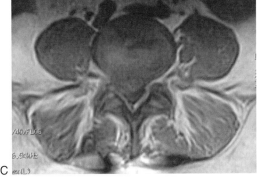

C

FIG. 12-9. Large subligamentous disc herniation. Sagittal T1-weighted (**A**), fast spin-echo T2-weighted (**B**), and axial T1-weighted (**C**) images demonstrate a large disc herniation at the L4-5 level, which is significantly effacing and displacing the thecal sac. Disc herniations can often be low signal intensity on fast spin-echo T2-weighted images.

Bulging of the annulus fibrosus is common and frequently asymptomatic (Fig. 12-12). Protrusions are also seen commonly in asymptomatic patients. Disc protrusions are characterized by a focal projection or asymmetry of the posterior disc margin beyond the posterior borders of the adjacent vertebral bodies. A disc protrusion is a contained disc herniation; the herniated nuclear material extends through a tear of the inner annulus but does not extend through the outermost annular fibers. Sagittal MR images are often not specific when differentiating an annular disc bulge from a protrusion. In such cases, axial images are better than sagittal images, because focal contour changes in the posterior disc margin are the key findings. A bulge is smooth, whereas a protrusion is nodular

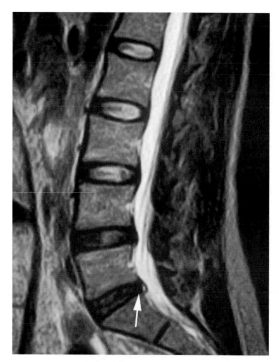

FIG. 12-10. Small subligamentous disc protrusion. T2-weighted sagittal image demonstrates low signal intensity disc with a small area (*arrow*) of high signal intensity, which represents disc material that has extended through the annulus. Even though these protrusions are small, they can be a source of pain and should be noted in the report.

(Fig. 12-13). Occasionally, underlying fissuring or tears may be identified on T2-weighted or gadolinium-labeled diethylenetriaminepentaacetic acid (Gd-DTPA)–enhanced T1-weighted sagittal images. Although, by definition, a disc protrusion is a herniated disc, partial tearing of inner annular fibers cannot be reliably identified with either computed tomography or MRI.

Extrusions are generally associated with acute symptoms. In an extruded disc, the gelatinous nucleus pulposus material extends through all layers of the annulus and produces an extradural mass that often indents the ventral aspect of the thecal sac. Extruded discs may extend superior (more commonly) or inferior to the intervertebral disc either in the midline or posterolaterally in the lateral recess (more commonly) (Fig. 12-14). Differentiation of a protrusion from an extrusion is not always possible.

A free fragment, or a sequestered disc, represents disc material that is no longer in continuity with its parent intervertebral disc of origin. It may be adjacent to the disc of origin or it may migrate cranially or caudally in the spinal canal. Sequestrations are often surrounded by epidural fibrosis, thus increasing the size and mass effect of the lesion and simulating tumors in some patients. Sequestered free fragments are best detected on sagittal scans showing migration along the dorsal surface of the vertebral bodies (Fig. 12-15).

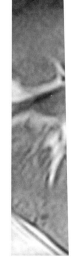

FIG. 12-11. La
T1-weighted im
ciated sequeste
Fourier transfo
which contrasts
Note that the le
is unaffected by

The free fragm
signal intensity

Midline disc
terolateral or pa
is more likely t

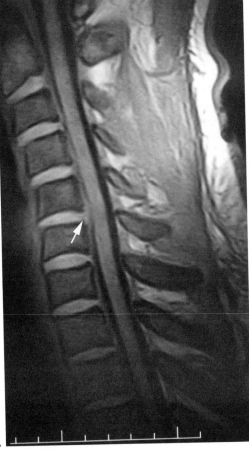
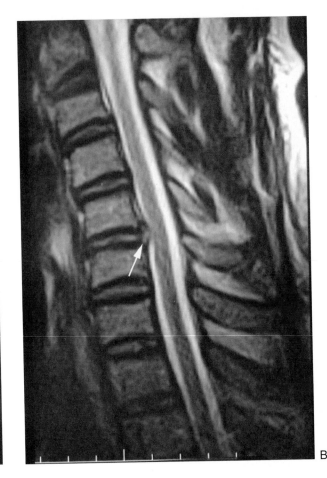
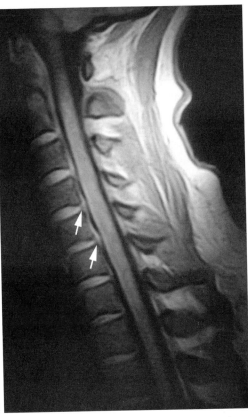
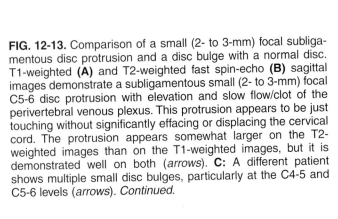

FIG. 12-13. Comparison of a small (2- to 3-mm) focal subligamentous disc protrusion and a disc bulge with a normal disc. T1-weighted **(A)** and T2-weighted fast spin-echo **(B)** sagittal images demonstrate a subligamentous small (2- to 3-mm) focal C5-6 disc protrusion with elevation and slow flow/clot of the perivertebral venous plexus. This protrusion appears to be just touching without significantly effacing or displacing the cervical cord. The protrusion appears somewhat larger on the T2-weighted images than on the T1-weighted images, but it is demonstrated well on both (*arrows*). **C:** A different patient shows multiple small disc bulges, particularly at the C4-5 and C5-6 levels (*arrows*). *Continued.*

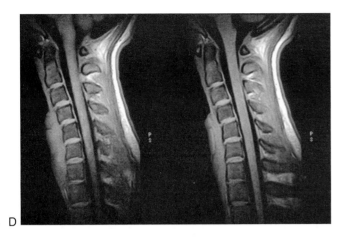

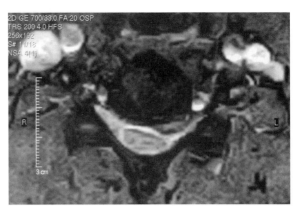

FIG. 12-14. Left paracentral disc herniation extending into the lateral recess. T2-weighted axial images show disc material extending into the lateral recess and intervertebral foramina, which is significantly narrowing the left intervertebral foramen and lateral recess and mildly effacing the left lateral aspect of the cervical cord.

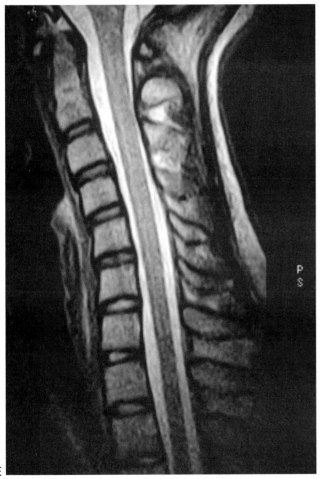

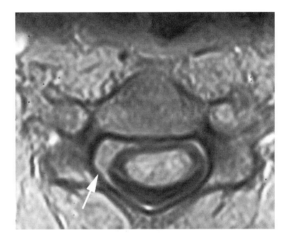

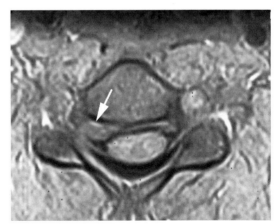

FIG. 12-13. *Continued.* **D:** Normal cervical spine with reversal of the normal lordotic curve. When a reversal of the normal lordotic curve is present, it can appear that there are small bulges, but these are secondary to the reversal of the curve and is normal. **E:** Corresponding T2-weighted fast spin-echo image to **D**.

FIG. 12-15. Sequestered disc fragment posterior to the vertebral body. Axial T1-weighted three-dimensional Fourier transform image of the cervical spine demonstrates a soft tissue mass in the right lateral recess posterior to the vertebral body. This was an extruded fragment (*arrows*), which can often be subtle on magnetic resonance imaging. High-resolution continuous slice axial imaging is helpful in identifying these subtle, but important, lesions.

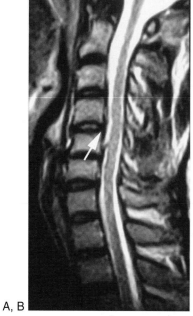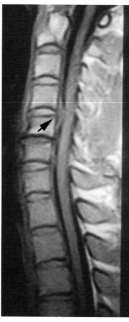

A, B

FIG. 12-16. Subligamentous disc herniation (*arrows*) at C4-5. Fast spin-echo T2-weighted **(A)** and two-dimensional T1-weighted **(B)** sagittal images of the cervical spine. **A:** Disc herniation tracks with cerebrospinal fluid (CSF) on the T2-weighted images. **B:** This lesion is easily identified on the T1-weighted images (*arrow*) secondary to the dark CSF and intermediate signal intensity of the herniated nucleus pulposus. T1-weighted images are extremely important in the spine and should not be skipped even if it means bringing the patient back for repeat examination. With open magnetic resonance imaging systems, it is best to alternate T1 and T2 sequences because many of these claustrophobic patients may only complete two sequences. Courtesy of General Electric Medical Systems, Milwaukee, WI.

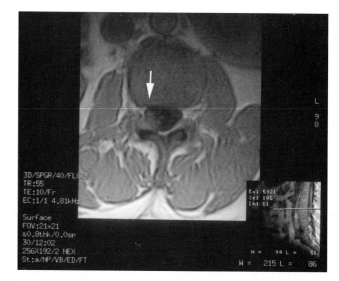

FIG. 12-18. Normal layering of the nerve roots in the dependent portion of the thecal sac with the patient lying on her side. Axial T1-weighted three-dimensional Fourier transform images demonstrate the nerve roots layering in the right lateral aspect of the thecal sac (*arrow*). Often, patients are in severe pain and cannot lie on their backs or are extremely claustrophobic and prefer to lie on their sides. These patients can be scanned using a solenoidal coil placed against the back. This also may be an excellent way to diagnose arachnoid scarring because, in theory, layering of the nerve roots in the dependent portion of the spinal canal should not occur with arachnoid scarring/arachnoiditis.

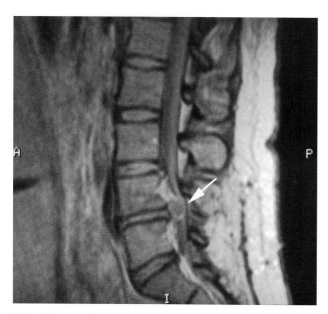

FIG. 12-17. Inflamed postoperative disc fragment with gadolinium. T1-weighted three-dimensional Fourier transform postcontrast sagittal image demonstrates a mass with rim enhancement (*arrow*) in a postoperative patient.

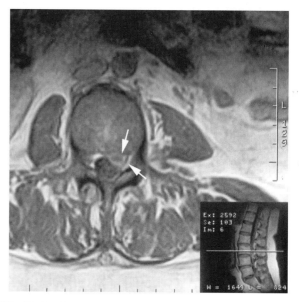

FIG. 12-19. Extruded disc fragment producing a bull's-eye enhancement pattern. T1-weighted axial three-dimensional Fourier transform postcontrast image demonstrates an enhancing rim around a soft tissue mass (*arrows*) in the epidural space that is compressing the thecal sac.

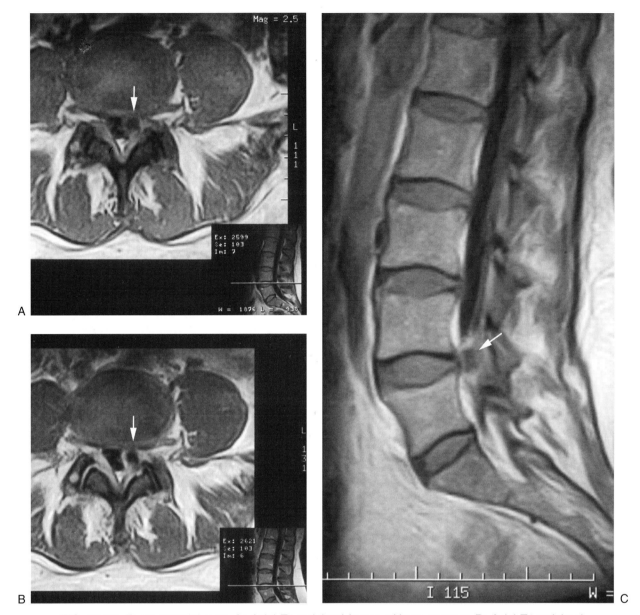

FIG. 12-20. Facet synovial cyst. **A:** Axial T1-weighted image without contrast. **B:** Axial T1-weighted image with contrast. **C:** Sagittal T1-weighted image with contrast. An extradural cystic lesion (*arrows*) is identified with peripheral enhancement adjacent to the left L-4 facet joint. This lesion can easily be mistaken for the bull's-eye enhancement pattern seen with large disc fragments.

weight-bearing surface of the end plate. Anterior and anterolateral spurs are generally not significant; however, if the spurs form posteriorly or posterolaterally, the neural foramina or spinal canal may become compromised. Posterolateral spurs and disc protrusions often cause a radiculopathy due to nerve entrapment, stretch, or compression. A myelopathy may develop owing to gradual compression of the arterial blood supply, direct compression of the cord, or a combination of the two factors.

Degenerative Thoracic Disc Disease

The MRI study must include a definitive way of accurately localizing the level of the disc herniation. Simply assuming that the suprasternal notch is opposite the T3 vertebral body and counting down from this point are not sufficiently accurate for surgical planning. MRI should include the entire cervical spine, which allows localization of the thoracic disc space by counting from the C-2 vertebral

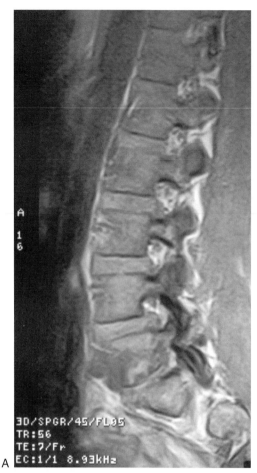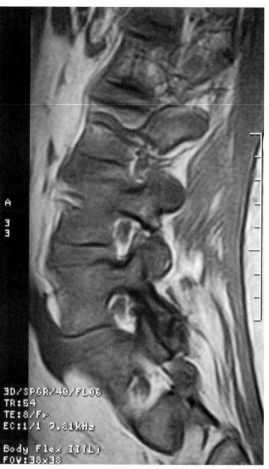

FIG. 12-21. Mild narrowing of the intervertebral foramina. **A:** Sagittal T1-weighted three-dimensional Fourier transform (3D FT) image demonstrates narrowing of the L4-5 intervertebral foramina secondary to ligamentum flavum hypertrophy and disc bulge. **B:** Sagittal T1-weighted 3D FT image of a normal intervertebral foramina in which the nerve root is identified surrounded by fat and is not compressed. Often, the intervertebral foramina are overlooked on the sagittal T1-weighted 3D FT image. This can be an important sequence to carefully review, especially the parasagittal images, to rule out intervertebral foraminal pathology.

body. Localizing a thoracic disc level by counting down from the cervical spine is more accurate than counting up from the sacrum, because anomalies of the lumbar spine (six lumbar vertebral bodies) are much more common than are anomalies of the cervical spine. Furthermore, accurate localization of the herniated disc at surgery involves counting from the first rib down.

The thoracic spine is not exempt from the effects of aging and degeneration. Kyphosis is a common finding, especially in elderly women. The thoracic spine is much less mobile than either the cervical or the lumbar spine; consequently, symptomatic degenerative disease is less common. Furthermore, the radiographic appearance of thoracic degenerative spinal disease is less obvious than that of cervical and lumbar spinal disease.

Although symptomatic degeneration in the thoracic spine is least common, relatively less compromise of the thoracic spine may result in neurologic deficits for two reasons:

1. The spinal cord occupies a relatively larger percentage of the canal throughout the thoracic spine, and compression may occur from relatively smaller osteophytes.
2. The vascular supply to the thoracic spinal cord comes primarily from segmental or radicular arteries. This supply places the thoracic cord at an even greater risk of ischemia from compression.

Degenerative Lumbar Disc Disease

Pathogenesis

The pathogenesis of intervertebral disc degeneration is not well understood. Trauma is not likely the major factor in degeneration. Repetitive cyclic loading of the disc may result in failure of annular fibers. Decreasing permeability of the vertebral end plates has been suggested as a cause for disc degeneration and annulus tear. The vertebral joints of adjacent vertebrae share three main articulations: the intervertebral disc and two apophyseal or facet joints (uncinate processes serve as minor articulations for stability). Any process that affects one of these joints also affects the others. From a histologic standpoint, multiple changes occur during aging in the subchondral bone, nucleus pulposus, and annulus fibrosus. The gradual loss of vascular channels in the end plates may lead to metabolic derangements within the disc and subsequently to desiccation of the disc with recurrent trauma. The axis of flexion and extension may become irregular, and abnormal movement combined with loss of disc-space height results in subluxation of the posterior joints, displacement of the facets, and stenosis of the lateral recesses and foramina (Figs. 12-21 and 12-22).

Despite the lack of consensus about the cause of disc degeneration, the morphologic features are herniations, bulging, loss of height, and loss of signal intensity. The radial tear of the annulus is a common characteristic of disc degeneration. The radial tear involves all layers of the annulus fibrosus in its anterior, posterior, or, possibly, lateral portion. The radial tear can be seen effectively with precise anatomic sectioning techniques such as cryomicrotomy.

A radial tear may be detected by MRI as a band of high–signal intensity tissue in the region of the disc normally characterized by low signal intensity. It may also be visualized on contrast-enhanced MRI as a band or patch of enhancement in the margin of the disc. The radial tear may therefore be a marker of disc degeneration.

Central stenosis can occur anteriorly from a bulging degenerative disc or posteriorly from an enlarged lamina, ligamentum flavum thickening and subluxation, and osteophyte formation in the facets (Fig. 12-23). With disc degeneration and loss of disc-space height, nerve root kinking can trap the nerve root between a bulging disc and a pedicle. Patients with degenerative spinal stenosis undergo gradual compression of the nerve roots of the cauda equina due to canal narrowing.

Spondylolisthesis and Spondylolysis

Spondylolisthesis is defined as the forward movement of the body of one lumbar vertebra on the vertebra below it or on the sacrum. *Spondylolisthesis* is a general term for a disease process of various causes in which slippage is the common end result. *Spondylolysis* is a specific term describing a defect in, or the absence of, the pars interarticularis (Fig. 12-24). When spondylolysis is present, spondylolisthesis may develop. Spondylolysis may result from dysplasia of the posterior elements, failure of pars interarticularis ossification, fractures through the pars, and degenerative changes. Fracture of other than the pars interarticularis may also cause spondylolisthesis, and certain metabolic diseases of bone are associated with a form of spondylolisthesis (Fig. 12-25).

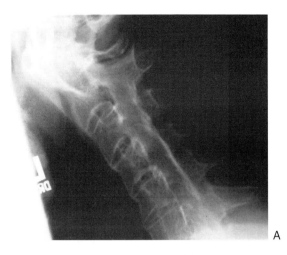

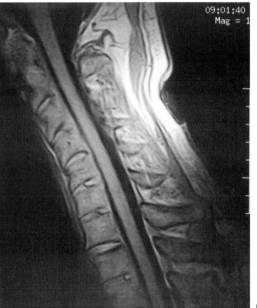

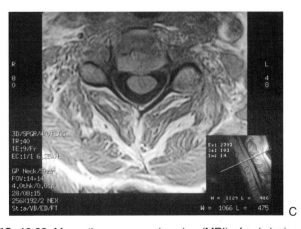

FIG. 12-22. Magnetic resonance imaging (MRI) of ankylosing spondylitis. Plain film **(A)**, T1-weighted three-dimensional Fourier transform (3D FT) sagittal **(B)**, and T1-weighted 3D FT axial **(C)** images of the cervical spine. The diagnosis of ankylosing spondylitis can be subtle on MRI; however, close evaluation of the sagittal T1-weighted images shows loss of the normal bony cortex along the posterior aspect of the vertebral bodies, and the discs do not appear to reach the cerebrospinal fluid. Obtaining corresponding plain films can be extremely beneficial in evaluating spinal MRI.

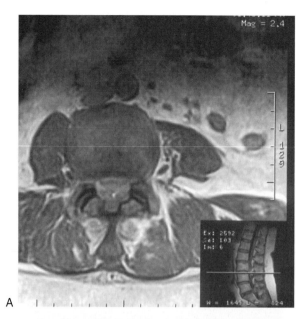

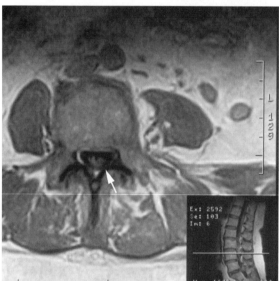

FIG. 12-23. Severe spinal stenosis. **A:** The T1-weighted axial three-dimensional Fourier transform image of the lumbar spine demonstrates a lack of cerebrospinal fluid (CSF) at this level. Extensive ligamentum flavum hypertrophy and associated disc bulge, which is severely narrowing the spinal canal and has essentially compressed out almost all of the CSF from this level, are seen. **B:** An axial image, from just below **A**, which demonstrates the nerve roots to be clumped centrally in the spinal canal (*arrow*). This is secondary to the spinal stenosis above and not evidence of arachnoid scarring.

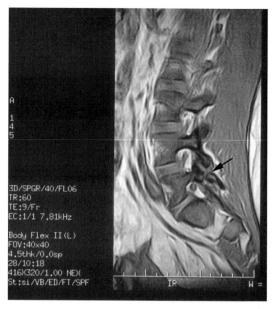

FIG. 12-24. Pars fracture at L-5. Sagittal T1-weighted three-dimensional Fourier transform image demonstrates a classic pars fracture in the L-5 vertebra (*arrow*). The parasagittal T1-weighted images are helpful to evaluate the intervertebral foramina for stenosis and posterolateral disc herniations and protrusions and are also good sequences to look for pars lesions.

intervention. MRI may be helpful in the initial evaluation to rule out other causes of low back pain in the spondylolisthetic patient, such as disc prolapse at the level above the listhesis. The fibrocartilaginous mass present at the pars defect in isthmic spondylolisthesis is often easily

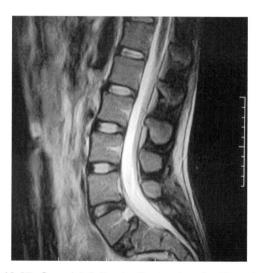

FIG. 12-25. Spondylolisthesis. Fast spin-echo T2-weighted sagittal image demonstrates anterior spondylolisthesis of L-5 on S-1 with pseudo-disc bulges at both L4-5 and L5-S1. Note that L-5 appears to be a transitional vertebral body, and it is important to mention that the last normal appearing lumbar disc is between L-5 and S-1. Therefore, if surgery is planned, accurate numbering of the disc levels on corresponding plain films can be more easily accomplished.

Despite advances in computed tomography and MRI, anteroposterior and lateral lumbosacral spinal x-rays are vital in the evaluation of spondylolisthesis and spondylolysis. Information gained from plain x-rays can aid in the decision for further imaging studies and possible surgical

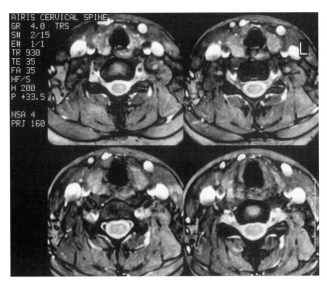

FIG. 12-26. Normal axial image. Axial T2-weighted images of the cervical spine nicely demonstrate widely patent intervertebral foramina and the H-shaped gray/white interface in the cord itself. (Image courtesy of Hitachi Medical Systems America, Inc., Twinsburg, OH.)

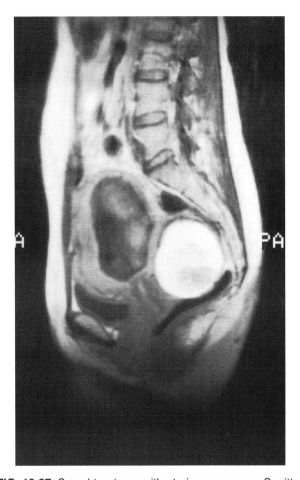

FIG. 12-27. Sacral teratoma with uterine pregnancy. Sagittal T1-weighted image demonstrates a high signal intensity lesion in the pelvis that is well circumscribed consistent with a teratoma. A large thick-walled mass with an oblong signal intensity inside is also present and is consistent with a fetus. When imaging the lumbar spine, it is important to evaluate the pelvis for masses that may be the source of the patient's back or radicular pain.

visualized on MRI. Parasagittal views are often helpful in assessing neural foraminal compromise. Axial views often delineate the degree of foraminal narrowing.

SPINAL CORD

Normal Spinal Cord Anatomy

The butterfly-shaped central gray matter of the spinal cord is the most conspicuous landmark on histologic sections (Fig. 12-26). Proton-weighted MR images revealed increased intensity in the gray matter (4). The surface of the cord is longitudinally indented by the median fissure, penetrates the cord for a depth of up to 3 mm, and contains branches of the anterior spinal artery and vein. The central core of the spinal cord contains the spinal cord gray matter, which comprises nerve cell bodies, demyelinated fibers, and dendrites. It has roughly the form of a butterfly or the letter H. The white matter is divided into three main columns known as *funiculi*. The dorsal funiculi are the prominent columns of white matter that carry the largest ascending tracts to the cerebral cortex. The cervical and lumbosacral cord is slightly enlarged at those levels at which the nerves supplying the extremities are associated. In the cervical cord, the enlargement is at approximately cord levels C-4 to T-1. The lumbosacral enlargement is found at vertebral levels T9-12, corresponding to cord levels L-2 to S-3.

Spinal Neoplasm

Spinal tumors are often categorized as extradural or intradural and extramedullary or intramedullary in location.

This classification is somewhat of an overgeneralization, because some lesions may reside in two compartments simultaneously (5). For example, a nerve root sheath tumor, such as a neurofibroma, may appear dumbbell-shaped and extend into both the extradural and intradural extramedullary spaces (Fig. 12-27).

Intramedullary Neoplasms

In the intramedullary space, primary tumors are far more common than are secondary tumors or metastases. Metastases to the cord itself are comparatively unusual. More than 90% of intramedullary tumors are gliomas, especially ependymoma and low-grade astrocytoma. Spinal cord glioblastomas are uncommon. Other primary spinal cord

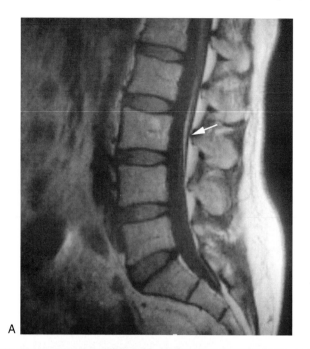

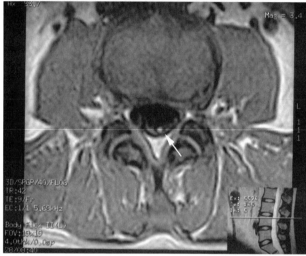

FIG. 12-28. Small lipoma in the filum terminale (*arrows*). T1-weighted spin-echo sagittal image **(A)** and T1-weighted axial three-dimensional Fourier transform image from a different patient **(B)**. Often, small lipomas in the filum can present a somewhat confusing picture on magnetic resonance imaging because they can appear to have different levels of brightness, depending on the pulse sequence used. When making this diagnosis, it is helpful to compare the brightness of the filum terminale with the surrounding fat.

tumors include hemangioblastoma, lipoma (Fig. 12-28), metastases, and paraganglioma.

Ependymoma

Ependymomas are the most common type of glioma of the spinal cord and filum terminale. The lumbosacral segments are most frequently involved, largely because spinal ependymomas appear to be almost equally divided between intramedullary tumors and those originating in the region of the conus medullaris. When the latter group is excluded, the distribution of intramedullary ependymomas at various spinal cord levels is approximately even. Ependymomas are interesting in their relationships between location, histology, and biological aggressiveness. Whereas cellular ependymomas can occur anywhere in the neuraxis including the conus, papillary tumors are confined to the spinal region, and the myxopapillary variant of papillary tumors is unique to the conus and filum terminale. The vast majority of spinal ependymomas have little infiltrative potential and exhibit slow biological growth. Ependymomas are seen in some patients with type II neurofibromatosis.

MRI shows a widened cord with isointense signal compared to T1-weighted images and mixed signal on T2-weighted images. Hemorrhage is common and is often apparent as a hemosiderin "tail" extending into the central canal of the spinal cord above and below the tumor. Tumor cysts and syrinx cavities are frequently present. Virtually all ependymomas enhance strongly after contrast administration; this is helpful to differentiate cystic areas and syrinx cavities from neoplasm (6). No reliable criteria exist to separate ependymoma from astrocytoma.

Astrocytoma

Unlike astrocytoma in the brain, most spinal cord astrocytomas are low-grade neoplasms. The tumors infiltrate the cord and are more difficult to resect than are ependymomas. Astrocytoma is less likely to hemorrhage than ependymoma. Tumor cysts are common, although syrinx is less common than with ependymoma (7). The cervical cord is the most common location (Fig. 12-29). On MRI, these tumors appear as multisegmental intramedullary masses, usually isointense to hypointense on T1-weighted images and hyperintense on T2-weighted images (8). More than 95% of spinal cord astrocytomas enhance (more than in the brain), but nonenhancing tumors do occur.

Hemangioblastoma

Hemangioblastomas are rare benign tumors that may be intramedullary or combined intramedullary and extramedullary in location. Approximately one-third occur in conjunction with von Hippel–Lindau syndrome (9). One or more enhancing vascular nodules are seen with an accompanying syrinx or focal cyst, often involving the cervicomedullary junction (Fig. 12-30).

Extramedullary Neoplasms

In the extradural space, metastases are far more common than are primary tumors, although numerous primary bone tumors can occur. However, with few exceptions, such as

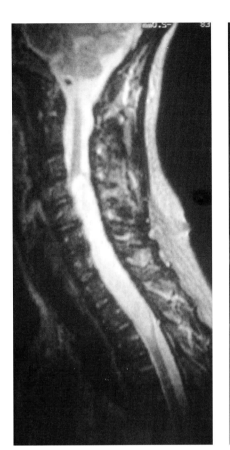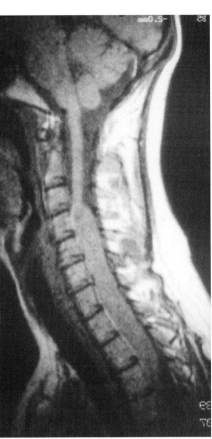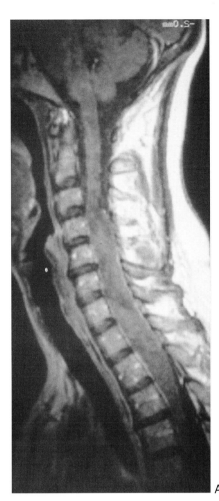

A–C

FIG. 12-29. Grade II glioma of the cervical and upper thoracic cord. T2-weighted **(A)**, proton density–weighted **(B)**, and postcontrast T1-weighted **(C)** sagittal images demonstrate an extensive infiltrative tumor with expansion of the cord. When imaging spinal tumors or syrinxes, it is important to see to the inferior aspect to know the full extent of the disease process.

hemangioma, most of the primary bone tumors are comparatively unusual (10,11).

In the intradural extramedullary space, primary tumors, such as neurofibroma and meningioma, are relatively common. Secondary tumors or leptomeningeal metastases are seen with increasing frequency as imaging and other tests assist clinicians in the diagnosis (Fig. 12-31).

Nerve sheath tumors and meningiomas account for more than 80% of all intradural extramedullary neoplasms. The most common intradural extramedullary masses involving the spine are nerve sheath tumors. More than 95% of these tumors are schwannomas or neurofibromas (Fig. 12-32). Other tumors include metastases, epidermoid and dermoid tumors, paraganglioma, and lipoma.

Nerve Sheath Tumors

Nerve sheath tumors may present as intradural extramedullary masses, dumbbell-shaped lesions, extradural masses, or rarely, as intramedullary lesions. Schwannoma is the most frequently occurring nerve sheath tumor and is usually a sporadic lesion. Neurofibromas occur in conjunction with type I neurofibromatosis, whereas meningioma and ependymoma are seen in neurofibromatosis type II. Almost all nerve sheath tumors enhance with gadolinium and are hyperintense on T2-weighted images. A small number of these tumors are slightly hyperintense on T1-weighted images, although the typical lesion is isointense.

Meningioma

Most meningiomas are benign. Aggressive meningiomas are less common in the spine than in the intracranial compartment. Meningiomas are second to nerve sheath tumors in frequency, and they are seen in peak incidence in women in the fifth and sixth decades of life. Multiple spinal meningiomas are seen in conjunction with neurofibro-

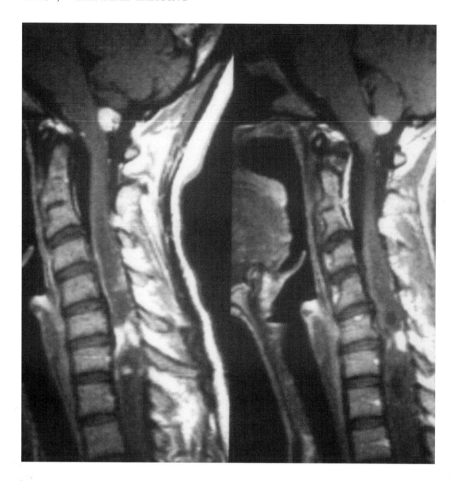

FIG. 12-30. Hemangioblastoma. Post-contrast T1-weighted images of the inferior brainstem and cervical cord demonstrate an enhancing tumor nodule at the craniocervical junction. An extensive syrinx extends from approximately C2-3 to the thoracic cord. In this syrinx, multiple enhancing neural nodules represent secondary seeding of the tumor. This study should not be viewed as complete, because the inferior aspect of the syrinx is not visualized. It is also important in such cases to image the entire spinal canal for other enhancing nodules.

matosis type II. These tumors have a broad-based dural attachment, show intense enhancement with contrast administration, and may show an enhancing dural "tail," as in the intracranial compartmental lesions. Approximately 5% of meningiomas are hypointense, and 5% are hyperintense on T1- and T2-weighted images, whereas most are isointense.

Syrinx

At least six categories of syringomyelia exist: congenital, traumatic (Fig. 12-33), neoplastic, compressive, postinflammatory (arachnoiditis), and idiopathic. The most common form is the congenital type, usually associated with a Chiari I malformation. This type makes up 40% to 50% of all cases. A presyringomyelic state of microcystic myelomalacia and edema is most often seen in patients who have suffered severe spinal cord trauma (12,13). Gadolinium is often used in the evaluation of these patients. Open MRI may be specifically requested because of the ease of MRI evaluation of patients in cervical halo fixation devices.

Demyelinating and Inflammatory Disease

Spinal cord involvement is considered by some to be inevitable at some stage of multiple sclerosis, producing motor, sensory, or sphincteric disturbance or a combination. Cervical cord lesions, particularly of the posterior column, may be associated with Lhermitte's sign, in which the patient experiences the sudden sensation of an electric shock running down his or her back when the head is flexed suddenly. The criterion requiring multiplicity in time and space for clinically definite multiple sclerosis (MS) can be satisfied by a gadolinium-enhanced MRI study if the study shows chronic nonenhancing lesions as well as acute enhancing lesions (14).

Cavitation in MS plaque in the spinal cord can rarely occur and is presumed to result from severe inflammatory changes occurring in some acute plaques (15). Large acute lesions may be associated with severe edema and cord swelling leading to vascular compression, ischemia, and acute necrotic myelopathy. Gadolinium contrast enhancement occurs in acute lesions (Fig. 12-34), but the duration of enhancement is variable, correlating with the variable course of disease in patients, and usually lasts less than 1

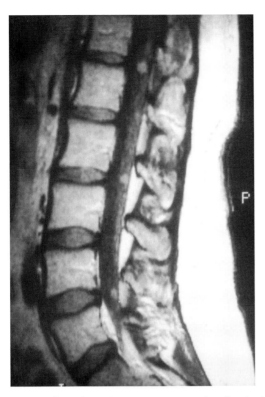

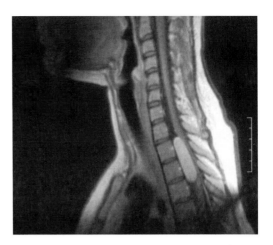

FIG. 12-32. Large enhancing neurofibroma. Sagittal T1-weighted postgadolinium image of the cervical and upper thoracic spine demonstrates a large, well-circumscribed enhancing mass that is consistent with a neurofibroma. It is important to look at the entire field of view of the sagittal images. Often, when obtaining sagittal images of the cervical spine, the technologist may crop out the upper thoracic spine. It can be helpful to make a second set of films that shows the entire field of view, as in this case, to identify lesions that may be in the upper thoracic spine.

FIG. 12-31. Spinal melanoma metastasis. Sagittal T1-weighted image without gadolinium demonstrates multiple nodules in the spinal canal, which has signal intensity similar to marrow fat. Melanoma is one of the few lesions with metastases that can be bright on T1-weighted images due to shortened T1 from the melanin content.

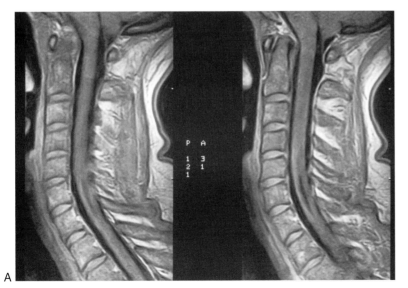

A

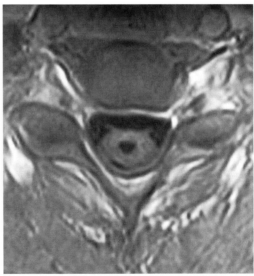

B

FIG. 12-33. Traumatic syrinx. Sagittal **(A)** and axial **(B)** T1-weighted three-dimensional Fourier transform images demonstrate cerebrospinal fluid signal intensity in the central portion of the cervical cord. The axial T1-weighted images are most helpful in identifying a syrinx. In patients without a history of trauma, all syrinx should be considered to be caused by tumors until proven otherwise, which is why gadolinium is essential whenever a syrinx is identified. The sagittal large field of view demonstrates the entire extent of this small syrinx.

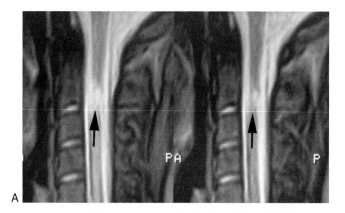

A

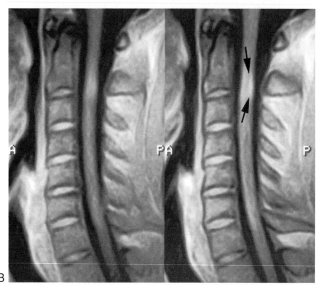

B

FIG. 12-34. Gadolinium-enhancing multiple sclerosis (MS) lesion of the upper cervical cord. T2-weighted **(A)** and T1-weighted postcontrast sagittal **(B)** gradient-echo images demonstrate a lesion that is bright on the T2-weighted images and enhances in the posterior region (*arrows*). This lesion at the C2-3 level is consistent with the patient's known history of MS. In patients who present with a cervical cord lesion, a T2-weighted and fluid attenuated inversion recovery image of the brain can be very helpful in making the diagnosis of MS.

month. Enhancement may occasionally show a small peripheral lesion that is obscured on T2-weighted imaging owing to its small size and proximity to high–signal intensity CSF. MS plaque enhancement is not likely in patients with clinically stable disease.

Chronic lesions cannot be differentiated from acute or subacute lesions on noncontrast images, unless a change in cord size occurs. Focal or diffuse spinal cord atrophy may occur in chronic MS. Short segment focal atrophic areas result from involution of a localized plaque. These areas often have a persistent high signal abnormality on T2-weighted MR images. Diffuse cord atrophy is a well known

result of chronic MS, and frequently no signal abnormality is seen.

Acute Transverse Myelitis

Transverse myelitis is an inflammatory intramedullary disorder of the spinal cord. The term is nonspecific in that a number of conditions and etiologic agents are associated with the clinical syndrome of transverse myelitis, including parainfectious and postvaccinial events, MS, paraneoplastic myelopathy, vascular insufficiency, and autoimmune disorders (16).

MRI may be normal in some patients who fulfill the clinical criteria of the disease. MRI may also appear falsely negative if performed very early in the disease. When positive, the MR appearance of acute transverse myelitis is variable and nonspecific. The affected area of the cord may appear swollen or normal in size. Cavitation rarely occurs, but hypointensity may be seen on T1-weighted images. T2-weighted images show abnormal increased intensity. Short or long segments of the cord may be affected (17). The entire transverse diameter of the cord is affected, and if an incomplete cord lesion is in the transverse dimension, the likelihood that the diagnosis will ultimately be MS is increased. Mild to moderate enhancement may be seen with gadolinium in contrast to the more intense enhancement noted with most cord tumors.

VASCULAR DISEASE AND SPINAL CORD ISCHEMIA

Because of the limited but critical sources of blood supply to the spinal cord, any pathologic processes that interfere with this crucial blood supply may result in spinal cord ischemia, infarction, or both.

Vascular Anatomy

The blood supply to the entire spinal cord is uniquely dependent on three longitudinal arterial trunks: a single anterior spinal artery and paired posterior spinal arteries. These spinal arteries extend from the medulla oblongata to the conus medullaris. Although these longitudinal trunks are usually continuous, the anterior spinal artery is narrowest in the midthoracic region and widest in the cervical region. Thirty-one pairs of radicular arteries penetrate the spinal canal through the intervertebral foramina. Of these 63 arteries, the number of anterior radiculomedullary arteries supplying the anterior spinal artery rarely exceeds nine but ranges from two to 17, defining cervicothoracic, midthoracic, and thoracolumbar territories (18). The cervicothoracic territory includes the cervical spinal cord, its brachial plexus enlargement, and the

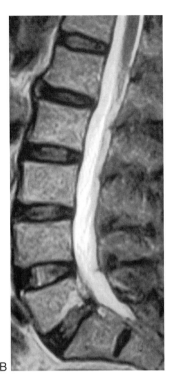 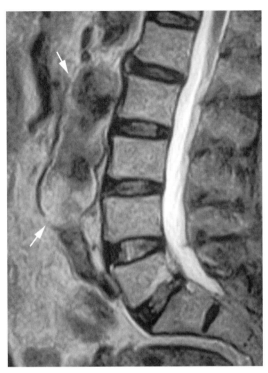

A, B

FIG. 12-35. Aortic aneurysm. T2-weighted sagittal fast spin-echo images. **A:** Filmed with the mid and anterior portion of the abdomen cropped off to present a more appealing picture to the referring physician. **B:** When the entire field of view is not evaluated, it can be easy to miss pathology in the abdomen and pelvis, such as this rather obvious aortic aneurysm (*arrows*), which most likely is the reason for this patient's severe low back pain.

first two or three thoracic segments. This territory is richly supplied by the anterior spinal artery arising from the intracranial vertebral arteries, the midcervical radicular branches of the vertebral artery, and the branches of the costocervical trunk. The midthoracic territory (T4-8) is usually supplied by a radicular branch arising at about the T-7 level. The thoracolumbar territory includes the lower thoracic segments and the lumbar enlargement. This area is supplied by the artery of Adamkiewicz, which is the largest anterior medullary feeder. The artery of Adamkiewicz occurs on the left side in 80% of subjects and can arise anywhere between the T5 and L4 levels (T9-L2 in 85%, T9-11 in 75%, L1-2 in 10%, and T5-8 in 15%) (18). When the artery of Adamkiewicz originates from a high intercostal vessel, a supplemental arterial supply to the conus medullaris from a smaller radicular branch originating more inferiorly usually exists. The radicular arteries form two distinct systems of intrinsic blood supply to the spinal cord. The first system is a posterolateral peripheral plexus formed primarily by the two posterior spinal arteries that run longitudinally along the posterolateral sulcus of the cord and are richly interconnected by anastomotic channels. The posterior medullary feeders (radiculomedullary arteries) supplying the posterior spinal artery are more numerous, usually ranging from ten to 23. (19). The posterior spinal arteries are also supplied by radicular arteries derived from segmental arteries or their regional equivalents (including several arteries and posterior inferior cerebellar arteries). In most cases, the artery of Adamkiewicz

supplies the entire lumbosacral cord, including the posterior spinal arteries.

Spinal Cord Ischemia

Spinal cord ischemia or infarction primarily affects the older age group, usually with a devastating outcome. One of the causes of cord infarction is aortic dissection. Rarely, spinal cord infarction is limited to the gray matter, and in these patients abrupt onset of muscle weakness in the legs occurs, but with no pain or sensory loss.

The causes of spinal cord ischemia are variable and include arteriosclerosis, dissection of an aortic aneurysm, infection, trauma, vasculitis, antiphospholipid syndrome, emboli, aortic surgery, decompression sickness, and radiation therapy (20). Most cases of spontaneous spinal cord ischemia occur in patients with a thoracoabdominal aortic aneurysm (Fig. 12-35). Most spinal cord infarctions occur in the upper thoracic region around the T-4 level or at the thoracolumbar junction. Infarctions in the latter site may result from occlusion of the artery of Adamkiewicz, which is frequently the only blood supply to the thoracolumbar junction. In the upper thoracic regions, medullary feeder arteries are sparse, the anterior spinal artery is narrow, sulcus arteries are fewer and smaller, the spinal canal is narrow, and the spinal cord is in a watershed area between major feeding arteries (19). The vertical extent of spinal cord infarction may vary from one to 15 segments, depending on the vascular anatomy of the cord and extent of occlusion. Single segmental infarction is frequently caused by ischemia in the watershed area, as occurs in hypotension. Single segmental infarction may also be seen in diseases that affect the small end arteries, such as emboli or focal vasculopathies.

Spinal cord swelling is typically seen in acute cord infarction. Spinal cord infarcts should be considered in the differential diagnosis of all patients with slightly expansile cord lesions associated with T1 and T2 prolongation in the appropriate clinical setting. Axial and sagittal images are useful in demonstrating the areas of abnormal signal. Signal abnormality may involve only the gray matter structures but, in more severely affected patients, extends throughout the entire cross section of the cord to affect gray and white matter, suggesting involvement of anterior and posterior spinal arterial vascular distributions. T1-weighted images are often normal or demonstrate only subtle cord enlargement in the acute stage. After administration of gadolinium, cord enhancement may occur, especially involving the gray matter. Serial imaging can document the evolution of hemorrhage and breakdown of the blood–cord barrier and can demonstrate evolving signal changes in nearby vertebral bodies that may also be associated with spinal ischemia. Abnormal signal, particularly a central triangular area near the end plate of the vertebral body, associated with a nonexpansile or slightly expansile cord lesion should suggest the possibility of spinal cord infarction (19,21).

Vascular Malformations of the Spinal Cord

Spinal arteriovenous malformations (AVMs) represent 3% to 4% of spinal cord masses. Spinal AVMs occur more commonly in men and are usually manifested between the fifth and seventh decades of life. Symon (22) noted a 9 to 1 male predominance with an age range of 29 to 75 years. Only 13% of all spinal AVMs occur in patients younger than age 20 (23). The lower thoracic spinal cord and conus are usually the most severely affected (Fig. 12-36), despite the locus of the fistula. The most common AVM is type I (i.e., dural arteriovenous fistula) (Fig. 12-37) (24).

Spinal AVMs have been broadly divided into two groups: intramedullary and extramedullary. Intramedullary AVMs are usually seen in young patients and are characterized by acute hemorrhage and primarily derived from the anterior spinal cord blood supply. Most spinal AVMs are extramedullary and seen in elderly men. These lesions are characterized by progressive neurologic deficits and a posterior blood supply.

Classification

Vascular malformations of the spinal cord have been classified into four types (25):

- *Type I* spinal vascular malformations are characterized by a single tortuous arterialized vein that trellises over the pia of the spinal cord.

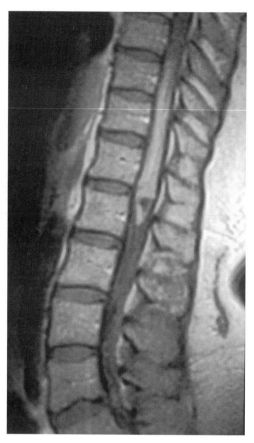

FIG. 12-36. Extensive vascular malformation of the distal thoracic cord and conus. Sagittal T1-weighted spin-echo image with contrast demonstrates extensive enhancing soft tissue extending from the lower thoracic cord into the conus. This was thought to be an astrocytoma or ependymoma. After biopsy, however, a vascular malformation was demonstrated. It is important to include vascular malformations in the differential diagnosis for spinal cord lesions.

- *Type II*, or glomus, spinal vascular malformation contain an identifiable focal *intramedullary* nidus of AVM supplied by multiple feeders from the anterior or posterior spinal arteries.
- *Type III*, or juvenile, spinal AVMs have multiple arterial feeders from several different vertebral levels.
- *Type IV intradural*, or perimedullary, arteriovenous fistulas lie completely outside the spinal cord and pia mater.

Another type of vascular lesion, the cavernous angioma, can best be described as a tumor. Cavernous angiomas are slow-flow vascular malformations without arteriovenous shunting (26) that displace neural tissue. These lesions are more common in the brain, and when they occur in the spine are most often intramedullary. Cavernous angiomas of the spine are pathologically identical to their intracranial counterparts and vary in diameter from several millimeters to more than a centimeter. Most commonly, they are well-demarcated lesions surrounded by hemosiderin-stained gliotic neural tissue. The constant presence of blood storage products suggests episodic leakage of blood or low-grade

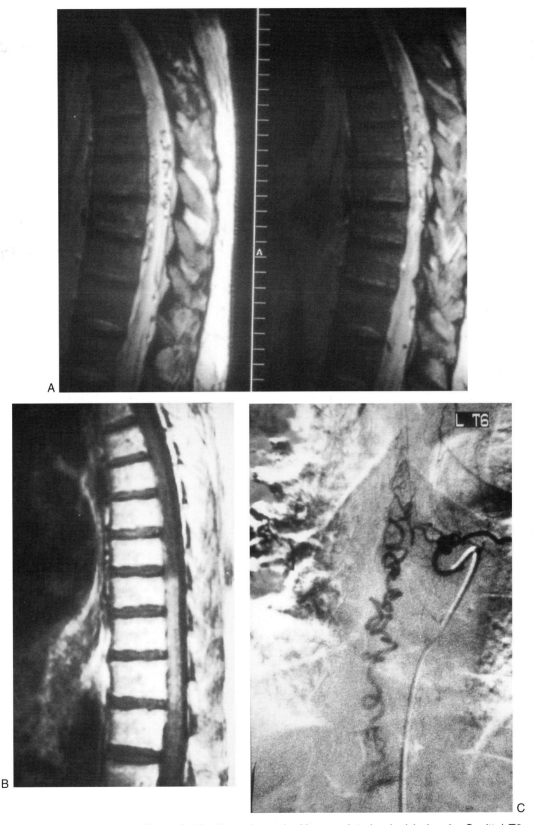

FIG. 12-37. Arteriovenous fistula in the thoracic cord with associated spinal ischemia. Sagittal T2-weighted images **(A)**, sagittal T1-weighted postgadolinium image **(B)**, and spinal angiogram **(C)** demonstrate an extensive serpentine signal void in the spinal canal outlined by the cerebrospinal fluid on the T2-weighted images. The angiogram confirms that these low signal intensity lesions are vessels. This appearance should be contrasted with dephasing artifacts, as demonstrated in Figure 12-39.

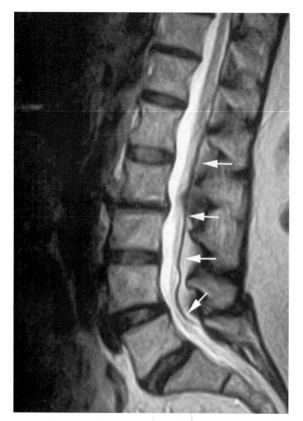

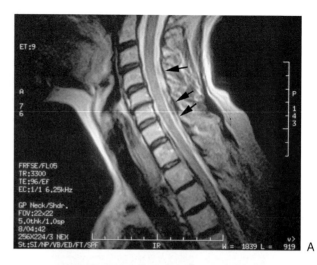

FIG. 12-38. Linear area of low signal intensity in the posterior aspect of the lumbar spine is consistent with chemical shift artifact (*arrows*). T2-weighted sagittal fast spin-echo image of the lumbar spine demonstrates a longitudinal low signal intensity posterior to the thecal sac at the junction with the epidural fat (*arrows*). The frequency-encoding axis is anterior to posterior. Therefore, the chemical shift artifact is anterior to posterior. This can be exaggerated with the lower bandwidths used in open magnetic resonance imaging. To confirm the diagnosis, simply swap the phase and frequency, and this black line disappears from its current location. It is important not to mistake this artifact for hemosiderin.

hemorrhage from the lesions. Acute hemorrhage within or adjacent to the lesions is present in some cases.

MRI findings are often characteristic and usually permit a relatively specific diagnosis. A rim of low signal intensity representing iron storage products completely surrounds the lesion (Fig. 12-38). Intrinsic heterogeneous signal abnormality is present on T1- and T2-weighted images representing blood products of various ages.

Foix-Alajouanine Syndrome

In 1926, Foix and Alajouanine described a process associated with enlarged vessels without thrombosis within the spinal cord. Since then, the term *Foix-Alajouanine syndrome* has been used to describe almost any type of necrosis or infarction in the spinal cord (27). Two forms of the disorder have been described. One is characterized by enlarged,

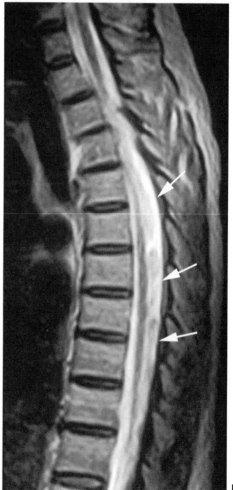

FIG. 12-39. Dephasing from flow artifact mimicking a spinal arteriovenous malformation (*arrows*). **A, B:** Sagittal fast spin-echo T2-weighted images. The dephasing of the cerebrospinal fluid (CSF) due to flow turbulence is commonly seen in open magnetic resonance imaging, especially with fast spin-echo images. This is exaggerated with atrophy of the cord **(B)**. To confirm that this is an artifact, flow compensation should be turned off or on—whichever is the opposite of its status during the examination. Also, other sequences with bright CSF, such as fast short tau inversion recovery, can be helpful to confirm that this is a simple dephasing artifact.

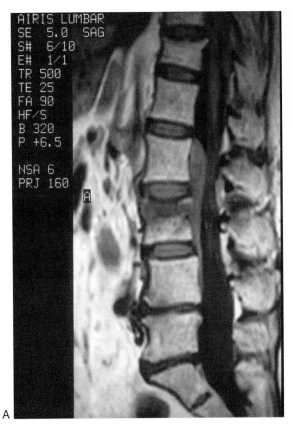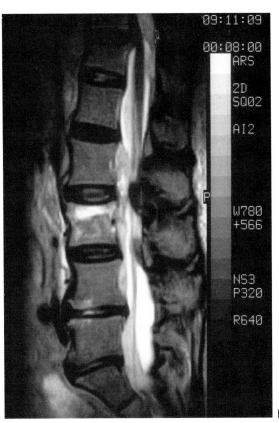

FIG. 12-40. Large hematoma in the epidural space compressing the thecal sac. T1-weighted **(A)** and T2-weighted **(B)** sagittal images demonstrate epidural fluid collections of mixed signal intensity that appear to be compressing the thecal sac. It is crucial to differentiate hematomas from other fluid collections such as abscesses. Computed tomography can be an excellent adjunct to magnetic resonance imaging to assist in this differential diagnosis.

hypertrophic vessels within the spinal cord and is considered idiopathic, although an associated carcinoma elsewhere has been noted in some cases. The pathologic processes that occur in Foix-Alajouanine syndrome may represent the final common pathway of a chronic progressive radiculomyelopathy of ischemic and exudative character due to a variety of local morphologic or functional vascular anomalies.

IMAGING

MRI is the primary modality for investigating spinal cord disorders. Axial and sagittal T1-weighted images should be obtained with and without contrast. Sagittal T2-weighted images are necessary, and axial T2-weighted images are advisable. Techniques such as 512 matrix data acquisition, 3- to 4-mm section thickness, and phased-array surface coils should be used whenever possible.

The MRI finding of spinal cord AVM consists of increased signal on T2-weighted images and normal or low signal on T1-weighted images. High signal in the lower cord and conus is a constant finding that is probably caused by venous hypertension of the lower spinal cord. The intramedullary changes can be nonspecific, especially

with small lesions, and must be distinguished from MS, trauma, ischemia, cyst, or transverse myelitis. The cord may be mildly enlarged along the affected segment. Serpiginous signal loss (flow void) and signal gain in small vessels may be seen along the posterior margin of the cord and within the cord. The flow-void signal due to enlarged vessels must be distinguished from CSF flow artifact (Fig. 12-39). Gadolinium enhancement is very helpful in further characterizing the nature of the signal abnormality in the spinal cord. Enhancement may be seen, indicating a breakdown in the blood–cord barrier associated with chronic or subacute ischemic damage. Enhancement intensifies over 45 minutes (28).

SPINAL CORD TRAUMA

Spinal cord injury is a devastating condition of major public health importance. The annual incidence of spinal cord injury in the United States has been estimated at more than 14,000 cases by the National Spinal Cord Injury Data Research Center, with 10,000 patients surviving the initial traumatic event. Approximately 10% of this group die while hospitalized; half of these deaths occur during the first month. Most spinal cord

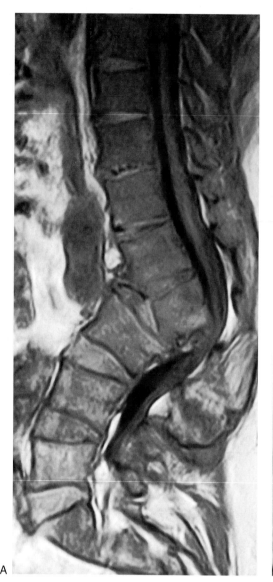
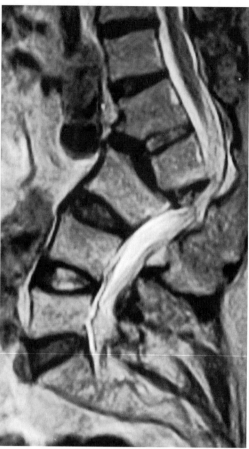

A   B

FIG. 12-41. Congenital kyphotic malformation of the lumbar spine. T1-weighted three-dimensional Fourier transform **(A)** and fast spin-echo T2-weighted **(B)** sagittal images of the lumbar spine demonstrate a disc space between the superior aspect of L-3 and the anterior aspect of L-1 and L-2. Severe canal stenosis is secondary to this congenital abnormality. No destruction of the vertebral bodies or collapse that would suggest trauma is noted. The marrow in the vertebral bodies is also normal in signal intensity, which also suggests a congenital abnormality. This patient complained of low back pain and was able to walk into the magnetic resonance imaging center. When presented with an unusual spine abnormality such as this, it is important to consider congenital origin and not just trauma or infection.

injuries occur in young individuals. Approximately 50% of patients are younger than 25 years, and 80% are male.

Motor vehicle accidents are the primary cause of spinal cord injury, accounting for 40% to 50% of cases. In descending order of frequency, falls, sporting accidents (especially diving), and penetrating injuries of the spinal column secondary to gunshot or knife wounds are responsible for almost all other spinal cord injuries.

The greatest impact MRI has had in the evaluation of spinal trauma has been in assessment of the intracanalicular and paraspinal soft tissues, especially the spinal cord. The integrity of the intervertebral discs and ligamentous complexes can be routinely evaluated after trauma (29). MRI permits direct visualization of the morphology of the injured cord parenchyma and the relationship of the surrounding structures to the spinal cord (Figs. 12-40 and 12-41) (30).

Spinal Cord Concussion

Concussion of the spinal cord refers to a temporary and reversible loss of function, with symptoms resolving over sev-

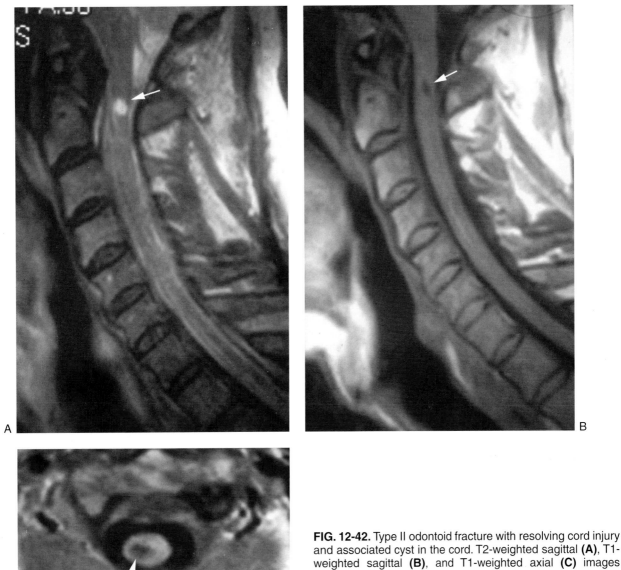

FIG. 12-42. Type II odontoid fracture with resolving cord injury and associated cyst in the cord. T2-weighted sagittal **(A)**, T1-weighted sagittal **(B)**, and T1-weighted axial **(C)** images clearly demonstrate the small cystic-appearing lesion in the cervical cord just posterior to the C-2 vertebral body (*arrows*). Whenever presented with a small cyst in the cord, attention should be paid to the surrounding vertebral structures to rule out fracture and to evaluate for ligamentous injury.

eral minutes to hours. No known histologic changes are associated with this injury. The loss of function most likely is due to reversible changes in the metabolism of the nerve cells, axons, or endothelial cells, produced by a mild jarring of the cord.

Spinal Cord Contusion

Contusion of the spinal cord refers to a bruise with mechanical damage to the tissue and varying degrees of hemorrhage. A further distinction is sometimes made between those injuries with an intact cord surface and those with tearing or maceration of the cord. Regardless of the severity, the

histologic changes are not completely reversible, and some degree of neurologic deficit usually persists. In the hyperacute phase, a contused cord may appear normal. Early edema formation may be seen and, in more severe cases, actual parenchymal disruption and petechial hemorrhage may occur. If a gross hematoma occurs during this stage, it is often located in the ventral part of the posterior horns or about the central canal. Within a few hours of injury, necrosis and hemorrhage begin to develop within the central gray matter of the cord, and, after approximately 24 hours, most lesions exhibit hemorrhagic necrosis. Ischemic lesions may also be seen in remote segments of the cord owing to injury to spinal arteries. Over the next few weeks to months, gliosis, cyst formation, and atrophy of the cord develop (Fig. 12-42). Scarring also occurs in the arachnoid and may produce cord tethering or arachnoid cysts (31).

Spinal Cord Maceration

Maceration of the cord may occur as a result of comminuted fractures when bony fragments are displaced into the cord or may be due to extreme dislocations that produce marked narrowing of the spinal canal. In addition to the generally more severe mechanical disruption caused by this type of injury, tearing of the cord surface and pia occurs. As a result, mesenchymal granulation tissue can grow into the cord and produce a larger fibrotic scar within the cord. Otherwise, many of the pathologic changes are similar to those seen in cord contusion.

Spinal Cord Laceration

Laceration of the cord is produced by penetrating injuries, such as stab or gunshot wounds, or by the sharp edges of bony fracture fragments. Because gunshot wounds and comminuted fractures usually also produce contusive effects, this discussion concentrates on stab wounds.

Spinal Cord Transsection

Complete transsection of the cord may be the result of stab or missile injuries but may also be caused by severe hyperextension of the cervical spine. In neonates, cord transsection may be the result of traction on the head during difficult deliveries. Although the cord becomes completely severed, the dura usually remains at least partially intact and can keep the margins of the cord opposed. Scar tissue may then be able to bridge the gap between the torn edges of the cord, but this does not result in any functional recovery (32).

SPINAL INFECTIONS

Spinal infections are uncommon. Infections of the spine can be separated into infections of the vertebral bodies and discs, epidural space, intradural space, and of the spinal cord itself.

Pyogenic infections of the spine involve primarily the disc space in children and the vertebral bodies in adults. The lumbar spine is most frequently involved.

Discitis and Osteomyelitis

The MRI findings of discitis and osteomyelitis closely match the pathologic findings. Bony destruction secondary to lytic enzymes and the associated increased water con-

tent are reflected by the increased signal intensity on T2-weighted images and decreased signal intensity on T1-weighted images (Fig. 12-43). The signal alterations often precede the destructive changes. Degenerative disease of the disc and vertebrae can simulate infection. Modic type I changes are characterized by low signal intensity on T1-weighted images and high signal intensity on T2-weighted images, which can mimic infection. A degenerated disc can also enhance even in its central portion or in the periphery adjacent to the vertebral end plates; however, the disc is usually of low signal intensity on T2-weighted images. A follow-up study in several weeks should demonstrate no change, in contrast to the progressive changes of discitis. The type II and III changes have signal characteristics that can easily be differentiated from discitis and osteomyelitis (33).

Infection of the Epidural and Subdural Spaces

Infection of the spinal epidural and subdural spaces is relatively uncommon. Yet, despite advances in medical imaging and diagnostic studies, when spinal epidural or subdural infections do occur, their diagnosis is often missed at the time of initial presentation. This delay in diagnosis and initiation of appropriate treatment accounts for the continued high morbidity and mortality rates associated with intraspinal abscesses. Increased awareness of the clinical picture of a spinal abscess and a high index of suspicion of spinal sepsis are essential for the physician to make an early diagnosis and prevent potential neurologic sequelae and death.

Various pyogenic, granulomatous, fungal, and parasitic infections have been reported to invade the spinal epidural and subdural spaces. The following paragraphs provide a brief review of these pathogenic organisms, the spinal infections they cause, and an outline of appropriate diagnostic management and treatment protocols.

The most common location for an epidural spinal infection is the lumbar spine, and the next most common locations are the thoracic and cervical spinal segments.

MRI may demonstrate very early changes, including decreased T1-weighted signal and increased T2-weighted signals of the vertebral bone marrow and disc. The STIR sequence is especially useful for demonstration of vertebral body changes by accentuating differences in water content seen on spin-echo sequences. Gadolinium enhancement is important, but precontrast scans are necessary because bone marrow enhancement due to inflammation may be isointense compared to normal fatty bone marrow. The disc space almost always is involved in pyogenic infections but rarely in neoplastic disease or very late in tuberculous infections. Loss of the vertebral end plate and generalized blurring of the margins between disc, end plate, and bone marrow are the key findings on noncontrast T1-weighted images. Large paraspinous masses often are associated with

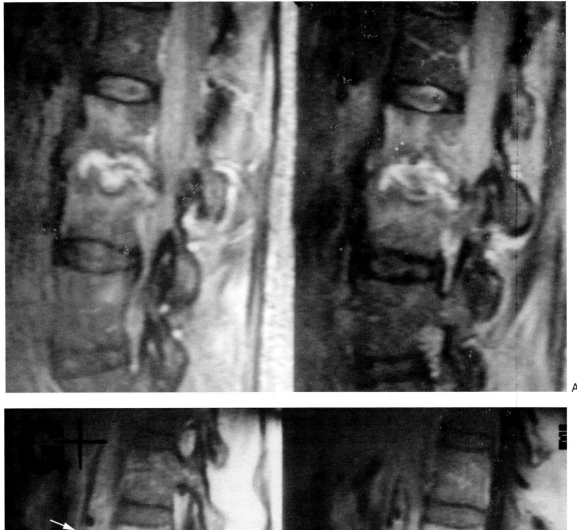

A

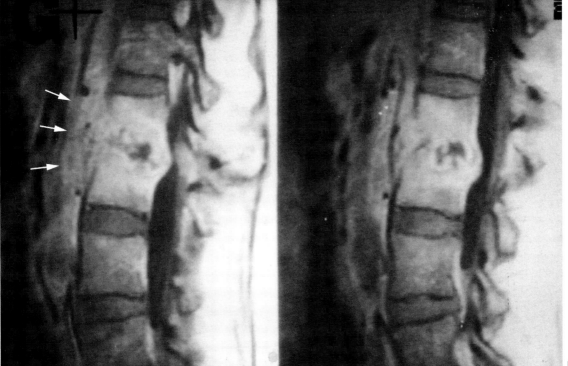

B

FIG. 12-43. Discitis at the L3-4 level. T2-weighted **(A)** and T1-weighted postcontrast **(B)** sagittal images demonstrate extensive loss of vertebral body end plates and marked contrast enhancement of the infected disc and surrounding vertebral bodies. A small ventral epidural extension of this infectious process is also seen. A perivertebral abscess is identified on the postgadolinium studies anterior to the vertebral bodies and appears to extend superior to the L-2 vertebral body (*arrows*).

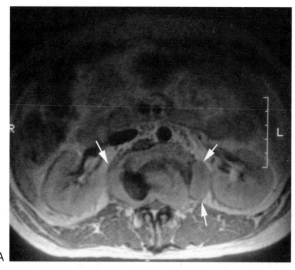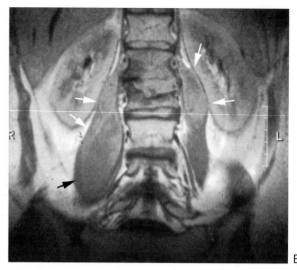

A

B

FIG. 12-44. Tuberculosis of the spine with extension into both psoas muscles. Axial **(A)** and coronal **(B)** T1-weighted images, both without contrast, demonstrate extensive soft tissue mass, which extends out through the intervertebral foramina and surrounds the vertebral body. Also, note is made of extension into both psoas muscles (*arrows*). These bilateral psoas muscle abscesses are classic features of tuberculosis. Whenever spinal magnetic resonance imaging exhibits a large soft tissue mass, infection should always be included in the differential diagnosis.

tuberculous infections (Fig. 12-44) (34). When epidural abscesses are present, they usually extend across several spinal segments, with an average extent of four vertebrae. Discitis or osteomyelitis is the preceding source of infection in most cases of spinal epidural abscess. A significant number of patients report a history of intravenous drug abuse (35,36).

Another common predisposing factor for a spinal epidural infection is a preceding invasive diagnostic or surgical procedure on the spine. An epidural infection is iso- or hypointense to the spinal cord on unenhanced T1-weighted images and hyperintense on T2-weighted and proton density–weighted images. Postcontrast MRI shows homogeneous or heterogeneous enhancement of the solid portion of the abscess, or peripheral enhancement around a central liquefied collection of purulent material, or both. Dural enhancement is noted in cases of abscesses spanning several vertebral segments, and engorgement of the epidural venous plexus and basivertebral veins is observed occasionally. Reactive paraspinous fluid collections are often seen in association with spinal epidural infections.

MRI can also be used successfully to follow the progression of the occasional abscess that is managed conservatively. The changes seen on follow-up MRI correlate well with the patient's clinical improvement or deterioration. Despite clinical improvement, persistent contrast enhancement is often observed at the site of discitis, osteomyelitis, or surgical drainage (37–40).

REFERENCES

1. Modic MT, Herfkens RJ. Devil's advocate: normal age-related changes in MR signal intensity. *Radiology* 1990;177:332–334.
2. Andersson GBJ, Brown MD, Dvorak J, et al. Consensus summary on the diagnosis and treatment of lumbar disc herniation. *Spine* 1996;21:755–786.
3. Teresi LM, Lufkin RB, Reicher MA, et al. Asymptomatic degenerative disk disease and spondylosis of the cervical spine: MR imaging. *Radiology* 1987;164:83–88.
4. Carvilin MJ, Asato R, Hackney DB, Kassab E, Joseph PM. High-resolution MR of the spinal cord in humans and rats. *AJNR Am J Neuroradiol* 1989;10:13–17.
5. Enzmann DR, DeLaPaz RL. Tumor. In: Enzman DR, DeLaPaz RL, Rubin JB, eds. *Magnetic resonance of the spine*. Baltimore: Mosby, 1990.
6. Sze G, Krol G, Zimmerman RD, Deck MDF. Intramedullary disease of the spine: diagnosis using gadolinium-DTPA enhanced MR imaging. *AJR Am J Roentgenol* 1988;151:1193–1204.
7. Valk J. Gadolinium-DTPA in MR of spinal lesions. *AJNR Am J Neuroradiol* 1988;9:345–350.
8. Goy AM, Pinto RS, Raghavenda BN, Epstein FJ, Kricheff II. Intramedullary spinal cord tumors: MR imaging with emphasis on associated cysts. *Radiology* 1986;161:381–386.
9. Browne TR, Adams RD, Roberson GH. Hemangioblastoma of the spinal cord. Review and report of five cases. *Arch Neurol* 1976;33:435–441.
10. Parizel PM, Baleriaux D, Rodesch G, et al. Gd-DTPA enhanced MR imaging of spinal tumors. *AJNR Am J Neuroradiol* 1989;10:249–258.
11. Dillon WP, Norman D, Newton TH, Bolla K, Mark A. Intradural spinal cord lesions: Gd-DTPA-enhanced MR imaging. *Radiology* 1989;170:229–237.
12. Sherman JL, Barkovich AJ, Citrin CM. The MR appearance of syringomyelia: new observations. *AJNR Am J Neuroradiol* 1986;7:985–995.
13. Kalfas I, Wilberger J, Goldberg A, Prostko ER. Magnetic resonance imaging in acute spinal cord trauma. *Neurosurgery* 1988;23(3):295–299.

14. Larsson E-M, Holtas S, Nilsson O. Gd-DTPA-enhanced MR of suspected spinal multiple sclerosis. *AJNR Am J Neuroradiol* 1989;10:1071–1076.
15. Ransohoff RM, Whitman G, Weinstein M. Detection of cavitary spinal cord lesions in multiple sclerosis patients by magnetic resonance imaging. *Neurology* 1990;39(Suppl):333.
16. Berman M, Feldman S, Alter M, Zilber N, Kahana E. Acute transverse myelitis: incidence and etiologic considerations. *Neurology* 1981;31:966–971.
17. Barakos JA, Mark AS, Dillon WP, Norman D. MR imaging of acute transverse myelitis and AIDS myelopathy. *J Comput Assist Tomogr* 1990;14:45–50.
18. El-Toraei I, Juler G. Ischemic myelopathy. *Angiology* 1979;30:81–94.
19. Yuh W, Marsh E, Wang A, et al. MR imaging of spinal cord and vertebral body infarction. *AJNR Am J Neuroradiol* 1992;13:145–154.
20. Hasegawa M, Yamashita J, Yamashima T, Kiyonobu I, Fujishima Y, Yamazaki M. Spinal cord infarction associated with primary antiphospholipid syndrome in a young child. *J Neurosurg* 1993;79:446–450.
21. Morgan MK. Outcome from treatment for spinal arteriovenous malformation. *Neurosurg Clin North Am* 1999;10(1):113–119.
22. Symon L, Kuyama H, Kendall B. Dural arteriovenous malformations of the spine. Clinical features and surgical results in 55 cases. *J Neurosurg* 1984;60(2):238–247.
23. Mikulis DJ, Ogilvy CS, McKee A, Davis KR, Ojeman RG. Spinal cord infarction and fibrocartilagenous emboli. *AJNR Am J Neuroradiol* 1992;13(1):155–160.
24. Beaujeux RL, Reizine DC, Casasco A, et al. Endovascular treatment of vertebral arteriovenous fistula. *Radiology* 1992;183:361–367.
25. Anson J, Spetzler R. Classification of spinal arteriovenous malformations. *Barrow Neurological Institute Q* 1992;8:2–8.
26. Ogilvy C, Louis D, Ojemann R. Intramedullary cavernous malformations of the spine. *Neurosurgery* 1992;31:219–230.
27. Wirth FP, Post KD, DiChiro G, et al. Foix-Alajouanine disease: spontaneous thrombosis of a spinal cord arteriovenous malformation: a case report. *Neurology* 1970;20:1114.
28. Terwey B, Becker H, Thron AK, et al. Gadolinium-DTPA enhanced MR imaging of spinal dural arteriovenous fistulas. *J Comput Assist Tomogr* 1989;13:30.
29. Chakeres DW, Flickinger F, Bresnahan JC, et al. MRI imaging of acute spinal cord trauma. *AJNR Am J Neuroradiol* 1987;8(1):5–10.
30. Flanders AE, Schaefer DM, Doan HT, Mishkin MM, Gonzalez CF, Northrup BE. Acute cervical spine trauma: correlation of MRI imaging findings with degree of neurologic deficit. *Radiology* 1990; 177(1):25–33.
31. Quencer RM, Sheldon JJ, Donovan Post MJ, et al. MRI of the chronically injured cervical spinal cord. *AJR Am J Roentgenol* 1986;147: 125–132.
32. Gelland FE, Paul KS, Geisler FH. Early sequelae of gunshot wounds to the spine: radiologic diagnosis. *Radiology* 1988;167:523–526.
33. Modic MT, Feiglan DH, Piraino DW, et al. Vertebral osteomyelitis: assessment using MR. *Radiology* 1985;157:157–166.
34. deRoos A, van Persijn van Meerten EL, Bloem JL, Bluemm RG. MRI of tuberculous spondylitis. *AJR Am J Roentgenol* 1986;147:79–82.
35. Donovan Post MJ, Sze G, Quencerr RM, Elsmont FJ, Green BA, Gahbauer H. Gadolinium-enhanced MR in spinal infection. *J Comput Assist Tomogr* 1990;14:721–729.
36. Thrush A, Enzmann D. MR imaging of infectious spondylitis. *AJNR Am J Neuroradiol* 1990;11:1171–1180.
37. Colombo N, Berry I, Norman D. Injections of the spine. In: Manelfe C, ed. *Imaging of the spine and spinal cord.* New York: Raven Press, 1992:489–512.
38. Sandhu FS, Dillon WP. Spinal epidural abscess: evaluation with contrast-enhanced MR imaging. *AJNR Am J Neuroradiol* 1991;12:1087–1093.
39. Numaguchi Y, Rigamonti D, Rothman MI, Sato S, Mihara F, Sadato N. Spinal epidural abscess: evaluation with gadolinium-enhanced MR imaging. *Radiographics* 1993;13:545–559.
40. Quencer RM. Spinal epidural abscess: evaluation with gadolinium-enhanced MR imaging: invited commentary. *Radiographics* 1993; 13:559.

Open MRI,
edited by Peter A. Rothschild and Debra Reinking Rothschild.
Lippincott Williams & Wilkins. Philadelphia © 2000.

CHAPTER 13

Open Magnetic Resonance Imaging of Cranial and Cervical Trauma

Kevin R. Moore, Blaine L. Hart, William W. Orrison, Jr., and Peter A. Rothschild

Trauma of the head and spine are among the most costly of injuries in terms of the financial burden to society and the morbidity and mortality. Open magnetic resonance imaging (MRI) offers a unique method of determining the extent of head and spinal injury and may allow for prevention of the severe sequelae that often accompany these traumatic disorders.

Of the approximately 7 million cases of traumatic brain injury (TBI) that occur annually, it is estimated that more than 500,000 of these patients are admitted to hospitals each year. Traumatic head injury results in lifelong debilitation for approximately 100,000 of these individuals. TBI results in more lost work days than any other disease process, accounting for an estimated 30 million missed work days each year. Trauma is the leading cause of death in young adults and children in the United States and the third leading cause of death for all age groups. More than 50% of these deaths are secondary to TBI (1–8).

Neuroimaging studies are often used to guide the management of patients with TBI and may play an essential role in determining the most appropriate form of treatment and intervention. The severity of TBI varies with the age of the patient, the type of object impacted, and the force and the direction of the assault to the head. Sophisticated imaging techniques, many of which are available in most hospital settings, can detect positive findings in even mild trauma. Certain more subtle types of neuropathologic changes occurring after head trauma may require neuroanatomic and neurophysiologic methods of analysis to identify dysfunctional foci within the brain. Abnormalities from TBI may be present even if gross structural pathology is not apparent. Computed tomography (CT) remains the most commonly used method of brain evaluation in patients with TBI; however, other brain imaging modalities, such as MRI, positron emission tomography, single photon emission CT, and magnetic source imaging, are beginning to play a vital role in the evaluation of patients with TBI, especially those with relatively minor TBI. Less severe TBI may be associated with prolonged symptoms, such as headache, memory loss, cognitive deficits, imbalance, psychological complaints, and personality changes.

Open MRI has allowed the evaluation of acutely injured or ill patients in a manner similar to that used for CT (1,2,9–15). Unlike typical high-field systems, the open magnet design permits closer monitoring of unstable patients and facilitates access for procedures.

Primary TBI refers to those insults to the brain that occur at the time of the initial impact, forces that directly strike or are transmitted to the brain during the instance of trauma. Head trauma may result in damage to the skull, scalp, sinuses, face, and neck—the same structures that can assist in absorbing the force of impact and in providing some protection to the brain tissue. Location of primary TBI may be intra- or extraaxial. Hemorrhages into the subdural, epidural, subarachnoid, or ventricular spaces are the most common forms of extraaxial primary TBI. Common types of intraaxial primary TBI include contusions, hematomas, and deep axonal injury, also known as *shear injury* (1,16–19).

EXTRAAXIAL HEMORRHAGE

In the evaluation of possible extraaxial hemorrhage, CT and MRI examinations are potentially important. CT is generally the first imaging study in this setting, in which it is important to exclude extraaxial fluid collections that have

K. R. Moore: Department of Radiology, Neuroradiology Section, University of Utah School of Medicine, Salt Lake City, Utah

B. L. Hart: Department of Radiology, University of New Mexico School of Medicine, Albuquerque, New Mexico

W. W. Orrison Jr.: Department of Radiology, University of Utah School of Medicine, Salt Lake City, Utah

P. A. Rothschild: Department of Radiology, University of California, San Francisco, San Francisco, California; Open MRI, Hayward, California; Open MRI, Louisville, Kentucky

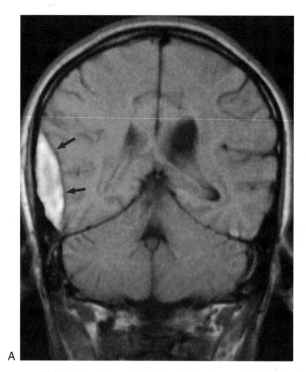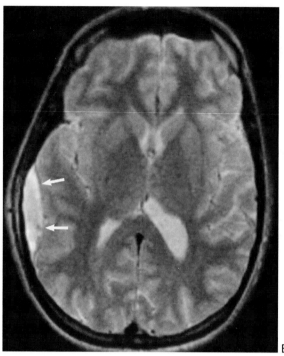

FIG. 13-1. Subacute epidural hematoma (EDH). **A:** Coronal T1-weighted spin-echo image [repetition time (TR), 500/echo time (TE), 3]. **B:** Axial T2-weighted conventional spin echo (TR 300/TE 80). The biconvex extraaxial collection (*arrows*) in the right middle fossa is hyperintense on T1- and T2-weighted images, representing a subacute EDH in this patient 10 days after closed-head injury.

caused significant pressure effects within the cranial vault. A negative CT does not rule out the presence of a significant extraaxial fluid collection. MRI may be required to exclude extraaxial fluid in the setting of head trauma, and open MRI is particularly of value in this setting. MRI is indicated in patients who exhibit unexplained neurologic symptoms after an injury to the head (20–23).

Epidural Hematoma

Epidural hematomas (EDHs), which are identified on less than 5% of the neuroimaging studies performed for acute head trauma, account for approximately 10% of fatal cranial injuries. EDH is seen most commonly during the second and third decades of life, with fewer of this type of extraaxial hematoma noted in early childhood or during the latter years of life. This decreased incidence of EDH in the very young and very old is a result in part of a lower overall frequency of head trauma in these age groups and may also be secondary to the compliance of the skull in early life and more adherent dura in later life (24–33).

Despite the fact that no intracranial epidural space exists normally, EDHs are located between the dura and the skull. The epidural space is a potential space. No true space is present, and the attachment of the dura to the inner table of the skull is commonly tightly adherent. In the presence of severe head trauma, the dura can be stripped away from its attachment to the inner table of the skull. When this occurs, the epidural space can fill with extravasated hemorrhage from adjacent meningeal blood vessels, diploic veins, or dural sinuses. The margins of the dura remain adherent to the inner table of the skull, leaving the EDH with a biconvex or lentiform appearance (Fig. 13-1). The EDH may cross dural attachments but typically does not cross a suture. The vast majority of EDHs are unilateral, with only 5% occurring bilaterally, and most occur above the tentorium (24,34). Up to 95% of all cases of EDH involve a fracture that results in direct injury to the middle meningeal artery or causes a tear in a dural venous sinus.

EDHs are in fact the most common posttraumatic space-occupying masses in the posterior fossa. Although subdural hematoma (SDH) is more prevalent than EDH above the tentorium, below the tentorium EDH is more common than SDH. The posterior fossa EDH still represents a relatively uncommon lesion (accounting for only approximately 10% of all EDHs). Whereas most supratentorial EDHs are arterial in origin, the majority of infratentorial EDHs are of venous origin. This is most likely due to the abundance of dural veins in the posterior fossa, as well as the greater force required for arterial rupture as compared to disruption of the relatively more fragile venous structures (30,35–43).

EDH is commonly accompanied by an adjacent skull fracture. On CT, the EDH typically appears as a well-defined

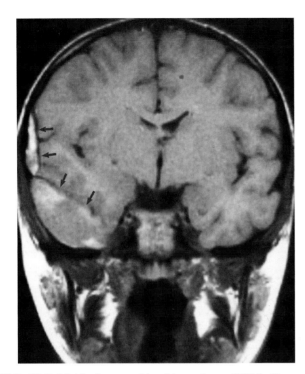

FIG. 13-2. Middle fossa epidural hematoma (EDH). Coronal T1-weighted spin-echo image [repetition time (TR), 500/echo time (TE), 40] shows a right extraaxial mixed isointense/hyperintense collection (*arrows*) exerting mass effect on the adjacent temporal lobe. Aside from mass effect, the temporal lobe appears uninjured. Unlike acute subdural hematoma, which frequently associates with an adjacent cerebral contusion, EDH often does not display an underlying brain injury.

biconvex or lentiform high-attenuation extraaxial mass that displaces the gray/white matter interface away from the skull and causes focal brain compression. EDHs located over the vertex may have less well-defined margins. Approximately two-thirds of EDHs are of uniformly high attenuation with Hounsfield unit (HU) values in the 50 to 70 range (normal brain is approximately 30 HU). Various episodes of hemorrhage are indicated by the one-third of lower attenuation EDHs commonly of mixed density. Because patients with EDH are often quite lucid for several hours after the trauma, this history, accompanied by a subsequent decline in the level of consciousness, is classically known as the *lucid interval*. Continued enlargement of the EDH during the first 24 to 48 hours postinjury probably results in delayed onset in the impaired level of consciousness. The fracture often present in EDH cases can result in laceration of the middle meningeal artery. This arterial insult is extremely likely to continue to bleed, and delayed impairment in the level of consciousness may lead to delayed referral, diagnosis, and treatment. It is possible for an EDH to resolve spontaneously; however, this is generally not the rule (24,44–46).

MRI of EDH demonstrates a biconvex or lentiform shape and is similar in configuration to the appearance on CT (Fig. 13-2). The acute EDH is typically isointense on T1-weighted images and of either increased or decreased signal on T2-weighted sequences. The signal intensity may be decreased acutely as a result of the extremely rapid clot formation that commonly occurs in EDH, making the diagnosis more difficult. Identification of epidural bleeding over the convexities on CT may be difficult. MRI may be necessary to demonstrate this abnormality. When the hemorrhage extends across the interhemispheric fissure, it is most likely epidural in location, because the superior sagittal sinus and falx represent a barrier to extension of SDHs across the midline (1,20,21).

Subdural Hematoma

An SDH is a hemorrhagic fluid collection below the meningeal layer of the dura but outside the arachnoid. Rupture of superficial cerebral veins on the convexities located near venous sinuses results in more than one-half of all SDHs. SDH formation may also result from disruption of cortical bridging veins between the temporal lobes and the sphenoparietal or petrosal sinuses. The superficial cortical veins are vulnerable to tearing during TBI, particularly in cases of high-strain or rotational forces that may spare the underlying brain. SDHs are therefore more commonly related to assaults and falls than to motor vehicle accidents, in which deep tissue contusions or shearing injuries are more often seen. An SDH may arise from hemorrhage within the underlying brain with subsequent extension through the pia and arachnoid into the subdural space. The arachnoid can also be torn during trauma, and the SDH may consist of a combination of blood and cerebrospinal fluid (CSF) (25,47–55).

SDH can be a life-threatening injury, and mortality rates are reported to be as high as 85%. SDH is identified in more than 25% of all cases of head trauma–related deaths, and up to 20% of all head trauma cases are found to have SDH. On CT, an acute SDH is typically noted as a high-density, crescent-shaped extraaxial fluid collection. The SDH has a concave inner margin and a convex outer margin that tends to follow the normal contour of the brain surface. An SDH may be quite extensive and occupy much of the cerebral cortical surface. Other than the nonaccidental trauma from child abuse, bilateral SDHs, isolated interhemispheric SDHs, and parafalcine SDHs are relatively uncommon injuries. Clinical suspicion of abuse should be high when such injuries are identified in a child (1,20,56,57).

MRI can be quite useful for identifying an SDH, regardless of the age of the bleed. Although many SDHs are readily identified on MRI, in problematic cases intravenous administration of contrast media may reveal enhancement in the margins of an SDH that make it more obvious. The SDH may be classified as hyperacute, acute, subacute, or chronic based on the age and signal intensity of the lesion (Fig. 13-3). The acute SDH is less than 7 days old. Between days 7 and 21, the SDH is in the subacute phase (Fig. 13-4). Chronic SDHs are those that are more than 21 days old.

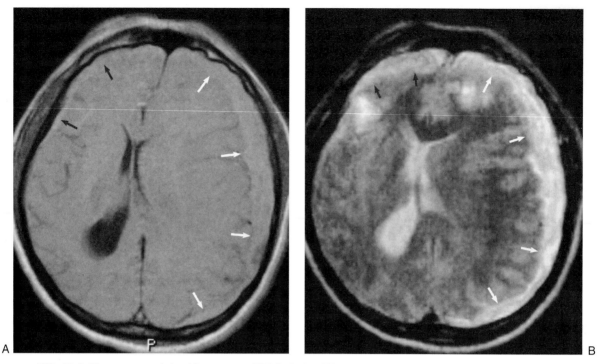

FIG. 13-3. Hyperacute subdural hematoma (SDH). **A:** Axial T1-weighted spin-echo image (TR 500/TE 30). **B:** Axial T2-weighted CSE image [repetition time (TR), 300/echo time (TE), 80]. A large left SDH (*white arrows*) is seen with mass effect that is isointense on T1-weighted imaging and hyperintense similar to cerebrospinal fluid signal on T2-weighted imaging, consistent with hyperacute (oxyhemoglobin predominant) subdural hemorrhage. A smaller collection is on the right with the same signal characteristics (*black arrows*). The subsequent change from T2 hyperintensity to hypointensity reflects progression of blood products from oxyhemoglobin to deoxyhemoglobin, which is characteristic of acute hemorrhage.

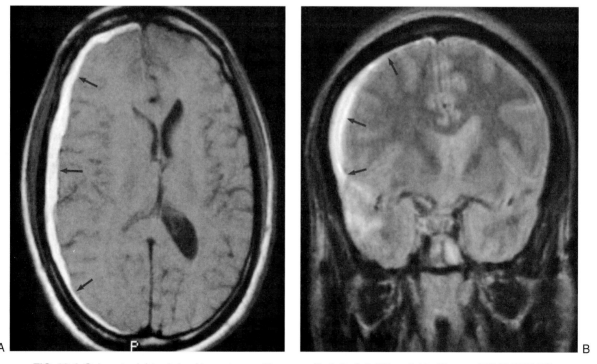

FIG. 13-4. Subacute right subdural hematoma with mass effect. **A:** Axial T1-weighted image (TR 500/TE 30). **B:** Coronal T2-weighted CSE [repetition time (TR), 2,080/echo time (TE), 90]. The presence of hyperintense signal intensity (*arrows*) on T1- and T2-weighted images is indicative of extracellular methemoglobin and subacute hemorrhage age.

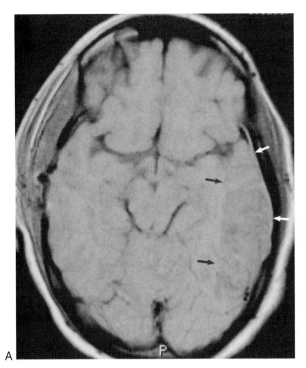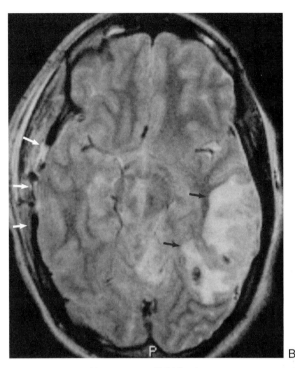

FIG. 13-5. Acute left temporal lobe contusion with hyperacute subdural hematoma (SDH) after evacuation of contralateral epidural hematoma (EDH). **A:** Axial T1-weighted spin-echo [repetition time (TR), 600/echo time (TE), 30] image shows a hypointense left temporal lobe mass lesion (*black arrows*) with small adjacent isointense SDH (*white arrows*). **B:** Axial T2-weighted CSE (TR 3,000/TE 90) image confirms a mixed hyperintense left temporal lobe contusion (*black arrows*) with edema and scattered areas of hypointensity representing acute deoxyhemoglobin, accompanied by a small hyperintense SDH. Note the right temporal craniotomy for prior evacuation of an EDH (*white arrows*).

Confusing the matter, imaging guidelines regarding the aging of SDHs are not absolute, and consideration must be given to circumstances such as a low hematocrit, coagulopathies, and rebleeding (1,20,21).

MRI can be useful for clarifying cases that are problematic on CT. For example, it is nearly impossible to distinguish between a chronic SDH and a subdural hygroma on CT. Both of these lesions are extraaxial fluid density masses and cause inward displacement of cortical veins against the surface of the brain. A true subdural hygroma is composed of CSF and frequently is due to laceration of the arachnoid, with CSF escaping into the subdural space. This creates a space-occupying, extraaxial, fluid-filled mass. Presumably, the torn arachnoid functions as a one-way valve, allowing the flow of CSF into but not out of the subdural space. MRI can determine the nature of the fluid occupying the subdural space. The diagnosis of a subdural hygroma is more assured when the signal intensity is that of CSF on all pulse sequences (1,20,21,58–60). In contradistinction, chronic SDH demonstrates signal intensity that does not follow CSF on one or more sequences. Frequently, it is higher signal on T1-weighted images, a key discriminating feature. Differences in T2 hyperintensity are often difficult to appreciate.

In cases of SDH and EDH, surgical intervention is relatively common. Because the decrease in pressure after surgical evaluation may permit accumulation of an extraaxial mass on the opposite side of the cranium (Fig. 13-5), a repeat CT or MRI examination must be done after surgical removal of an SDH or EDH. A follow-up scan may also be important for excluding residual hematoma, expanding hemorrhage, or new areas of hemorrhage or infarction. Ventricular shunting procedures predispose to SDH, which has been shown to occur in up to nearly one-third of patients undergoing ventriculostomy, and SDH in shunted patients is more common in adults than in children. The decrease in intracranial pressure that often accompanies shunting procedures decreases the likelihood that bleeding will tamponade, and, as the brain falls away from the cranial vault, increased tension on the bridging veins leads to vessel disruption and hemorrhage into the subdural space. Motion artifact can mimic SDH (Fig. 13-6) (1,20,21,61–63).

Subarachnoid Hemorrhage

In most cases of posttraumatic subarachnoid hemorrhage (SAH), the volume of hemorrhage into the subarachnoid space is not clinically significant. SAH is the most common form of hemorrhage in head trauma, accompanies the majority of cases of significant TBI, and is massive in 12% of cases. SAH may

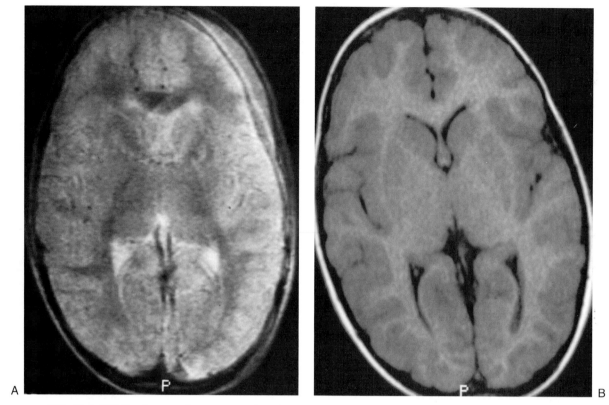

FIG. 13-6. Pitfalls of magnetic resonance imaging: motion artifact mimicking subdural hematoma (SDH). **A:** Patient motion artifact on the axial T2-weighted CSE [repetition time (TR), 2,800/echo time (TE), 80] image implies a left SDH. **B:** Axial T1-weighted spin-echo (TR 300/TE 25) imaging performed immediately after the T2-weighted imaging confirms the absence of hemorrhage.

be associated with multiple other forms of TBI; in some instances of TBI, SAH is the only finding. The origin of the SAH can be several sources, including minor injury to the small bridging cortical veins that pass through the subarachnoid space; direct laceration of surface veins and arteries, such as occurs when accompanied by a fracture or penetration from a projectile; dissection of an intraparenchymal hematoma into the subarachnoid space or ventricular system; and lysis of vessels and adhesions owing to violent brain motion. The very young and the very old are most vulnerable to SAH, because the subarachnoid space in these populations is typically significantly larger than in other age groups (64,65).

The interpeduncular cistern, the sylvian fissures, and the apex of the tentorium are classic sites of SAH. SAH manifests as areas of high attenuation on CT located in the basal cisterns, sylvian fissures, superior cerebellar cisterns, and the sulci over the cerebral convexities. The narrow high-density collections of blood that represent the SAH on CT may be very difficult to recognize for the uninitiated and sometimes for even more experienced readers when the hemorrhage is symmetric and diffuse. The entire brain may appear quite normal, because no distortion or asymmetry may be present.

It has been previously reported that SAH is difficult to image with MRI. It has since been demonstrated that acute SAH is as easy or in some cases easier to identify with

MRI than with CT. This is particularly true using gradient-echo (GRE) or fluid attenuated inversion recovery (FLAIR) techniques on low-field strength magnets (Fig. 13-7). SAH becomes increasingly obvious on MRI as it ages and less readily identified on CT. SAH clears over time through phagocytosis and erythrocyte lysis. Often, at least some degree of residual hemosiderin deposition occurs within the subarachnoid spaces as the hemorrhagic CSF is replaced. This may be identified on MRI as regions of markedly decreased signal, especially on T2-weighted or GRE sequences, and is called *superficial hemosiderosis*. It can be seen after a single episode of SAH, but it more commonly follows multiple hemorrhages into the subarachnoid spaces. Because of this, MRI may be able to demonstrate that SAH has been present months or years after the offending event (66–80).

Most commonly, the complications that occur after traumatic SAH are related to CSF flow dynamics. Although uncommon, vasospasm is by far the most ominous and often the most critical complication of SAH. Left untreated, it can cause severe cerebral ischemia or infarction. Hydrocephalus resulting from decreased CSF absorption or flow blockage is the most common sequelae of SAH. The level of the cerebral aqueduct is a common location for CSF flow to be decreased. However, CSF absorption defects occur at the

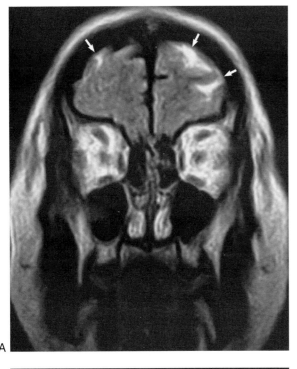

A

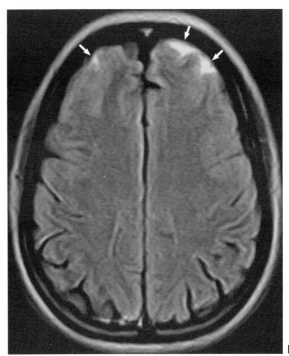

B

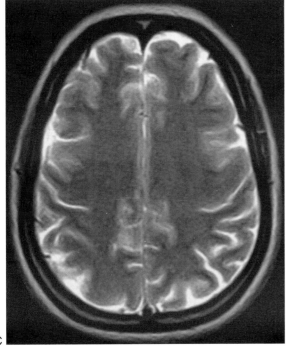

C

FIG. 13-7. Conspicuity of subarachnoid hemorrhage (SAH) on fluid attenuated inversion recovery (FLAIR) imaging. **A:** Coronal FLAIR image [repetition time (TR), 6,000/echo time (TE), 116/T1 1400]. **B:** Axial FLAIR image (TR 6,000/TE 98/T1 1400). Prior computed tomographic scan (not shown) demonstrated small bifrontal areas of SAH. Coronal and axial FLAIR images clearly show bifrontal subarachnoid high signal intensity characteristic of SAH (*white arrows*). **C:** A comparable axial T2-weighted fast spin-echo (TR 5,200/TE 87) slice shows mild bifrontal prominence of the subarachnoid spaces that is within normal allowable limits. No discernible signal abnormality suggests the SAH.

same physiologic level. Apparently, a direct relationship exists between the extent of SAH and the probability of obstructive hydrocephalus. A loss of normal CSF absorption at the level of the arachnoid villi of the pacchionian granulations occurs after SAH. The arachnoid villi become clogged with phagocytes, and this eventually results in proliferation of connective tissue fibroblasts and obliteration of the affected pacchionian granulations. Ventriculoperitoneal

shunting is not of benefit in all cases but may be effective in treating patients with posttraumatic hydrocephalus (81–83).

Intraventricular Hemorrhage

Intraventricular hemorrhage (IVH) is an ominous sign on neuroimaging. The prognosis is generally poor; however, when

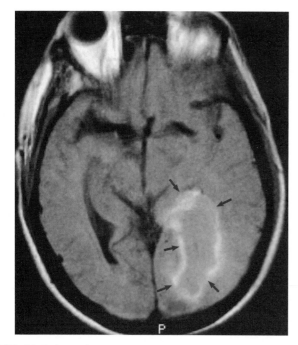

FIG. 13-8. Acute intraventricular hemorrhage (IVH). Axial T1-weighted spin-echo [repetition time (TR), 600/echo time (TE), 30] image reveals marked distension of the left ventricular atrium by isointense IVH (*arrows*), with a peripheral rim of high signal intensity reflecting early subacute hemorrhage (methemoglobin).

the IVH is relatively isolated and unaccompanied by other significant TBI, the outcome may not be as severe. IVH is generally found in fewer than 5% of patients with TBI, and most cases of IVH are accompanied by multiple additional forms of posttraumatic brain insult. Hemorrhage into the ventricular system usually occurs by means of extension from intraparenchymal bleeding, deep penetrating wounds, tearing of subependymal veins, or diffusion from SAH. An association exists between shearing injury of the corpus callosum and IVH, with an IVH incidence of 60% when corpus collosal shear injury is present. IVH is typically cleared from the ventricular system within 1 to 2 weeks. This occurs unless hemorrhage recurs or a hemorrhagic "ventricular cast" is formed (84–88).

The MRI appearance of IVH is highly variable and can change in minutes. Blood-fluid layering within the ventricular system is frequently observed on MRI and can be seen within minutes of the bleeding incident. IVH on MRI typically demonstrates increased signal in the regions of hemorrhage on T1-weighted sequences, with decreased signal on T2-weighted images. If the patient rebleeds, the signal intensity of the intraventricular hemorrhage can change rapidly. Intraventricular blood collections also demonstrate more rapid progression through the stages of intraparenchymal hemorrhage (IPH), with correspondingly more rapid changes in perceived signal intensity (1,20,21,83) (Figs. 13-8 and 13-9).

Accumulation of blood within the ventricular system can result in obstructive hydrocephalus, particularly at the level of the cerebral aqueduct. IVH can cause irritation of the

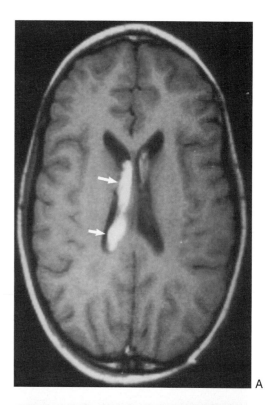

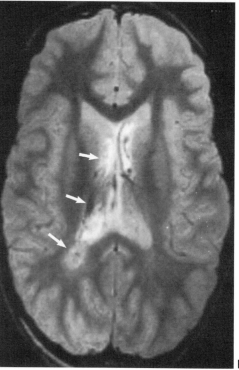

FIG. 13-9. Subacute subependymal hemorrhage into choroid plexus. **A:** Axial T1-weighted spin-echo [repetition time (TR), 600/echo time (TE), 17] image. **B:** Axial T2-weighted CSE (TR 3000/TE 60) image. The right lateral ventricle choroid plexus demonstrates T1 hyperintensity and mixed T2 hypo- and hyperintensity reflective of intra- and extracellular methemoglobin (*arrows*), markers of subacute hemorrhage.

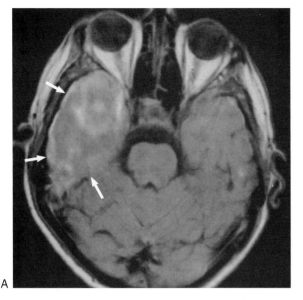

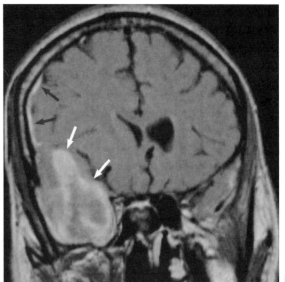

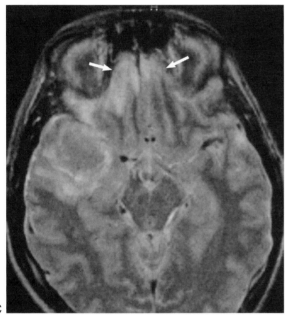

FIG. 13-10. Temporal lobe contusion with subdural hematoma (SDH). Axial T1-weighted spin-echo [repetition time (TR), 600/echo time (TE), 30] **(A)** and coronal T1-weighted spin-echo (TR 750/TE 30) **(B)** images reveal a mixed hypo- and isointense right temporal contusion (*white arrows*) with mass effect but no herniation. The peripheral T1 hyperintensity reflects early subacute blood. A small adjacent hyperintense subacute SDH (*black arrows*) is also present. A comparable axial T2-weighted imaging slice also demonstrated subacute T2 hyperintensity (not shown). **C:** Axial T2-weighted conventional spin echo (TR 3,000/TE 80) image slightly higher reveals hyperintense edema extending into the inferior frontal lobe (*arrows*), a classic location for traumatic brain injury.

ependymal lining of the ventricular system. Delayed obstruction can also occur at the level of the aqueduct, resulting from prolonged irritation of the ependyma with resulting ventriculitis. The obstructive hydrocephalus that occurs is most often apparent at the levels of the third and lateral ventricles, implicating the aqueduct as the area of most probable obstruction. This type of hydrocephalus is most often responsive to ventriculoperitoneal shunting performed within a reasonable period (1,20,21,83).

Intraparenchymal Hemorrhage

One of the most common findings in TBI is IPH. IPH is found in cerebral contusions (see Fig. 13-5), diffuse axonal

injury (DAI), and brainstem injury and when the cerebral arteries or veins have sustained direct injury. IPH is also invariably present in cases of penetrating head injury, particularly when high-velocity projectiles are involved. On CT, IPH appears as diffuse or focal areas of increased density that are easily identified in most cases. The appearance of IPH is strikingly similar, regardless of the exact nature of the insult. As the bleeding resolves, the high density decreases over time on CT images. After the initial insult, the density gradual decreases until the region becomes isodense with surrounding brain tissue. Usually in 10 days to 2 weeks, the attenuation decreases to the level of the surrounding brain. At this stage, CT contrast enhancement surrounding the lesion is common. In fact, contrast enhancement may be necessary to convincingly demonstrate the pathology during this time.

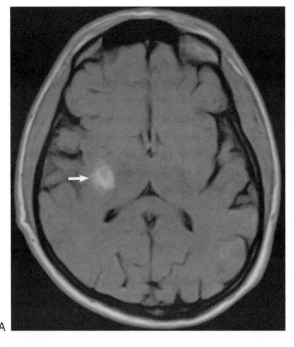

A

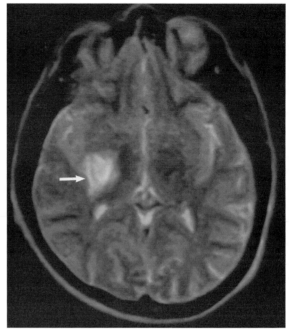

B

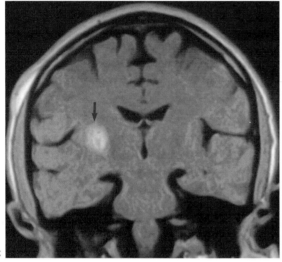

C

FIG. 13-11. Subacute intraparenchymal hemorrhage (IPH). **A:** Axial T1-weighted [repetition time (TR), 58/time echo (TE), 22; flip angle, 60 degrees] image. **B:** Axial T2-weighted conventional spin echo (TR 3,000/TE 105) image. **C:** Coronal T1-weighted (TR 58/TE 22, FA 60) image. The T1- and T2-weighted images reveal hyperintensity in the right putamen (*arrows*), reflecting subacute IPH. The area of hyperintensity is larger on the T2-weighted image, which reflects surrounding edema that is hypointense and less obvious on the T1-weighted images.

This type of CT enhancement may be present approximately 1 week after the injury (17,57,66).

Continued aging of the IPH results in a focal area of decreased density on CT, which may continue to decrease for up to 6 months before the final level of attenuation is reached. A delay in formation of IPH is not uncommon, especially with contusions, which often demonstrate more hemorrhage in the first few hours to days after injury. Axial GRE imaging techniques can reveal subtle areas of hemorrhage in cases of diagnostic uncertainty. Also, lesions that later manifest hemorrhage on CT frequently can be characterized by edema on MRI at an earlier stage. The size and total number of IPH lesions are also known to increase with time after the TBI, and such a delay often indicates a poor prognosis (17,57,66,89–92).

The variations in the appearance of IPH result from a combination of the time from ictus, hemorrhage source, location of

the hemorrhage, field strength of the magnet used, and the clinical state of the patient. Clinical conditions that directly affect the MRI appearance of the lesion include hematocrit, clotting time, blood oxygenation, intracellular protein concentrations, rates of red blood cell settling, and amount of red blood cell packing. IPH can be readily identified on MRI; MRI is frequently positive when the CT is negative or inconclusive. The MRI characteristics of IPH can be highly variable; however, the identification of focal hemorrhage on MRI has been assisted dramatically by the addition of GRE and FLAIR sequences to traditional imaging protocols (1,20,21,72,93–101). FLAIR sequences often increase sensitivity to the edema that often accompanies small areas of hemorrhage.

On MRI, IPH begins as an area of slight hyperintensity or isointensity that becomes hypointense within the first 12 to 24 hours on T1-weighted images (Fig. 13-10). The T2-

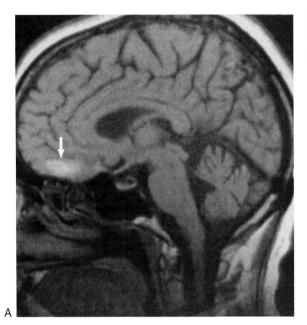
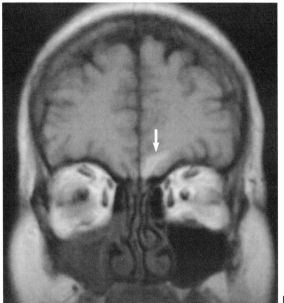

FIG. 13-12. Subacute intraparenchymal hemorrhage (contusion). **A:** Sagittal T1-weighted spin-echo [repetition time (TR), 500/echo time (TE), 40] image. **B:** Coronal T1-weighted spin-echo (TR 500/TE 30) image. Sagittal and coronal T1-weighted images show hyperintense signal intensity (*arrows*) in the classic left inferior frontal location consistent with a subacute contusion.

weighted sequences in this very early (hyperacute) period initially show a hyperintense lesion that rapidly becomes hypointense. The early appearance of hyperintensity in IPH may reflect the longer T2 of oxygenated blood and the effect of increased proton density on T1-weighted sequences. The hypointensity seen in the acute phase of IPH is characteristic on T1- and T2-weighted sequences, but is most obvious on T2, probably because of the presence of a combination of deoxyhemoglobin, red blood cell dehydration, and clot matrix formation (72,102–105). Subacute IPH usually has signal characteristics similar to subacute hemorrhage in other areas of the brain (Fig. 13-11).

Cerebral contusions represent regions of primary neuronal injury and are frequently identified in TBI. These lesions are made up of punctate parenchymal hemorrhages, or "microhemorrhages," that may become confluent "macrohemorrhages." Cerebral contusions are common in the anterior temporal and frontal lobes, as well as the occipital poles. They have been noted to be composed of linear zones of hemorrhage that tend to be found along the cortical gyri; and are often centered around the gyral crests under the calvarium (20–23,57,95) (Fig. 13-12). A common MR imaging pitfall is mistaking ossification in the falx as a medial parenchymal contusion (Fig. 13-13). Chronic contusions are characterized by encephalomalacia and T1 and T2 signal after fluid (Fig. 13-14).

Given the multiple complex stages of evolution common to these lesions, the imaging findings in cerebral contusions tend to be variable. Whereas the CT may be normal or minimally abnormal initially, MRI typically demonstrates the lesions from the onset of injury. CT frequently shows progression over time in the size, number, and amount of hemorrhage within the contusions. Such changes are most obvious over the first 24 to 48 hours, with one-fourth of cases demonstrating delayed hemorrhage in areas that were previously free of perceptible hemorrhage (20–23,57).

Diffuse Axonal Injury

DAI (also known as *shearing injury*, *deep white matter injury*, or *deep axonal injury*) is caused by rapid deceleration or acceleration events. These events are often combined with rotational forces acting simultaneously on the brain. DAI lesions occur in predictable locations and are usually identified in a diffuse bilateral pattern. DAI is found at the corticomedullary junction, corpus callosum, internal capsule, deep gray matter, and brainstem regions. A predilection exists for the corticomedullary junction of the frontotemporal region, posterior body and splenium of the corpus callosum, caudate nuclei, thalamus, internal capsule, and dorsolateral tegmentum (1,25,106–108).

The DAI injury can be seen as a tear at the nonuniform regions of the brain, such as the gray/white matter interfaces of the cerebral cortex, the internal capsule, the deep gray matter, the upper brainstem, and the corpus callosum (Fig. 13-15). Pathologically, DAI has been described as microscopic axonal bulbs or retraction balls representing small hemorrhagic lesions. When combined with cerebral contusions, DAI represents the most significant cause of morbid-

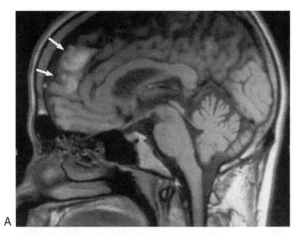

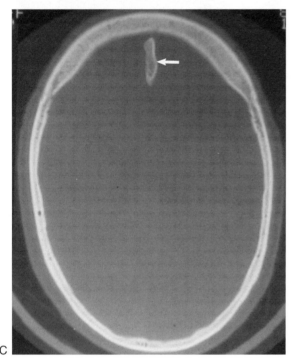

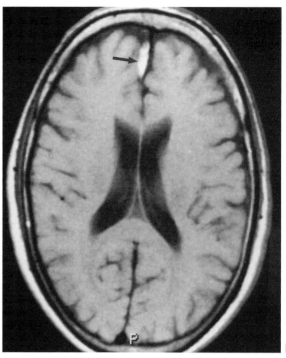

FIG. 13-13. Pitfalls of magnetic resonance imaging: ossification in the falx mimicking hemorrhage. Axial [repetition time (TR), 500/echo time (TE), 30] **(A)** and sagittal (TR 500/TE 40) **(B)** T1-weighted spin-echo images show hyperintensity (*arrows*) in the anterior interhemispheric fissure resembling blood in this patient who sustained head trauma. **C:** Axial bone window computed tomography reveals that this is ossification (*arrow*) along the falx cerebri in the interhemispheric fissure rather than the expected blood products.

ity in patients with TBI. DAI is uncommon without a history of severe closed-head injury and accounts for nearly 50% of all intraaxial TBI. Patients with DAI usually lose consciousness and become comatose at the time of the initial TBI (20–23,57,95,106,107,109,110).

Fewer than one-half of the patients who are ultimately shown to have DAI demonstrate discernible abnormalities on the initial CT scan. In fact, the initial CT scan may be normal even when DAI is the prevalent pathologic process. Delayed CT imaging often demonstrates the DAI that was not seen on earlier CT studies. The appearance of DAI on CT varies over time and is dependent on the amount of bleeding that has occurred and the extent of surrounding edema.

The MRI findings in DAI include little or no signal change on T1-weighted sequences, focal areas of increased signal on T2-weighted and FLAIR imaging, and variable signal on gradient recalled sequences depending on the stage of hemorrhage. The various stages of hemorrhage discussed under Intraparenchymal Hemorrhage apply to DAI as well. It is important to remember that the timing of the imaging is critical to understanding the anticipated appearance of DAI on MRI.

Imaging Selection

A correct and complete clinical diagnosis often provides the most important information when choosing an imaging modality in the setting of TBI. The goal of imaging in the acute trauma setting is to assist in the management and

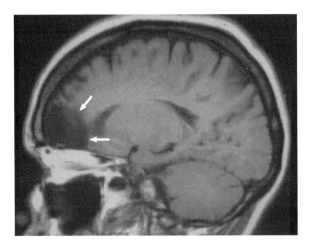

FIG. 13-14. Chronic encephalomalacia after inferior frontal lobe contusion. Sagittal T1-weighted spin-echo [repetition time (TR), 600/echo time (TE) 17] image reveals volume loss and T1 hypointensity (*arrows*) that follows cerebrospinal fluid signal in the classic inferior frontal lobe location.

treatment of the patient. Selection of the imaging modality is often critical and may be complicated by a severely injured or impaired patient. Additionally, the problems of managing the acutely injured patient often include multiple organ systems and cross the boundaries of medical disci-

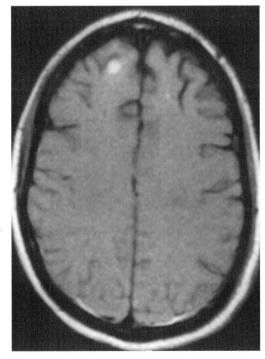

FIG. 13-15. Subacute frontal lobe diffuse axonal injury. Axial T1-weighted spin-echo [repetition time (TR), 600/echo time (TE), 25] image reveals a hyperintense subacute shear hemorrhage in the right frontal lobe at the gray/white matter interface, a classic location for shear injuries. Gradient-echo imaging (not performed) would show a hypointense lesion larger than on the conventional sequences ("blooming" artifact).

plines. A complete understanding of each of the imaging modalities available, as well as the relative advantages and limitations of each, is critical. Only through rapid and accurate use of the medical imaging tools available can neuroimaging facilitate patient care in the setting of acute head trauma. Moreover, it is important to remember that whenever a significant head injury has been sustained, the cervical spine is also at risk.

SPINAL TRAUMA

The incidence of spinal cord injury (SCI) in the United States is approximately 40 per million. This represents approximately 10,000 new cases each year, with more than 200,000 people thought to have SCI. Spinal injuries are a major source of death and disability. Often, the victim of a spine insult is a young or middle-aged adult. Young men are disproportionately affected, with approximately 60% of spinal injuries occurring between the ages of 16 and 30 years. Eighty percent are men. The social and economic costs of spinal injury are significant. For example, the estimated lifetime cost of injury for a 25-year-old rendered paraplegic from a spinal injury is more than $400,000 (111–113).

Spinal trauma frequently results in some form of neurologic damage, disability, or pain. Diagnostic imaging is important in the evaluation of spinal injuries, and plain film x-ray studies are often used as the primary means of initial evaluation. However, CT and MRI are increasingly being used as one of the first-line methods in the evaluation of a potential spinal injury. These modalities are now quite often seen as necessary to complete the imaging evaluation, because the consequences of missed injuries can be serious. Therefore, careful attention to a complete radiologic evaluation is necessary, and the appropriate use of CT and MRI studies is paramount (111,114–125).

Injuries to the spinal cord, nerve roots, and spinal nerves represent the major cause of severe morbidity and mortality from spine injury. However, persistent pain and limitation of movement may result from bone and joint involvement. In most cases, the initial management of the spinal injured patient is directed toward prevention or minimizing the progression of neural injury. The radiologist must remember to evaluate not only the skeletal components of the spine but also the soft tissue and neural elements in patients who have suffered potential spine injury (111,121,122).

Spinal injuries are often referred to clinically in terms related to the mechanism of injury, such as *flexion, extension, axial loading, rotation,* and *lateral bending.* The extent of soft tissue injury varies depending on the mechanism. Life expectancy is directly related to the level of injury (111,121).

Neurologic complications result primarily from injury to the spinal cord and nerve roots. The posttraumatic canal diameter seen on radiologic studies is probably as much as three times the actual diameter of the spinal canal at the instant of the insult, which means that, in addition to any residual compression that may be seen on imaging studies, there may also have been direct injury to the spinal cord or nerve roots at the instant of injury out of proportion to the degree of canal compromise. This initial transient force that may be applied to the soft tissues and neural elements can contribute significantly to the extent of injury. MRI may be the only method currently available to image these types of insults. Because treatment using high-dose methylprednisolone as a spinal cord protectant in the acute stages of spinal injury is increasing, the ability to image the initial injury may be very important in the management of the patient. Aging the injury is also important, because high-dose corticosteroids can be detrimental in the subacute phase. MRI is potentially the most valuable imaging method in this regard (111,112,121–123).

Conventional Imaging Assessment

MRI can be used to assess the extent of spinal injury and assist in the determination of management strategies, and it may also prove valuable in evaluating the prognosis. Plain film radiography has historically been the most widely used method for imaging the injured spine. Current alignment of the skeletal elements is typically well demonstrated with plain films. Alterations in bone contour can often be seen, and in many institutions plain films remain the initial imaging test of choice for acute spinal trauma. It is important to remember that an adequate evaluation of the lateral cervical spine radiograph begins with full visualization of the cervical spine, including the relation of C-7 to T-1. A "swimmer's view" may be necessary to appreciate this relationship. Assessment for abnormal widening of the prevertebral soft tissues and for splaying of the spinous processes is also important. The soft tissue thickness anterior to C-3 should not exceed 4 mm in a normal adult. Alignment is evaluated along the normally lordotic curves of the cervical spine, and the skeletal elements should be closely evaluated for cortical disruption or evidence of displacement (111,121,124–126).

Motion or dynamic studies, such as the lateral flexion and extension view, are often used to evaluate the stability of the spine and to assess the integrity of the ligamentous soft tissues. In many institutions, the flexion-extension radiograph remains the standard for the evaluation of instability, despite the significant limitations in the use of the lateral flexion and extension view in the setting of acute trauma. Optimal flexion and extension views are performed in an upright position and under *patient, not physician*, control. The acutely injured patient is frequently unable to cooperate for this optimal examination. Therefore, there is a risk of exacerbating or causing an injury when instability is present (111,121,127–129). Pursuing dynamic flexion-extension imaging of an acutely injured patient under fluoroscopy can be frustrating and difficult.

Even in cooperative patients, flexion and extension radiographs are further compromised by the fact that the acutely injured patient has poor movement due to guarding or spasm. During flexion-extension radiography for acute spinal trauma, approximately one-fourth to one-third of patients show minimal movement. This finding can be regarded as suspicious for injury but is a nondiagnostic result. Lack of movement can be secondary to muscle spasm or guarding. Patients with significant ligamentous injury can be misconstrued as normal if guarding due to pain obscures identification of instability or fracture. These patients are typically treated as though they are at risk of instability and are often placed in a cervical collar. A repeat flexion-extension examination is then performed after approximately 2 weeks (111,127–129), at which time instability may be identified when the protection of muscle spasm is no longer present.

Therefore, flexion-extension views are most beneficial when delayed 7 to 10 days after injury and are of extremely limited value in the acute setting. However, triaging these patients with multiple injuries often is significantly modified if a spine injury is confirmed early in treatment. MRI offers a method of assessing ligamentous damage that may accompany the acute injury without the risk of movement. MRI is a safer method than flexion-extension when urgent assessment of spinal stability is required (111,127–133).

Magnetic Resonance Imaging Assessment

In some cases, MRI is consistently used for the acute evaluation of soft tissue injury, spinal cord compromise, and the other complications of spinal trauma. MRI is far more sensitive to soft tissue injury than are plain films or CT. MRI has been shown to have statistically significant greater sensitivity for the detection of ligamentous injury, disc protrusion, disc herniation, spinal canal compromise, and EDH compared to plain films or CT. MR angiography (MRA) also provides a noninvasive method to evaluate for arterial injury, such as dissection that may accompany spinal injury. More rapid pulse sequences have lowered the time of scanning, making MRI more practical for use in the acute trauma setting. Open magnet designs have allowed expanded use in patients with severe injuries that require closer monitoring or concurrent therapy. MRI-compatible ventilators and monitoring equipment are widely available and permit invasive monitoring during imaging. Coil placement may be a problem for some patients, but flexible coils can often be creatively used even with immobilization devices in place (111,134–138).

Typically, a minimum of two pulse sequences are used in the sagittal plane, including one with T1 weighting and another with T2 weighting. Tailored axial images are beneficial for closer evaluation of suspected disc protrusion and spinal cord compression from disc or bone fragments identified on sagittal images. The persistent bright appearance of fat on fast spin-echo techniques and sometimes even on conventional spin-echo techniques can complicate interpretation of the examination. Because fat near the coil may also be bright on T2-weighted images, it can be more difficult to detect hemorrhage or edema in the dorsal soft tissues. This is addressed by using fat suppression or inversion recovery sequences, which suppress fat and thus highlight edema. Short tau inversion recovery sequences are particularly effective at higher fields (111,134,139–143).

Plain films and CT are of very limited value in soft tissue evaluation, and MRI is vastly superior in this regard. MRI is of benefit when extensive degenerative changes are present or in the setting of congenital anomalies or old trauma. MRI can confidently confirm or exclude soft tissue injury in most cases, and a normal MRI substantially decreases the likelihood that an acute injury is present. MRI is particularly helpful in the evaluation of patients who are uncooperative, comatose, or intubated. Significant ligamentous injury and occult fractures may appear normal on plain radiographs and can be overlooked in noncommunicating injured patients who cannot verbally express the full extent of their sensory deficits or pain. A normal MRI can have a profound effect and facilitate nursing care including early termination of stabilization procedures. A positive MRI can prevent premature termination of such precautions (111,134,136–140).

MRI is a time-efficient method for acute evaluation of the cervical spine. A limited screening trauma cervical spine MRI in our institution consists of sagittal T1-weighted and fast short tau inversion recovery sequences. If this examination is abnormal, it can be followed by axial T2-weighted fast spin-echo sequences. The sagittal short tau inversion recovery is particularly important, because it nullifies the fat signal, allowing adequate evaluation for occult marrow or ligamentous edema. The presence of a spinal cord hematoma significantly affects prognosis, and a GRE sequence can be added when cord contusion is suspected clinically (111,141,142).

On MRI, as with CT and plain radiographs, it is important to assess the alignment of the spine. A major advantage of MRI is the ability to assess the ligamentous structures for edema or disruption. Because esophageal and pharyngeal fluid may be confused with prevertebral edema in intubated patients, it is important to note when these devices are present. This concern can often be addressed by careful evaluation of the prevertebral region on axial images. Evidence of fluid signal within the region of the anterior or posterior longitudinal ligaments suggests injury or disruption to these structures. These dense ligaments normally have very low signal intensity on MRI so that disruption of these ligaments can be relatively easily detected (111,134–144).

The ligamenta flava and interspinous and supraspinous ligaments located dorsal to the spinal canal are assessed

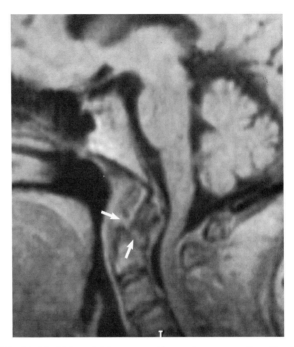

FIG. 13-16. Odontoid fracture with cord compression. Sagittal T1-weighted [repetition time (TR), 68/echo time (TE), 24; flip angle, 45 degrees] imaging reveals a displaced odontoid base fracture (*arrows*) involving the body of C-2 (type III). The dens has been retropulsed, causing distortion of the cord and narrowing of the central canal. Hypointense signal within the dens reflects marrow edema.

similarly. Edema in the interspinous ligaments may represent true ligamentous injury, edema related to ruptured blood vessels, or generalized edema. When fluid is seen in the facet joints or significant subluxation of the facets is present, capsular disruption with possible accompanying facet fracture should be suspected. The sagittal images should extend sufficiently lateral to include the facets to assess the integrity of the capsular ligaments. Edema in the supraodontoid bursa is indicative of possible craniocervical or upper cervical injury (111,143).

On MRI, the bone marrow signal can be assessed for edema that indicates either bone contusion or fracture (Figs. 13-16 and 13-17). Because a relative paucity of marrow exists within the neural arches, including at the level of C-1, injury at this level results in relatively minimal edema. Therefore, MRI can be less sensitive at this level compared to other regions of the spine. It is important to additionally perform a CT scan whenever craniocervical junction injury is suspected. In addition, avulsion injuries tend to result in less edema when compared to compression- or burst-type fractures. The intervertebral disks can be assessed for shear and traumatic herniation. The spinal canal should be closely evaluated for the presence of hematoma, and the spinal cord should be evaluated for the presence or absence of contusion or hemorrhage. In addition, the extent of any compression of

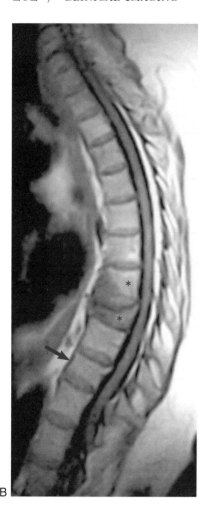 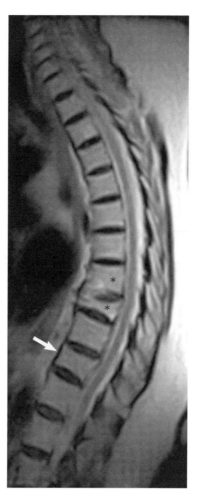

A, B

FIG. 13-17. Discriminating between acute and chronic vertebral fractures. **A:** Sagittal T1-weighted spin-echo image. **B:** Sagittal T2-weighted fast spin-echo image. Sagittal T1- and T2-weighted images show compression fractures at T-8, T-9, and T-11. The anterior wedge compression fracture at T-11 (*arrows*) reveals normal marrow signal on both sequences and remodeling changes of the end plates consistent with a chronic fracture. In contrast, the anterior-inferior body of T-8 and anterior body of T-9 show hypointensity (*asterisks*) relative to marrow on the T1-weighted imaging and isointensity to slight hyperintensity to marrow signal on the T2-weighted imaging, indicative of marrow edema in an acute fracture. The patient's symptoms were referable to T-9 level. The spinal cord signal is normal, supporting the absence of long tract signs on physical examination.

the spinal cord and possible decrease in spinal canal diameter can be noted (111,115,134,144).

We believe that MRI is the procedure of choice for evaluation of SCI. Although CT-myelography may be used when MRI cannot be performed, it predominantly outlines the spinal cord without displaying internal anatomy. MRI demonstrates the size and position of the spinal cord as well as evidence of any impingement. It also provides information regarding the integrity of the spinal cord. It has been reported that the edema and spinal cord hemorrhage detected on MRI directly correlate with patient prognosis. Long-term outcome for recovery is decreased for patients with worse spinal cord swelling and edema. It is the worst for those patients with MRI evidence of intramedullary hemorrhage (111,134,137,139,140).

The late sequelae of SCI are also better assessed by MRI. The presence of a syrinx is common after SCI and is easily identified as a region of fluid signal intensity on all pulse sequences within the cord. MRI can also demonstrate compromise of neural foramina when nerve root damage is present (111,134,140,142,145).

The vascular damage that may accompany spinal trauma may result in brain injury. This is most frequently secondary to vertebral artery injury, and as many as 50%

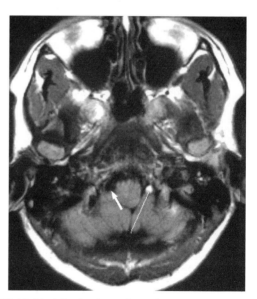

FIG. 13-18. Vertebral artery dissection and occlusion. Axial T1-weighted spin-echo image reveals abnormal hypertense signal without hypointense flow void in the left vertebral artery (*marker*) indicative of very slow flow or occlusion. The right vertebral artery (*arrow*) demonstrates a normal hypointense flow void.

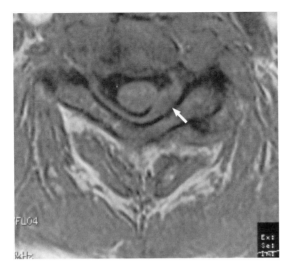
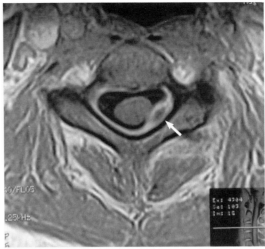
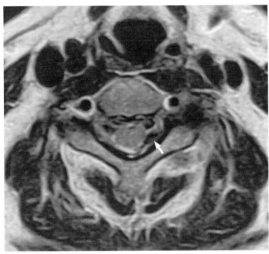

FIG. 13-19. Chronic spinal epidural hematoma. **A:** Axial T1-weighted three-dimensional (3D) spoiled gradient echo (SPGR) image. **B:** Axial T1-weighted 3D SPGR image with contrast. **C:** Axial T2-weighted fast recovery fast spin-echo image from a febrile, otherwise healthy patient with abrupt onset of neck pain that persisted, prompting later imaging referral. A T1 hypointense biconvex epidural collection (*arrows*) is noted in the left dorsal canal at C2-3 with rim enhancement after contrast administration. T2-weighted imaging shows central hypointensity in the area questioned (*arrows*), reflecting chronic hematoma.

of patients with fractures that involve the foramen transversarium have angiographic evidence of vertebral artery injury. Most cases involve only a unilateral vertebral artery injury. These patients may not manifest clinical evidence of posterior fossa damage, presumably because adequate blood supply from the contralateral vertebral artery is present. Nonetheless, when posterior fossa ischemic changes are present, they are best evaluated by MRI. MRA represents a reasonable screening test for vertebral artery injury. Routine MR images should always be inspected for the presence of normal flow voids in the vertebral arteries (Fig. 13-18). Arterial dissection with intimal tear typically produces an eccentric crescent of altered flow or increased signal thrombus in the arterial wall (111,146–148) that is frequently more easily appre-

ciated on the axial images or MRA source images than on the reconstructed MRA images.

CONCLUSION

Imaging studies are an extremely important part of the evaluation of cranial and spinal injury. MRI is increasingly becoming the modality of choice for the exclusion of significant head and spine injury (Figs. 13-19 and 13-20) regardless of the initial type of radiologic evaluation that may have been performed. However, it is vital that the radiologist be able to accurately interpret all types of neuroimaging procedures to limit the often very severe consequences of cranial and spinal trauma (1,20–23,111,149–151).

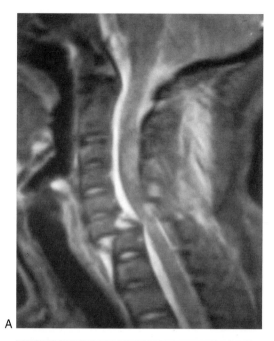

A

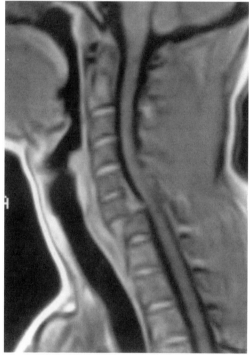

B

FIG. 13-20. Fracture dislocation at C6-7. **A:** T1-weighted sagittal image. **B:** T2-weighted sagittal image. C-6 is anteriorly dislocated with respect to C-7. The anterior longitudinal ligament is separated from the C-7 vertebral body, and the posterior longitudinal ligament is separated from the C-6 vertebral body. The superior posterior lip of C-7 effaces the anterior aspect of the cervical cord. Magnetic resonance imaging is an excellent modality to evaluate the cord in acute trauma.

REFERENCES

1. Orrison WW Jr, Lewine JD. Magnetic source imaging. In: Orrison WW Jr, ed. *Neuroimaging.* Philadelphia: WB Saunders, 2000 (*in press*).
2. Gean AD. *Imaging of head trauma.* New York: Raven Press, 1994:2.
3. Goldstein M. Traumatic brain injury: a silent epidemic. *Ann Neurol* 1990;27:327.
4. Cooper PR. Epidemiology of head injury. In: Cooper PR, ed. *Head injury.* Baltimore: Williams & Wilkins, 1982:1–14.
5. Frankowski RF. Descriptive epidemiology studies of head injury in the United States: 1974–1984. *Adv Psychosom Med* 1986;16:153–172.
6. Jennett B. Disability after head injury: observations on the use of the Glasgow Outcome Scale. *J Neurol Neurosurg Psychiatry* 1981;44:285–293.
7. Federle MP, Brant-Zawadski M. Trauma: CT and emergency. *Diagn Imag* 1982;4:34–38.
8. Gean AD. *Imaging of head trauma.* New York: Raven Press, 1994:16.
9. Levin HS, Benton AI, Grossman RG, eds. *Neurobehavioral consequences of closed head injury.* New York: Oxford University Press, 1982.
10. McLaurin RL, Titchener JL. Post-traumatic syndrome. In: Youmans JR, ed. *Neurological surgery,* 2nd ed. Philadelphia: WB Saunders, 1982:2175–2187.
11. Annegers JF, Grabow JD, Kurland LT, et al. The incidence, causes, and secular trends of head trauma in Olmsted County, MN 1935–1974. *Neurology* 1980;30:912–919.
12. Kooper KD, Tabaddor K, Hauser WA, et al. The epidemiology of head injury in the Bronx. *Neuroepidemiology* 1983;2:70–88.
13. Leninger BE, Gramling SE, Farrell ED, et al. Neuropsychological deficits in symptomatic minor head injury patients after concussion and mild concussion. *J Neurol Neurosurg Psychiatry* 1990;53:293–296.
14. McNemer Q. Note on the sampling error of the differences between correlated proportions or percentages. *Psychometrika* 1947;12:153–157.
15. Rutherford WH, Merrett JD, McDonald JR. Sequelae of concussion caused by minor head injuries. *Lancet* 1977;1:1–4.
16. Orrison WW Jr, Lewine JD. Neuroimaging in closed head injury. In: Rizzo M, Tranel D, eds. *Head injury and postconcussive syndrome.* New York: Churchill Livingstone, 1996.
17. Orrison WW. *Introduction to neuroimaging.* Boston: Little, Brown and Company, 1989:61–63.
18. Fong YT, Teal JS, Hieshima GB. *Neuroradiology of head trauma.* Baltimore: University Park Press, 1984.
19. Gean AD. *Imaging of head trauma.* New York: Raven Press, 1994:4.
20. Orrison WW Jr, Lewine JD. Neuroimaging in closed head injury. In: Rizzo M, Tranel D, eds. *Head injury and postconcussive syndrome.* New York: Churchill Livingstone, 1996.
21. Orrison WW Jr, Gentry LR, Stimac GK, Tarrel RM, Espinosa MC, Cobb LC. Blinded comparison of cranial CT and MR in closed head injury evaluation. *AJNR Am J Neuroradiol* 1994;15:351–356.
22. Gentry LR, Godersky JC, Thompson B, Dunn VD. Prospective comparative study of intermediate-field MR and CT in the evaluation of closed head trauma. *AJNR Am J Neuroradiol* 1988;9:91–100.
23. Gentry LR, Godersky JC, Thompson GH. MR imaging of head trauma: review of the distribution and radiopathologic features of traumatic lesions. *AJNR Am J Neuroradiol* 1988;9:101–110.
24. Osborn AG. *Diagnostic neuroradiology.* St. Louis: Mosby–Year Book, 1994:204.
25. Adams JH. Pathology of nonmissile head injury. *Neuroimag Clin North Am* 1991;1:397–410.
26. Gean AD. *Imaging of head trauma.* New York: Raven Press, 1994:109.
27. Jennett B, Teasdale G. *Management of head injuries.* Philadelphia: FA Davis, 1981.
28. Galbraith SL. Age-distribution of extradural hemorrhage without skull fracture. *Lancet* 1973;1:1217–1218.
29. Rivas JJ, Lobato RD, Sarabia R, et al. Extradural hematoma: analysis of factors influencing the courses of 161 patients. *Neurosurgery* 1988;23:44–51.
30. Lobato RD, Rivas JJ, Cordobes F, et al. Acute epidural hematoma: an analysis of factors influencing outcome of patients undergoing surgery in coma. *J Neurosurg* 1988;68:48–57.
31. Seelig JM, Becker DP, Miller JD, Greenberg RP, Ward JD, Choi SC. Traumatic acute subdural hematoma. Major mortality reduction in comatose patients treated within four hours. *N Engl J Med* 1981;304:1511–1518.

32. Hoff J, Barnes E, Barnes B, et al. Traumatic subdural hygroma. *J Trauma* 1973;13:870–876.

33. Baykaner K, Alp H, Ceviker N, Keski S, Seckin Z. Observation of 95 patients with extradural hematomas and review of the literature. *Surg Neurol* 1988;30:339–341.

34. Dharker SR, Bhargava N. Bilateral epidural hematoma. *Acta Neurochir (Wien)* 1991;110:29–32.

35. Gean AD. *Imaging of head trauma.* New York: Raven Press, 1994:110.

36. Reed D, Robertson WD, Graeb DA, et al. Acute subdural hematomas: atypical CT findings. *AJNR Am J Neuroradiol* 1986;7:417–421.

37. French BN, Cobb CA III, Corkill G, et al. Delayed evolution of post-traumatic subdural hygroma. *Surg Neurol* 1978;9:145–148.

38. Ford LE, McLaurin RL. Mechanisms of extradural hematomas. *J Neurosurg* 1963;20:760–769.

39. Fisher RG, Kim JK, Sachs E Jr. Complications in posterior fossa due to occipital trauma and their operability. *JAMA* 1958;167:176–182.

40. Servadei F, Faccani G, Roccella A, et al. Asymptomatic extradural haematomas: results of a multicenter study of 158 cases in minor head injury. *Acta Neurochir (Wien)* 1989;96:39–45.

41. Knuckey NW, Gelbard B, Epstein MH. The management of "asymptomatic" epidural hematomas: a prospective study. *J Neurosurg* 1989;70:392–396.

42. Milo R, Razon N. Schiffer J. Delayed epidural hematoma: a review. *Acta Neurochir (Wein)* 1987;84:13–23.

43. Pozzati E, Tognetti F, Cavallo M, Acciarri N. Extradural hematomas of the posterior cranial fossa: observations on a series of 32 consecutive cases treated after the introduction of computed tomographic scanning. *Surg Neurol* 1989;32:300–303.

44. Bricolo AP, Pasut LM. Extradural hematoma: toward zero mortality. *Neurosurgery* 1984;14:8–12.

45. Smith HK, Miller JD. The danger of an ultra-early computed tomographic scan in a patient with an evolving acute epidural hematoma. *Neurosurgery* 1991;29:258–260.

46. Kuroiwa T, Tanabe H, Takatsuka H, et al. Rapid spontaneous resolution of acute extradural and subdural hematomas. *J Neurosurg* 1993;78:126–128.

47. Gean AD. *Imaging of head trauma.* New York: Raven Press, 1994:76–78.

48. Teasdale G, Galbraith S. Acute traumatic intracranial hematomas. *Prog Neurol Surg* 1981;10:66–99.

49. Gennarelli TA, Thibault LE. Biomechanics of acute subdural hematoma. *J Trauma* 1982;22:680–685.

50. Ommaya AK, Yarnell P. Subdural haematoma after whiplash injury. *Lancet* 1969;2:237–239.

51. Chambers JW. The acute SDH. *J Neurosurg* 1951;8:263–268.

52. Laudig GH, Browder DER, Watson RA, et al. Subdural hematomas: a study of 143 cases. *Ann Surg* 1941;113:170–188.

53. Gennarelli TA, Thibault LE. Biomechanics of acute subdural hematoma. *J Trauma* 1982;22:686.

54. Shenkin HA. Acute subdural hematoma: review of 39 consecutive cases with a high incidence of cortical rupture. *J Neurosurg* 1982;57:254–257.

55. Osborn AG. *Diagnostic neuroradiology.* St. Louis: Mosby–Year Book, 1994:205.

56. Wilberger JE, Harris M, Diamond DL. Auto subdural hematoma: morbidity, mortality, and operative timings. *J Neurosurg* 1991;74:212–218.

57. Osborn AG. *Diagnostic neuroradiology.* St. Louis: Mosby–Year Book, 1994.

58. Reed D, Robertson WD, Graeb DA, et al. Acute subdural hematomas: atypical CT findings. *AJNR Am J Neuroradiol* 1991;12:341–343.

59. Hashimoto N, Sakakibara T, Yamamoto K, et al. Two fluid-blood density levels in chronic subdural hematoma. *J Neurosurg* 1992;77:310–311.

60. Wilms G, Marchal G, Guesens E. Isodense subdural haematomas on CT: MR findings. *Neuroradiology* 1992;34:497–499.

61. Gean AD. *Imaging of head trauma.* New York: Raven Press, 1994:80.

62. Black PM, Ojemann RG, Tzouras A. CSF shunting for dementia, incontinence, and gait disturbance. *Clin Neurosurg* 1985;32:632–651.

63. Naidich TP, Schott LH, Baron RL. Computed tomography in the evaluation of hydrocephalus. *Radiol Clin North Am* 1982;20:143–167.

64. Freytag E. Autopsy findings in head injuries from blunt forces. *Arch Pathol* 1963;75:402–413.

65. Gean AD. *Imaging of head trauma.* New York: Raven Press, 1994.

66. Orrison WW Jr, Lewine JD. Neuroimaging in closed head injury. In: Rizzo M, Tranel D, eds. *Head injury and postconcussive syndrome.* New York: Churchill Livingstone, 1996.

67. Yeakley JW, Mayer JS, Patchell CC, et al. The pseudodelta sign in acute head trauma. *J Neurosurg* 1988;69:867–868.

68. Osborn AG, Anderson RE, Wing SD. The false falx sign. *Radiology* 1980;134:421–425.

69. Modesti LM, Binet EF. Value of computed tomography in the diagnosis and management of subarachnoid hemorrhage. *Neurosurgery* 1978;3:151–156.

70. Gean AD. *Imaging of head trauma.* New York: Raven Press, 1994:132.

71. Bank WO, Baleriauz D, Matos C, et al. Subarachnoid hemorrhage into pre-existing arachnoid cysts: a potential pitfall in the interpretation of MRI and CT. In: *Proceedings of the annual meeting of the American Society of Neuroradiology.* Washington: American Society of Neuroradiology, 1991:63.

72. Chaney RK, Taber KH, Orrison WW Jr, Hayman LA. Magnetic resonance imaging of intracerebral hemorrhage at different field strengths: a review of reported intraparenchymal signal intensities. *Neuroimag Clin North Am* 1992;2(1):25–51.

73. Barfuss H, Fisher H, Hentschel D, et al. Whole-body MR imaging and spectroscopy with a 4-T system. *Radiology* 1988;169:811–816.

74. Mitchell MD. Efficacy studies of low-field-strength MR imaging: feast or famine. *Radiology* 1996;200(1):284.

75. Drejer J, Thomsen HS, Tanttu J. Low-field imaging of the spine: a comparative study of a traditional and a new, completely balanced gradient-echo sequence. *Acta Radiol* 1995;36:505–509.

76. Tsuchiya K, Mizutani Y, Hachiya J. Preliminary evaluation of fluid-attenuated inversion-recovery MR in the diagnosis of intracranial tumors. *AJNR Am J Neuroradiol* 1996;17:1081–1086.

77. Lotz H, Ekelund L, Hietala SO, Wickman G. Low-field (0.02) MR imaging of the whole body. *J Comput Assist Tomogr* 1988;12(6):1006–1013.

78. Sipponen RE, Sipponen JT, Sivula A. Low-field (0.02) nuclear magnetic resonance imaging of the brain. *J Comput Assist Tomogr* 1985;9:237–241.

79. Sipponen JT, Sipponen RE, Tantu JL, Sivula A. Intracranial hematomas studied by MR imaging at 0.17 and 0.02 T. *J Comput Assist Tomogr* 1985;9:698–704.

80. Fagerlund M, Björnebrink J, Elelund L, Toolanen G. Ultra low field MR imaging of cervical spine involvement in rheumatoid arthritis. *Acta Radiologica* 1992;33(2):89–92.

81. Gean AD. *Imaging of head trauma.* New York: Raven Press, 1994: 134–135.

82. Bagley C Jr. Blood in the cerebrospinal fluid: resultant functional and organic alterations in the central nervous system. *Arch Surg* 1928;17:18–38.

83. Timming R, Orrison WW Jr, Mikula JA. Computerized tomography and rehabilitation outcome after severe head trauma. *Arch Phys Med Rehabil* 1982;63:154–159.

84. Osborn AG. *Diagnostic neuroradiology.* St. Louis: Mosby–Year Book, 1994:221.

85. LeRoux PD, Haglund MM, Newell DW, et al. Intraventricular hemorrhage in blunt head trauma: an analysis of 43 cases. *Neurosurgery* 1992;31:678–685.

86. Lee JP, Lui TN, Change CN. Acute post-traumatic intraventricular hemorrhage analysis of 25 patients with emphasis on final outcome. *Acta Neurol Scand* 1991;84:89–90.

87. Gean AD. *Imaging of head trauma.* New York: Raven Press, 1994:124–125.

88. Gentry LR, Thompson B, Godersky JC. Trauma to the corpus callosum: MR features. *AJNR Am J Neuroradiol* 1988;9:1129–1138.

89. Zimmerman RD, Leeds NE, Nadich TP. Ring blush associated with intracerebral hematoma. *Radiology* 1977;122:707–711.

90. Tsai FY, Huprich JE, Gardner FC, et al. Diagnostic and prognostic implications of computed tomography of head trauma. *J Comput Assist Tomogr* 1978;2:323–331.

91. Kishore PRS, Lipper MIT, Becker DP, et al. Significance of CT in head injury: correlation with intracranial pressure. *AJNR Am J Neuroradiol* 1981;2:307–311.

92. Weisburg LA. Computerized tomography in intracranial hemorrhage. *Arch Neurol* 1979;36:422–426.

93. Dolinskas CA, Bilaniuk LT, Zimmerman RA, et al. Computed tomography of intracerebral hematomas. I. Transmission CT observations on hematoma resolution. *AJR Am J Roentgenol* 1977;129:681–688.

94. Dolinskas CA, Bilaniuk LT, Zimmerman RA, et al. Computed tomography of intracerebral hematomas. II. Radionuclide and transmission CT studies of the perihematoma region. *AJR Am J Roentgenol* 1977;129:689–692.

95. Orrison WW Jr, Lewine JD. Neuroimaging in closed head injury. In: Rizzo M, Tranel D, eds. *Head injury and postconcussive syndrome.* New York: Churchill Livingstone, 1996.

96. Atlas SW, Grossman RI, Gomori JM, et al. Hemorrhagic intracranial malignant neoplasms: spin-echo MR imaging. *Radiology* 1987;164: 71–77.

97. Atlas SW, Mark AS, Grossman RI, Gomori JM. Intracranial hemorrhage: gradient-echo MR imaging at 1.5 T. *Radiology* 1988;168:803–807.

98. Barkovich AJ, Atlas SW. Magnetic resonance imaging of intracranial hemorrhage. *Radiol Clin North Am* 1988;26(4):801–820.

99. Dooms AC, Uske A, Brant-Zawadzki M, et al. Spin-echo MR imaging of intracranial hemorrhage. *Neuroradiology* 1986;28:132–138.

100. Hardy PA, Kucharczyk W, Henkelman RM. Cause of signal loss in MR images of old hemorrhagic lesions. *Radiology* 1990;174:549–555.

101. Hayman LA, Taber KH, Ford JJ, Bryan RN. Mechanisms of MR signal alteration by acute intracerebral blood: old concepts and new theories. *AJNR Am J Neuroradiol* 1991;12:899–907.

102. Brooks RA, DiChiro G, Petronas N. MR imaging of cerebral hematomas at different field strengths: theory and applications. *J Comput Assist Tomogr* 1989;13(2):194–206.

103. DiChiro G, Brooks RA, Girton ME, et al. Sequential MR studies of intracerebral hematomas in monkeys. *AJNR Am J Neuroradiol* 1986;7:193–199.

104. Zimmerman RD, Heier LA, Snow RB, et al. Acute intracranial hemorrhage: intensity changes on sequential MR scans at 0.5 T. *AJR Am J Roentgenol* 1988;150:651–661.

105. Gomori JM, Grossman RI, Goldberg HI, et al. Intracranial hematomas: imaging by high-field MR. *Radiology* 1985;157:87–93.

106. Orrison WW Jr. *Introduction to neuroimaging.* Boston: Little, Brown and Company, 1989.

107. Osborn AG. *Diagnostic neuroradiology.* St. Louis: Mosby–Year Book, 1994:212.

108. Hosoda K, Tamaki N, Masumura M, et al. Magnetic resonance images of chronic subdural hematomas. *J Neurosurg* 1987;67:677–683.

109. Hesselink JR, Dowd CF, Healy ME, et al. MR imaging of brain contusions: a comparative study with CT. *AJNR Am J Neuroradiol* 1988;9:269–278.

110. Gentry LR. Head trauma. In: Atlas SW, ed. *Magnetic resonance imaging of the brain and spine.* New York: Raven Press, 1991:439–466.

111. Hart BL, Butman JA, Benzel EC. Spine trauma. In: Orrison WW Jr, ed. *Neuroimaging.* Philadelphia: WB Saunders, 2000 (*in press*).

112. DeVivo MJ, Rutt RD, Black KJ, et al. Trends in spinal cord injury demographics and treatment outcomes between 1973 and 1986. *Arch Phys Med Rehabil* 1992;73:424–430.

113. National Spinal Cord Injury Statistical Center. *Spinal cord injury facts and figures at a glance.* Birmingham, AL: National Spinal Cord Injury Statistical Center, 1998.

114. Harris JH Jr, Mirvis SE. *The radiology of acute cervical spine trauma.* Baltimore: Williams & Wilkins, 1996.

115. Effendi B, Roy D, Cornish B, Dussault RG, Laurin CA. Fractures of the ring of the axis: a classification based on the analysis of 131 cases. *J Bone Joint Surg [Br]* 1981;63:319–327.

116. Miller MO, Gehweiler JA, Martinez S, Charlton OP, Daffner RH. Significant new observations on cervical spine trauma. *AJR Am J Roentgenol* 1978;130:659–663.

117. Shaffer MA, Doris PE. Limitation of the cross table lateral view in detecting cervical spine injuries: a retrospective analysis. *Ann Emerg Med* 1981;10:508–513.

118. Streitweiser DR, Knopp R, Wales LR, et al. Accuracy of standard radiographic views in detecting cervical spine fractures. *Ann Emerg Med* 1983;12:538–542.

119. Ross SE, Schwab CW, David ET, et al. Clearing the cervical spine: initial radiologic evaluation. *J Trauma* 1987;27(9):1055–1060.

120. Penning L. Roentgenographic evaluation: obtaining and interpreting plain films in cervical spine injury. In: Bailey RW, ed. *The cervical spine.* Philadelphia: JB Lippincott Co, 1983.

121. Stover SL, Whiteneck GG, DeLisa JA. *Spinal cord injury: clinical outcome from the model systems.* Gaithersburg, MD: Aspen, 1995.

122. Bracken MB, Shepard MJ, Collins WF, et al. A randomized, controlled trial of methylprednisolone or naloxone in the treatment of acute spinal-cord injury. Results of the Second National Acute Spinal Cord Injury Study. *N Engl J Med* 1990;322:1405–1411.

123. Chang DG, Tencer AF, Ching RP, et al. Geometric changes in the cervical spine canal during impact. *Spine* 1994;19(8):973–980.

124. Benzel EC, Hart BL, Ball PA, et al. Fractures of the C-2 vertebral body. *J Neurosurg* 1994;81:206–212.

125. Hay PD. Measurement of the soft tissues of the neck. In: Lusted LB, Keats TE, eds. *Atlas of roentgenographic measurement,* 3rd ed. Chicago: Year Book, 1972.

126. Harris JH Jr. Abnormal cervicocranial retropharyngeal soft-tissue contour in the detection of subtle acute cervicocranial injuries. *Emerg Radiol* 1994;1:15–23.

127. Lewis LM, Docherty M, Ruoff BE, et al. Flexion-extension views in the evaluation of cervical-spine injuries. *Ann Emerg Med* 1991;20: 117–121.

128. Bohrer SP, Chen YM, Sayers DG. Cervical spine flexion patterns. *Skeletal Radiol* 1990;19:521–525.

129. Taylor AR, Blackwood W. Paraplegia in cervical injuries with normal radiographic appearance. *J Bone Joint Surg [Br]* 1948;30: 245–248.

130. Juhl JH, Miller SM, Roberts GW. Roentgenographic variations in the normal cervical spine. *Radiology* 1962;78:591–597.

131. Webb JK, Broughton RBK, McSween T, et al. Hidden flexion injury of the cervical spine. *J Bone Joint Surg [Br]* 1976;68:322–327.

132. Olerud C, Jonsson H. Compression of the cervical spine cord after reduction of fracture dislocation: report of 2 cases. *Acta Orthop Scand* 1991;62:599–601.

133. Robertson PA, Ryan MD. Neurological deterioration after reduction of cervical subluxation: mechanical compression by disc tissue. *J Bone Joint Surg [Br]* 1992;74:224–227.

134. Orrison WW, Benzel EC, Willis BK, Hart BL, Espinosa M. Magnetic resonance imaging evaluation of acute spine trauma. *Emerg Radiol* 1995;2:120–128.

135. Davis JW, Phreaner DL, Hoyt DB, Mackersie RC. The etiology of missed cervical spine injuries. *J Trauma* 1993;34:342–346.

136. Beers GJ, Raque GH, Wagner GG, et al. MR imaging in acute cervical spine trauma. *J Comput Assist Tomogr* 1988;12:755–761.

137. Chakeres DW, Flickinger F, Bresnahan JC, et al. MR imaging of acute spinal cord trauma. *AJNR Am J Neuroradiol* 1987;8(1):5–10.

138. Goldberg AL, Rothfus WE, Deeb ZL, et al. The impact of magnetic resonance on the diagnostic evaluation of acute cervicothoracic spinal trauma. *Skeletal Radiol* 1988;17:89–95.

139. Hackney DB, Asato R, Joseph PM, et al. Hemorrhage and edema in acute spinal canal compression: demonstration by MR imaging. *Radiology* 1986;161:387–390.

140. McArdle CB, Crofford MJ, Mirjakhraee M, et al. Surface coil MR of spinal trauma: preliminary experience. *AJNR Am J Neuroradiol* 1986; 7:886–893.

141. Mirvis SE, Geisler FH, Jelinek JJ, et al. Acute cervical spine trauma: evaluation with 1.5T MR imaging. *Radiology* 1988;166: 807–816.

142. Tarr RW, Drolshagen LF, Kerner TC, et al. MR imaging of recent spinal trauma. *J Comput Assist Tomogr* 1987;11:412–417.

143. Warner J, Shanmuganathan K, Mirvis SE, Cerva D. Magnetic resonance imaging of ligamentous injury of the cervical spine. *Emerg Radiol* 1996;3:9–15.

144. Benzel EC, Hart BL, Ball PA, Baldwin NG, Orrison WW, Espinosa MC. Magnetic resonance imaging for the evaluation of patients with occult cervical spine injury. *J Neurosurg* 1996;85:824–829.

145. Rizzolo SJ, Piazza MR, Cotler JM, et al. Intervertebral disc injury complicating cervical spine trauma. *Spine* 1991;16:S187–S189.

146. Keiper MD, Zimmerman RZ, Bilaniuk LT. MRI in the assessment of the supportive soft tissues of the cervical spine in acute trauma in children. *Neuroradiology* 1998;40:359–363.

147. Flanders AE, Schaefer DM, Doan HT, et al. Acute cervical spine trauma: correlation of MR imaging findings with degree of neurologic deficit. *Radiology* 1990;177:25–33.

148. Willis BK, Greiner F, Orrison WW, Benzel EC. The incidence of vertebral artery injury after midcervical spine fracture or subluxation. *Neurosurgery* 1994;34:435–441.

149. Kulkarni MV, McArdle CB, Kopanicky D, et al. Acute spinal cord injury: MR imaging at 1.5T. *Radiology* 1987;164:837–843.

150. Schaefer DM, Flanders AE, Osterhold JL, Northrup BE. Prognostic significance of magnetic resonance imaging in the acute phase of cervical spine injury. *J Neurosurg* 1992;76:218–223.

151. Silberstein M, Tress BM, Hennessy O. Prediction of neurologic outcome in acute spinal cord injury: the role of CT and MR. *AJNR Am J Neuroradiol* 1992;13:1597–1608.

Open MRI,
edited by Peter A. Rothschild and Debra Reinking Rothschild.
Lippincott Williams & Wilkins. Philadelphia © 2000.

CHAPTER 14

Open Magnetic Resonance Imaging of the Musculoskeletal System

Joseph Triolo

Imaging the musculoskeletal system on open magnetic resonance imaging (MRI) systems requires a strong understanding of the various pulse sequences and careful decision making when choosing sequences to maximize the potential of open MRI. Unlike high-field systems in which signal is abundant, lower field open systems require careful tailoring of the various pulse sequences to maximize signal and optimize resolution and contrast. Also, the longer scan times on open systems demand care when determining which pulse sequences to use. These considerations are important when demonstrating the wide range of pathology encountered in the musculoskeletal system.

Numerous anatomic structures need to be identified when imaging the musculoskeletal system, including the fibrocartilaginous menisci and labrum, hyaline cartilage, tendons, ligaments, bone marrow, and soft tissues. All of these anatomic structures have different appearances on the various pulse sequences. Choosing the appropriate pulse sequences and performing the study in a timely fashion are goals of every radiologist and MRI technologist.

For open MRI to complement or compete in a predominantly high-field environment, open systems must emphasize their advantages over high-field closed MRI systems when it comes to patient comfort and selection, while providing high-quality images. Open MRI users must also understand the challenges they face. Lower inherent signal is a battle that must be continually fought. Pertinent to the musculoskeletal system, however, is the current inability to suppress fat signal with presaturation techniques. Chemical fat saturation is an extremely useful technique on higher field strength systems, producing high-contrast, high-resolution images. Lower field open systems can produce high-contrast images

on short tau inversion recovery (STIR) sequences, but at the price of lower resolution. Open systems can produce high-resolution T1-weighted images, but at the cost of longer scan times and no fat suppression. These trade-offs between contrast, resolution, and scan time underscore the importance of using the appropriate pulse sequences.

SIGNAL AND NOISE

The constant challenge for open systems is to improve the signal-to-noise ratio (SNR). Because signal is proportional to field strength, all lower field open systems are at an inherent disadvantage in comparison to high-field closed MRI; therefore, attempts must constantly be made to maximize the SNR. Doing so requires a thorough understanding of the factors that contribute to the SNR and the trade-offs necessary to obtain high resolution and high SNR.

Three major factors affect the SNR: bandwidth, voxel size, and number of excitations (NEX). Bandwidth determines over what range of frequencies signal and noise are sampled. Voxel size determines the amount of tissue sampled (size of the net magnetization vector), and NEX determines how many times the voxel is sampled. In all aspects of MRI, almost every factor that is adjusted to improve SNR has a costly effect, predominantly on resolution and scan time. These effects can be more detrimental at lower field strengths, in which the SNR is often in short supply. The only methods for improving SNR that do not affect resolution or scan time are the use of dedicated small parts coils and postprocessing filters to reduce noise.

Improved coil technology can improve SNR without affecting scan time or resolution and, as a result, higher resolution scans can be performed in a similar or even shorter period. Noise reduction filters are used on all open magnets and are discussed later in the section Postprocessing Noise Reduction.

J. Triolo: Ocean Medical Imaging Center, Community Medical Center, Toms River, New Jersey

Bandwidth

Lowering or narrowing the bandwidth can be used to improve SNR by sampling a narrow range of frequencies. Lower bandwidths decrease the amount of noise sampled relative to signal, and the overall SNR improves. Lowering the bandwidth increases the sampling time (i.e., the time the frequency readout gradient is turned on). As a result, the echo times (TEs) become longer, because the echo is centered over the longer readout gradient. Fewer slices can be acquired during each repetition time (TR); therefore, scan time increases. For routine spin-echo (SE) and gradient-echo (GRE) imaging, no other significant downsides exist except for increased chemical shift artifact. Chemical shift artifact has its greatest effect at higher field strengths but can be seen on lower field open systems with very narrow bandwidths. Bandwidths in the range of 3 to 6 kHz are commonly used for routine SE and GRE imaging.

During fast spin-echo (FSE) imaging, lowering the bandwidth widens the distance between each echo of the echo train because the readout gradient is on for a longer period. The number of slices for each TR decreases and echo spacing widens, resulting in blurring artifact. The blurring artifact with wider echo spacing is more dramatic at shorter TEs (see Chapter 9, Fast Spin-Echo Imaging).

Voxel Size

Voxel size plays a significant role in determining the amount of signal acquired. The size of the signal vector (net magnetization vector) is proportional to the field strength and the amount of tissue sampled (voxel size). Voxel size is the product of the pixel size and the slice thickness. Pixel size, in turn, is determined by the field of view (FOV) and number of frequency- and phase-encoding steps. The disadvantage of increasing the voxel size is loss of resolution. FOV is the largest determinant of pixel size, and increasing the FOV has the greatest effect on improving the SNR. When imaging large patients, increasing the FOV is probably the simplest and most dramatic means of improving the SNR.

Phase-Encoding Steps

The phase-encoding steps not only affect the voxel size but also the scan time. Reducing the number of phase-encoding steps results in an increase in signal (as the voxel size is larger) and reduces scan time. Reducing the phase-encoding steps is a helpful technique when shorter scan times are needed, as with an uncooperative patient. The downside is decreased resolution. The degree of resolution needed for a particular scan should be determined before the particular pulse sequence. For example, STIR sequences have low inherent signal but have high contrast, as fat is essentially nullified. Although the signal is low, contrast is high, and lower resolution scans are very informative and acceptable. High-resolution STIR scans are difficult to perform even on high field strengths, as there is very little inherent signal, but high resolution is not necessary for STIR imaging. To successfully perform STIR scans on lower field open systems, lowering the phase matrix increases signal and shortens scan time, so more NEX can be acquired to compensate for the lack of signal from fat. On T1-weighted scans [which are two-dimensional (2D) SE or three-dimensional (3D) T1-weighted GRE], signal is inherently high, and the phase matrix can be increased because less NEX are required and high-resolution scans can be successfully performed, which is crucial for T1-weighted images.

Frequency-Encoding Steps

Adjusting the frequency-encoding steps has little effect on scan time but can be helpful in adjusting resolution and signal. Higher frequency-encoding steps do stress the gradients and slightly increase the minimum TE, but not to the same degree as lowering bandwidth. On pulse sequences with inherently high signal, as with T1-weighted SE or 3D volume GRE, the frequency encoding can be increased to improve resolution and still produce high SNR images without increasing scan time. When less signal is available, as with inversion recovery or heavily T2-weighted sequences, lower frequency-encoding steps do improve signal by forming a larger voxel. Also, square pixel acquisition can be formed, often resulting in better resolution.

Slice Thickness

Slice thickness has a linear relationship with respect to signal. When trying to improve signal by increasing slice thickness, one should always consider the initial slice thickness prescribed. It is important to remember that increasing slice thickness has a much greater effect on SNR if the original slices were thin. Changing from 3 to 4 mm results in a 33% increase in SNR, whereas changing from 7 to 8 mm only results in a 14% increase in SNR. Also, the appropriate imaging plane should be considered when attempting thinner slices, because the thinner slice scans require longer scan times. When a large superior to inferior surface needs to be covered, thinner slices can be more efficiently performed in the sagittal or coronal plane than in the axial plane.

Number of Excitations

Increasing the NEX has the obvious downside of increasing scan time, with no improvement of resolution. Increasing NEX is more helpful at lower NEX scans, because doubling the NEX increases the SNR by approximately 40%. An increase in NEX from 1 to 2 has a much greater effect on the SNR than an increase from 6 to 7. Thus, at higher NEX, increasing the NEX becomes time consuming and is associated with little improvement in the SNR. Higher NEX, however, can be useful to average out motion. An NEX above 6 or 7 is not very helpful. Higher NEX scans are required on FSE inversion recovery and T2-weighted images because bandwidths cannot be lowered dramatically as can be done with SE or GRE sequences, and the only means of increasing signal is to increase the NEX.

PULSE SEQUENCES

Choosing the appropriate pulse sequence is critical in open MRI. Keeping in mind the importance of the SNR and contrast-to-noise ratio (CNR), the best sequence should be chosen to achieve the goal of the selected series. On high-field systems, SNR is high primarily due to field strength; also, contrast can be dramatically increased by applying chemical fat-saturation pulses. Thus, on high-field strength systems, both high SNR and CNR can be achieved with the same pulse sequence, especially with fat-saturated T1-weighted images with intraarticular gadolinium.

On lower field open systems, the luxury of both high SNR and CNR cannot be achieved on the same pulse sequence. Currently, fat-saturation pulses cannot be successfully performed because the resonant peaks of fat and water are too close together, and the peaks cannot be separated to selectively suppress the fat. As a result, the signal from fat on FSE sequences cannot be suppressed and higher contrast scans are more difficult to obtain. The best technique for producing high-contrast images is to nullify fat with STIR sequences. This can be successfully accomplished on open systems in the same manner it is accomplished at high-field strengths, because STIR takes advantage of different T1 relaxation times of fat and other tissues and not its resonant frequency.

To create high-resolution images, one must take advantage of the predominantly short T1 values of various musculoskeletal structures, such as subcutaneous fat, cartilage, and bone marrow, which have higher inherent signal. T1-weighted images can be obtained using conventional SE or 3D spoiled (T1) GRE sequences. The 3D spoiled GRE sequences are the most useful in open MRI because thinner and higher resolution slices can be obtained compared to those that can be obtained with 2D imaging techniques.

As a rule of thumb in musculoskeletal imaging, certain pulse sequences with inherently higher signal, such as T1-weighted SE, proton density–weighted SE, and 3D T1-weighted GRE sequences, should be performed to maximize SNR, whereas T2-weighted FSE and STIR sequences are best used to maximize the CNR. By combining high SNR and high CNR sequences, open MRI can create high-quality, diagnostic examinations.

T1-Weighted and Proton Density–Weighted Sequences

The high quantity of fat in the musculoskeletal system (subcutaneous soft tissues and bone marrow) makes it relatively easy to obtain high-quality images from T1-weighted scans. T1-weighted images demonstrate excellent contrast between these high signal structures and the low signal from tendons and ligaments, as well as with intermediate signal from muscle. With an inherently higher SNR, the parameters of T1-weighted and proton density–weighted sequences can be adjusted to produce high-resolution images.

T1-weighted 3D GRE imaging requires special mention. Because of less chemical shift and susceptibility artifacts at lower field strengths, 3D imaging is a useful technique on open MRI as volume imaging exhibits inherently higher signal. On 3D scans, a whole volume of tissue is excited and additional phase-encoding steps are applied in the slice selection axis (slice encoding) to localize the slices. Increasing the number of slices with 3D scans results in a higher SNR, and signal is less dependent on slice thickness than with 2D scans. As a result, thinner slices, smaller FOVs, and higher matrices can be acquired. 3D T1-weighted (spoiled) GRE sequences use short TRs of 50 to 70 ms and flip angles of approximately 45 degrees.

On 3D T1-weighted GRE sequences, the lower bandwidths of 3 to 4 kHz allow low NEX scans of 0.75 to 1.50, depending on whether "no phase wrap" is used. Artifacts, however, are more problematic with GRE images as susceptibility artifact is increased, as is chemical shift artifact. Out-of-phase TEs should be avoided. Throughout the musculoskeletal chapters (Chapters 15 to 20), all T1 images are labeled as 2D or 3D so the reader can judge for him- or herself.

T2-Weighted Fast Spin-Echo Sequences

T2-weighted FSE is a very important pulse sequence for musculoskeletal imaging. With T2-weighted FSE, multiple echoes are used to acquire information from a single TR, which dramatically reduces scan time. Contrast between tissues (other than fat) and fluid is better demonstrated on FSE than T1, which is important for the detection of musculoskeletal pathology. Fluid coursing with or extending into the tendons and ligaments is the most useful sign when identifying pathology. T2-weighted FSE and STIR images best demonstrate fluid; however, STIR scans are limited in resolution, and the higher resolution T2 scans are often more informative when imaging the musculoskeletal system. To provide heavily T2-weighted images, longer TEs are required to demonstrate fluid as high signal and differentiate it from fat. The TE controls contrast on T2-weighted images, and TEs in the range of 110 to 140 ms provide excellent T2 contrast. At longer TEs, however, less signal is available and higher NEX scans of 5 to 7 are often required.

Blurring or distortion artifact may be problematic on FSE with longer echo train lengths and narrow bandwidths. Blurring artifact is exaggerated at shorter TEs, and many radiologists therefore avoid proton density–weighted FSE, especially when evaluating the menisci. Using longer TEs on T2-weighted images, higher echo train lengths can be used to allow faster scanning, T2 contrast is increased, and blurring artifact is minimized. Carefully choosing the bandwidth is important, because lower bandwidths widen the echo spacing.

Inversion Recovery

STIR pulse sequences are an essential tool for musculoskeletal imaging on open systems. STIR sequences take advantage of the short T1 time of fat to suppress its signal, which differs from fat-saturation techniques in which the resonating frequency peak of fat is suppressed. The resonating frequency peaks of fat and water are determined by a multiple of the magnetic field strength. At lower field strengths, the peaks of fat and water are close together, and with current technology, fat cannot be suppressed without suppressing water. With STIR techniques, the T1 time of fat is much shorter than that of water and the two can be successfully separated at all field strengths.

STIR sequences have low signal because the inherent signal of fat is essentially nullified, much of the scanning time is spent acquiring signal, and higher NEX scans are required. To increase signal, larger voxel sizes and thicker slices are required and, as a result, resolution is lost. Slice thicknesses generally have to be greater than 5 mm to produce quality images. Nullification of fat creates images that are very sensitive to fluid, which is very bright relative to background. The bright signal from fluid is a very helpful sign in identifying musculoskeletal pathology. The combination of FSE and STIR allows faster scanning and is the most common method used for inversion recovery imaging (fast STIR).

Gradient Echo

2D GRE scans are best performed with T2 weighting. T2 contrast depends on longer TEs and shorter flip angles. Longer TRs are also useful because they allow full recovery of the longer T2 substances such as fluid. The longer TRs make 3D GRE scans with T2 weighting very time consuming. With GRE scans, low bandwidths in the 3- to 5-mHz range allow for an improved SNR, and TEs that are out of phase should be avoided to minimize artifacts. T2-weighted GRE scans provide useful information when evaluating the labrum, cartilage, and smaller ligaments.

Postprocessing Noise Reduction

Another way to improve image quality without a penalty in time or resolution is to postprocess out noise in the image with advanced mathematical algorithms, thereby increasing the SNR, a technique called *image enhancement* or *image filtering*. This technique works for all types of sequences and all types of MRI examinations.

In this method, the image is analyzed regarding the location of structures (edges and lines) and their orientation and curvature. In image segment areas in which no structures are found, noise reduction is automatically performed. Yet, unlike the low-pass and standard statistical filtering processes, the enhancement process, with its use of artificial intelligence, can distinguish image segments that contain structures. In those segments, it takes into account the detected location, orientation, and curvature of structures (including the weakest structures) and maintains image sharpness by preserving these structures. This method not only keeps edges and lines in their original form but can also enhance the edges and lines in the image, unlike less sophisticated noise filters. As a result, open MR images can be made sharper while noise is simultaneously reduced, in contrast to other algorithms that blur the image. This method allows increased patient through-put because scan times can be shortened (i.e., NEX) while maintaining image quality. Additionally, with the use of postprocessing image enhancement for musculoskeletal imaging, high-resolution imaging using an FOV of 10 cm $\times$ 10 cm or smaller can be obtained with adequate SNR.

The images seen in the musculoskeletal chapters (Chapters 15 to 20) and most images in the other chapters were postprocessed to decrease noise. The use of the postprocessing enhancement technique has made high-resolution, pristine images possible with lower field strength open MRI. This, and the advances in open MRI technology, have led to the wide acceptance of open MRI by radiologists and referring physicians, especially orthopedic surgeons, when only a few years ago, low-field open MRI was thought of as a last resort.

CONCLUSION

The role of open MRI of the musculoskeletal system is increasing. Patient requests for open systems and the ability to serve a wider range of patients have encouraged many radiologists to include open systems in their practices.

With numerous applications for the musculoskeletal system, MRI has evolved into a unique subspecialty requiring a strong understanding of musculoskeletal pathology and the ability to demonstrate specific abnormalities with the various MRI techniques. Musculoskeletal imaging is challenging at all field strengths. Numerous anatomic structures need to be demonstrated, and the pathology is diverse. In addition to the traumatic injuries encountered in the musculoskeletal system, inflammatory, infectious, and neoplastic conditions all may be encountered. MRI has clear advantages over other imaging modalities, with its soft tissue contrast and multiplanar imaging capabilities, making it the best diagnostic examination for the musculoskeletal system.

To perform high-quality examinations on open systems, radiologists and MRI technologists must possess a sound understanding of parameters such as bandwidth, NEX, and voxel size to fully exploit the capabilities of open MRI. Understanding techniques such as FSE, fast STIR, 3D spoiled GRE, and postprocessing is equally important. Application of these concepts fully maximizes the potential of open MRI systems to produce the high-resolution and high-contrast images necessary to demonstrate the wide range of pathology encountered in the musculoskeletal system.

Open MRI,
edited by Peter A. Rothschild and Debra Reinking Rothschild.
Lippincott Williams & Wilkins. Philadelphia © 2000.

CHAPTER 15

Open Magnetic Resonance Imaging of the Shoulder

Joseph Triolo, Peter A. Rothschild, and Elizabeth J. DuBose

Quality imaging of the shoulder is critical on the open magnetic resonance imaging (MRI) system. Open systems can serve a wider range of patients than closed systems. Imaging the shoulder requires placing patients headfirst into the magnet; this is often difficult for anxious patients and intolerable for claustrophobic patients in closed systems. The tunnel shape of high-field systems also makes it difficult, if not impossible, for broad-shouldered patients to enter the magnet. Open systems serve a unique role for imaging these patients.

Closed high-field strength systems are limited not only in their patient selection, but they also are subject to many artifacts that are less problematic on lower field open systems. Ghosting artifact may result from any type of motion that occurs during scanning. This artifact propagates along the phase axis, and the amount of artifact is proportional to the field strength of the magnet. Motion from high signal structures creates more artifact than is seen from structures with low signal. As a result, fat, which has increased signal on T1-weighted images and on T2-weighted fast spin-echo (FSE) sequences, creates the greatest artifact. Respiratory motion is a major cause of ghosting artifact when imaging the shoulder, owing to its close proximity to the chest wall. The coronal images are most affected with this type of artifact.

Motion of the shoulder joint itself, with respiration as well as vessel pulsation, also contributes to ghosting artifact and results in image degradation. Again, the amount of artifact is related to field strength, and ghosting artifact is less problematic on lower field open systems.

Susceptibility artifact caused by local field inhomogeneities is also related to the field strength of the magnet and greater on high-field strength systems. This artifact may be seen after procedures such as decompression surgery, labral repairs, and capsular shift procedures. Respiratory artifact, pulsation artifact, and field inhomogeneity are all less problematic on lower field systems.

Chemical fat saturation, which is an advantage of high-field systems, may be difficult to perform in closed MRI systems because the shoulder cannot be placed at isocenter. In fact, if one is not careful on closed high-field systems, water can be suppressed—instead of fat—and doing so may obscure pathology. As a result, the artifacts from ghosting and susceptibility, as well as the inconsistency in fat saturation, make imaging the shoulder on closed high-field systems difficult at times, thus providing a unique opportunity for open systems to play a major role in imaging of the shoulder.

ANATOMY

The glenohumeral articulation is a dynamic joint consisting of a ball-in-socket joint with a wide range of motion, the powerful muscles of the shoulder girdle, and a capsular complex. These structures all contribute to the complexity of this joint.

Rotator Cuff

The tendons of the supraspinatus, infraspinatus, teres minor, and subscapularis muscles fuse distally to form the rotator cuff (Figs. 15-1, 15-2, and 15-3). The supraspinatus, infraspinatus, and teres minor tendons insert on the greater tuberosity from anterior to posterior, respectively. The subscapularis tendon inserts on the lesser tuberosity. The biceps tendon courses between the subscapularis muscle and the

J. Triolo: Ocean Medical Imaging Center, Community Medical Center, Toms River, New Jersey

P. A. Rothschild: Department of Radiology, University of California, San Francisco, San Francisco, California; Open MRI, Hayward, California; Open MRI, Louisville, Kentucky

E. J. DuBose: Open MRI, Hayward, California; Open MRI, Louisville, Kentucky

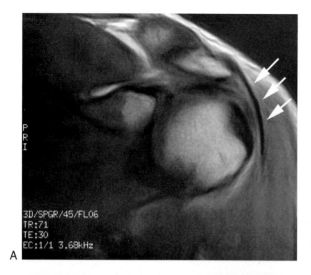

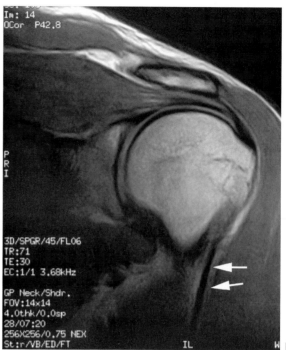

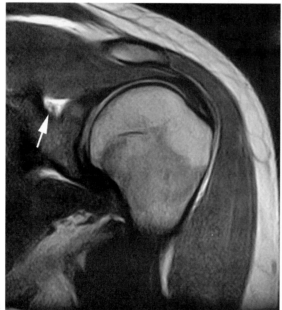

FIG. 15-1. Normal sagittal shoulder. Sagittal T1-weighted three-dimensional (3D) gradient-echo (GRE) high-resolution images with a 14-cm field of view. The supraspinatus muscle and tendon are well identified. Articular cartilage of normal thickness is identified over the glenoid and humeral head. To determine whether the images have high enough resolution to identify detailed pathology, one should attempt to identify the articular cartilage. **A:** The deltoid ligament attaching to the acromion (*arrows*) is demonstrated. **B:** The long head of the biceps is identified just below the humeral head (*arrows*). The superior glenoid labrum is also well seen. **C:** The suprascapular notch with the suprascapular artery and nerve surrounded by normal fat (*arrow*) is demonstrated. This is an important area to evaluate in every patient for ganglion/paralabral cyst as seen in Figure 15-11. On lower field open magnets using T1-weighted 3D GRE, the normal supraspinatus tendon appears black.

supraspinatus tendon; this space is termed the *rotator interval*, and a capsule covers this interval. The coracohumeral ligament extends from the coracoid process to insert on the greater tuberosity (1). As the biceps tendon courses through the joint capsule, joint fluid may extend along the biceps tendon and through the rotator interval; this should not be confused with a rotator cuff tear.

The supraspinatus muscle and tendon complex is the most important component of the rotator cuff, as it is the most frequently affected by pathology. The supraspinatus and infraspinatus essentially act as pulleys for abduction of the shoulder. The supraspinatus takes an oblique course, extending anteriorly to attach to the most anterior aspect of the greater tuberosity (Fig. 15-4). Identifying the biceps as it courses between the greater and lesser tuberosities is

helpful in locating the anterior attachment of the supraspinatus tendon on the greater tuberosity. This attachment is important to identify because small or partial tears may be missed in this region. The infraspinatus muscle inserts on the scapula, and the muscle can be distinguished from the supraspinatus muscle by its more inferior to superior orientation.

The subscapularis muscle and tendon form the anteriormost portion of the rotator cuff, inserting on the lesser tuberosity. The teres minor muscle and tendon form the posterior portion of the rotator cuff, inserting on the posterior-most aspect of the greater tuberosity. Other important muscles that support the shoulder include the deltoid, pectoralis major and minor, and the latissimus dorsi. Pathology involving these structures may mimic rotator cuff symptoms.

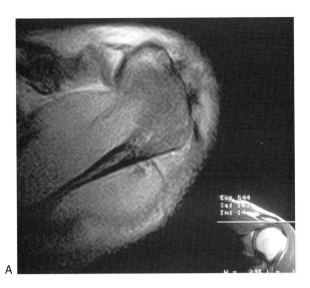

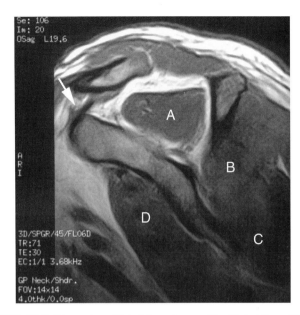

FIG. 15-3. Normal sagittal oblique image. Sagittal oblique T1-weighted three-dimensional gradient-echo image. It is important in shoulder imaging to identify the muscle belly of the muscles that make up the rotator cuff specifically to look for atrophy. Muscles identified are the supraspinatus (*A*), the infraspinatus (*B*), teres minor (*C*), and subscapularis (*D*). Also identified is the coracoclavicular ligament (*arrow*).

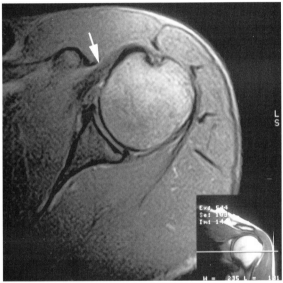

FIG. 15-2. Normal axial T2-weighted gradient-echo images. **A:** The normal-appearing belly of the supraspinatus muscle and normal appearance of the acromion. Axial images in the superior aspect of the shoulder can be very helpful for identifying atrophy or retraction of the supraspinatus muscle. Note the reference image, which identifies the exact location of this axial image, in the lower corner of the film. **B:** The subscapularis muscle and tendon are demonstrated anteriorly (*arrow*), as are the infraspinatus muscle and tendon posteriorly. The anterior and posterior glenoid labrum are normal in appearance.

Glenohumeral Ligament–Labral Complex

The inferior glenohumeral ligament is the largest of the three glenohumeral ligaments. It consists of anterior and posterior bundles and is believed to be the most important ligament to maintain stability of the glenohumeral joint (2). The middle glenohumeral ligament (Fig. 15-5) is more variable in its appearance and may be thickened with an absent anterior labrum (Buford complex) (3). The smaller superior glenohumeral ligament is more constant in its appearance.

The fibrocartilaginous labrum covers the rim of the glenoid, creating a deeper glenoid fossa and adding to stability of the glenohumeral joint. Anteroinferiorly, the inferior glenohumeral ligament attaches to the labrum, creating a support against anteroinferior dislocations. The middle glenohumeral ligament attaches more superiorly along the labrum, and superiorly the long head of the biceps tendon attaches to the superior labrum.

Osseous Structures

Acromial shape is believed to play an important role in impingement. The acromion may be flat (type 1), curved (type 2), or hooked (type 3). Types 2 and 3 are believed to contribute to impingement (Fig. 15-6) (4). An unfused acromion ossification center, *os acromialis*, is also believed to have a strong association with rotator cuff pathology (Fig. 15-7) (5). Downsloping of the lateral aspect of the acromion may also play a role in impingement.

The supraspinatus tendon courses through an outlet formed by the coracoid process, the coracoacromial ligament, and the acromion, termed the *coracoacromial arch*. The acromioclavicular joint also forms a superior border to the myotendinous region supraspinatus more medially. The humeral head is a caplike structure delineated by the anatomic neck that extends

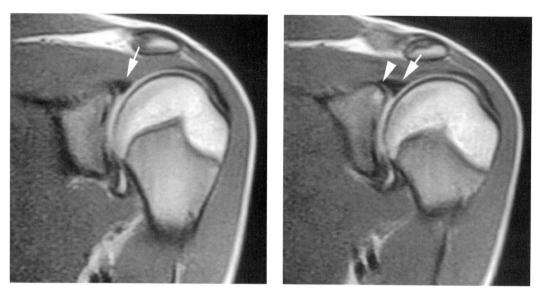

FIG. 15-4. Normal shoulder magnetic resonance arthrogram. T1-weighted coronal oblique spin-echo two-dimensional images demonstrate normal supraspinatus muscle and tendon. Notice the smooth myotendinous junction and normal low signal of the tendon. The superior labrum have smooth and regular appearances (*arrows*). A small amount of contrast may normally extend under the superior labrum as in this case (*arrowhead*).

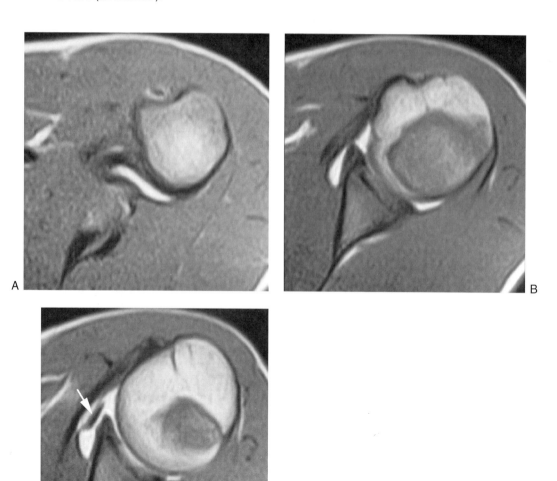

FIG. 15-5. A–C: Normal shoulder arthrogram. Axial T1-weighted spin-echo two-dimensional images after contrast injection. The inferior glenohumeral ligament complex is demonstrated. The normal anterior and posterior glenoid labrum are well delineated, as is the middle glenohumeral ligament (*arrow*), seen best in **C.**

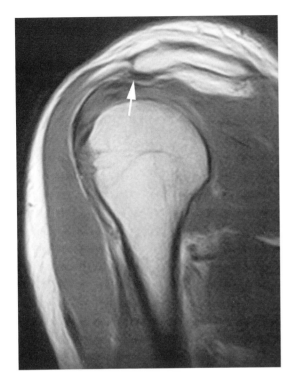

FIG. 15-6. Hooked acromion (type III). Sagittal oblique T1-weighted three-dimensional gradient-echo image demonstrates a hooked (type III) acromion. The small area of low signal intensity just inferior to the hooked part of the acromion is the normal attachment of the deltoid muscle (*arrow*) and should not be mistaken for a spur.

laterally from the superior aspect of the tuberosities to the medial margin of the humeral neck. Fractures along the anatomic neck place the humeral head at greater risk for avascular necrosis. The surgical neck is at the junction of the rounded humeral head and the sticklike humeral shaft. This is the most common location for fractures (6).

The scapula is a complex bone that provides strength and range of motion to the shoulder girdle. The flat-bone portion

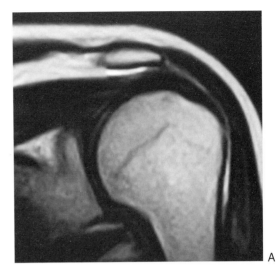

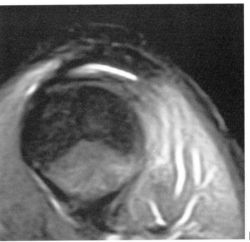

FIG. 15-8. Subacromial bursitis. **A:** Coronal oblique T2-weighted fast spin-echo image. **B:** Fast short tau inversion recovery (STIR) sagittal oblique image. Both images clearly demonstrate a small amount of fluid in the subacromial bursa. It is clear that the rotator cuff is intact, which is consistent with a small bursitis.

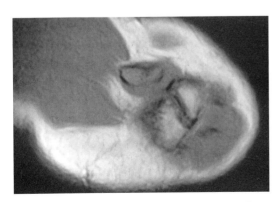

FIG. 15-7. Os acromialis. Axial T1-weighted gradient-echo image clearly demonstrates a separate ossification center of the acromion, which is consistent with os acromialis. Patients with os acromialis are believed to have higher incidence of impingement, and this should be mentioned in the magnetic resonance imaging report.

of the scapula provides important muscular attachments for the muscles of the rotator cuff. Other muscular attachments include the deltoid, trapezium, latissimus dorsi, and the flexors and extensors of the arm. The glenoid portion of the scapula is a cuplike attachment that provides mobility of the glenohumeral joint.

The coracoid process extends anteriorly from the scapula and has numerous ligamentous attachments. The coracoacromial ligament extends posteriorly and laterally to attach to the anterior acromion. This acromial attachment is the site for anterior subacromial spur formation. Other ligamentous attachments include the coracoclavicular and coracohumeral ligaments.

Two important bursae cover the rotator cuff: the subacromial and subdeltoid bursae. These bursae act as a cushion to protect the supraspinatus tendon from the coracoacromial arch. They may become inflamed (bursitis) (Fig. 15-8) and present with symptoms mimicking a rotator cuff tear, or they may fill with fluid in the presence of a full-thickness rotator cuff tear, which creates a communication between the bursae and the joint. Fluid may also be present in the subacromial bursa due to recent parenteral injection.

Two important recesses within the scapula are the suprascapular notch and the spinoglenoid notch. The suprascapular nerve courses through the suprascapular notch to supply the supraspinatus and infraspinatus muscles. The transverse ligament forms a superior border over this groove. The spinoglenoid notch lies more inferiorly between the spine of the scapula and the posteroinferior glenoid. A branch of the suprascapular nerve, which supplies the infraspinatus muscle, courses though this groove. The inferior transverse scapular ligament forms a superior border of this space. Ganglia of this region may compress the branch of the suprascapular nerve that supplies the infraspinatus muscle, causing an entrapment neuropathy (7).

TECHNIQUE

A protocol for the shoulder should be designed to focus on the intricate rotator cuff and the capsular complex, as well as to cover the muscles and scapula of the shoulder girdle. Pulse sequences must be tailored to define normal anatomic structures, as well as demonstrate the wide range of pathology that may be encountered in the shoulder.

T1-weighted images should be performed in the coronal and sagittal oblique planes. T1-weighted images may consist of a simple spin-echo T1 sequence or a three-dimensional (3D) gradient-echo (GRE) sequence. Both sequences have advantages and disadvantages. The spin-echo sequence is less affected by susceptibility artifacts. However, volume or 3D sequences have the advantages of higher signal, higher resolution, thinner slices, and no slice gap. Images can be reconstructed and viewed in any plane. They are best performed as T1-weighted scans to take advantage of the inherent signal from bone marrow, subcutaneous fat, and the musculature. A T1-weighted 3D GRE is the most commonly used volume scan in open MRI.

T1-weighted images are useful to identify tendinopathy, in which loss of the normal low signal from the tendon is seen. T1-weighted images also best identify subacromial spurs, acromial morphology, myotendinous retraction, muscle atrophy, and bone marrow abnormalities. Subacromial spurs and acromial morphology are best demonstrated on the sagittal oblique images.

T2-weighted images are most commonly performed in the coronal oblique plane. Radiologists and orthopedic surgeons are most comfortable with this imaging plane. The T2-weighted FSE technique is essential because scan times can be significantly reduced and scans with a higher number of excitations (NEX) can be performed to improve the signal-to-noise ratio. On open systems, efforts must be taken to make these images as heavily T2 weighted as pos-

sible, because fat saturation is currently not possible. Echo time (TE) controls contrast on T2-weighted images, and TEs in the 120- to 140-ms range are most helpful. Such TEs also help reduce blurring from the wider echo spacing encountered on low-field strength magnets. Bandwidths should be kept in the 6- to 7-mHz range. Higher NEX scans are required to compensate for the higher bandwidths and the loss of signal needed with longer TE sequences. Higher NEX scans also help reduce respiratory artifact because more signals are averaged together. These long TE sequences are useful in separating fat from fluid because, as the TE increases, fluid exhibits higher signal intensity relative to fat.

T2-weighted images are useful for demonstrating rotator cuff tears, marrow edema, and soft tissue pathology. Marrow edema or replacement may be difficult to detect on T2-weighted scans because fat and edema are increased in signal intensity. Inversion recovery sequences are useful to help prevent confusion.

Short tau inversion recovery (STIR) sequences are essential to perform on lower open field systems. These scans should also be performed with FSE technique (fast STIR) to reduce scan time, so more NEX can be acquired to improve the signal-to-noise ratio. This sequence is best performed in the sagittal oblique plane, in which the low-signal rotator cuff is seen in cross section, so that partial- and full-thickness tears are readily identified (Fig. 15-9). Furthermore, coronal STIR sequences are helpful for identifying tendinopathy of the rotator cuff. The field of view can be increased not only to increase signal but also to include as much of the surrounding soft tissues as possible, because muscle injuries of the shoulder girdle may mimic rotator cuff pathology. STIR in the sagittal plane is very sensitive to fluid and is useful for identifying cuff tears, tendinitis, bursitis, marrow edema, soft tissue edema, and fluid collections.

GRE images are most useful in differentiating the labrum from cartilage and the overlying tendons and muscle. Evaluating the anterior labrum is best performed in the axial plane. Heavily T2-weighted GRE images are most useful because joint fluid can provide an arthrographic effect. Axial GRE sequences are currently best performed as a two-dimensional sequence with high resolution.

Evaluation of the Rotator Cuff

The most common reason for MRI evaluation of the shoulder is pain. Although it is necessary to identify rotator cuff tears, an attempt to determine the etiology must be made. In the nonathlete, impingement is believed to be the greatest contributing factor to rotator cuff tears (7); however, other possible factors include the avascular region of the critical zone and partial degenerative tears leading to abnormal mechanics of the shoulder joint. Because impingement is a clinically important entity, describing findings suggestive of impingement syndrome is helpful to the referring orthopedic surgeon.

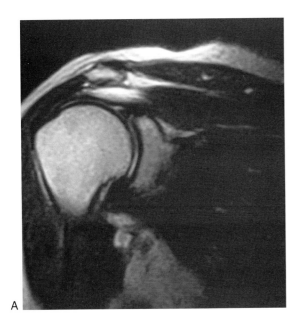

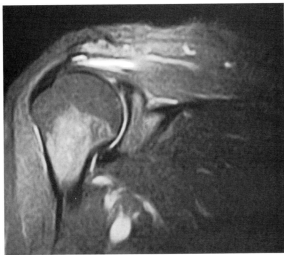

FIG. 15-9. Partial tear and associated tendinitis of the supraspinatus. **A:** Coronal oblique T2-weighted fast spin-echo image. **B:** Coronal oblique fast short tau inversion recovery (STIR) image. On both images, high signal intensity is identified in the distal supraspinatus muscle and appears to extend into the beginning of the supraspinatus tendon. No evidence of retraction is present. The STIR images are very sensitive for tendinitis and small tears as identified in this case.

Impingement

Evaluation of impingement and rotator cuff pathology are the most common reasons for MRI of the shoulder. Impingement is a clinical diagnosis referring to pain during certain provocative movements of the shoulder including pain with abduction from 60 to 90 degrees of motion and pain during internal rotation of the flexed arm. The diagnosis of impingement cannot be made with any imaging modality alone, as findings suggestive of impingement may be present in an asymptomatic patient (8). Also, patients are usually not symptomatic when lying in the magnet with the arm in adduction, so a discrete finding of impingement on MRI may not correspond to the abnormality that is producing symptoms. MRI, however, serves a very important role as it can identify findings that may suggest impingement. These findings include tendinopathy, acromial morphology, subacromial spurs, acromioclavicular joint disease, and subchondral cystic changes of the greater tuberosity.

Tendon pathology occurs in stages, with the initial changes resulting in tendinosis or tendinitis. Tendon thickening may be seen with or without edema. Edema is more suggestive of the active process of tendinitis, whereas low signal on T1- and T2-weighted sequences is more suggestive of fibrosis and chronic changes of tendinosis. Changes of tendinopathy are probably best identified on open MRI with T1-weighted images, in which the homogeneous low signal of tendon is lost. The location in which this is best identified is the critical zone, 5 mm to 1.5 cm proximal to the greater tuberosity attachment of the supraspinatus. However, T1-weighted images do not distinguish between edema, fibrosis, and a tendon tear. T2-weighted images are essential to detect edema and to identify fluid within a rotator cuff tear. Because T1-weighted images better demonstrate anatomy, T1 SE and 3D GRE images are helpful to demonstrate myotendinous retraction and muscle atrophy, significant findings that can affect the surgical management.

With fraying and partial tears, thinning of the tendon is seen, whereas with tendinitis and tendinosis, the tendon is often thickened. It is often difficult to separate tendinitis and partial tears, and areas of tendon thinning should be reviewed with scrutiny. Myotendinous retraction is a clear sign of a full-thickness rotator cuff tear (Fig. 15-10).

The acromion is an important structure to evaluate in patients with suspected impingement or rotator cuff tears. The acromial shape of flat, curved, or hooked is best defined on the sagittal oblique images. Type 3 has the greatest association with impingement (see Fig. 15-6) (4). An os acromialis is best visualized on the axial images (see Fig. 15-7).

Lateral downsloping of the acromion narrows the supraspinatus outlet and may play a role in impingement and rotator cuff pathology. Subacromial spurs that form along the undersurface of the acromion at the attachment of the coracoacromial ligament are another contributing factor to impingement. Subacromial spurs are best demonstrated on sagittal oblique images by following the coracoacromial ligament. Acromioclavicular pathology also plays a role in impingement, with inferior osteophytes being the most important finding because of the possibility of compression of the myotendinous junction or muscle belly of the supraspinatus.

The greater tuberosity is the site for attachment of the supraspinatus (most anteriorly), infraspinatus, and teres minor (most posteriorly) tendons. Subchondral cystic changes, subchondral marrow edema, and erosive changes all may be associated with impingement syndrome. Most often, these changes occur along the more posterior aspect of the greater tuberosity.

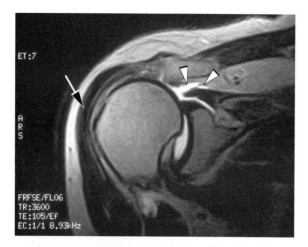

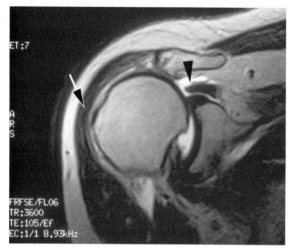

FIG. 15-10. Full-thickness rotator cuff tear with retraction. Coronal oblique T2-weighted fast spin-echo image demonstrates a complete tear with tendinous retraction and superior migration of the humeral head. The deltoid muscle is identified and overlies the greater tuberosity (*arrows*), which may simulate an intact rotator cuff. However, the torn and retracted supraspinatus tendon is clearly delineated by fluid (*arrowheads*).

Rotator Cuff Tears

Rotator cuff tears most commonly involve the anterior aspect of the distal supraspinatus tendon, often known as the *critical zone.* Identifying the anterior-most portion of the rotator cuff is important because this area must be scrutinized for small tears. The biceps tendon is a helpful marker as it courses just anterior to the supraspinatus tendon at the greater tuberosity attachment.

Tears should be characterized as partial or full thickness. Acute full-thickness tears are fairly easy to identify, because fluid extends through the full thickness of the tendon. Full-thickness rotator cuff tears should be classified according to size. Small tears are less than 1 cm, large tears are 3 to 5 cm (see Fig. 15-10), and massive tears are larger than 5 cm (9). Coronal T2-weighted images most readily demonstrate tears

of the rotator cuff. Full-thickness tears may be difficult to detect when they extend obliquely through the tendon or parallel the course of the tendon. In these cases, tears will not be seen extending through the full thickness of the tendon on a single coronal oblique image. Sagittal oblique images best demonstrate this type of full-thickness tear because the image is perpendicular to the direction of the tear.

A second type of tear that is difficult to detect on the coronal oblique series is a small peripheral tear at the attachment of the supraspinatus tendon. On the coronal views, it is difficult to determine whether the fluid lies within the course of the tendon or over the tendon, as is seen with peritendinitis and bursitis. Again, sagittal oblique images best demonstrate the full thickness of the rotator cuff out to its bony attachment.

Partial tears (see Fig. 15-9) are also best demonstrated on sagittal oblique plane images. Because the sagittal oblique plain is perpendicular to the course of the supraspinatus tendon, partial tears involving the bursal surface, articular surface, or intrasubstance portion of the supraspinatus tendon are best identified. Identifying partial tears in coronal and sagittal oblique planes helps confirm the diagnosis.

The myotendinous junction is an important landmark on the coronal oblique images. Myotendinous retraction is a clear sign of full-thickness rotator cuff tears, and the degree of retraction should be determined. Identifying myotendinous retraction also helps prevent confusion in cases of massive rotator cuff tears. Massive, chronic tears may be confusing when retraction of the supraspinatus and infraspinatus tendons results in superior migration of the humeral head (see Fig. 15-10). As a result, the deltoid muscle overlays the greater tuberosity. Fluid may be displaced, and the lack of fluid with an overlying deltoid muscle can simulate an intact rotator cuff. Identifying the retracted muscle belly and recognizing the superior migration of the humeral head easily prevent confusion when identifying chronic rotator cuff tears.

The biceps tendon may also be dislocated or torn, especially in cases of massive rotator cuff tears. Axial images are helpful to identify these changes of the biceps and surrounding pathology (Fig. 15-11).

When a supraspinatus tear is identified, the infraspinatus tendon should be carefully scrutinized to identify pathology. The infraspinatus tendon can be identified by its change in orientation with a more oblique course when compared to the horizontal orientation of the supraspinatus tendon. Thinning and degeneration of the infraspinatus tendon are often seen in association with supraspinatus tears. The infraspinatus may be torn in the presence of a massive supraspinatus tear. This is best identified on the sagittal oblique images, in which the full anterior to posterior dimension of the greater tuberosity can be identified on a single slice. Also, tears of the posterior rotator cuff may be seen as an isolated finding in patients with internal impingement. This has been reported in the overhead throwing athlete (10).

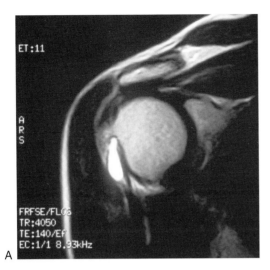

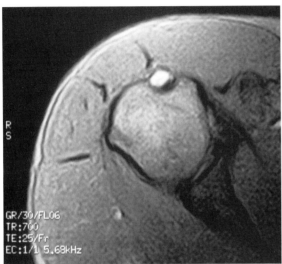

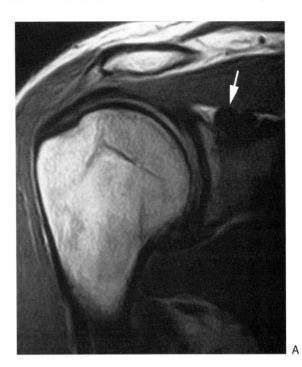

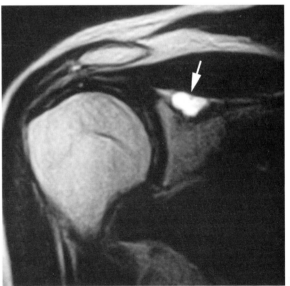

FIG. 15-11. Ganglion cyst. Fast spin-echo coronal oblique **(A)** and axial two-dimensional gradient-echo **(B)** T2-weighted images demonstrate a high-signal-intensity, well-circumscribed lesion in the bicipital groove. The biceps tendon appears normal in size and thickness, and no evidence is found of fluid extending down the synovial sheath around the biceps. Ganglion cysts are easily identified on T2-weighted and short tau inversion recovery images and can be a source of pain.

FIG. 15-12. Suprascapular notch ganglion. **A:** T1-weighted coronal oblique three-dimensional gradient-echo image demonstrates a low-signal-intensity, well-circumscribed lesion in the suprascapular notch (*arrow*). **B:** The fluid in this ganglion becomes bright on the T2-weighted fast spin-echo coronal oblique image (*arrow*), making this lesion much easier to identify. One should be diligent to ensure that technologists do not crop out the scapular notch region when filming.

Miscellaneous Disorders

Ganglia and paralabral cysts are two lesions about the shoulder joint that have significant clinical symptoms. Ganglia typically occur in two locations, the suprascapular and spinoglenoid notches. Through the suprascapular notch courses the suprascapular nerve, which supplies motor and sensory fibers to the supraspinatus and infraspinatus muscles. Ganglia in this region may compress the suprascapular nerve.

The spinoglenoid notch lies more inferiorly, between the spine of the scapula and the posteroinferior glenoid. Ganglia in this region may compress the branch of the suprascapular nerve that supplies the infraspinatus muscle (Fig. 15-12) (11). Entrapment neuropathies may result from ganglia in

either of these two regions because they are bordered by an overlying ligament. Edema within the corresponding muscle group is the earliest MRI finding. These changes are best demonstrated on T2-weighted and fast STIR images. Chronic nerve entrapment may progress to muscle atrophy.

Paralabral cysts are fluid collections that communicate with the joint through a weakness in the capsulolabral complex or

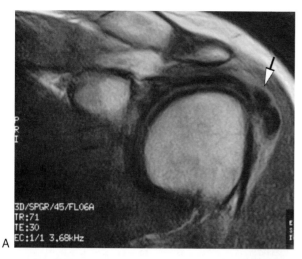

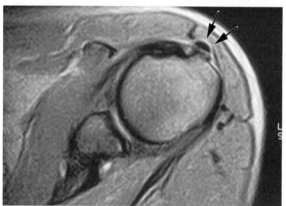

FIG. 15-13. Calcific tendinitis. **A:** Coronal oblique T1-weighted three-dimensional gradient-echo (GRE) image demonstrates a low-signal-intensity, well-circumscribed lesion just lateral to the humeral head (*arrow*). **B:** Axial T2-weighted two-dimensional GRE image demonstrates that this lesion is also low signal intensity on the T2-weighted images. This low signal intensity is from calcific deposits. Minimal surrounding edema is also identified (*arrows*). Every attempt should be made to obtain plain films when interpreting musculoskeletal images.

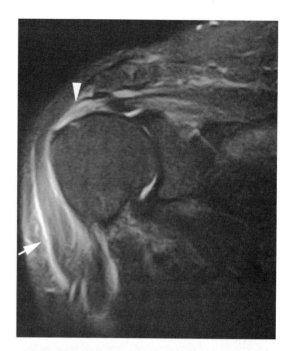

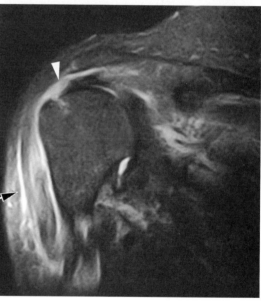

FIG. 15-14. Deltoid partial tear/sprain. Coronal oblique fast short tau inversion recovery (STIR) images demonstrate high signal intensity in the deltoid muscle itself as well as focal high signal intensity between the muscle belly and the surrounding subcutaneous fat (*arrows*). Also identified are tendinitis and associated tear in the supraspinatus tendon (*arrowheads*). Fast STIR images are the best sequence for identifying muscle damage and tendinitis.

labral tear. Patients may have symptoms of pain or instability, or a paralabral cyst may be an incidental finding in an asymptomatic patient. The most common locations are posterior or superior, but they may be seen at any site of a labral tear (12).

Calcific tendonitis is a common cause of shoulder pain and can be diagnosed with MRI. Calcific deposits are low signal foci on T1- and T2-weighted sequences (Fig. 15-13). Calcium is most conspicuous on GRE examinations because greater susceptibility artifact results in marked decreased signal. Calcific deposits may be associated with adjacent tendon edema identified on T2-weighted images suggesting associated tendinitis. Many patients, however, may still be symptomatic from calcific deposits and lack changes of tendinitis.

Other intraarticular abnormalities include intraarticular bodies and infectious or inflammatory arthropathies. *Intraarticular body* is probably the most appropriate term,

because cartilage fragments, pieces of the fibrocartilaginous labrum, or cortical bone may be present. The smaller nonossified fragments are most difficult to detect. They are best diagnosed on heavily T2-weighted FSE or GRE sequences when a joint effusion, which provides an arthrographic effect, is present. GRE sequences are particularly helpful

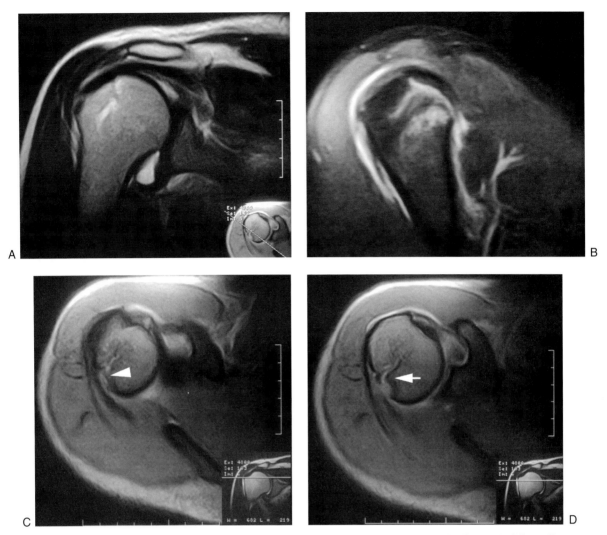

FIG. 15-15. Nondisplaced fracture and bone contusion of the humeral head. **A:** Coronal oblique T2-weighted fast spin-echo (FSE) image. **B:** Sagittal oblique fast short tau inversion recovery (STIR) image. The extent of the fracture, which is of high signal intensity, is demonstrated. **C,D:** Axial gradient-echo (GRE) T2-weighted images. This patient suffered relatively minor trauma; however, the patient developed a fracture of the humeral head. The break in the cortex with high signal intensity extending along the cortex and into the subcortical bone (*arrowheads, arrow*) is demonstrated. The image in **A**, however, does not show the fracture line to be as bright in comparison with the surrounding marrow as the STIR or T2-weighted GRE images. Fractures, especially nondisplaced types, can be difficult to identify on the FSE T2-weighted images; thus, fast STIR images are preferred over T2-weighted images in patients with trauma. Also, GRE T2-weighted images have higher resolution than STIR; therefore GRE sequences can be helpful in identifying breaks in the bony cortex, as in this case.

because ossified or calcified bodies demonstrate low signal. Fragments may also contain bone marrow, and these are easily identified on T1-weighted images with high signal from fatty marrow. Typical locations in which intraarticular bodies can be identified include the subscapularis recess, the axillary pouch, and posteriorly within the joint capsule.

Other entities that may mimic rotator cuff pathology include pathology in adjacent muscles. Deltoid strains and injuries to the latissimus dorsi muscle may simulate rotator cuff pathol-

ogy. Also, injury to these muscles may be associated with rotator cuff pathology. STIR is the most useful sequence to diagnose soft tissue pathology because it provides the greatest soft tissue contrast by nullifying signal from fat (Fig. 15-14).

Fractures may be incidental findings on MRI in patients with shoulder pain and normal radiographs. MRI is the best modality to detect nondisplaced shoulder fractures, because trabecular disruption and marrow edema are easily identified (Fig. 15-15). Lower field open field systems are extremely useful, because fast STIR sequences readily demonstrate marrow edema and T1- and T2-weighted GRE images provide information on trabecular disruption. Fractures may not be detected on T2-weighted images because marrow edema and normal fatty marrow are increased in signal, which may obscure fracture or other marrow-related disorders. T1-weighted 3D GRE sequences demonstrate the trabecular meshwork extremely well and can detect subtle fractures. Subtle fractures that may not be readily identified on plain film radiographs include nondisplaced anatomic neck fractures, Salter 1 and 2 fractures in adolescents, small Hill-Sacks and bony Bankart lesion.

ARTHROGRAPHY AND INSTABILITY

The glenoid labrum has always been recognized as an important structure for stability. The labrum creates a deep fossa, providing a larger articulating surface with the humeral head (Fig. 15-16). The glenohumeral ligaments, the biceps tendon, and the muscles of the rotator cuff are also believed to play an important role in the maintenance of joint stability (13). The complex mechanics and interaction of these structures lead to difficulty in determining the etiology of instability. Similar to impingement, instability is a clinical diagnosis. Many patients have so-called joint laxity, but many of these patients are asymptomatic and have an examination similar to patients with true instability. These patients do not suffer from pain, subluxation, or frank dislocation, which are symptoms seen in the unstable shoulder.

As the mechanics of instability are difficult to understand, so is the diagnosis. Arthrography is the best means to evaluate the labrum and glenohumeral ligaments. Without distending the joint, soft tissue structures collapse on each other and the thin, smaller structures, which are important for stability, are difficult to identify. In fact, many abnormalities, such as SLAP (superior labral injury that extends from anterior to posterior) and Bankart-type lesions, appear normal at initial visualization during arthroscopy, and the lesion is only identified when the labrum is displaced by probing at arthroscopy. Distending the joint is the best means of separating and identifying the structures important for instability. Using diluted gadolinium creates the best images because T1-weighted sequences with high inherent signal can be performed. Saline arthrograms are also useful; however, pathology needs to be demonstrated on T2-weighted images, which does not provide the same resolution as higher signal-to-noise T1-weighted images.

Technique

When using intraarticular gadolinium, patient consent should be obtained. The role of intraarticular gadolinium should be discussed with the patient, because the intraarticular administration of gadolinium has not been approved by the U.S. Food and Drug Administration. Intraarticular gadolinium, however, has been used safely since the early 1990s without known complications. In the hospital setting, the procedure should be approved by an internal review board.

Intraarticular placement of a needle should be confirmed with fluoroscopy, MRI, computed tomography, or whatever means available. Distension of the joint requires approximately 10 to 15 mL of fluid. In patients with adhesive capsulitis, the joint capsule may only hold 10 mL or less with normal injection pressures. Care should be taken not to overdistend the joint and extravasate into the soft tissue. If gadolinium is used, it should be diluted with saline in a dilution of approximately 1:200 to 1:300 when scanning on lower field open MRI. After arthrography, the shoulder joint should be exercised, especially with abduction and external rotation, in an attempt to fill subtle defects in the labrum.

T1-weighted images, either SE or 3D GRE, should be performed in all three planes to demonstrate the labrum, ligaments, and rotator cuff. A T2-weighted sequence should be performed in the coronal oblique and possibly the sagittal oblique plane, because small and partial-thickness rotator cuff tears may be difficult to detect on T1-weighted images when fat signal is not suppressed. Bursal surface and intrasubstance tears do not communicate with the joint and are not identified on T1-weighted sequences. Fast STIR sequences are of little use in evaluating the ligaments, labrum, and rotator cuff, because the T1 shortening of gadolinium results in nullification of the signal from joint fluid, similar to the effect seen on fat from the inversion pulse.

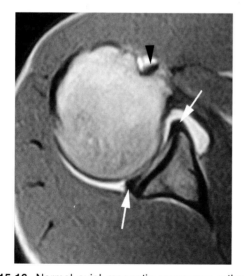

FIG. 15-16. Normal axial magnetic resonance arthrogram. T1-weighted two-dimensional spin-echo postgadolinium arthrogram demonstrates a normal triangular appearance of the anterior and posterior labrum (*arrows*). The underlying articular cartilage is also well identified. Note the fluid along the biceps tendon (*arrowhead*).

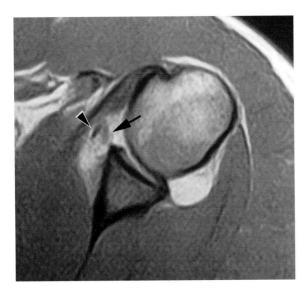

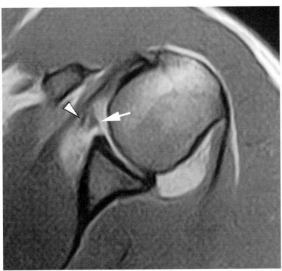

FIG. 15-17. Bankart lesion in a patient with instability. Axial T1-weighted spin-echo postgadolinium images demonstrate an avulsed anterior labrum (*arrows*). Note the middle glenohumeral ligament coursing anterior to the avulsed labrum (*arrowheads*).

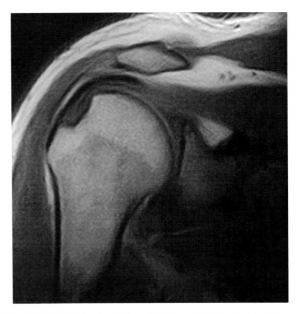

FIG. 15-18. Hill-Sachs deformity. Sagittal T1-weighted three-dimensional gradient-echo image demonstrates a depression in the cortical margin along the posterolateral aspects of the humeral head. No associated low signal intensity exists in the subcortical bone to suggest acute bone contusion, and this lesion appears well delineated, suggesting this is old.

Pathology

Instability may be broadly grouped into unidirectional or multidirectional instability. Unidirectional instability is typically posttraumatic in nature, usually anterior in direction, and often has a Bankart lesion that requires surgery. Unidirectional instability may be posterior, but this accounts for less than 5% of cases (14). Recurrent subluxations or dislocations are often seen with Bankart lesions, and a corresponding Hill-Sachs defect almost always is present (15). Many descriptions of the Bankart lesion exist; however, it is most commonly known as an *anterior labral tear* at the attachment of the inferior glenohumeral ligament (Figs. 15-17 and 15-18).

Multidirectional instability is generally considered to be atraumatic and may often be bilateral. Discrete findings are often not identified with MR arthrography and the diagnosis is more difficult than in unidirectional instability. Conservative management with rehabilitation is the initial treatment, and cases that are refractory to rehabilitation require an inferior capsular shift surgical procedure.

Internal impingement is another form of instability and is believed to result from weakness of the anterior joint capsule from repetitive microtrauma during an overhead throwing motion. The posterior rotator cuff (posterior supraspinatus and infraspinatus) abuts the superior and posterior glenoid, and posterior rotator cuff tears are typically seen in these patients (16).

SLAP lesion refers to a superior labral injury that extends from anterior to posterior. These tears typically involve the biceps attachment and are best demonstrated at MR arthrography. A sublabral foramen, which is a normal variation, is also present, and a small amount of fluid may extend under the superior labrum. Visualizing fluid extending under the labrum on multiple slices or identifying separation of the labrum helps confirm the diagnosis (Fig. 15-19).

MR arthrography is also a very useful means to identify intraarticular bodies and cartilage defects. Intraarticular bodies are readily identified in the distended joint as free fragments to fall into the dependent aspects of the joint. Intraarticular bodies should not be confused with artifact from accidental injection of air during arthrography. Air lies in the most ventral aspect of the joint when the patient

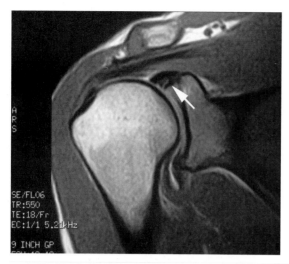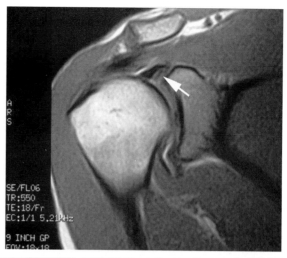

FIG. 15-19. SLAP lesion. T1-weighted spin-echo two-dimensional coronal oblique postgadolinium arthrograms demonstrate contrast extending under the superior labrum (*arrows*). Loss of the normal triangular appearance of the labrum is seen (compared to normal Fig. 15-1). The articular cartilage is well delineated in this shoulder magnetic resonance arthrogram. The overlying rotator cuff is intact and normal.

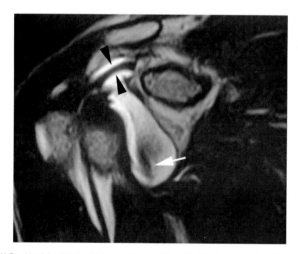

FIG. 15-20. Air bubble artifact. T2-weighted coronal oblique fast spin-echo post gadolinium arthrogram demonstrates low signal from air in the axillary pouch (*arrow*). Notice the biceps tendon coursing through the joint space (*arrowheads*). It is important to remember that the patient is lying supine, and any air that may have been injected into the joint during the arthrogram tends to float anteriorly.

is supine (Fig. 15-20). Cartilage defects can be identified during arthrography because the bright signal from contrast fills gaps in the cartilage. Contrast may even extend into subcortical bone, raising the concern for an unstable osteochondral lesion.

REFERENCES

1. Ferrari DA. Capsular ligaments of the shoulder. Anatomical and functional study of the anterior superior capsule. *Am J Sports Med* 1990;18:20.
2. Chandnani VP, Gagliardi JA, Murnane TG, et al. Glenohumeral ligaments and shoulder capsular mechanism: evaluation with MR arthrography. *Radiology* 1995;196:27.
3. Tirmann PFJ, Feller JF, Palmer WE, et al. The Buford complex—a variation of normal shoulder anatomy: MR arthrographic imaging features. *AJR Am J Roentgenol* 1996;166:869.
4. Bigliani LU, Morrison DS, April EW. The morphology of the acromion and its relationship to rotator cuff tears. *Orthop Trans* 1986;10:228.
5. Mudge MK, Wood VE, Frykman GK. Rotator cuff tears associated with os acromiale. *J Bone Joint Surg [Am]* 1984;66:427.
6. Rose SH, Melton J III, Morrey BF, et al. Epidemiologic features of humeral fractures. *Clin Orthop* 1982;168:24.
7. Neer CS. Impingement lesions. *Clin Orthop* 1983;173:70.
8. Sherman OH. MR imaging of impingement and rotator cuff disorders. *Magn Reson Imag Clin North Am* 1997;5:721.
9. Post M, Silver R, Singh M. Rotator cuff tears. Diagnosis and treatment. *Clin Orthop* 1983;173:78.
10. Jobe C. Superior glenoid impingement. *Clin Orthop* 1996;330:98.
11. Skirving AP, Kosak TKW, Davis SJ. Infraspinatus paralysis due to spinoglenoid notch ganglion. *J Bone Joint Surg [Br]* 1994;76:588.
12. Steiner E, Steinbach LS, Schnarkowski P, et al. Ganglia and cysts around joints. *Radiol Clin North Am* 1996;34:395.
13. Matsen FA, Harryman DT, Sidles JA. Mechanics of glenohumeral instability. *Clin Sports Med* 1991;10:783.
14. Sykhar MJ, Warren RF, Altchek DW. Instability of the shoulder. In: Nicholas JA, Hershman EB, Posner MA, eds. *The upper extremity in sports medicine.* St. Louis: Mosby, 1990:181.
15. Danzig LA, Greenway G, Resnick D. The Hill-Sachs lesion: an experimental study. *Am J Sports Med* 1980;8:328.
16. Tirman PFJ, Bost FW, Garvin GJ, et al. Posterosuperior glenoid impingement of the shoulder: findings at MR imaging and MR arthrography with arthroscopic correlation. *Radiology* 1994;193:431.

Open MRI,
edited by Peter A. Rothschild and Debra Reinking Rothschild.
Lippincott Williams & Wilkins. Philadelphia © 2000.

CHAPTER   16

Open Magnetic Resonance Imaging of the Elbow

Joseph Triolo and Peter A. Rothschild

Imaging the elbow can be successfully performed on open magnetic resonance imaging (MRI) systems, and it carries many of the same advantages that imaging the shoulder enjoys. On high-field closed systems, the elbow is preferably placed over one's head, so it can be positioned at isocenter. This position is difficult to maintain for long periods, and motion artifact is often a problem. Also, larger patients do not fit into the closed high-field systems in this position. Positioning the elbow at one's side on high-field systems results in artifacts from field inhomogeneity, because the elbow is not at isocenter, to ghosting and aliasing artifact from the adjacent torso. Also, chemical fat saturation is often inconsistent on high-field systems due to the position of the elbow in relationship to the isocenter of the magnet.

Open MRI systems allow positioning of the elbow comfortably at the patient's side and at isocenter. The elbow can be at an appropriate distance from the body to minimize aliasing and ghosting artifact. Patient motion and susceptibility artifact are also less problematic. As a result, high-quality diagnostic imaging of the elbow can be performed on open MRI systems.

ANATOMY

The elbow primarily functions as a hinge-type joint with the flexion and extension as the primary motion. This motion is supported by the olecranon abutting the olecranon fossa of the humerus in full extension and by the proximal radioulnar joint pivoting on the trochlear and capitellar surfaces of the humerus. The trochlea is spindle shaped, allowing for rotation of the ulna. The capitellum is a convex

structure that functions like a ball-in-socket joint with the smaller radial head (Fig. 16-1). Being a convex structure, the capitellum is prone to osteochondral injuries.

Pronation and supination are allowed by the radial head rotating against the radial notch of the ulna and by the complex mechanics of translation and rotation of the distal radioulnar joint. The radial tuberosity is an important structure that serves as the distal attachment of the biceps tendon. The coronoid process is the attachment of the brachialis muscle. The medial and lateral epicondyles of the humerus serve as attachments for the common flexor and extensor tendons, as well as the collateral ligaments (Fig. 16-2; see also Fig. 16-1).

The predominant muscles of the anterior compartment are the biceps and brachialis muscles. The biceps tendon arises from two heads that attach to the superior glenoid and the coracoid process of the scapula, and the distal tendon inserts onto the radial tuberosity of the proximal radius (Fig. 16-3). Because the distal biceps tendon is a common location for injury, axial images of the elbow should include the radial tuberosity. The bicipital aponeurosis extends from the myotendinous junction of the biceps and extends onto the flexor muscles of the forearm.

The brachialis tendon courses deep to the biceps muscle and attaches to the anterior aspect of the coronoid process and the ulnar tuberosity (Fig. 16-4). This muscle is also a strong flexor of the elbow and maintains strength when the biceps is injured. The brachialis tendon is injured less frequently than the biceps tendon (1).

Posteriorly, the triceps is essentially the only muscle, except for the small anconeus muscle, that is located posteriorly at the elbow joint. The anconeus arises from the lateral epicondyle and primarily inserts onto the olecranon. The triceps muscle extends the elbow and is the only muscle located dorsally along the humeral shaft. The long head arises from the inferior glenoid, and the medial and lateral heads arise from the proximal humerus. The distal tendon has a broad attachment on the proximal olecranon. The distal triceps tendon, unlike the Achilles and biceps tendon, is

J. Triolo: Ocean Medical Imaging Center, Community Medical Center, Toms River, New Jersey

P. A. Rothschild: Department of Radiology, University of California, San Francisco, San Francisco, California; Open MRI, Hayward, California; Open MRI, Louisville, Kentucky

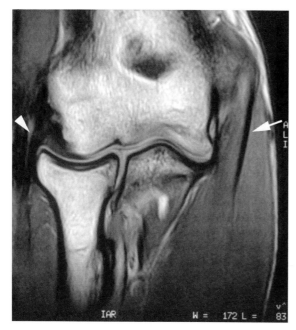

FIG. 16-1. Normal elbow. Coronal T1-weighted gradient-echo three-dimensional image demonstrates normal articulation of the radiocapitellar joint. The normal articular cartilage is well visualized on this high-resolution image. The posterior aspect of the common extensor tendon (*arrowhead*) and the common flexor tendon (*arrow*) are well visualized.

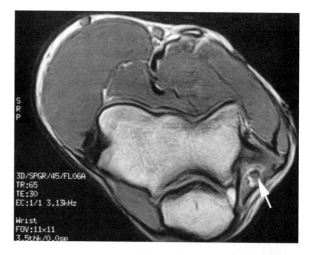

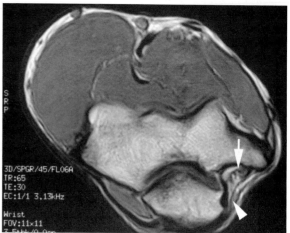

FIG. 16-2. Normal ulnar nerve in the cubital tunnel. Axial T1-weighted high-resolution gradient-echo three-dimensional images demonstrate the ulnar nerve (*arrows*); just below the ulnar nerve is the cubital tunnel retinaculum (*arrowhead*). On open magnetic resonance imaging (MRI) in the past, this was an area that was often overlooked owing to poor resolution. However, in today's advanced open MRI with high-resolution sequences such as this 11-cm field of view, it is possible to thoroughly evaluate the cubital tunnel in the elbow.

not homogeneously low in signal intensity; instead, it has a striated appearance.

Arising from the medial epicondyle is the common flexor tendon and ulnar collateral ligament (UCL). The UCL is composed of the three bands: the anterior, intermediate, and posterior bands. The anterior band is the most important clinically and the most readily identified on coronal images. The UCL resists valgus stress (2). The common flexor tendon is the proximal attachment of several superficial flexors of the forearm.

From the lateral epicondyle arise the common extensor tendons and the lateral collateral ligament (see Fig. 16-2). The lateral collateral ligament has a radial attachment to the annular ligament and an ulnar attachment to the lateral ulna. The lateral collateral resists varus stress. The annular ligament loops over the radial head and maintains the proximal radioulnar joint.

Lateral muscular attachments include the supinator, brachioradialis, extensor carpi radialis longus, and the common extensor tendon, on which the remainder of the extensor muscles originate. The collateral ligaments and common tendons should be evaluated in two planes. The coronal oblique plane is the best plane to evaluate the ligaments and tendons. The coronal oblique plane should be oriented parallel to the epicondyles (see Fig. 16-1). Heavily T2-weighted fast spin-echo images are often most useful in providing resolution to identify the small ligaments and con-

trast to demonstrate ligament and tendon tears. The axial plane is also extremely useful to identify abnormalities within the epicondyle and tendons. Fast short tau inversion recovery (STIR) imaging provides the greatest contrast and helps confirm abnormalities suspected on the coronal oblique images.

The course of the ulnar and median nerves is important to understand at the level of the elbow, because the elbow is a common site for nerve entrapment. MRI findings of nerve entrapment need to be correlated with clinical history and electromyographic studies. The ulnar nerve courses through the cubital tunnel, which is posterior to the medial epicondyle and is covered by the cubital tunnel retinaculum proximally and the arcuate ligament (flexor carpi ulnaris

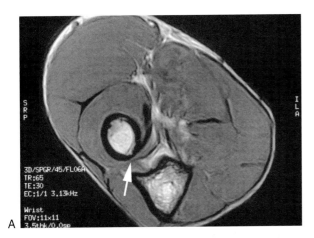

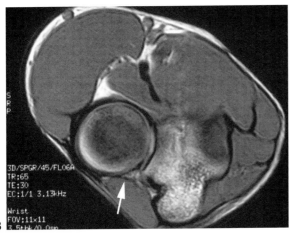

FIG. 16-3. Normal elbow. Axial T1-weighted three-dimensional gradient-echo images. **A:** Normal biceps attachment at the radial tuberosity (*arrow*) is demonstrated. **B:** More proximally, the biceps tendon is identified anteriorly and the normal annular ligament encircles the radial head (*arrow*).

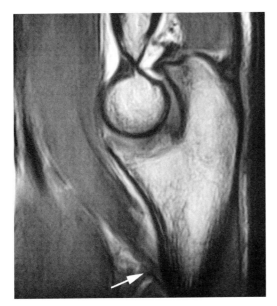

FIG. 16-4. Normal elbow. Axial T1-weighted images demonstrate normal brachialis attachment onto the ulna (*arrow*).

aponeurosis) posteriorly (see Fig. 16-2). The arcuate ligament extends from the olecranon to medial epicondyle. The cubital tunnel is a possible site of compression of the ulnar nerve, and the superficial course of the ulnar nerve at the elbow makes it prone to injury (3).

The median nerve courses anteriorly though the cubital fossa, deep to the biceps aponeurosis, and exits between the two heads of the pronator. The aponeurosis and pronator heads are two common sites for entrapment of the median nerve (4).

TECHNIQUE

Sagittal T1-weighted and fast STIR sequences are extremely useful when evaluating the biceps, brachialis, and triceps tendons. T1-weighted images can be obtained as spin-echo or three-dimensional gradient-echo (GRE) sequences. These images help identify osseous abnormalities, normal muscles and tendons, and myotendinous retraction in cases of tendon tears. The fast STIR sequence is very sensitive to soft tissue and osseous pathology and helps give an overall assessment of pathology involving the elbow joint. As with the ankle, the sagittal plane is useful when performing fast STIR sequences because the greatest coverage can be performed with the fewest slices, minimizing the scan time on longer STIR techniques. Intraarticular bodies are also best demonstrated in the sagittal plane. Intraarticular bodies are frequently located in the coronoid or olecranon fossa.

In the axial plane, a STIR sequence is very useful. High-resolution images are not necessary in this plane because the intricate collateral ligaments are not well depicted, and high contrast from STIR is very useful to evaluate the epicondyles as well as the biceps and triceps tendon attachments. T1-weighted axial images should be performed if concern for ulnar nerve pathology exists, because higher resolution scans are needed in such cases.

At least two sequences should be performed in the coronal plane because high resolution is required to demonstrate the collateral ligaments, and contrast is required to identify soft tissue and osseous abnormalities. The coronal images should be oriented parallel to the epicondyles to best demonstrate the epicondyles, capitellum, collateral ligaments, and common tendons. T2-weighted fast spin-echo images can provide resolution and contrast to demonstrate tendon and ligament abnormalities. A T2-weighted GRE or T-1 three-dimensional gradient can also be very useful to demonstrate the collateral ligaments as well as cartilage and osteochondral abnormalities.

PATHOLOGY

Tendon injuries are probably the most common reason for an MRI examination of the elbow. A distal biceps tendon tear is the most common tendon injury encountered in the elbow. The biceps tendon usually tears at the radial tuberos-

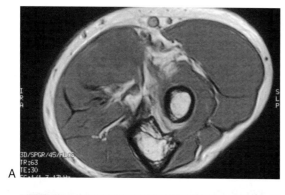

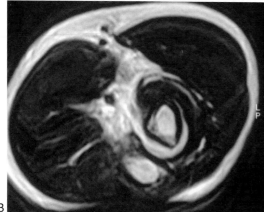

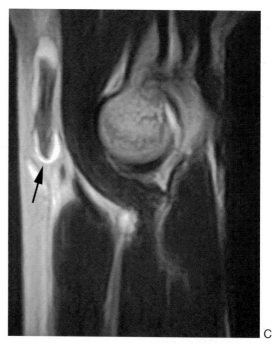

FIG. 16-5. Complete tear of the biceps tendon. **A:** Axial T1-weighted high-resolution three-dimensional gradient-echo image. **B:** Axial T2-weighted fast spin-echo (FSE) image. Compared with Figure 16-3A, which demonstrates a normal biceps attachment to the radius, this region **(A)** is replaced with amorphous soft tissue that is bright on the T2-weighted FSE images. The biceps tendon is not identified in its normal region of insertion on the axial images **(A,B)**. **C:** Sagittal T2-weighted FSE image. The retracted biceps tendon (*arrow*), which is capped with a small amount of fluid, is demonstrated. Careful evaluation of the bony cortex in the region of insertion of the biceps on both the T1- and T2-weighted images is of great assistance in ruling out avulsion-type fractures.

ity (Figs. 16-5 and 16-6). Axial STIR is the best sequence and plane to image the tear and also helps distinguish partial- from full-thickness tears. Sagittal images best demonstrate muscle belly retraction. Triceps tendon tears can be evaluated in a similar fashion, combining sagittal and axial images (Fig. 16-7).

The common flexor and extensor tendons can be difficult to evaluate because they are smaller structures than the biceps and triceps and they are obliquely oriented. Tendinitis and partial tears may be difficult to distinguish, and both entities may also coexist. Laterally, the common extensor tendon may demonstrate edematous changes representing tendinitis, commonly termed *tennis elbow* (Fig. 16-8) (5). However, repetitive occupational activity is probably the most frequent etiology. Edema may be seen in the adjacent soft tissues as well as in the underlying bone marrow of the lateral epicondyle.

Medially, similar changes of tendinitis may be seen in the common flexor tendon, adjacent soft tissues, and medial epicondyle. A variety of terms exist for medial epicondylitis, because it is seen in pitchers, golfers, and tennis players. Medial epicondylitis is less common than lateral epicondyli-

tis. Common flexor and extensor tendon tears usually occur in an already diseased tendon; however, a severe single trauma, such as a fracture-dislocation, may also be the etiology.

Ligaments

UCL injury is usually the result of valgus stress on the elbow. This usually occurs during a throwing motion and is commonly seen in pitchers. The injury can also be the result of severe elbow trauma. UCL injury may result in medial elbow instability, which can be demonstrated with stress radiographs. Tears usually involve the larger anterior bundle and occur in the midsubstance (6). UCL tears are identified on coronal oblique images. The radial collateral ligament is less frequently injured.

Osteochondral Lesions

Osteochondral fractures and osteochondritis dissecans are injuries that can be encountered in any joint. In the elbow,

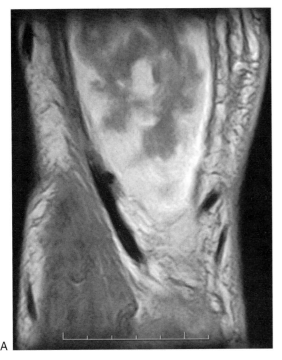

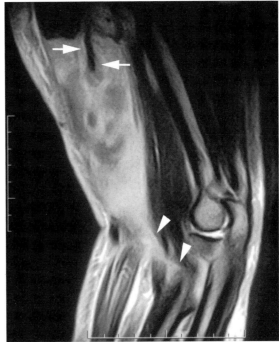

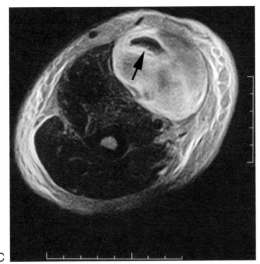

FIG. 16-6. Traumatic complete tear of the biceps tendon with a large hematoma. **A:** Coronal T1-weighted gradient-echo three-dimensional image. **B:** Sagittal T2-weighted fast spin-echo (FSE) image. **C:** T2-weighted axial image. These images show a large hematoma with mixed signal intensity on both T1- and T2-weighted images. The retracted tendon is identified in the superior aspect of **B** (*arrows*) and as a thick band of low signal intensity on **C** (*arrow*). The T2-weighted image FSE **(B)** provides excellent detail and pathologic information. High signal intensity can be seen extending down to the region of the anatomic insertion of the biceps in the proximal radius (**B**; *arrowheads*).

osteochondritis dissecans most frequently involves the capitellum (Fig. 16-9). Two-dimensional T1-weighted GRE and high-resolution three-dimensional T1-weighted GRE coronal oblique sequences are most useful, and attempts should be made to identify fluid within a lesion. This finding may suggest an unstable fragment. Complications of any osteochondral lesion include loss of cartilage promoting early osteoarthritis and the development of intraarticular bodies.

The elbow is a common site for intraarticular bodies. The knee is the only other joint more frequently involved (7). Intraarticular bodies may become loose and move within the joint capsule. They may also grow as they are bathed in

synovial fluid. Intraarticular bodies are best detected when a joint effusion is present, and they commonly lie anteriorly within the coronoid fossa or posteriorly in the olecranon fossa. Intraarticular bodies are more difficult to detect in the trochlear-ulnar articulation. Intraarticular bodies are best demonstrated on T2-weighted GRE or fast spin-echo examinations, because a joint effusion provides an arthrographic effect. T1-weighted images are useful when the loose bodies contain bone marrow and are increased in signal intensity.

As with other joints, lower field open systems are useful in identifying fractures as well as soft tissue pathology. Nondisplaced radial head fractures, as well as capitellar or

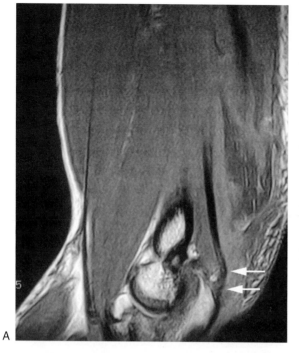

A

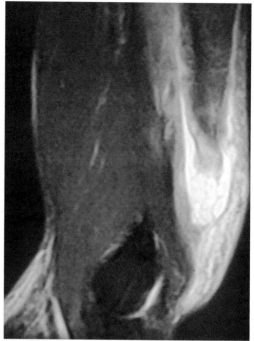

B

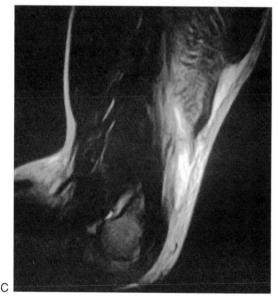

C

FIG. 16-7. Complete tear of the medial head of the triceps with retraction. **A:** Sagittal T1-weighted three-dimensional gradient-echo image. **B:** Sagittal fast short tau inversion recovery (STIR) image. **C:** Sagittal T2-weighted fast spin-echo image. These images demonstrate complete retraction of the medial head of the triceps with fluid signal intensity surrounding the distal portion of the medial head of the triceps. In this case, the anatomy is much better demonstrated on the T2-weighted and STIR images **(B,C)** than on the T1-weighted image **(A)**. The triceps tendon is identified inserting on the olecranon on the T1-weighted image **(A**; *arrows*), thus confirming that this is only a partial tear of the triceps.

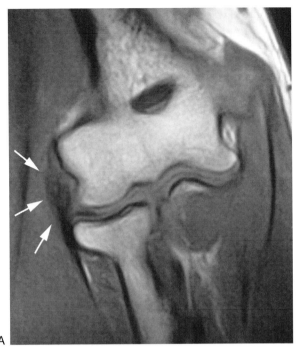

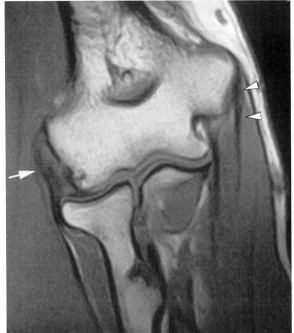

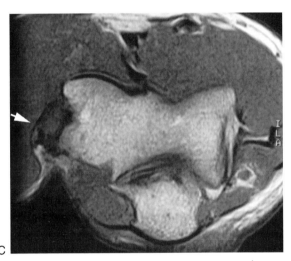

FIG. 16-8. Common extensor tendinitis. **A,B:** Coronal T1-weighted two-dimensional spin-echo (SE) image. **C:** Axial T1-weighted two-dimensional SE image. These images demonstrate abnormal thickening of the common extensor tendon at the attachment on the lateral epicondyle (*arrows*). Notice the normal appearance of the common flexor tendon at its attachment to the medial epicondyle (*arrowheads*). On lower field open magnetic resonance imaging, one must become comfortable diagnosing tendon abnormality on T1-weighted images as well as on T2-weighted and short tau inversion recovery (STIR) sequences because at lower field strengths, one can obtain high-resolution T1-weighted images; however, it is somewhat more difficult to obtain high resolution with adequate signal-to-noise ratios in images from STIR and fast SE T2-weighted sequences.

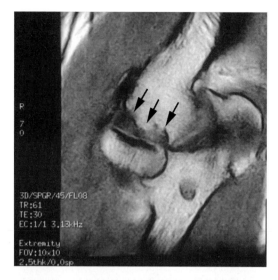

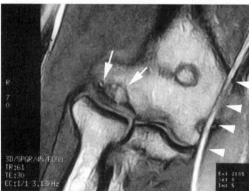

FIG. 16-9. Osteochondritis dissecans of the capitellum. Coronal oblique T1-weighted gradient-echo three-dimensional high-resolution image with a field of view of 10 cm and a slice thickness of 2.5 mm. High-resolution thin-slice T1-weighted images clearly demonstrate the irregularity along the anterior distal capitellum with loss of the normal articular cartilage (*arrows*) when compared with a normal elbow (see Fig. 16-1). Incidental note is made of wraparound along the medial aspect of the elbow joint (*arrowheads*) due to the use of a small field of view and no use of "no phase wrap."

supracondylar fracture, can be easily detected on fast STIR sequences. Open systems serve a unique role in pediatric patients when trying to identify capitellar or supracondylar fractures, which are difficult to detect on radiographs. MRI can easily evaluate these fractures, and the open system allows parents to be at the child's side during the examination.

REFERENCES

1. Ho CP. MR imaging of tendon injuries in the elbow. *Magn Reson Imag Clin North Am* 1997;5:529.
2. Morrey BF, An KN. Functional anatomy of the ligaments of the elbow. *Clin Orthop* 1995;201:84.
3. McPherson SA, Meals RA. Cubital tunnel syndrome. *Orthop Clin North Am* 1992;23:111.
4. Spinner M, Linscheid RL. Nerve entrapment syndromes. In: Morrey BF, ed. *The elbow and its disorders*, 2nd ed. Philadelphia: WB Saunders, 1993:813.
5. Pattern RM. Overuse syndromes and injuries involving the elbow: MR imaging findings. *AJR Am J Roentgenol* 1995;164:1205.
6. Conway JE, Jobe FW, Glousman RE, et al. Medial instability of the elbow in throwing athletes. Treatment by repair or reconstruction of the ulnar collateral ligament. *J Bone Joint Surg [Am]* 1992;74:67.
7. Morrey BF. Loose bodies. In: Morey BF, ed. *The elbow and its disorders*, 2nd ed. Philadelphia: WB Saunders, 1993:860.

Open MRI,
edited by Peter A. Rothschild and Debra Reinking Rothschild.
Lippincott Williams & Wilkins. Philadelphia © 2000.

CHAPTER 17

Open Magnetic Resonance Imaging of the Wrist

Joseph Triolo and Peter A. Rothschild

Magnetic resonance imaging (MRI) serves a unique role in imaging of the wrist, because it can detect subtle pathologic changes of the carpal bones and provide the soft tissue contrast necessary to visualize the interosseous ligaments. Carpal bone evaluation is difficult with computed tomography and conventional radiography, because subtle fractures and early changes of avascular necrosis (AVN) cannot be detected. Also, aside from MRI, arthrography is the only means of evaluating the interosseous ligaments. In addition to these advantages, MRI has multiplanar imaging capabilities, which allow depiction of abnormalities in the most useful imaging plane.

Similar to the elbow, the wrist is difficult to position on closed MRI systems. Large or broad-shouldered patients may not fit into the closed systems, and claustrophobia is a major problem because the patient needs to be placed far into the magnet to be imaged. Placing the arm overhead allows positioning of the wrist at isocenter and results in the best images; however, this is a difficult position to maintain for many patients, and motion artifact can be a significant problem. Placing the wrist at the patient's side is more comfortable for patients, but the wrist is not at isocenter, resulting in problems ranging from difficulty in localizing the wrist, to wrap and ghosting artifact from the adjacent torso, to the inability to consistently fat saturate on high-field systems. Additionally, artifacts such as aliasing, ghosting, and susceptibility are all less problematic on lower field open systems. Also, open MRI systems allow positioning of the wrist comfortably at the patient's side, appropriately spaced from the adjacent torso, and, most important for image quality, at isocenter of the magnet. These factors combine to produce musculoskeletal images that are competitive with those obtained in closed high-field MRI systems.

ANATOMY

Osseous

The carpal bones and ligaments function together to provide stability and motion of the wrist. The eight carpal bones can be divided into proximal and distal rows. The proximal carpal row forms an arch that rotates about the distal radioulnar joint to provide not only flexion and extension but also rotation in the coronal plane. The scaphoid bone is the largest and bears the greatest axial load of the proximal carpal row. The scaphoid bone is most prone to fracture and runs the risk of AVN involving the proximal pole. The adjacent lunate bone is crescent shaped with a large articular surface covered by hyaline cartilage. The lunate bone is very mobile (Fig. 17-1), making it more susceptible to dislocation than fracture (1). The triquetrum has many ligamentous and tendinous attachments. It also bears the axial load on the ulnar side of the wrist and is prone to fracture.

The distal carpal row functions as a pivot for flexion and extension of the metacarpophalangeal joints. The capitate bone is largest and also carries a greater axial load, making it prone to fracture. The trapezium and hamate bones are important attachments of the flexor retinaculum. The hook of the hamate forms the floor of Guyon's canal, which contains the ulnar artery and nerve (Fig. 17-2). The hamate bone, like the cuboid bone in the foot, articulates with the fourth and fifth metacarpals.

Ligaments

Alignment of the carpal bones and their relationship with the distal radioulnar joint (DRUJ) are maintained by several important ligaments. The triangular fibrocartilage complex (TFCC) is an important stabilizer of the DRUJ. The TFCC also acts as a cushion for the ulnocarpal articulation. The TFCC is composed of the triangular fibrocartilage (TFC) and several other components connecting the distal ulnar and carpal bones along the

J. Triolo: Ocean Medical Imaging Center, Community Medical Center, Toms River, New Jersey

P. A. Rothschild: Department of Radiology, University of California, San Francisco, San Francisco, California; Open MRI, Hayward, California; Open MRI, Louisville, Kentucky

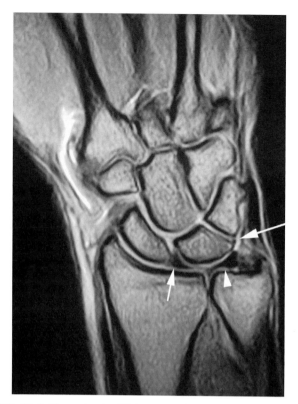

FIG. 17-1. Normal wrist. High-resolution coronal T2-weighted gradient-echo image demonstrates normal alignment of proximal carpal row. The TFCC (*arrowhead*) is well visualized. The meniscal homologue is often heterogeneous in signal intensity. The scapholunate ligament (*arrow*) has a normal triangular appearance, and the small lunate triquetral ligament is also visualized (*long arrow*).

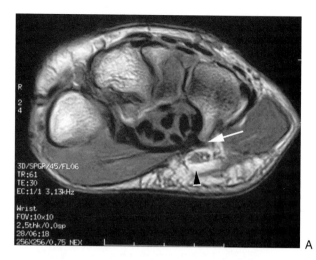

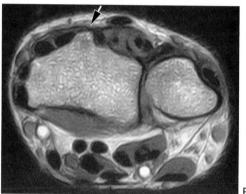

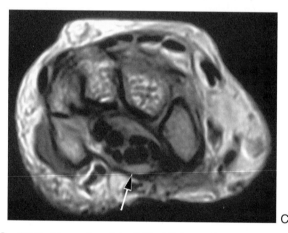

FIG. 17-2. Normal wrist. **A,B:** High-resolution axial T1-weighted three-dimensional gradient-echo image with 10 × 10 field of view; 2.5-mm slice thickness; 6 minutes, 18 seconds. **A:** Normal hamate hook and flexor retinaculum attachment (*arrow*). The ulnar neurovascular bundle extends along the volar soft tissues in Guyon's canal (*arrowhead*). **B:** More proximally, the dorsal projection of Lister's tubercle is an attachment of the extensor retinaculum (*arrow*). **C:** Axial proton density–weighted two-dimensional spin-echo image demonstrates normal low signal from the flexor and extensor tendons with intermediate signal from the median nerve (*arrow*), which is volar in the carpal tunnel.

ulnar aspect of the wrist (see Fig. 17-1) (2). The TFC is a disc-shaped structure extending from the ulna styloid to the ulnar aspect of the distal radius. Other components include the meniscal homologue, radioulnar ligaments, the ulnar-collateral ligament, and the sheath of the extensor carpi ulnaris.

The proximal carpal row is maintained by two important interosseous ligaments: the scapholunate ligament (SLL) and the lunotriquetral ligament (LTL) (3). The SLL connects the proximal aspects of the scaphoid and lunate bones and maintains their relationship. The ligament is often linear or triangular in shape and is consistently seen on lower field open MRI (see Fig. 17-1). The LTL is a smaller structure that is not consistently visualized on open MRI. High-field closed MRI can only consistently visualize the LTL with the use of phased-array coils. The LTL connects the proximal aspects of the lunate and triquetral bones, maintaining their alignment.

The TFCC and interosseous ligaments are considered extremely important in maintaining function and stability of the proximal carpal row. These ligaments cannot be directly visualized with MRI, and arthrography is invasive and only indirectly visualizes these ligaments.

The wrist is also stabilized by numerous dorsal and volar capsular ligaments. Numerous classification systems exist

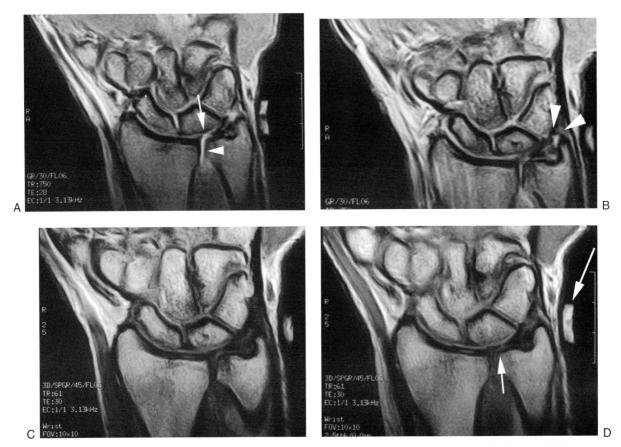

FIG. 17-3. Triangular fibrocartilage (TFC) tear. **A,B:** Coronal oblique T2-weighted gradient-echo (GRE) images demonstrate a tear at the radial attachment (*arrow*). Fluid extends into the distal radioulnar joint (*arrowhead*). The TFC also appears torn at the ulnar styloid attachment (*double arrowhead*). (Compare to Fig. 17-1A with normal low signal TFC.) **C,D:** Coronal three-dimensional T1-weighted GRE images, with 10 × 10 field of view and 2.5-mm slice thickness, on same patient demonstrates intermediate signal at radial attachment (*arrow*). Notice the normal scapholunate ligament. An oil marker was placed over the area of pain on the ulnar side (*long arrow*).

that further divide these ligaments into extrinsic and intrinsic ligaments. The volar ligaments are believed to be stronger and more important, but these ligaments have variable courses and are inconsistently visualized with MRI.

Tendons and Nerves

The extensor tendons course over the dorsal radius and ulna at the wrist. They are covered by the extensor retinaculum, which has several attachments to the dorsal radius and ulna and thus divides the extensor tendons into six compartments. The best visualized bony attachment is to Lister's tubercle on the dorsum of the wrist (see Fig. 17-2). The extensor tendons are covered by synovial sheaths to reduce friction, and the communicating sheaths may allow spread of inflammation (tenosynovitis) or infection.

The deep and superficial flexor tendons course through the carpal tunnel between the carpal bones and the thick flexor retinaculum. The flexor retinaculum has medial attachments to the pisiform and hook of the hamate and lateral attach-

ments to the trapezium and scaphoid. The median nerve also courses superficially in the carpal tunnel (see Fig. 17-2).

The ulnar nerve courses superficial to the flexor retinaculum along the ulnar aspect of the wrist, over the hook of the hamate. This region is called *Guyon's canal* and is a potential site of ulnar nerve compression or injury. Like the elbow, the ulnar nerve takes a superficial course, can also be injured by direct trauma, and may be compressed by the hook of the hamate.

TECHNIQUE

The wrist should be localized in the axial plane to allow the obtainment of coronal oblique sequences first. The coronal oblique images best demonstrate the interosseous ligaments and carpal bones. These sequences are the most informative and time consuming, because detailed images are required. With the wrist placed comfortably at the patient's side and in pronation, the carpal bones are slightly angulated. The coronal images should be angulated to the DRUJ. Doing so best demonstrates the TFCC, SLL, LTL, and carpal bones (see Fig. 17-1). Keeping the patient comfortable is essential to the prevention of motion artifact.

At least two sequences should be performed in the coronal oblique plane. A T1-weighted three-dimensional (3D) spoiled gradient reversal echo is preferable because thin slices, usually 1.0 to 2.5 mm, can be performed without an interval gap. Phase and frequency matrices of 244 or 256 can be performed with fields of view of less than 12 cm for high resolution (Fig. 17-3). Routine spin-echo (SE) sequences can only be performed with 3-mm slices, which may not be adequate for evaluating the smaller structures of the wrist.

A coronal T2-weighted fast spin-echo (FSE) or gradient-echo sequence should also be performed if the study is directed at evaluating the ligaments. This sequence should be heavily T2 weighted with a long repetition time and echo time. Longer echo train lengths can be helpful because fewer slices are needed, allowing faster scanning. Higher echo times, as well as a greater bandwidth, should be used to narrow the echo spacing and reduce blurring artifact. T2-weighted FSE provides better resolution than do fast short tau inversion recovery (STIR) sequences. If the study is indicated to evaluate for fracture or AVN, a coronal STIR is essential, because fat is nullified and marrow edema is easily identified. On T2-weighted FSE images, fat and edema are increased in signal intensity, making marrow changes less conspicuous. Also, coronal STIR allows the greatest coverage with the fewest number of slices, minimizing scan time.

In the axial plane, T1-weighted SE or T1-weighted 3D gradient-echo sequences are useful to provide the needed resolution, which is helpful in identifying the contents of the carpal tunnel and as well as the dorsal tendons. High resolution is not as critical in the axial plane as it is in the coronal plane. As a result, T1-weighted SE sequences may be more practical in the axial plane. An axial STIR sequence is also useful, because this is probably the best plane to identify ganglia and soft tissue abnormalities. Images in this plane also best demonstrate the hook of the hamate, if concern for a hamate hook fracture is present. If carpal tunnel syndrome is a concern, proton density– and T2-weighted FSE images are more helpful than STIR images, because higher resolution helps identify the contents of the carpal tunnel.

Always remember that a STIR should be performed in at least one plane, because signal from fat needs to be nullified to identify subtle osseous and soft tissue abnormalities. Also, when imaging the wrist, it is more useful to perform a few high-resolution scans than to perform several less detailed images, especially when imaging the small interosseous ligaments and carpal bones.

PATHOLOGY

Ligaments

The TFC is probably the ligament of the wrist most frequently submitted for evaluation by MRI. TFC tears may be degenerative or traumatic, and they frequently present with pain. The incidence of degenerative tears increases with age, and many may be asymptomatic and even bilateral. As a result, TFCC tears need to be viewed in the appropriate clinical setting. TFCC tears usually involve the radial or ulnar attachments of the TFC attachments; however, the classification of TFCC tears is broad (see Fig. 17-3) (4).

Disruption of the normal disc appearance on T1-weighted images is helpful; however, demonstrating fluid extending through the ligament on T2-weighted images is a clear indication of a tear. Fluid on both sides of the TFC (the DRUJ and radiocarpal joint) does not always indicate a tear. Also, when a TFC tear is present, fluid may not be seen in both of these joint spaces. Intraarticular gadolinium in the radiocarpal joint is extremely useful when evaluating the interosseous ligaments, and 3D SPGR sequences can be used because on these sequences gadolinium is increased in signal intensity (Fig. 17-4).

SLL tears can result in widening of the scapholunate joint space, which may lead to carpal instability and a progressive arthritis. Patients with scapholunate instability present with pain and weakness (5). On MRI, the SLL does not exhibit its normal triangular or linear appearance on T1-weighted images, and again, identifying fluid on T2-weighted imaging extending through the SLL at the base of the scapholunate articulation helps to confirm the diagnosis (Fig. 17-5). Identifying fluid in the radiocarpal joint and midcarpal row does not always indicate a tear of the SLL, and this finding may also be present with LTL tears.

Osseous

Fractures can be readily identified on lower field open MRI and most commonly involve the scaphoid, capitate, triquetrum, and hook of the hamate. Subtle distal radius or ulnar fractures may also be detected . Open systems can successfully use fast STIR, which nullifies the background signal from fatty marrow and demonstrates marrow edema as increased signal. T1-weighted images may be helpful in detecting trabecular disruption and providing anatomic detail, which is lacking on STIR images. Because the carpal bones of the wrist are small, a volume 3D T1-weighted gradient-echo technique is again the most useful sequence because thin (1- to 2-mm) slices can be obtained without an interval gap. T2-weighted sequences may be misleading, because fat and edema exhibit increased signal, obscuring the detection of subtle fractures.

The DRUJ and ulnar variance should be evaluated because they may provide information on carpal pathology. Ulnar positive variance should raise the concern for TFC injury and ulnar impaction syndrome. In this syndrome, the ulna abuts the lunate bone, injuring the TFC and resulting in degenerative changes along the proximal articular surface of the lunate, in which subchondral cystic changes may be identified (6). Negative ulnar variance

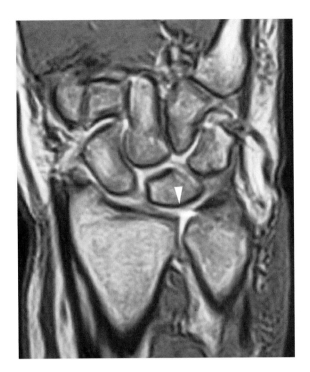

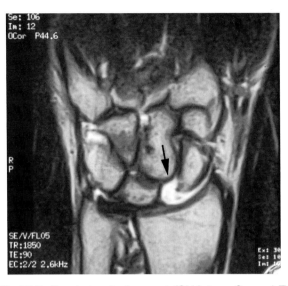

FIG. 17-5. Scapholunate ligament (SLL) tear. Coronal T2-weighted images demonstrate bright fluid filling the location of the SLL, which is not visualized (*arrow*). Widening of the scapholunate joint space is seen.

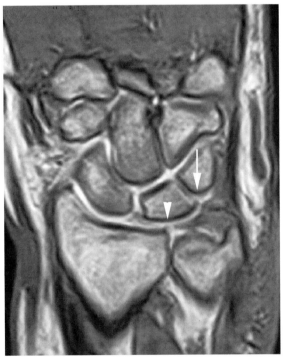

FIG. 17-4. Triangular fibrocartilage (TFC) tear. Three-dimensional T1-weighted gradient-echo image after intraarticular administration of dilute gadolinium. Notice bright fluid from T1 shortening effects of gadolinium filling tear at radial attachment of TFC (*arrowheads*). Bright signal is also present in the midcarpal row. The patient also has a tear of the lunotriquetral ligament (*arrow*).

may be seen with AVN of the lunate bone (Kienbock's disease) (Fig. 17-6).

In addition to AVN of the lunate bone, the proximal pole of the scaphoid may also develop AVN in cases of scaphoid waist fractures. Nonunion is also a complication (7). Open systems can readily identify changes of AVN by combining information obtained on STIR and T1-weighted sequences.

Tendons and Soft Tissues

The multiple tendons of the wrist and their associated synovial sheaths may become inflamed, representing tendinitis and tenosynovitis (Fig. 17-7). These changes are usually the result of overuse or repetitive microtrauma, but they may also be seen in cases of inflammatory or infectious arthropathies.

Changes are best demonstrated on T2-weighted images, in which improved resolution over STIR images allows better visualization of the individual tendons. Thickening and abnormal morphology, as well as edema extending along or within the tendon, is readily identified on heavily T2-weighted FSE images (see Fig. 17-7). Because subcutaneous fat and edema exhibit increased signal on T2-weighted FSE images, STIR, in the axial plane, should be used to confirm changes on edema.

The tendons of the wrist are compartmentalized, and several tendons may be involved simultaneously. These compartments may allow for the spread of inflammation or infection. General tendon groups include the flexor tendons, which course through the carpal tunnel and are bordered by the flexor retinaculum, and the extensor tendons. The extensor tendons are divided into six individual com-

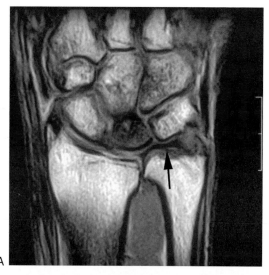

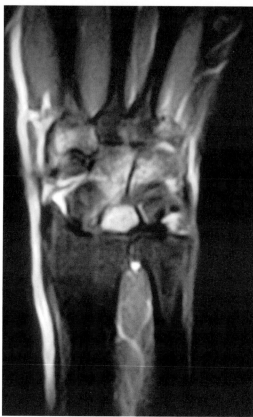

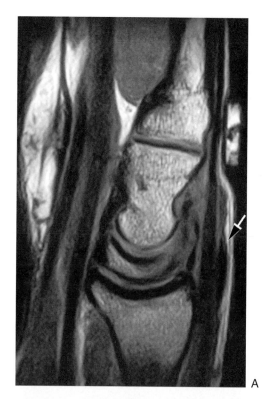

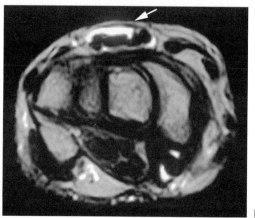

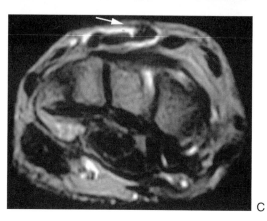

FIG. 17-6. Avascular necrosis of the lunate. Coronal three-dimensional T1-weighted gradient-echo **(A)** and coronal fast short tau inversion recovery **(B)** images demonstrate marrow edema of the lunate bone but no evidence of collapse. A minimal degree of positive ulnar variance is seen, but the triangular fibrocartilage complex appears intact (*arrow*).

FIG. 17-7. Extensor tenosynovitis confined to the dorsal compartment. Sagittal T1-weighted three-dimensional gradient-echo **(A)** and axial T2-weighted fast spin-echo **(B,C)** images demonstrate several extensor tendons with adjacent fluid (*arrows*). The fluid is dark on the T1 sequence (*arrows*), as are the tendons, making the T2 sequences necessary to arrive at the correct diagnosis.

partments on the dorsum of the wrist by the extensor retinaculum. Compartment changes are best identified in the axial plane.

Ganglia are the most common masses in the wrist. They usually occur on the dorsum of the wrist but can occur along the volar aspect or may be intraosseous. Ganglia are more commonly seen in female patients and usually present in the young adult ages. Clinically, patients may be asymptomatic, or they may present with a palpable mass, pain, or tendon dysfunction (8). Ganglia are fluid filled and are best demonstrated on T2-weighted and STIR sequences. The course and extent of ganglia should be described, because MRI may be used as a guide for surgery.

REFERENCES

1. Prendergast N, Rauschning W. Normal anatomy of the hand and wrist. *Magn Reson Imag Clin North Am* 1995;3:197.
2. Palmer AK, Werner FW. The triangular fibrocartilage complex of the wrist—anatomy and function. *J Hand Surg* 1981;6:153.
3. Ruby LK. Carpal instability. *J Bone Joint Surg [Am]* 1995;77:476.
4. Palmer AK. Triangular fibrocartilage complex lesions: a classification. *J Hand Surg* 1989;14:594.
5. Linscheid RL, Dodyns JH. Treatment of scapholunate dissociation: rotary subluxation of the scaphoid. *Hand Clin* 1992;8:645.
6. Escobedo EM, Bergman AG, Hunter JC. MR imaging of ulnar impaction. *Skel Radiol* 1995;24:85.
7. Gelberman RH, Wolock BS, Siegel DB. Fractures and non-union of the carpal scaphoid. *J Bone Joint Surg [Am]* 1989;71:1560.
8. Cardinal E, Buckwalter KA, Braunstein EM, et al. Occult dorsal ganglion: comparison of US and MR imaging. *Radiology* 1994;193:259.

Open MRI,
edited by Peter A. Rothschild and Debra Reinking Rothschild.
Lippincott Williams & Wilkins. Philadelphia © 2000.

CHAPTER 18

Open Magnetic Resonance Imaging of the Hip

Peter A. Rothschild and Joseph Triolo

Evaluation of hip pain is a diagnostic challenge because a wide range of pathology affects the hip. Clinically, disc disease of the lumbar spine can easily be confused with hip pathology. Magnetic resonance imaging (MRI) is well suited to demonstrate changes ranging from osteoarthritis (OA) to stress fractures and avascular necrosis (AVN). Conventional radiography and nuclear medicine examinations often have subtle or nonspecific changes. MRI is advantageous because it can demonstrate marrow changes of the femoral head at an earlier stage than bone scans and computed tomography (1,2). Furthermore, MRI's superior soft tissue contrast and multiplanar capabilities make it the single best modality for imaging of the hips.

TECHNIQUE

Open systems can successfully evaluate marrow pathology using a variety of pulse sequences. Short tau inversion recovery (STIR) is probably the most useful pulse sequence, because signal from fatty bone marrow is nullified and underlying marrow edema is readily identified. STIR is usually combined with fast spin-echo (FSE) to produce high-contrast images in a timely fashion. Even on high-field systems, fast STIR sequences are preferable because it is difficult to successfully perform chemical fat suppression over larger fields of view with presaturation pulses. As a result, producing images with similar contrast on both hips at the same time can be difficult with T2-weighted FSE fat-suppressed images alone.

T1-weighted sequences are easily performed and provide excellent anatomic detail. T2-weighted images are useful when it is necessary to combine higher resolution with higher contrast, which is helpful when visualizing the soft tissues of the hips and pelvis. By using the various pulse sequences, MRI is the diagnostic study of choice for evaluating disease processes such as AVN, congenital hip dislocation, tumor, infection, or fracture.

When evaluating hip pathology with MRI, the hips and the pelvis should be included on the same series. Processes such as AVN of the femoral heads and pelvic fractures can be bilateral. Metastatic bone disease and Paget's disease may be diffuse processes that are more easily diagnosed when more than one focus is identified. In the coronal plane, T1-weighted and fast STIR images should be obtained. These sequences are most useful when evaluating fractures, metastatic disease, and the early changes of AVN. T1-weighted images provide anatomic detail, whereas fast STIR images are extremely sensitive for pathology (Fig. 18-1). Combining the information from both sequences helps differentiate between benign lesions, such as bone islands and Paget's disease, and more aggressive processes, such as metastatic disease (Fig. 18-2). Soft tissue abnormalities may be an isolated finding, or they may indicate an underlying osseous pathology (Fig. 18-3).

In the axial plane, T2-weighted FSE images are useful because they provide improved resolution over STIR images and T2 weighting to evaluate soft tissue changes (Fig. 18-4). Again, heavy T2 weighting is necessary to obtain the required contrast. This is achieved by using long repetition time (TR) and long echo time (TE) sequences. Because TE has greater effect on contrast, TEs in the 120 to 140 ms range are useful. Long TEs are also beneficial with FSE techniques to minimize blurring artifact.

In the axial plane, T1-weighted sequences can also be extremely helpful. Three-dimensional spoiled gradient-echo images are very useful for demonstrating trabecular bone and are best used when evaluating the pelvis for subtle rami fractures. T1-weighted SE images in the axial plane should be used when evaluating the pelvic side walls for masses or adenopathy.

P. A. Rothschild: Department of Radiology, University of California, San Francisco, San Francisco, California; Open MRI, Hayward, California; Open MRI, Louisville, Kentucky

J. Triolo: Ocean Medical Imaging Center, Community Medical Center, Toms River, New Jersey

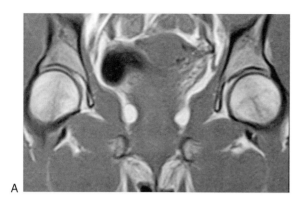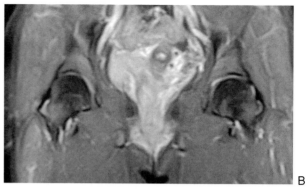

A   B

FIG. 18-1. Normal hip examination. T1-weighted **(A)** and fast short tau inversion recovery (STIR) **(B)** coronal images demonstrate normal articular cartilage and normal marrow signal. **A:** Fat pad in acetabular fossa is bright on T1-weighted images. **B:** Fast STIR images have essentially no signal from fat.

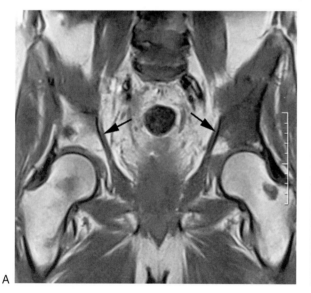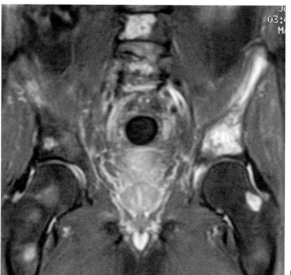

A   B

FIG. 18-2. Metastatic lymphoma to the pelvis and hip. **A:** Coronal T1-weighted spin-echo image. **B:** Coronal fast short tau inversion recovery (STIR). **A:** The T1-weighted images give nice anatomic definition, especially of the bony cortex (*arrows*). **B:** The STIR images better show the pathology (which is very bright) and extension into the surrounding soft tissues. However, the T1-weighted high-resolution images can often better define bony cortical destruction. When imaging the pelvis, it is important to perform T1-weighted and STIR imaging. Also notice the involvement of the lumbar vertebral bodies.

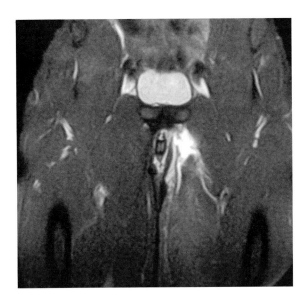

FIG. 18-3. Complete tear with retraction of the biceps femoris muscle and tendon. Fast short tau inversion recovery (STIR) image demonstrates fluid signal intensity between the top of the biceps femoris muscle and the inferior pubic rami. Note the increased signal intensity in the entire biceps femoris muscle. STIR images are excellent for identifying soft tissue abnormality that may be the source of the patient's hip or groin pain.

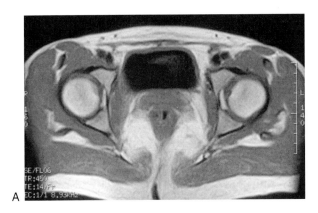

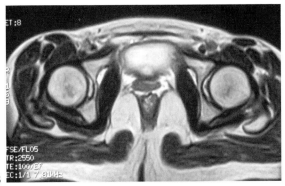

FIG. 18-4. Normal hip examination. T1-weighted **(A)** and T2-weighted **(B)** axial images. T2 images can provide the best combination of resolution and contrast. However, marrow signal is still relatively bright, which makes this sequence less than optimal for identifying marrow replacement processes.

PATHOLOGY

The most frequent indication for MRI of the hip in an outpatient setting is to identify changes of AVN. AVN (also called *osteonecrosis, aseptic necrosis, ischemic necrosis*) is a process that results from an insufficient blood supply to the subchondral bone in the epiphyseal region. The most common site for AVN is the hips (3). The causes of AVN can be divided into traumatic and nontraumatic, with trauma (e.g., fracture or dislocation) being the most frequent cause (4).

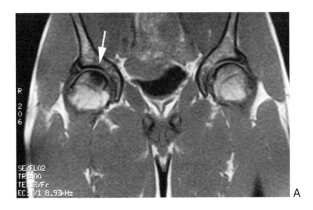

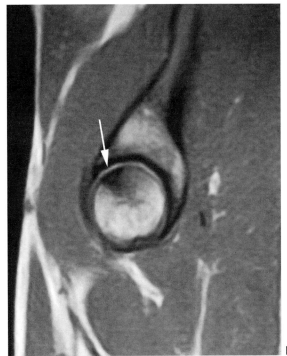

FIG. 18-5. Small area of early avascular necrosis at right femoral head. Coronal **(A)** and sagittal **(B)** T1-weighted spin-echo images demonstrate a wedge-shaped area of low signal intensity that appears to abut the bony cortex; however, the articular cartilage is intact over this lesion (*arrows*). Because of the intact articular cartilage over the lesion, this patient was treated conservatively. Lower field open magnets using high-resolution T1-weighted sequences can clearly demonstrate articular cartilage over the femoral head, which is important in the clinical evaluation of certain types of pathology such as avascular necrosis.

TABLE 18-1. *Mitchell's classification of avascular necrosis (AVN) of the hip*

Class A
  Fatlike MRI appearance
  Bright on T1-weighted images
  Intermediate to bright on T2-weighted scans depending
    on field strength, with dark signal intensity rim
  Early AVN before revascularization of the central region
Class B
  Bloodlike MRI pattern (similar to subacute blood)
  High signal intensity on long and short TR/TE images
  Due to inflammation or vascular engorgement or if
    subacute blood is present
  Least common appearance
Class C
  Fluidlike appearance
  Low signal intensity on short TR/TE images
  High signal intensity on long TR image
  Due to inflammation, hyperemia, fibrosis, or sclerosis
  Decreased lipid content in the femoral head
  Late stage of AVN
Class D
  Fibrouslike appearance on MRI
  Low signal intensity on all pulse sequences
  Fibrosis and sclerosis predominant
  Advanced AVN
  Often complicated by secondary collapse and osteoarthritis

MRI, magnetic resonance imaging; TE, echo time; TR, repetition time.
From ref. 6, with permission.

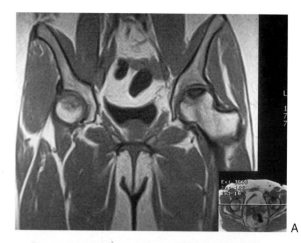
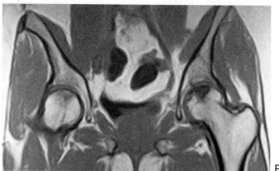
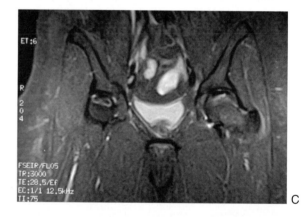
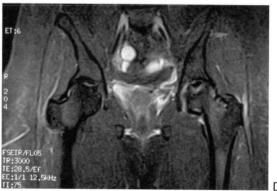

The current theory is that trauma causes a disruption in the nutrient retinacular and periosteal vessels that supply the femoral head, thereby resulting in necrosis.

Nontraumatic causes of AVN tend to present with bilateral involvement. These patients usually have predisposing conditions such as sickle cell disease, alcoholism, corticosteroid use, Gaucher's disease, postirradiation syndrome, Caisson's disease, gout, or iron overload. Often, nontraumatic AVN is idiopathic, without predisposing factors.

The normal femoral head on MRI has a high-signal-intensity marrow surrounded by a dark rim of cortical bone on T1-weighted images (short TR/TE). The best imaging plane to evaluate AVN and other hip pathology is the coronal plane. Because the femoral head is composed primarily of fat, any marrow-replacing process will lengthen the T1 relaxation time, thereby decreasing the signal intensity on short TR/TE sequences. The earliest finding with AVN is a focal area of decreased signal intensity on the T1-weighted image (Fig. 18-5). The most frequent area of involvement is the superior weight-bearing surface of the femoral head (5). Mitchell (6) has devised four classes of AVN according to the MRI appearance of the central region of the femoral head (Table 18-1 and Fig. 18-6). These classes may not have direct correlation with x-ray findings, because the bone marrow changes seen with MRI do not necessarily parallel the bony changes seen on x-rays.

A classic finding of AVN of the head is the "double line" sign. In a study by Mitchell (6), this sign was present in 80%

FIG. 18-6. Avascular necrosis. Coronal T1-weighted **(A,B)** and fast short tau inversion recovery **(C,D)** images demonstrate bilateral avascular necrosis. The changes are older and more extensive on the left side. The right side is class B and the left side is class D.

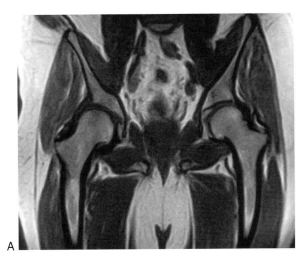
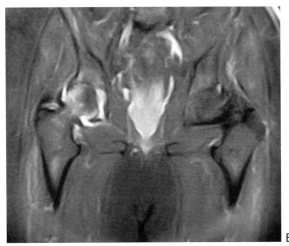

FIG. 18-7. Transient osteoporosis of the right hip. **A:** Coronal T1-weighted spin-echo image demonstrates vague low signal intensity throughout the femoral head, neck, and proximal shaft. **B:** Coronal fast short tau inversion recovery image demonstrates mild increased signal intensity in the femoral head and neck with associated joint effusion. This constellation of findings should not be misinterpreted for avascular necrosis. Often, follow-up examinations in 2 to 3 months can be helpful in confirming the diagnosis of transient osteoporosis, because transient osteoporosis should resolve over time and avascular necrosis tends to progress.

of the hips with AVN. This sign consists of a decreased signal intensity rim on T1- and T2-weighted images, with an inner band of increased signal intensity only on the T2-weighted images. The dark rim is believed to represent the reactive interface between dead and viable bone. This area consists of inflammatory changes and fibroblastic tissue and may also have sclerosis due to the thickening of the trabecular bone. The bright interzone is believed to be caused by hyperemia in the granulation tissue.

Treatment for AVN of the hips has been controversial. The most frequent procedures are core decompression, rotational osteotomy, and decreased weight bearing. For severe AVN, a total hip replacement may become necessary.

When interpreting hip MRI for AVN, one must be aware of a condition called *transient osteoporosis of the hip* (Fig. 18-7). Transient osteoporosis can mimic AVN clinically and on MRI. The cause of transient osteoporosis is uncertain (7), and it most commonly affects young or middle-aged men. These patients present with pain severe enough to produce a limp and restrict joint motion. Plain films demonstrate osteoporosis of the femoral head, and bone scans show increased uptake in the affected femoral head. The symptoms and x-ray and MRI findings normally resolve in 6 to 12 months without late sequelae. MRI demonstrates a circumscribed area of decreased signal intensity in the femoral heads on T1-weighted images and increased on the T2-weighted images, often with a joint effusion. When compared to AVN, this disease process is self-limiting and does not require treatment unless complicated by a fracture. Therefore, if transient osteoporosis (transient synovitis) is considered in the differential diagnosis, a follow-up MRI should be pursued.

FRACTURES

MRI is an extremely useful study to evaluate hip fractures in emergency department patients as well as stress fractures in the outpatient setting. MRI plays a vital role in elderly patients in whom plain films and computed tomography may not detect nondisplaced subcapital hip fractures. Furthermore, in the elderly, a bone scan may not be positive for 2 to 3 days (8). Excluding hip fractures can help prevent a costly hospitalization, and diagnosing the appropriate type of hip fracture assists in planning a prompt treatment course. Fractures are best evaluated on fast STIR images in the coronal plane (Fig. 18-8).

MRI is also useful in the evaluation of sacral fractures. Insufficiency fractures in the elderly can be easily diagnosed with bone scintigraphy and MRI. However, MRI can accurately locate one or more fractures involving the pelvic ring. Furthermore, because fractures of the pelvis may be pathologic in nature, MRI demonstrates soft tissue masses and marrow replacement processes.

Stress fractures in younger patients can also be demonstrated on MRI (Fig. 18-9). MRI has the added benefit over bone scintigraphy of not only being a more specific examination but also being able to identify other etiologies of hip pain, such as synovitis, bursitis, or tendonitis.

Osteoarthritis

OA is an important finding when evaluating patients with hip pain. Because lumbar disc disease may also present with

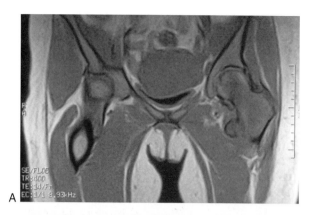

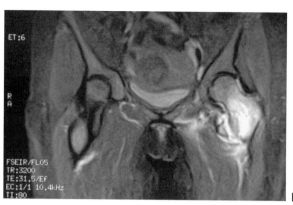

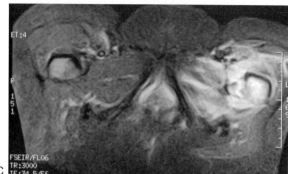

FIG. 18-8. Hip fracture. A: Coronal T1-weighted image demonstrates a fracture extending through the inter-trochanteric portion of the left hip with avulsion of the lesser trochanter. Marrow edema results in low signal on T1-weighted images. **B:** Coronal fast short tau inversion recovery (STIR) demonstrates high signal marrow edema and avulsed lesser trochanter. **C:** Axial fast STIR demonstrates fracture with adjacent soft tissue hematoma. Soft tissue changes extend to the obturator externus muscle.

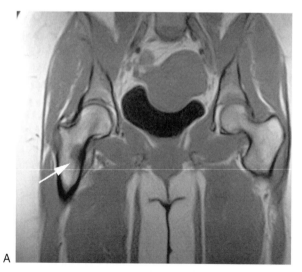

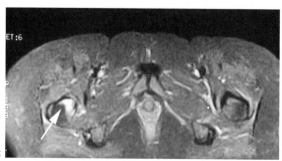

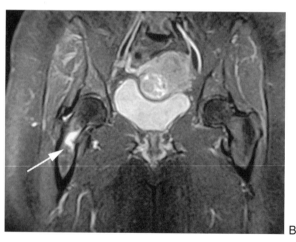

FIG. 18-9. Stress fracture of the proximal femur. A: Coronal T1-weighted spin-echo image. **B:** Coronal fast short tau inversion recovery (STIR) image. **C:** Axial fast STIR image. The T1-weighted image **(A)** demonstrates a well-circumscribed low signal intensity lesion that could be easily mistaken for metastasis (*arrow*). However, on closer examination, the bony cortex is intact over this lesion, even though it appears somewhat thickened. The STIR images **(B,C)** demonstrate a well-circumscribed high-signal-intensity lesion along the medial aspect of the bony cortex (*arrows*). Note that the high signal intensity does not extend into the surrounding soft tissues. When faced with a patient with severe hip pain and a solitary lesion, it is important to include stress fracture in the differential diagnosis and obtain follow-up images to evaluate the progress of this lesion.

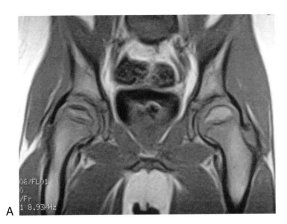

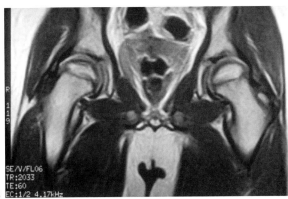

FIG. 18-10. Legg-Calvé-Perthes disease in an 8-year-old boy. Coronal T1-weighted **(A)** and T2-weighted **(B)** spin-echo images demonstrate asymmetry of the right superior capital femoral epiphysis. The right epiphysis is smaller than the left and also demonstrates subchondral changes of sclerosis. The right femoral head may go on to collapse or fragmentation.

hip pain, identifying OA of the hip, or its absence, allows early institution of appropriate treatment. Articular cartilage changes are best demonstrated on T1-weighted images (see Fig. 18-1). However, secondary findings of OA are extremely useful and readily identified on STIR and T2-weighted

sequences. These changes include subchondral marrow edema, joint space narrowing, subchondral cysts, osteophytes, and subchondral sclerosis.

Marrow edema may be confused with AVN. In AVN, marrow edema involves the normal weight-bearing surface, whereas in OA, edema involves an asymmetric portion of the joint, usually the superior and lateral aspects of the joint. Acetabular surface changes are also helpful in diagnosing OA. However, changes may also be seen in late stages of AVN when superimposed OA is present.

MRI is also used to evaluate a wide range of pathologic changes that involve the pediatric hip. Legg-Calvé-Perthes disease (Fig. 18-10), congenital hip dislocation, and osteomyelitis are all effectively demonstrated with MRI. Open systems are extremely useful in the pediatric population, providing comfort for the child and parent, because the parent may be by the child's side during the examination. The parent's presence reduces the child's anxiety and limits the need for sedation.

REFERENCES

1. Beltran J, Herman LJ, Burk JM, et al. Femoral head avascular necrosis: MR imaging with clinical pathologic and radionuclide correlation. *Radiology* 1988;166:215–220.
2. Mitchell MD, Kundel HL, Steinberg ME, et al. Avascular necrosis of the hip: comparison of MR, CT, and scintigraphy. *AJR Am J Roentgenol* 1986;147:67–71.
3. Wolf CR, Runge VL. Musculoskeletal system. In: Runge VL, ed. *Clinical magnetic resonance imaging.* Philadelphia: Lippincott, 1990: 419–428.
4. Solomon L. Mechanisms of idiopathic osteonecrosis. *Orthop Clin North Am* 1985;16:655–667.
5. Bassett LW, Gold RH, Reicher M, et al. Magnetic resonance imaging in the early diagnosis of ischemic necrosis of the femoral head. *Clin Orthop* 1987;214:237.
6. Mitchell DG, Rao VM, Dalinka MK, et al. Femoral head avascular necrosis: correlation of MR imaging, radiographic staging, radionuclide imaging, and clinical findings. *Radiology* 1987;162:709–715.
7. Bloem JL. Transient osteoporosis of the hip: MR imaging. *Radiology* 1988;167:753–755.
8. Matin P. Bone scintigraphy in the diagnosis and management of traumatic injury. *J Nucl Med* 1983;13:104.

Open MRI,
edited by Peter A. Rothschild and Debra Reinking Rothschild.
Lippincott Williams & Wilkins. Philadelphia © 2000.

CHAPTER 19

Open Magnetic Resonance Imaging of the Knee

Joseph Triolo and Peter A. Rothschild

The knee is probably the easiest of all the musculoskeletal structures to image on open magnetic resonance imaging (MRI) systems. The cylindric-type solenoidal coils are efficient because they can be placed around the knee, which provides an improved signal to noise ratio. Coils for the shoulder are less efficient because the shoulder cannot be encircled in a similar fashion. Furthermore, the knee is easily immobilized to prevent motion artifact, and no significant artifact from adjacent structures occurs. Artifacts, such as ghosting from respiratory motion and aliasing from adjacent anatomic structures, are less problematic when compared to those encountered when imaging the upper extremity.

Although imaging of the knee may be easier than that of the shoulder and upper extremity, pathology of the knee can be more difficult to demonstrate. Meniscal tears and cartilage defects can be subtle lesions, and their detection requires high-resolution imaging. These structures are important because they are critical to the weight-bearing function of the knee. Cartilage abnormalities are less important to shoulder function, and rotator cuff tears tend to be more conspicuous than meniscal tears. These differences underscore the different approaches to open MRI of the knee and shoulder.

ANATOMY

The knee is a major weight-bearing joint and has the largest articulating surfaces of any joint. The large condyles increase the articulating surface area, and the menisci act as cushions and function to increase the contact between the articulating surfaces of the femoral condyles and tibial plateaus. As a result, careful meniscal and cartilage evaluation is crucial on MRI of the knee.

J. Triolo: Ocean Medical Imaging Center, Community Medical Center, Toms River, New Jersey

P. A. Rothschild: Department of Radiology, University of California, San Francisco, San Francisco, California; Open MRI, Hayward, California; Open MRI, Louisville, Kentucky

Menisci

The medial meniscus has a larger posterior horn than anterior horn, and in cross section, it has a triangular appearance. On sagittal images, the body of the medial meniscus should have a bow-tie appearance (Fig. 19-1). A truncated appearance or deformity of the normal triangular meniscal shape should suggest a tear or postoperative changes. The medial meniscus has a firm attachment to the joint capsule, especially posteriorly. A small potential bursa does exist between the medial collateral ligament (MCL) and the body of the medial meniscus. Signal from fat or a small amount of fluid may be seen in this location. More posteriorly, fluid between the posterior horn of the medial meniscus and the joint capsule should raise concern for meniscocapsular separation (1).

Anteriorly, the transverse ligament, which is not adherent to the joint capsule, joins with the anterior horns of the medial and lateral meniscus. Because the transverse ligament is not adherent to the joint capsule, fluid is normally visualized extending along the transverse ligament (Fig. 19-2). This appearance should not be confused with a tear of the anterior horn of either the medial or lateral meniscus.

The lateral meniscus has anterior and posterior horns that are similar in size and have a triangular shape. The body of the lateral meniscus, like the medial meniscus, should have a bow-tie appearance on sagittal images (Fig. 19-3). The lateral meniscus is more loosely attached to the joint capsule and, posteriorly, the popliteus tendon courses through the joint capsule. Fluid is normally seen extending along the popliteus tendon between the posterior horn of the lateral meniscus and the joint capsule. The anterior horn of the lateral meniscus joins the transverse ligament, and posteriorly, the meniscofemoral ligaments may extend from the posterior horn of the lateral meniscus to the medial femoral condyle (Fig. 19-4). These ligaments can course anterior or posterior to the posterior cruciate ligament (PCL) and should not be confused with a displaced meniscal fragment. One, both, or none of the meniscofemoral ligaments may be present.

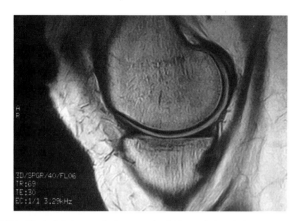

FIG. 19-1. High-resolution sagittal T1-weighted three-dimensional gradient-echo Fourier transformation. The bow-tie appearance of the anterior and posterior horn of the medial meniscus is visualized. The meniscus abuts the articular cartilage along the femoral condyle. The thin black line underlying the articular cartilage is the bony cortex, and below that is the bone marrow with the normal-appearing trabecular pattern.

Cartilage

Three articulating surfaces of the knee exist: the medial and lateral compartments and the patellofemoral joint. These joints are lined with thick hyaline cartilage. Abnormalities of the articular cartilage are important to identify because carti-

lage does not heal particularly well and defects in the articular promote further cartilage injury. Superimposed osteoarthritic changes, with osteophyte proliferation, may also contribute to injury and denude the articular cartilage. Cartilage abnormalities and superimposed osteoarthritis mimic the pain of a meniscal tear.

Numerous pulse sequences are used to evaluate cartilage. Numerous articles in the literature describe the best sequences to evaluate articular cartilage. However, no single sequence is agreed on as the best. On high-field systems, virtually all sequences use chemical fat saturation (2). Proton density–weighted, T2-weighted, and three-dimensional (3D) spoiled gradient reversal echo fat-saturated sequences are most commonly used on high-field systems. On lower field systems, fat saturation is not currently an option, and the 3D gradient-echo (GRE) is probably the best single pulse sequence to evaluate cartilage (Fig. 19-5). However, on lower field systems, all pulse sequences should be used to identify cartilage abnormalities accurately and consistently. If detecting a cartilage defect is an absolute necessity, MR arthrography with intraarticular gadolinium can be extremely helpful (Fig. 19-6).

Cruciate Ligaments

The cruciate ligaments are intracapsular and extrasynovial. The anterior cruciate ligament (ACL) is composed of a smaller anteromedial bundle and a larger posterolateral

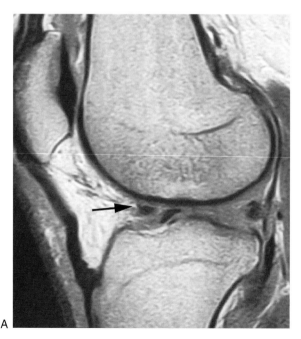

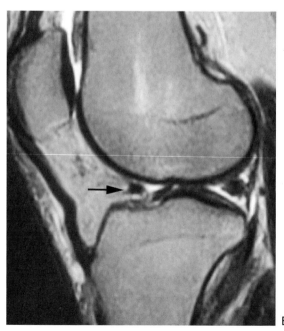

FIG. 19-2. A: Proton density–weighted sagittal image. **B:** Sagittal T2-weighted image. These images demonstrate three black structures in the knee joint. The posterior structure is the posterior horn of the lateral meniscus. The next structure anteriorly is the anterior horn of the lateral meniscus. The next structure anteriorly is the transverse ligament (*arrows*). Fluid can be visualized between the transverse meniscal ligament and the anterior horn of the lateral meniscus on the T2-weighted image. This should not be mistaken for a meniscal tear.

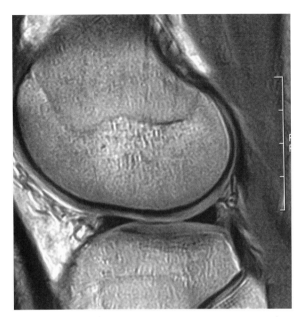

FIG. 19-3. Sagittal T1-weighted three-dimensional gradient-echo image. The anterior and posterior horns of the lateral meniscus are well visualized, giving a bow-tie appearance. The articular cartilage is of normal thickness and signal intensity. The thin black line midway up the femoral condyle is simply the epiphyseal plate and should not be mistaken for a fracture.

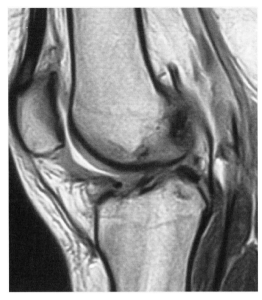

FIG. 19-5. Sagittal T1-weighted two-dimensional spin-echo image with intraarticular contrast. The band of high signal intensity just anterior to the distal femur is intraarticular gadolinium. This contrast nicely delineates the normal contour of the articular cartilage.

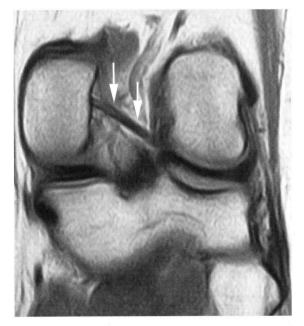

FIG. 19-4. Coronal T1-weighted two-dimensional spin-echo image. The posterior aspects of both the medial and lateral menisci are visualized. The linear band that extends from the posterior medial aspect of the lateral meniscus to the lateral aspect of the medial femoral condyle is the meniscal femoral ligament (*arrows*) and should not be mistaken for pathology.

bundle. The bundles extend from the medial aspect of the lateral femoral condyle and insert on the anteromedial aspect of the intercondylar portion of the tibia. Fluid may course in between and along the bundles, but fluid should not extend vertically through the bundles.

Compared to the ACL, the PCL appears as a thicker, more homogeneous low signal structure, extending from the lateral aspect of the medial femoral condyle to the anterolateral aspect of the intercondylar portion of the tibia. The PCL has a curvilinear orientation with the knee in extension, and its entire course is often visualized on a single sagittal image (Fig. 19-7). The PCL should not demonstrate any signal changes on T2-weighted images.

Collateral Ligaments

The MCL is composed of superficial and deep fibers. The ligament extends from the medial femoral condyle to the proximal medial tibial plateau (Fig. 19-8). Anterior to the MCL, the tendons of the gracilis, sartorius, and semitendinosus form the pes anserinus, which inserts onto the anterior medial tibial plateau. A potential bursa, the pes anserine bursa, may become inflamed and fill with fluid. This may mimic the pain of a medial meniscal tear. Posteriorly, the MCL blends with fibers of the semimembranosus to support the posteromedial corner of the knee.

Laterally, several important tendons need to be identified. Anteriorly, the iliotibial tract attaches to Gerdy's tubercle on the anterolateral tibial plateau (see Fig. 19-8). Portions of the iliotibial tract also form part of the lateral

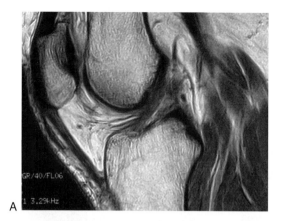

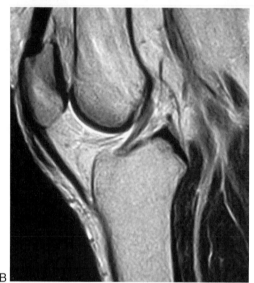

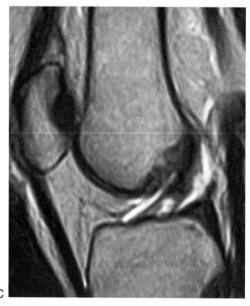

FIG. 19-6. A: Sagittal T1-weighted three-dimensional gradient-echo image. **B:** Sagittal T2-weighted image. **C:** Sagittal T2-weighted image from a different patient. T2-weighted images better delineate the anterior cruciate ligament at lower field strengths. Also, the fluid seen just anterior to the anterior cruciate ligament adds contrast, which improves visualization of the anterior cruciate ligament.

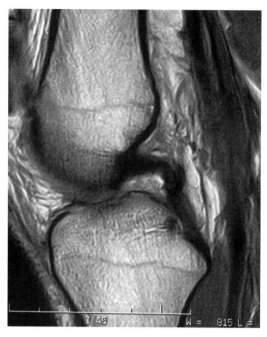

FIG. 19-7. Sagittal T1-weighted three-dimensional gradient-echo image. The posterior cruciate ligament is visualized in its entirety and is normal. Depending on positioning of the knee, it is not uncommon to see slight buckling of the posterior cruciate ligament, as in this case.

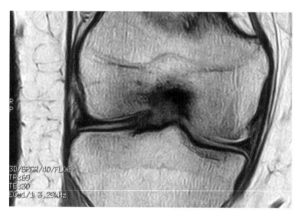

FIG. 19-8. Coronal T1-weighted three-dimensional (3D) gradient-echo image. The medial collateral ligament is demonstrated as a thin black band extending from the superior portion of the medial femoral condyle to the medial aspect of the tibial plateau. Also identified along the lateral aspect of the knee joint is a somewhat thicker band that extends inferiorly and attaches to the lateral tibial plateau; this is the iliotibial band. The 3D T1 images nicely demonstrate the tibial plateau articular cartilage.

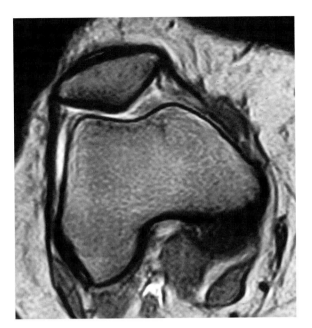

FIG. 19-9. Axial T2-weighted two-dimensional gradient-echo (GRE) image of the patella. A small amount of joint fluid is present, and narrowing of the patellofemoral joint is consistent with mild patellofemoral degenerative changes. The medial and lateral patellar retinacula are normal and well visualized on these GRE images.

retinaculum. Laterally, the fibular collateral ligament (FCL), which arises from the lateral femoral condyle, joins the biceps femoris tendons to form a common tendinous attachment on the fibular head. Posteriorly, the popliteus tendon courses through the joint capsule, posterior and lateral to the lateral meniscus, and inserts on the lateral femoral condyle, near the origin of the FCL. The popliteus tendon, joint capsule with the arcuate ligament (focally thickened portion of the capsule), and the lateral gastrocnemius muscle stabilize the posterolateral corner of the knee (3).

The extensor mechanism includes the quadriceps tendon, the patellar tendon, and the medial and lateral retinaculum (Fig. 19-9). The quadriceps muscle group forms a common quadriceps tendon, which extends around the sesamoid-like patella, to form the patellar tendon. The patellar tendon attaches to the tibial tubercle. The medial and lateral retinaculum maintains the position of the patella through the motions of flexion and extension. The hamstring muscle group includes the sartorius, gracilis, semimembranosus, semitendinosus, and biceps femoris muscles. These muscles function to flex the knee.

TECHNIQUE

When approaching an MRI examination of the knee, attention should first be paid to evaluating the menisci. Pain related to meniscal tears can be confused with many entities,

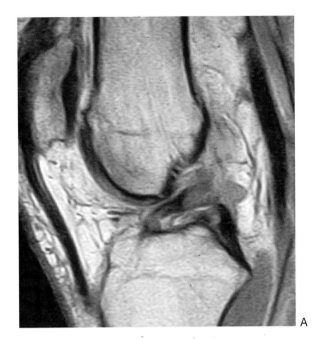

A

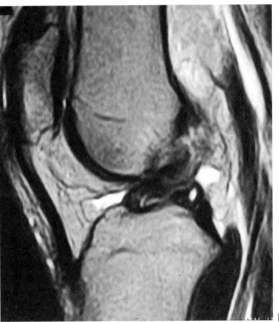

B

FIG. 19-10. A: Sagittal proton density–weighted spin-echo image. **B:** Sagittal T2-weighted spin-echo image. The anterior cruciate ligament is almost horizontal in position instead of its normal vertical course. The proximal portion of the anterior cruciate ligament is not visualized and consistent with a complete tear of the femoral attachment.

such as osteoarthritis, pes anserine bursitis, ganglia, and chondromalacia. Furthermore, complications of meniscal tears, such as meniscal cysts and displaced fragments, are important to recognize.

A high-resolution proton density– or T1-weighted scan should be performed in the sagittal oblique and coronal planes. The sagittal oblique plane is best angled at approxi-

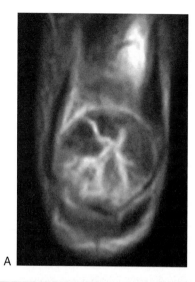

A

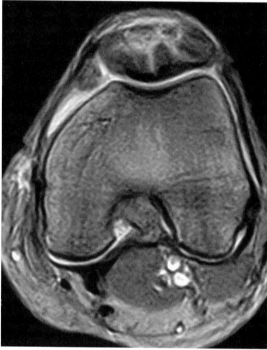

B

FIG. 19-11. A: Coronal fast short tau inversion recovery image through the patella. B: Axial T2-weighted gradient-echo image. Multiple linear high-signal-intensity bands extend through the patella, reaching a cortical surface, which is consistent with a complex fracture of the patella.

mately 5 to 10 degrees medially to better demonstrate the ACL. A field of view of 16 cm or less with a matrix of at least 256 (frequency) × 192 (phase) should be used. Slice thickness should be 4 mm or less with a skip of 1 mm or less. Routine spin-echo (SE) sequences are most commonly used. Fast (or turbo) spin-echo (FSE) sequences with proton density or T1 weighting tend to produce blurring artifact related to wide echo spacing. Even on high-field systems, SE sequences are usually preferred when evaluating the menisci to prevent the

blurring artifact that occurs with FSE at lower echo times (TEs). With lower field strengths, the lower bandwidths result in longer sampling times and longer TEs, which further widens the echo spacing and increases blurring artifact.

Sagittal T2-weighted images are essential for evaluating the cruciate ligaments, large meniscal tears, meniscal cysts, meniscocapsular separation, marrow edema, and paraarticular collections. The angled sagittal slices help to identify the proximal attachment of the ACL, which is a common site for an ACL tear (Fig. 19-10). Frequency direction should be anterior to posterior to prevent artifact from popliteal vessel pulsation. FSE sequences are extremely useful because multiple echoes can be acquired from a single repetition time, significantly decreasing scan time. TEs should be above 100 ms, preferably approximately 120 ms, which would provide heavy T2 weighting and minimize the effects of blurring artifact on FSE images.

An fast short tau inversion recovery (STIR) sequence (fast STIR) is an essential part of any musculoskeletal protocol on lower field systems. STIR sequences can overcome many of the disadvantages lower field open systems face because chemical fat saturation techniques are not currently available. STIR is extremely helpful in evaluating bone marrow pathology, ligament injury, and soft tissue abnormalities. These sequences are best performed in the coronal plane, which is helpful in identifying bone contusions and collateral ligament injuries. The field of view should be increased to 18 or 20 cm, which not only improves signal but also allows for greater coverage of the lower femur and proximal tibia. The inversion time should not be chosen at the exact null point of fat, because this will result in noisy images. At 0.2 T, 70 to 75 ms is a useful inversion time. Also, choosing a slightly longer TE not only adds T2 weighting, it also minimizes the blurring artifact on FSE images (Fig. 19-11). Shorter echo trains of 4 to 6 also help to tighten the echo spacing and decrease blurring artifact.

An axial pulse sequence is the most helpful plane when evaluating the patellar cartilage. This plane can also provide useful information on cruciate ligament, collateral ligament, and retinacular injury. A 3D GRE sequence is probably the most useful, because it best demonstrates the patellar cartilage. These T1-weighted images can be performed with high resolution. A two-dimensional GRE sequence is also useful for evaluating patellar cartilage, especially when a joint effusion is present, which provides an arthrographic effect (Fig. 19-12). The T2-weighted GRE image has the added benefit over T1-weighted images for better visualization of a cruciate ligament or a retinaculum injury. However, in younger patients with knee pain, a 3D GRE in the axial plane is the sequence of choice to evaluate for chondromalacia.

Meniscal Pathology

Meniscal tears can be described as vertical, horizontal, and radial. Meniscal tears are identified as a signal focus extend-

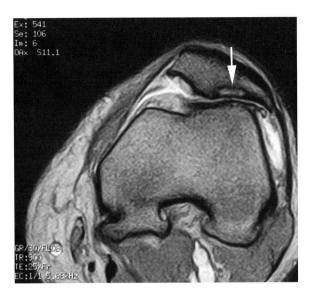

FIG. 19-12. Axial two-dimensional gradient-echo image. The patellofemoral joint is extremely narrowed, and essentially no articular cartilage is seen along the lateral facet of the patella. A thin area of high signal intensity is identified just below the bony cortex (*arrow*), which is consistent with extensive chondromalacia, grade IV.

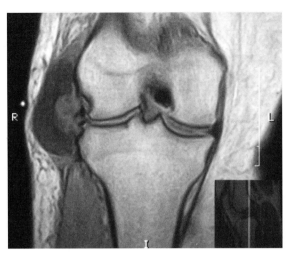

FIG. 19-14. Coronal T1-weighted three-dimensional gradient-echo image. The lateral meniscus is subluxed laterally, a band of (increased) signal intensity extends laterally through the meniscus, and a large parameniscal cyst is present. This patient presented with a knee mass. Large parameniscal cysts can mimic knee tumors clinically.

ing to an articular surface (Fig. 19-13) (4). Visualizing articular extension on two or more slices gives more confidence in the diagnosis. Furthermore, visualizing high signal fluid on T2-weighted images suggests the diagnosis, because degenerative changes should not contain fluid signal. Secondary signs

that indicate a meniscal tear include fluid surrounding the entire meniscus on T2 images, a deformity ("notch sign") along the articular surface of the meniscus, truncated appearance of the meniscus, complete replacement of the menisci with increased signal, and an associated meniscal cyst (Fig. 19-14). These findings suggest the diagnosis of a meniscal tear when meniscal signal itself is inconclusive.

Complications of meniscal tears include displaced meniscal fragments and meniscal cysts (Fig. 19-15). Bucket handle (flap) tears are vertically oriented, and displaced fragments may extend into the intercondylar notch, anterior to the PCL (double PCL sign). Bucket handle tears of the lateral meniscus tend to result in a "flipped meniscus," in which the posterior horn flips anteriorly and results in the "double meniscus sign" (5).

A discoid meniscus is a deformed, globular-appearing meniscus. Many variations of the shape of a discoid meniscus occur, in which the whole meniscus or a portion of the meniscus is abnormally enlarged. Discoid meniscus more commonly involves the lateral meniscus, is more common in men, and usually presents in the early adult years (6). The discoid meniscus has a higher incidence of tears than normal menisci (Fig. 19-16).

Meniscocapsular separation can be detected by identifying fluid between the medial meniscus and joint capsule. Between the MCL and body of the medial meniscus is a small bursa that may contain fluid or fat and should not be misinterpreted as meniscocapsular separation. The posterior horn of the medial meniscus has a firm capsular attachment, and fluid should not extend to this space. Posteriorly and laterally, recesses from the intercondylar region may carry fluid to the intercondylar edge of the posterior horn, and this should not be misinterpreted as meniscocapsular separation.

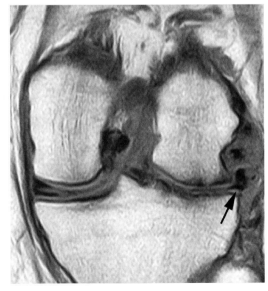

FIG. 19-13. Coronal T1-weighted spin-echo image. The linear area of signal in the medial meniscus reaches a free surface and is consistent with a tear. Narrowing of the articular cartilage and associated degenerative changes in the lateral compartment are seen. Lateral subluxation of a degenerated abnormal lateral meniscus is also demonstrated (*arrow*).

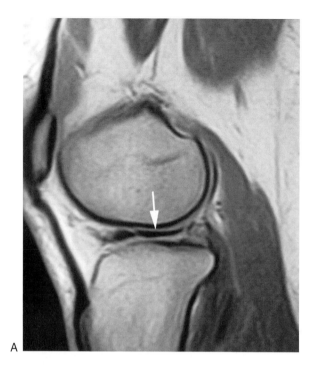

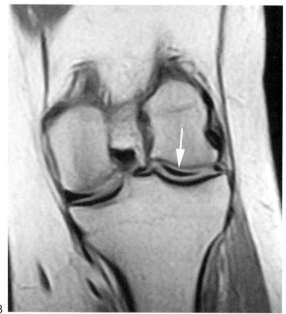

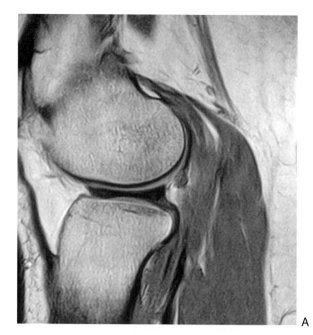

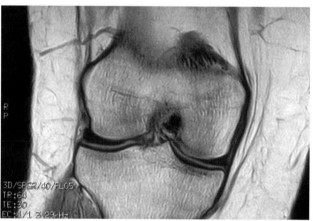

FIG. 19-16. A: Sagittal T1-weighted three-dimensional (3D) gradient-echo (GRE) image. **B:** Coronal T1-weighted 3D GRE image. These images demonstrate a discoid lateral meniscus. Before making this diagnosis, one must review the T2-weighted images to make sure that this is not joint fluid giving the appearance of a discoid meniscus.

FIG. 19-15. A: Sagittal proton density–weighted two-dimensional image demonstrates three black structures in the joint space. The structure anteriorly is the anterior horn. The long structure in the middle is the flap (*arrow*) of the posterior horn, which has flipped anteriorly. The small black structure posteriorly in the joint space is the slim remnant of the posterior horn. **B:** Coronal T2 proton density–weighted image demonstrates this flap tear interposed between the femoral condyle and tibial plateau (*arrow*). Proton density– and T2-weighted images are crucial because on T1-weighted three-dimensional images, fluid in the knee has the same signal intensity as the meniscus. Therefore, one must be extremely diligent in comparing the T1 with proton density and T2 images to accurately identify flap-type tears.

The lateral meniscus is loosely attached to the joint capsule. Fluid often extends between the lateral meniscus and the joint capsule, especially posteriorly, where the popliteus tendon courses through the joint capsule. The FCL and iliotibial band do not have a meniscal attachment.

Cruciate Ligaments

The cruciate ligaments are easier to evaluate than the menisci. The sagittal images should be angled 5 to 15 degrees to better visualize the ACL as it extends from lateral to medial. Fluid may extend between the bundles of the

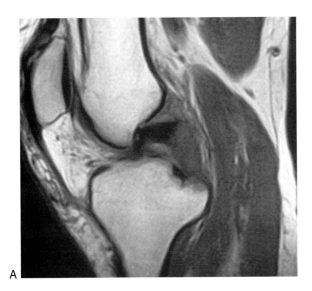

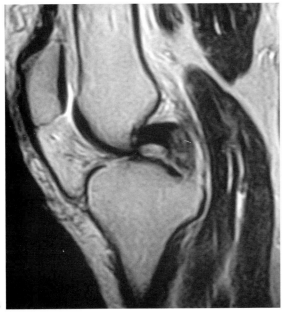

FIG. 19-17. A: Sagittal T1-weighted two-dimensional (2D) spin-echo image. **B:** Sagittal T2-weighted 2D spin-echo image. Only the proximal posterior cruciate ligament has normal low signal intensity on both the T1- and T2-weighted images. The mid and distal portion of the posterior cruciate ligament is abnormal in contour and signal intensity, consistent with a posterior cruciate ligament tear.

ACL, and this should not be confused with a partial tear or hemorrhage. Findings that may be seen with an ACL tear include fluid signal extending horizontally through the entire width of the ACL; a change in the orientation of the fiber of the ACL (a more horizontal course), which suggests a tear at the femoral attachment; and a lack of visualization of the ACL (see Fig. 19-10) (7). Tears are most often intrasubstance or occur at the femoral attachment. Tibial attachment tears are less frequent, because the ACL has a broad

attachment onto the tibial surface. Tibial attachment ACL tears are more frequently seen in adolescent patients.

PCL tears are less common than ACL tears. Various mechanisms of injury exist, but PCL tears usually result when the knee is flexed and the tibia is forced posteriorly. The PCL is more readily visualized on T2-weighted sagittal images as a thick homogeneous low signal structure. Tears of the PCL are more conspicuous than those of the ACL, because no fluid or edema should be seen within the substance of the PCL (Fig. 19-17). The tendon should have a normal curvilinear orientation and should not be abnormally thickened. Most PCL tears are intrasubstance, but avulsion can occur at the tibial or femoral attachment sites (8).

Collateral Ligaments

MCL tears are often categorized as grade 1, 2, or 3. Grade 1 strains show edematous changes, grade 2 strains show more extensive edematous changes with partial tearing, and grade 3 strains demonstrate a complete tear with retraction (Fig. 19-18).

Tears more commonly involve the superficial fibers than the deep fibers and are more frequent near the femoral attachment. Although isolated MCL tears may be seen with valgus stress of the knee, many associated findings may be seen with MCL tears (9). Associated findings include tears of one or both menisci, ACL or PCL tears, and femoral condylar or tibial plateau contusions.

The lateral ligaments include the biceps femoris tendon, the FCL, popliteus tendon, and iliotibial band. These tendons are less frequently injured when compared to the medial, especially as an isolated injury (10). Injuries to the lateral ligaments are more frequently associated with other injuries, such as ACL or MCL tears.

Extensor Mechanism

The quadriceps tendon is formed by the rectus femoris muscle and the three vastus muscles, medialis, lateralis, and intermedius. Complete quadriceps tears are very uncommon, and injuries tend to involve only a portion of the large tendon. The injury is usually the result of forced flexion and tends to occur at the myotendinous junction. Tears at the more distal patellar attachment tend to have an associated avulsion of the superior pole of the patella.

The patellar tendon is often affected by tendinitis but may also be torn. Partial tears at the proximal patellar attachment are seen in athletes who undertake repetitive jumping maneuvers (Fig. 19-19). The patellar tendon less commonly tears at the attachment to the tibial tubercle because this is a broad attachment.

The medial and lateral retinaculum maintain the position of the patella during flexion and extension. The medial retinaculum is supported by the vastus medialis muscle, and the lateral retinaculum is supported by the vastus lateralis

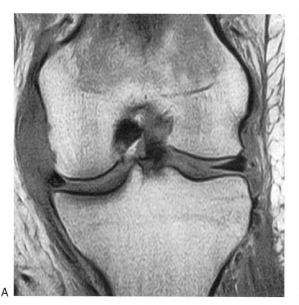
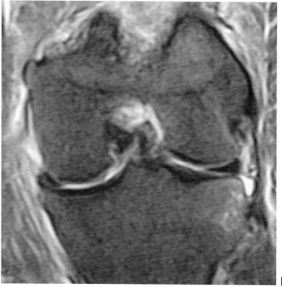

FIG. 19-18. A: Coronal T1-weighted two-dimensional spin-echo image demonstrates extensive soft tissue just medial to the femoral condyle. This is a combination of edema and granulation tissue. **B:** Coronal fast short tau inversion recovery (STIR) image nicely demonstrates the remnant of the proximal medial collateral ligament (MCL) and shows the area of tear of the MCL.

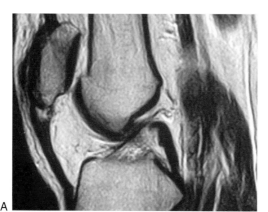
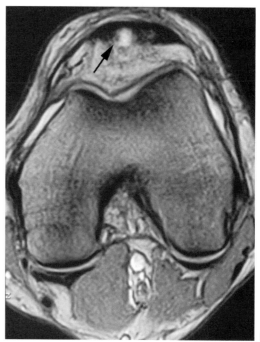
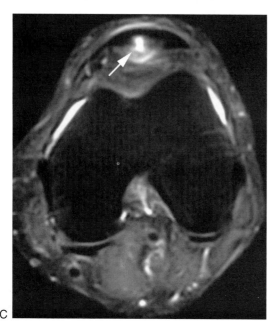

FIG. 19-19. A: Sagittal T2-weighted spin-echo image. **B:** Axial T2-weighted gradient-echo image. **C:** Axial fast short tau inversion recovery (STIR) image demonstrates increased signal intensity in the patellar tendon just inferior to the patella in the region of the insertion (*arrow*). It also demonstrates a linear area of increased signal intensity in the mid-tendon consistent with a small partial tear and associated acute tendinitis "jumper's knee" (*arrow*). These partial tendon tears (*arrows*) most often involve the proximal fibers of the patellar tendon and occur in athletes such as basketball players. STIR imaging is clearly the superior method to detect tendinitis or other processes in and around the knee joint.

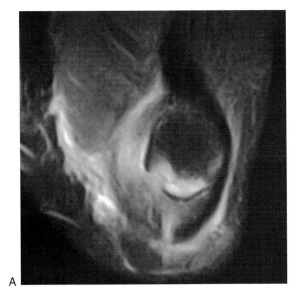

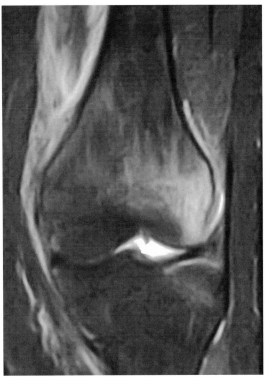

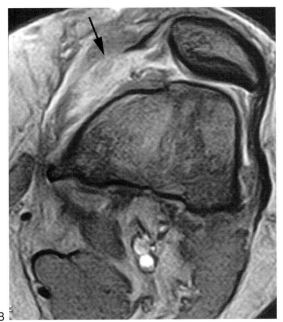

FIG. 19-20. A: Coronal fast short tau inversion recovery (STIR) image. **B:** Axial T2-weighted gradient-echo image. **C:** Coronal fast STIR image. These images demonstrate a complete tear of the medial retinaculum of the patella with femoral bone contusions/osteochondral fracture from lateral subluxation of the patella. An osteochondral fracture is identified along the medial and inferior aspect of the patella **(A)**, and the lateral femoral condyle bone contusion is identified on the coronal STIR **(C)**. The disruption in the medial retinaculum with fluid interspersed where the patellar retinaculum should be located is identified in **B** (*arrow*). Residual lateral tilting and subluxation to the patella are present.

and iliotibial tract. The lateral supporting structures are stronger than the medial structures, and the medial femoral condyle is larger than the lateral condyle. As a result, lateral dislocations occur more frequently than medial dislocations, and the medial retinaculum is more frequently torn (Fig. 19-20) (11).

Cartilage

Evaluating the articular cartilage is an essential part of a knee MRI examination. This is challenging on lower field open systems, which currently are not able to perform fat saturation techniques. Cartilage signal must be separated from the signal of joint fluid and from the signal of the underlying cortex and bone marrow. As a result, the combination of several pulse sequences must be used to reliably identify cartilage defects (Fig. 19-21).

On open MRI, the 3D GRE sequence is probably the single best pulse sequence to evaluate cartilage. However, limitations exist to its T1 weighting. On GRE sequences, fluid is very low in signal intensity (dark), whereas cartilage is increased in signal, and the underlying cortex is low signal on all pulse sequences. However, in the absence of a joint effusion, it may be difficult to separate the higher signal cartilage from adjacent fibro-fatty tissue. Another disadvantage of the GRE sequence is that subchondral marrow changes, such as cystic changes or marrow edema, can sometimes be

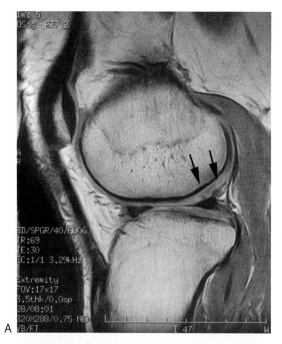

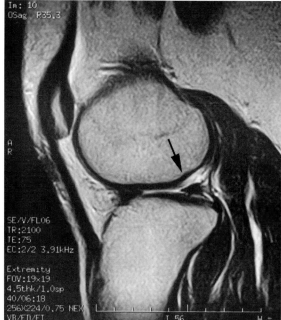

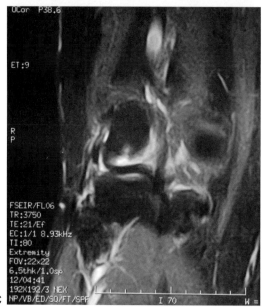

FIG. 19-21. A: Sagittal T1-weighted three-dimensional gradient-echo image shows mild thickening and low signal intensity in the femoral articular cartilage overlying the posterior horn of the lateral meniscus (*arrows*). **B:** Sagittal T2-weighted spin-echo image shows this area of articular cartilage to be edematous and becomes bright (*arrow*). **C:** Coronal fast short tau inversion recovery (STIR) image demonstrates an area of grade I chondromalacia of the femoral condyle and the medial lateral extent of the chondromalacia. The lower field strengths used in open magnetic resonance imaging present distinct advantages when evaluating the articular cartilage because susceptibility artifact from the bony cortex is not as much of a problem at lower field strengths. Therefore, the articular cartilage appears much closer to its true thickness and is easier to evaluate. One of the most common areas overlooked by radiologists interpreting knee images are subtle areas of chondromalacia, which are easily identified and treated by the orthopedic surgeon. Extreme diligence and high-resolution images are needed to evaluate the entire joint cartilage—not just of the patellar cartilage but also of the femoral and tibial cartilage for chondromalacia.

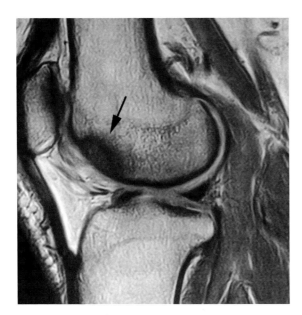

FIG. 19-22. Sagittal T1-weighted three-dimensional gradient-echo images demonstrate a large area of osteonecrosis along the anterior aspect of the lateral femoral condyle (*arrow*). These lesions are easily identified on the high-resolution T1-weighted images.

difficult to identify on a T1-weighted image. This may be the only indication of a cartilage abnormality. T1-weighted images also provide little information with regard to other abnormalities, such as ligament or soft tissue pathology.

T2-weighted images can be very useful in evaluating cartilage when fluid is present, because the joint effusion provides an arthrographic effect. Fluid extending through

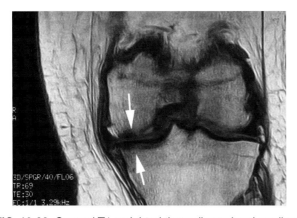

FIG. 19-23. Coronal T1-weighted three-dimensional gradient-echo image demonstrates severe joint space narrowing and degenerative changes in the medial compartment with medial subluxation of a degenerated and torn medial meniscus. It is easy to compare the thickness of the articular cartilage in the medial compartment (*arrows*) with the relatively normal thickness of the articular cartilage in the lateral compartment.

an area of articular cartilage to the underlying cortex is a clear indication of a cartilage defect. Subchondral edema and cystic changes are also easily identified on T2-weighted images.

Osteochondral lesions can involve any cartilaginous surface. The size of the lesion and the potential for an unstable fragment should be noted. Joint fluid extending into the osteochondral lesion suggests the possibility that the lesion may become loose and result in an intraarticular body. This finding is best identified on T2-weighted or STIR sequences, in which fluid is bright.

Osteochondritis dissecans (OD) and osteonecrosis are two entities that can be identified when imaging the knee. OD most commonly occurs on the lateral aspect of the medial femoral condyle. OD is more commonly seen in younger patients. Even though it is most likely posttraumatic in etiology, patients may not be symptomatic (Fig. 19-22) (12).

Osteonecrosis most commonly is seen in the elderly and in women. No history of injury is associated; nevertheless, patients are often symptomatic with a sudden onset of pain and tenderness. Osteonecrosis involves the weight-bearing surface of the knee with the medial femoral condyle being the most common location, although any weight-bearing surface may be involved (Fig. 19-23). Many of these patients have an associated meniscal tear or superimposed osteoarthritis (1). Osteonecrosis may "burn-out" over time and not show any marrow edema, suggesting an old area of necrosis. Acute changes of spontaneous osteonecrosis demonstrate subchondral marrow edema, which should not be confused with subchondral marrow edema from osteoarthritis.

Stability of the fragments in both osteonecrosis and OD should be assessed. Larger fragments or fluid extending into and out of an osteochondral lesion should raise concern for an unstable fragment. Cartilage defects and loose osteochondral fragments result in progressive osteoarthritic changes.

Marrow Pathology

A wide range of pathology affects the bone marrow. Fast STIR sequences are the most sensitive for marrow pathology. Fast STIR uses the same principle on high- and low-field systems, taking advantage of the difference in relaxation times of fat and water. Because separating signal from fat and water does not depend on their resonant frequencies, fast STIR can be successfully performed on lower field open systems.

Marrow pathology is seen in a wide range of disease processes. The most common setting is osteoarthritis, in which subchondral marrow edema and subchondral cystic changes are present. Contusions are also frequently seen in a subchondral location but may have a rounded appearance and can be at any subcortical site. Marrow edema associated with stress fractures tends to occur in weaker areas of bone,

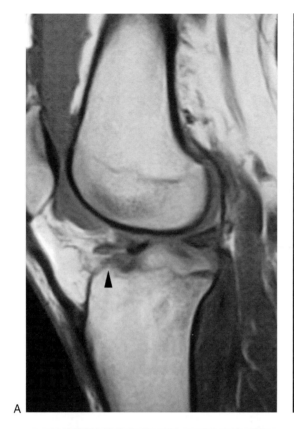

A

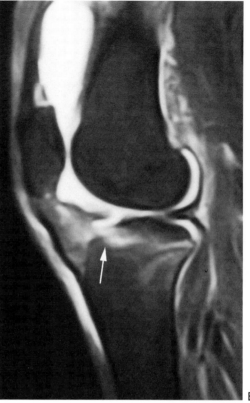

B

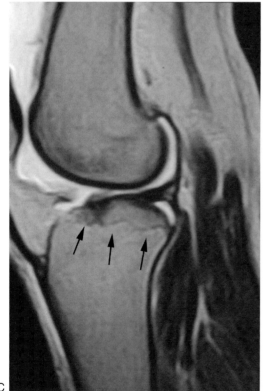

C

FIG. 19-24. A: Sagittal T1-weighted two-dimensional spin-echo image. **B:** Sagittal fast short tau inversion recovery (STIR) image. **C:** Sagittal T2-weighted spin-echo image demonstrates a fracture of the tibial plateau (*arrows*). Tibial plateau fractures are often missed on plain film and are very easily identified on T1 and STIR images. However, on the T2 spin-echo images, these fractures can be very subtle. Therefore, STIR images should be standard in the extremities for identifying fractures and bone contusions. Note that the break in the cortex (**A**, *arrowhead;* **B**, *arrow*) is also easily identified on the T1 and STIR images.

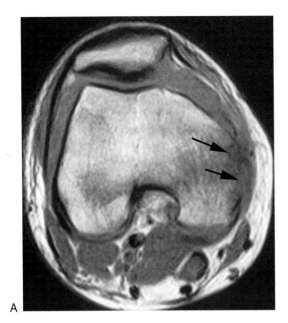

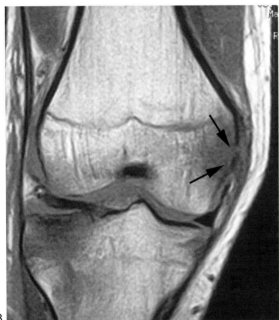

FIG. 19-25. A: Axial T1-weighted two-dimensional (2D) spin-echo image. **B:** Coronal T1-weighted 2D spin-echo image demonstrates an avulsion fracture of the medial aspect of the medial femoral condyle with associated bone contusion of the lateral tibial plateau. **A,B:** Magnetic resonance imaging shows a loss of the normal black cortex (*arrows*). It is important to follow the black band of the bony cortex along any area of bone contusion to identify a break in the cortex that would suggest an osteochondral fracture. At lower field strength, bone contusions are also easily identified on the T1-weighted images.

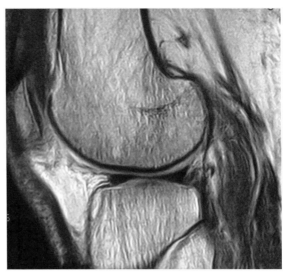

FIG. 19-26. Sagittal T1-weighted three-dimensional image demonstrates severe osteoporosis. This prominent trabecular pattern seen in the distal femur and proximal tibia on these high-resolution T1-weighted images should not be confused for a bone contusion or marrow-replacing process.

such as diametaphyseal locations, and not in the enlarged articulating areas of the femoral condyles or tibial plateaus. Trabecular microfractures demonstrate a linear orientation of the marrow edema, and the trabecular disruption is best demonstrated on T1-weighted SE or 3D SPGR images (Figs. 19-24 and 19-25). Fractures extending to cortical or intraarticular locations are best demonstrated on T1-weighted images. All of these marrow changes can be nicely demonstrated on open MRI. By understanding the pattern of marrow edema, the appropriate diagnosis is easily reached.

Marrow replacement, as seen with metastatic disease, tends to have more geographic areas of involvement (Fig. 19-26). Cortical destruction and periosteal reaction may be seen and can help to suggest a more aggressive process (Fig. 19-27). Bone sclerosis that may be seen with chronic osteomyelitis or bone-producing tumor (i.e., osteosarcomas) can also be readily identified on lower field open systems as low signal foci on both T1 and fast STIR sequences.

Articular and Paraarticular Fluid Collections

Within the joint, ganglia are typically associated with the cruciate ligaments or, anteriorly, extending from the alar folds into Hoffa's fat pad (13). These are easily identified on T2-weighted images. The ganglia associated with the alar fold are clinically important, because they may mimic symptoms of a meniscal tear.

Baker's cyst or synovial cysts are also easily identified on T2-weighted or fast STIR sequences. Debris or associated osseous bodies should be described. Prepatellar bursitis, pes anserine bursitis, and iliotibial band friction syndrome or

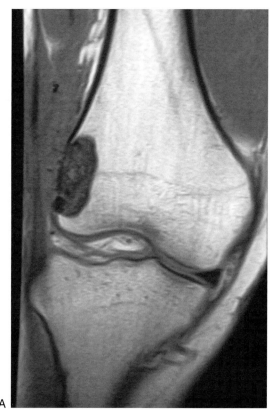
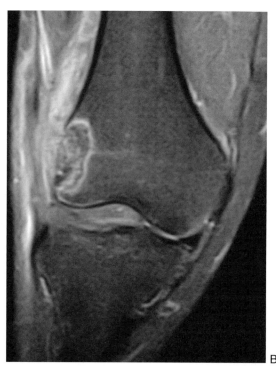

A

B

FIG. 19-27. A: Coronal T1-weighted two-dimensional spin-echo image. **B:** Coronal fast short tau inversion recovery (STIR) image demonstrates an approximately 3-cm bone tumor that is associated with a break in the bony cortex and extension of high signal intensity into the surrounding soft tissues best identified on the STIR image. The first thought may be a malignant tumor with extension into the surrounding soft tissues; however, this patient has recently undergone biopsy for benign enchondroma. Whenever evaluating an image, especially of a bone tumor, it is crucial to have an accurate history for any type of invasive procedure. Courtesy of General Electric Medical Systems, Inc., Milwaukee, WI.

bursitis all may mimic pain that can be confused with meniscal pathology. These findings can be nicely demonstrated using T2-weighted FSE or fast STIR sequences.

REFERENCES

1. Resnick D, Kang HS. Knee. In: *Internal derangements of joints.* Philadelphia: WB Saunders, 1997:555.
2. McCauley TR, Kier R, Lynch KJ, et al. Chondromalacia patellae: diagnosis with MR imaging. *AJR Am J Roentgenol* 1992;158:101.
3. De Lee JC, Riley MB, Rockwood CA Jr. Acute posterolateral rotary instability of the knee. *Am J Sports Med* 1983;11:199.
4. Stoller DW, Martin C, Crues JV III, et al. Meniscal tears: pathologic correlation with MR imaging. *Radiology* 1987;163:731.
5. Wright DH, DeSmet AA, Noris M. Bucket-handle tears of the medial and lateral menisci of the knee: value of MR imaging in detecting displaced fragments. *AJR Am J Roentgenol* 1995;165:621.
6. Nathan PA, Cole SC. Discoid meniscus—a clinical and pathologic study. *Clin Orthop* 1969;64:107.
7. Vahey TN, Broome DR, Kaye KJ, et al. Acute and chronic tears of the anterior cruciate ligament: differential features at MR imaging. *Radiology* 1991;181:251.
8. DeLee JC, Bergfeld JA, Drez D Jr, et al. The posterior cruciate ligament. In: De Lee JC, Drez D Jr, eds. *Orthopaedic sports medicine: principles and practice.* Philadelphia: WB Saunders, 1994:1374.
9. Schweitzer M, Tran D, Deely D. Medial collateral ligament injuries. *Radiology* 1995;194:825.
10. Ruiz ME, Erickson SJ. Medial and lateral supporting structures of the knee: normal MR imaging anatomy and pathologic findings. *Magn Reson Imag Clin North Am* 1994;2:381.
11. Lance E, Deutsch AL, Mink JH. Prior lateral patellar dislocation: MR imaging findings. *Radiology* 1993;189:905.
12. Schenck RC Jr, Goodnight JM. Osteochondritis desiccans. *J Bone Joint Surg [Am]* 1996;78:439.
13. Brown MF, Dandy DJ. Intra-articular ganglions of the knee. *J Arthrosc Rel Res* 1990;6:322.

Open MRI,
edited by Peter A. Rothschild and Debra Reinking Rothschild.
Lippincott Williams & Wilkins. Philadelphia © 2000.

CHAPTER 20

Open Magnetic Resonance Imaging of the Ankle

Joseph Triolo and Peter A. Rothschild

Although claustrophobia is not a significant problem when imaging the ankle on a closed magnet, anxious or very large patients often request the open system when they need a magnetic resonance imaging (MRI) examination of the ankle. Patients may even find an ankle MRI examination enjoyable, because they can read a book or magazine during the examination. This experience may also build the patients' comfort with open MRI systems, which may prove helpful if the patient needs to return for a more difficult MRI study, such as a cervical spine or shoulder examination.

Quality imaging of the ankle can be successfully performed on open MRI systems using a standard extremity coil, but better image quality can be obtained using a dedicated small parts coil. Additionally, the ankle can be easily immobilized to prevent motion artifact, and significant artifact from aliasing or ghosting is rarely a problem.

ANATOMY

Osseous

The osseous structures of the ankle have complex articulations to provide weight-bearing functions and a wide range of motion. The tibiotalar joint has a large articular surface, with the ankle mortise formed by the tibial plafond and medial and lateral malleolus (Fig. 20-1). The subtalar joint consists of a posterior talocalcaneal articulation and an anterior talocalcaneonavicular articulation (Figs. 20-2 and 20-3). A supporting middle facet adds to stability of the subtalar joint and is formed by the medial talocalcaneal ligament

joining the medial tubercle of the posterior of the talus with the sustentaculum tali portion of the calcaneus.

The midfoot also has complex articulations, with multiple connecting ligaments joining the hindfoot (talus and calcaneus) with the navicular and cuboid bones. The cuneiform and cuboid, considered part of the midfoot, articulate with the metatarsals. The cuboid bone articulates with the fourth and fifth metatarsals.

Ligaments

Ligaments that support the lateral ankle mortise include the anterior and posterior talofibular ligaments (ATFL and PTFL) and the calcaneofibular ligament (CFL) (Fig. 20-4). The distal tibiofibular syndesmosis is maintained by the interosseous ligament and the anterior, posterior, and transverse tibiofibular ligaments.

Medially, the deltoid ligament is a broad fan-shaped ligament composed of deep and superficial fibers. The deltoid ligament has strong attachments to navicular bone and sustentaculum, as well as to the anterior and posterior aspects of the talus. Other important ligaments of the foot include the spring ligament (plantar calcaneonavicular ligament) and the interosseous talocalcaneal ligaments, which course through the sinus tarsi.

Tendons

The tendons can be divided into three compartments. The anterior compartment contains the tibialis anterior, the extensor digitorum longus, and extensor hallucis longus tendons. A small peroneal tertius muscle is also present, coursing just lateral to the extensor digitorum longus muscle and tendon. Posteriorly, essentially two compartments are found: (a) A superficial posterior compartment contains the Achilles tendon and (b) more medially, the deep posterior compartment

J. Triolo: Ocean Medical Imaging Center, Community Medical Center, Toms River, New Jersey

P. A. Rothschild: Department of Radiology, University of California, San Francisco, San Francisco, California; Open MRI, Hayward, California; Open MRI, Louisville, Kentucky

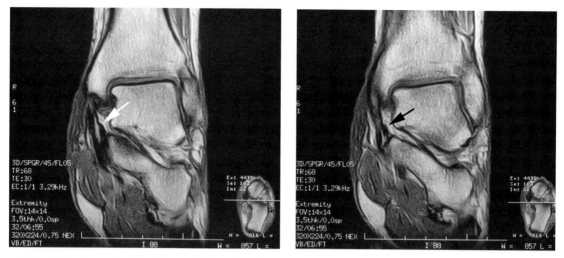

FIG. 20-1. Normal ankle. Coronal T1-weighted three-dimensional gradient-echo image demonstrates normal articular cartilage. The deltoid ligament (*arrows*) and interosseous ligaments are well visualized.

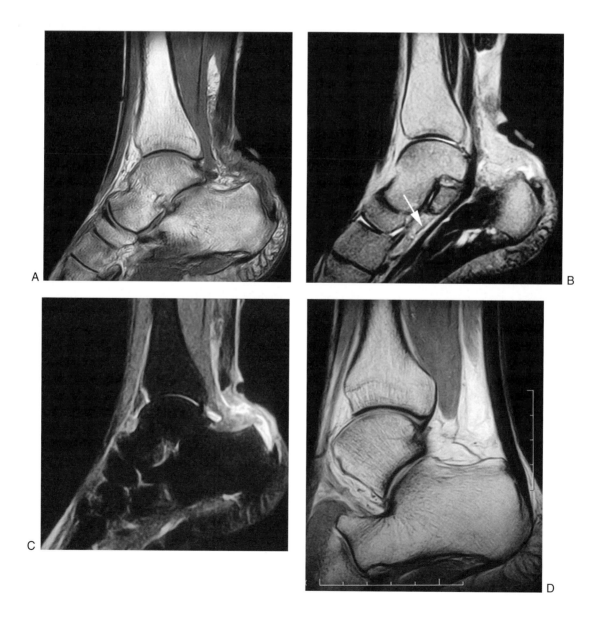

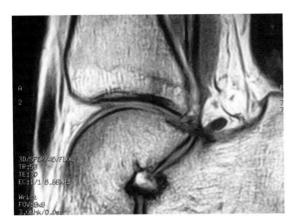

FIG. 20-3. Sagittal high-resolution T1-weighted three-dimensional (3D) gradient-echo image with an 8-cm field of view (FOV) and 3-mm slice thickness. High resolution can be obtained on open magnets using specialized coils and 3D sequences that demonstrate the bony trabecular pattern and show the articular cartilage extremely well. To rule out small areas of chondromalacia, these high-resolution small FOV sequences can be extremely helpful.

contains the posterior tibial tendon (PTT), flexor hallucis longus (FHL), and flexor digitorum longus (FDL) tendons. The PTT has numerous attachments onto the cuneiforms, cuboid, and metatarsals, with the largest and most important attachment to the navicular bone. The FHL is the most posterior and easiest to identify as it courses under the sustentaculum. The FHL also courses through the joint capsule and is commonly surrounded by a small amount of fluid.

The posterior tibial artery and nerve, as well as several veins, are contained within the deep posterior compartment and are located between the FHL and FDL. A flexor retinaculum covers the tendons and neurovascular structures of the deep posterior compartment just below the level of the medial malleolus. This forms the tarsal tunnel. Narrowing of the tarsal tunnel may compress the posterior tibial nerve and result in tarsal tunnel syndrome (1).

Laterally, the peroneus brevis and longus tendons course under the fibula. The peroneus brevis tendon attaches to the base of the fifth metatarsal, and the peroneus longus tendon

◄ **FIG. 20-2.** Normal subtalar joints. **A:** Sagittal T1-weighted three-dimensional (3D) gradient-echo (GRE) image demonstrates the posterior subtalar joint and the anterior talocalcaneonavicular joint. **B:** Sagittal T2-weighted fast spin-echo image demonstrates normal flexor hallucis longus (FHL) tendon extending under the sustentaculum. A small amount of fluid (*arrow*) normally is associated with the FHL. **C:** In a sagittal fast short tau inversion recovery image, a full-thickness Achilles tendon tear with retraction is identified on the same patient. **D:** Sagittal high-resolution T1-weighted 3D GRE image in another patient shows a normal Achilles tendon. With higher resolution, one can obtain better articular cartilage and trabecular definition.

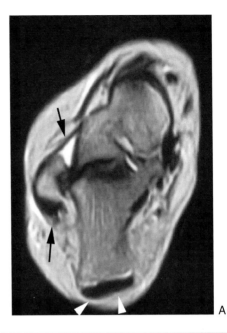

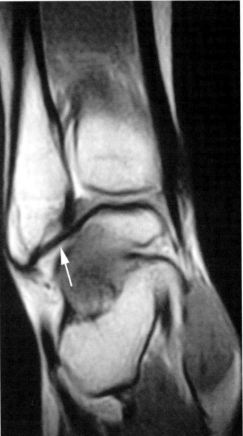

FIG. 20-4. Normal lateral ligaments. **A:** Axial T2-weighted fast spin-echo image demonstrates normal anterior talofibular ligament (*arrow*), normal distal Achilles tendon (*arrowheads*), and normal peroneal tendons coursing posterior to distal fibula (*long arrow*). **B:** Coronal proton density–weighted image demonstrates normal posterior talofibular ligament (*arrow*). *Continued.*

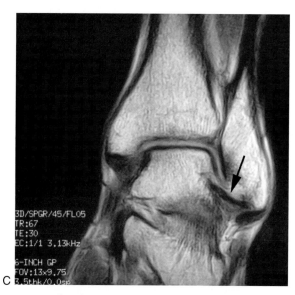

FIG. 20-4. *Continued.* **C:** Coronal T1-weighted three-dimensional gradient-echo image from a different patient nicely demonstrates the posterior talofibular ligament in its entirety (*arrow*). The T2- and T1-weighted images are useful in identifying normal versus pathologic ligamentous anatomy.

courses under the cuboid bone and extends along the bottom of the foot to attach to the base of the first metatarsal.

Along the plantar aspect of the foot, the plantar fascia has attachments to the sides of the first and fifth metatarsals, forming compartments of the great toe, small toe, and central compartment. The plantar aponeurosis, composed of thick fibrous connective tissue, covers the central compartment of the foot. The plantar aponeurosis arises from the inferior calcaneous and extends to each of the five distal digits. The central compartment of the foot consists of the flexor digitorum brevis muscle, tendons of the FDL and FHL, and the quadratus plantae muscles.

TECHNIQUE

Proper positioning of the ankle is important when demonstrating the ligaments of the ankle. Positioning the ankle in slight plantar flexion best demonstrates the ATFL. The axial images should be angled parallel to the talus. Visualization of the PTFL is more difficult, because it blends with the posterior tibiofibular ligament when the ankle is in plantar flexion. The PTFL, however, is a larger and stronger ligament than the ATFL, and PTFL tears rarely occur without the ATFL being initially torn.

Sagittal T1-weighted and fast short tau inversion recovery (STIR) sequences are useful sequences for demonstrating the tarsal bones and their alignment. The peroneal, FHL, and Achilles tendons are also well demonstrated in this plane. The STIR sequence is very sensitive for bone marrow pathology, and the sagittal plane provides the greatest cov-

erage for the least number of slices, which helps reduce scan time. The T1-weighted sequence can be performed with high-resolution technique by using a three-dimensional spoiled gradient-echo (GRE) sequence.

Although many of the tendons can be identified in the sagittal plane, axial images are very useful in identifying tendon pathology, especially when differentiating partial- from full-thickness tears. The sagittal plane is also not very useful when evaluating the ligaments of the ankle, except for the interosseous ligament, which can be identified in the sinus tarsi.

In the axial plane, T2-weighted fast spin-echo (FSE) and STIR are the most useful sequences. T2-weighted FSE provides better resolution than the STIR technique when evaluating the ATFL and Achilles tendon morphology and when identifying the individual tendons of each compartment. STIR images provide useful information when evaluating tears of the PTT and Achilles tendon.

In the coronal plane, T2-weighted FSE images provide the anatomic detail needed to evaluate the talar dome, deltoid ligament, medial malleolus, and CFL. Two-dimensional GRE images, which are T2 weighted, and T1-weighted three-dimensional GRE images can be most useful when evaluating the talar domes for osteochondral lesions. If concern for a subtle osteochondral injury exists, a STIR sequence is the most sensitive sequence to identify bone marrow pathology.

PATHOLOGY

Achilles Tendon

The Achilles tendon is probably the tendon most commonly evaluated when imaging the ankle. Abnormalities can involve a long segment of the Achilles tendon from the myotendinous junction to the calcaneal attachment. Degeneration and tendon tears are most commonly seen 2 to 6 cm from the calcaneal attachment. The normal Achilles tendon should slightly taper as it extends inferiorly, then broaden slightly as it attaches to the posterior calcaneous. On axial images, the Achilles tendon should have a smooth semilunar configuration and should be well delineated from the adjacent fascia. A rounded or oval shape of the tendon on axial images is abnormal. Thickening is best demonstrated on axial T2-weighted FSE images. Tendinosis appears as low signal on T1- and T2-weighted sequences. Increased signal within the Achilles tendon on T2-weighted images suggests tendonitis. Xanthoma deposits in patients with hypercholesterolemia demonstrate increased signal on T1- and T2-weighted images.

Partial- or full-thickness tears of the Achilles tendon usually occur in an already diseased tendon (Fig. 20-5) (2). Men are affected more commonly, and patients usually present between the ages of 30 and 50 years. Tears usually occur within the midsubstance of the tendon, approximately 2 to 6 cm from the calcaneal attachment. Care should be taken not to overdiagnose full-thickness tears. Full-thickness tears are

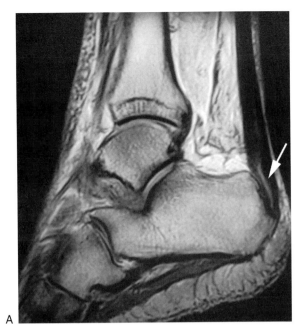

A

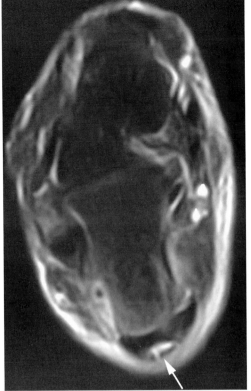

B

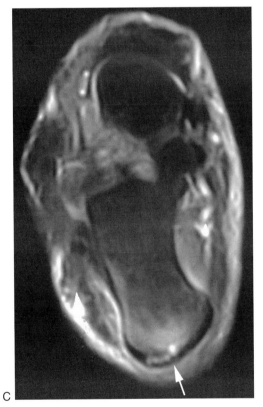

C

FIG. 20-5. Partial intrasubstance tear of the distal Achilles tendon. **A:** Sagittal high-resolution T1-weighted three-dimensional gradient-echo image demonstrates a linear area of increased signal intensity in the distal Achilles tendon (*arrow*) consistent with a small intrasubstance tear. **B,C:** The axial fast short tau inversion recovery sequences confirm a focal area of high signal intensity in the distal Achilles tendon (*arrows*). High-resolution T1-weighted images on open magnetic resonance imaging can be very useful in seeing abnormalities in ligaments and tendons.

best demonstrated in the axial plane. Myotendinous retraction may be seen with extensive partial-thickness tears as well as with full-thickness tears (see Fig. 20-2).

Aside from chronic tendinitis, Achilles tendon tears may be seen in patients with underlying systemic diseases, such as rheumatoid arthritis, lupus, and diabetes. The Achilles tendon is not surrounded by a synovial sheath, and adjacent soft tissue changes are known as *para-* or *peritendinitis.*

Fluid may also collect within the retrocalcaneal bursa, representing bursitis (Fig. 20-6).

Posterior Tibial Tendon

The PTT is important for plantar flexion and inversion. The PTT stabilizes the hindfoot. PTT tears classically occur in

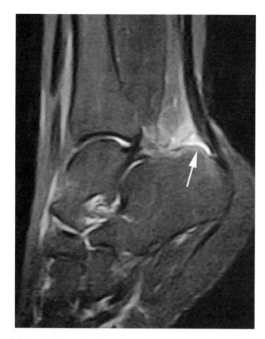

FIG. 20-6. Retrocalcaneal bursitis. Sagittal fast short tau inversion recovery image demonstrates fluid in the retrocalcaneal bursa (*arrow*) consistent with bursitis and mild thickening of the Achilles tendon consistent with tendonitis.

women in their fifth and sixth decades (3). Findings that are often identified on plain film radiographs include an accessory navicular bone and a pes planus deformity of the hindfoot.

The PTT normally has a thin, oblong appearance and is homogeneously low in signal intensity on all pulse sequences.

Partial tears, which tend to be chronic, demonstrate thickening and may be heterogeneous in signal intensity. Acute partial tears may be longitudinal in orientation, and the only indication may be fluid extending along the length of the tendon. Fluid coursing along the PTT may also be seen with large joint effusions, adjacent subcutaneous edema, and tenosynovitis (Fig. 20-7).

The remainder of the tendons of the ankle are less likely to demonstrate pathologic changes. Tendinitis, tenosynovitis, ganglia, and tears may involve any of the other tendons. The FHL is the only tendon that can normally demonstrate fluid coursing with the tendon. This can occur without pathology, because the FHL extends through the joint capsule.

Ligaments

Of the lateral ligaments, the ATFL is the weakest and most commonly torn. The ATFL normally appears as a thin low signal focus, extending from the inferior aspect of the fibula and attaching to the lateral talus. Thickening, or lack of visualization, is abnormal and suggests a tear. Chronic tears may be associated with fibrosis or hypertrophic changes. These changes may impinge on the anterolateral aspect of the tibiotalar joint (anterolateral impingement syndrome). Impingement can be seen involving various aspects of the ankle joint, especially posteriorly, where an enlarged os trigonum may result in pain or limitation of motion during plantar flexion.

The CFL is best demonstrated on coronal images. The CFL is stronger than the ATFL, and CFL tears are usually

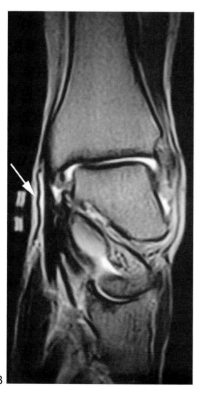
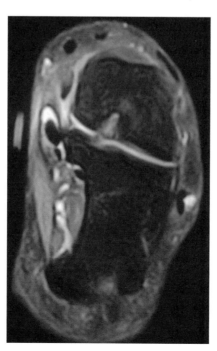

A, B

FIG. 20-7. Posterior tibial tendon (PTT) tenosynovitis. **A:** Coronal T2-weighted fast spin-echo image with a normal PTT with adjacent fluid in the synovial sheath (*arrow*). **B:** Axial fast short tau inversion recovery image at the same level eliminates signal from subcutaneous fat, and the normal signal intensity PTT and fluid in the sheath are easily identified.

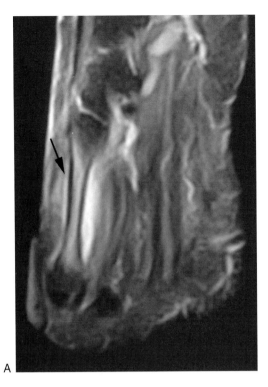

A

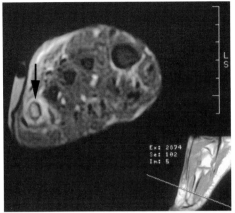

B

FIG. 20-8. Stress fracture of the fifth metatarsal shaft. Coronal **(A)** and axial **(B)** fast short tau inversion recovery (STIR) images demonstrate high signal intensity in the metatarsal (*arrows*) with extensive high signal intensity in the surrounding soft tissues extending along the dorsum of the foot. Stress fractures and associated stress reaction can easily be identified with magnetic resonance imaging, using STIR techniques.

seen only when the ATFL is torn. Due to the small size and posterior direction of the CFL, the CFL may be difficult to identify, especially when torn. Fluid extending along the peroneal tendon is a secondary finding of CFL tears, especially in association with an ATFL tear. The PTFL is the strongest of the lateral ligaments and is the last to be torn (4).

Medially, avulsions of the medial malleolus or tears of the deltoid ligament are clinically apparent and result in ankle instability and may widen the medial ankle mortise. These changes can be demonstrated with stress radiographs, and MRI is usually not necessary. Deltoid injuries are usually the result of eversion-type injuries. Trauma severe enough to injure the deltoid ligament is often associated with injuries of the lateral compartment of the ankle as well.

Stress Fracture

Stress fractures can involve any bone in the ankle, as well as the distal tibia and metatarsals (Fig. 20-8). The talus and calcaneous are the most common sites. Stress fractures are best identified on STIR sequences in which signal from fatty marrow is nullified. Edema may be difficult to detect on T2-weighted FSE images, because edema and fatty marrow are increased in signal intensity. On T1-weighted images, low signal from bone marrow may be identified with stress fractures, but this is not a consistent finding. Trabecular disruption is usually best seen on T1-weighted images. When imaging the metatarsal bones, a coronal oblique STIR

angled parallel to the metatarsals provides the greatest coverage with the fewest slices. This reduces scan time, which is helpful on the inversion recovery sequences because they can be very time consuming.

Osteochondral Lesions

With osteochondritis dissecans and osteochondral injuries of the talar dome (Fig. 20-9), it is critical to identify loose fragments in the tibiotalar joint because they can lead to early osteoarthritis. Talar dome injuries are best identified using a combination of sagittal STIR, sagittal T1-weighted three-dimensional GRE, and coronal T2-weighted FSE sequences. Coronal T2-weighted FSE and two-dimensional GRE are probably the most useful sequences, combining T2 weighting with anatomic detail. These sequences may also provide information on stability of an osteochondral lesion and identified fluid with the lesion.

Sinus Tarsi

Sinus tarsi syndrome results in pain along the lateral aspect of the foot and a sensation of instability of the hindfoot. Sinus tarsi syndrome is often associated with injuries of the lateral collateral ligaments or the PTT (5). Loss of the normal fat signal within the sinus tarsi or difficulty visualizing the interosseous ligaments may suggest the diagnosis (Fig. 20-10).

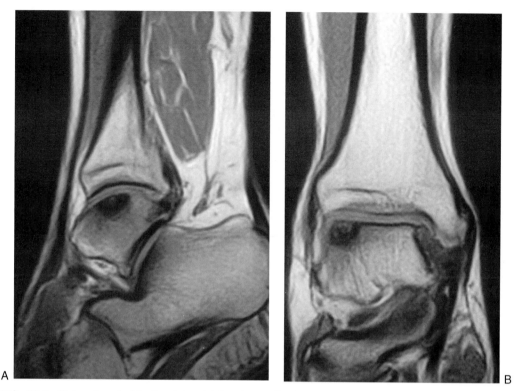

FIG. 20-9. Osteochondral lesion lateral talar dome. Sagittal **(A)** and coronal **(B)** T1-weighted two-dimensional spin-echo images demonstrate a well-circumscribed area of low signal intensity in the talar dome, extending into the subchondral bone. The articular cartilage appears intact over this area of osteochondritis dissecans.

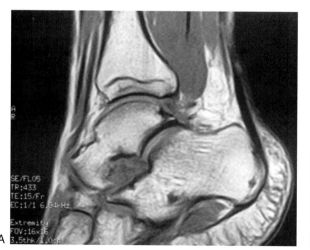
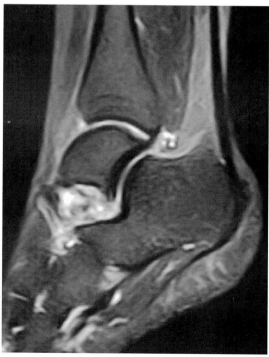

FIG. 20-10. Sinus tarsi syndrome. T1-weighted spin-echo **(A)** and fast short tau inversion recovery (STIR) sagittal **(B)** images demonstrate loss of normal fat signal on the T1-weighted and STIR images from the sinus tarsi and difficulty in visualizing the interosseous ligaments.

Plantar Fasciitis and Fibromatosis

Plantar fasciitis is a common cause of heel pain, and its diagnosis is important because many etiologies for heel pain exist. Plantar fasciitis is usually related to abnormal mechanics, such as a pes cavus deformity and pronated foot or degenerative changes. Systemic diseases are less common causes and include rheumatoid arthritis and seronegative arthropathies (6).

Plantar fasciitis is best demonstrated on sagittal STIR sequences with thickening or edema of the plantar fascia at the calcaneal attachment. Edema may be seen in the adjacent subcutaneous or deep soft tissues and at the calcaneal attachment. The plantar fascia may also tear.

Plantar fibromatosis represents excessive fibrotic changes involving the plantar fascia. Patients usually present with a painless lump or lumps along the bottom of the foot. Plantar fibromatosis is very variable in its aggressiveness and may invade the central compartment of the foot. Plantar fibromatosis tends to be low signal on all pulse sequences and often demonstrates enhancement with gadolinium (7).

REFERENCES

1. Erickson SJ, Quinn SF, Kneeland JB, et al. MR imaging of the tarsal tunnel and related spaces: normal and abnormal findings with anatomic correlations. *AJR Am J Roentgenol* 1990;155:323.
2. Reinig JW, Dorwart RH, Roden WC. MR imaging of a ruptured Achilles tendon. *J Comput Assist Tomogr* 1995;9:1131.
3. Johnson KA. Tibialis posterior tendon rupture. *Clin Orthop* 1983; 177:140.
4. Marder RA. Current methods for evaluation of ankle ligament injuries. *J Bone Joint Surg [Am]* 1994;76:1103.
5. Lowe A, Schilero J, Kanat IO. Sinus tarsi syndrome: a postoperative analysis. *J Foot Surg* 1985;24:108.
6. Bordelon RL. Subcalcaneal pain. *Clin Orthop* 1983;177:49.
7. Morrison WB, Schweitzer ME, Wapner KL, et al. Plantar fibromatosis: a benign aggressive neoplasm with a characteristic appearance on MR images. *Radiology* 1994;193:841.

Open MRI,
edited by Peter A. Rothschild and Debra Reinking Rothschild.
Lippincott Williams & Wilkins. Philadelphia © 2000.

CHAPTER 21

Body Imaging with Open Magnetic Resonance Imaging

Robert Berkenblit

An in-depth review of magnetic resonance imaging (MRI) of the abdomen and pelvis is beyond the scope of this chapter. Instead, this chapter discusses the more common entities encountered in the abdomen and pelvis and how to optimize examinations of the abdomen and pelvis at lower field strengths. A number of cases are presented to illustrate abdominal and pelvic anatomy and pathology as manifested on an open MRI system. All images, unless otherwise specified, are from a 0.3-T system (Hitachi Medical Systems America, Twinsburg, OH).

ABDOMEN

Liver

The liver is a common site for both benign and malignant disease. MRI is an excellent modality for evaluating the liver. On T1-weighted images, the liver is typically of increased signal intensity (SI) relative to the spleen. On T2-weighted images, the liver is typically of decreased SI relative to the spleen. On all sequences, the liver and spleen are typically of increased SI relative to skeletal muscle (Fig. 21-1). Adequate T1 weighting is necessary for lesion detection in the liver, whereas adequate T2 weighting is necessary for lesion characterization and detection. Contrast agents can also help to characterize and detect lesions. T2-weighted images with long TEs (preferably at least 120 to 150 ms) are necessary because cysts and hemangiomas are of high SI, whereas other solid lesions (i.e., metastases) are not as intense as these longer TEs (1).

Common focal hepatic lesions encountered on MRI include cysts, hemangiomas, metastases, and hepatocellular

R. Berkenblit: Albert Einstein College of Medicine of Yeshiva University, and Montefiore Medical Center, Bronx, New York; Montefiore Imaging Center, Bronx, New York

carcinoma (HCC). Hepatic cysts are benign developmental processes. Cysts are usually asymptomatic and are seen in approximately 2.5% of patients referred for ultrasound (2,3). On MRI, these cysts are well circumscribed, and they show decreased SI on T1-weighted images and increased SI on short tau inversion recovery (STIR) and T2-weighted images. Hepatic cysts do not enhance after administration of gadolinium chelates (Fig. 21-2).

Cavernous hemangiomas are the most common benign tumor in the liver. They are made up of numerous vascular channels with fibrous septae (3). Hemangiomas are seen in up to 20% of the population (2,3). These lesions are usually asymptomatic. On MRI, hemangiomas are well circumscribed, often with lobular borders, and they exhibit decreased SI on T1-weighted images and increased SI on T2-weighted images. Enhancement is typically slow and in a nodular, peripheral to central pattern, with very delayed washout. Enhancement may be rapid for small lesions or may be incomplete for large lesions (4). Differences in connective tissue content may cause variable appearances on STIR and T2-weighted images (1,2) (Fig. 21-3).

The liver is the most common site in the body for hematogenous metastases (1). A number of primary tumors may metastasize to the liver, most commonly those arising in the colon and breast. Because cysts and hemangiomas are common in the general population, distinguishing these benign entities from malignant lesions is a major role of liver MRI. Metastatic lesions demonstrate variable signal and enhancement features but are usually of decreased SI on T1-weighted images and moderate to high SI on T2-weighted images—often similar in SI to the spleen (1). Enhancement is also variable. Metastases may have irregular enhancement with gradual filling of the lesion and peripheral washout (2) (Fig. 21-4).

Liver damage due to any of a number of factors, including alcohol abuse, viral hepatitis (B and C), and excess iron deposition, may lead to cirrhosis. Early in the disease

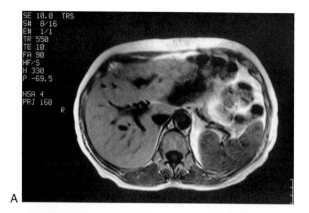

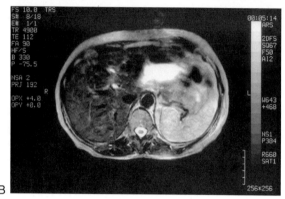

FIG. 21-1. Normal appearance of liver. **A:** In this T1-weighted spin-echo image [repetition time (TR), 550 ms; echo time (TE), 10 ms], the liver is of increased signal intensity (SI) relative to the spleen. **B:** In this T2-weighted fast spin-echo image (TR, 4,900 ms; TE, 112 ms), the liver is of decreased SI relative to the spleen. Notice the liver and spleen are of increased SI relative to skeletal muscle on both sequences.

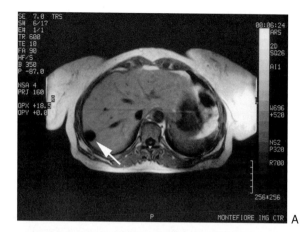

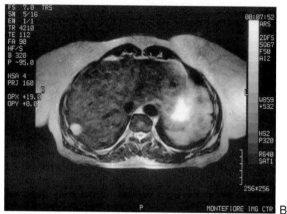

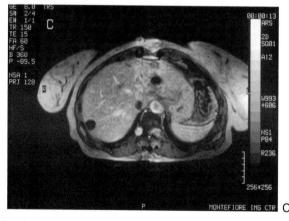

FIG. 21-2. A liver cyst is present in the right lobe of the liver demonstrating decreased signal intensity (SI) on a T1-weighted spin-echo image (*arrow*) **(A)** [repetition time (TR), 600 ms; echo time (TE), 10 ms], increased SI on a T2-weighted fast spin-echo image **(B)** (TR, 4,210 ms; TE, 112 ms), and no enhancement after administration of gadolinium on a T1-weighted gradient-echo image **(C)** (TR, 150 ms; TE, 15 ms; flip angle, 60 degrees).

process, the liver morphology may be normal. As the disease progresses, the right lobe may atrophy and the caudate and left lobes may enlarge (1). The MRI appearance of cirrhosis can be quite variable, due to differing degrees of fibrosis and edema. Cirrhotic livers may have a nodular appearance further complicating the appearance (2). Patients with cirrhosis are at increased risk for HCC. Regenerative nodules occur as a reparative response to hepatocyte injury. Adenomatous hyperplasia represents enlarged regenerative nodules and is considered premalignant (2). HCC tends to demonstrate decreased SI on T1-weighted images and increased SI on T2-weighted images (Table 21-1). However, increased SI on T1-weighted images may be seen. A fibrous capsule is common and is usually of decreased SI on T1-weighted images and may show increased SI peripherally on T2-weighted images. HCC may be unifocal, multifocal, or, rarely, diffuse in distribution (1,2).

Other focal hepatic lesions include focal nodular hyperplasia (FNH), adenoma, and cholangiocarcinoma. FNH is a benign tumor that is isointense to hypointense to liver on T1-weighted images and slightly hyperintense on T2-

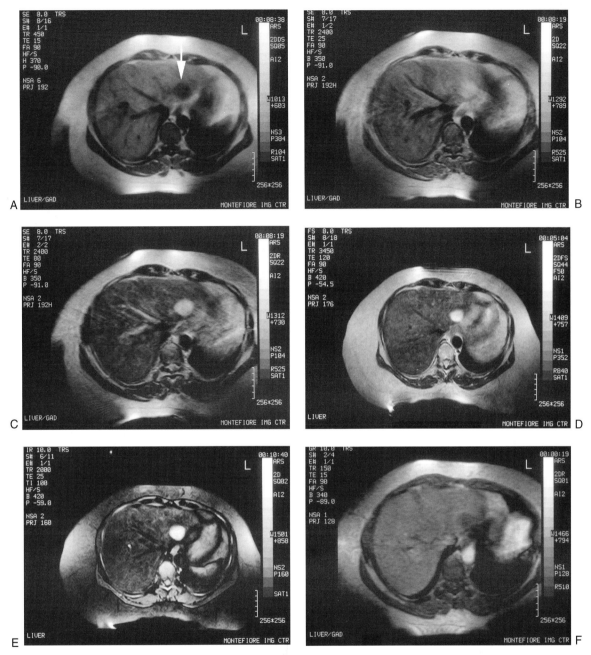

FIG. 21-3. Hemangioma in the left lobe of the liver. **A:** The lesion is of decreased signal intensity (SI) on a T1-weighted spin-echo (SE) image (*arrow*) [repetition time (TR), 450 ms; echo time (TE), 15 ms]. The lesion increases in SI with increased T2 weighting as the TE increases: SE **(B)** (TR, 2,400 ms; TE, 25 ms), SE **(C)** (TR, 2,400 ms; TE, 80 ms), and fast spin-echo **(D)** (TR, 3,450 ms; TE, 120 ms). **E:** The lesion is of high SI on a short tau inversion recovery sequence (TR, 2,000 ms; TE, 25 ms; inversion time, 100 ms). Pre- and postgadolinium T1-weighted gradient-echo images (TR, 150 ms; TE, 15 ms; flip angle, 90 degrees) show increasing peripheral to central nodular enhancement. **F:** Before gadolinium administration. *Continued.*

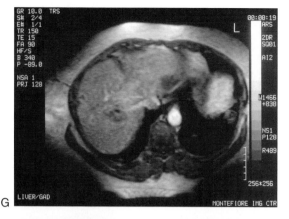

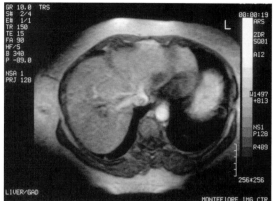

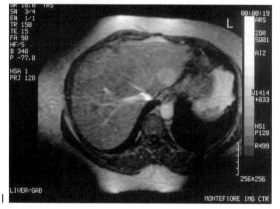

FIG. 21-3. *Continued.* **G:** Thirty-five seconds after gadolinium administration. **H:** One minute and 45 seconds after gadolinium administration. **I:** Almost 8 minutes after gadolinium administration.

weighted images. A central scar is often present and is of decreased SI on T1-weighted images and increased SI on T2-weighted images relative to the remainder of the lesion. After the administration of gadolinium, the lesion becomes rapidly hyperintense and, later, isointense or slightly hyperintense. The central scar becomes hyperintense on later images. Approximately two-thirds of FNH contain significant amounts of Kupffer cells, and therefore iron oxide agents may be helpful in evaluating these lesions (1,2).

Hepatic adenoma is a benign lesion composed of hepatocytes that is isointensive to hyperintense to liver on T1-weighted images and mildly hyperintense on T2-weighted images. Variable enhancement may occur, but hepatic adenomas often show rapid early enhancement. Hepatic adenoma may be difficult to distinguish from FNH (2).

Cholangiocarcinoma is a malignant tumor of the bile ducts that is usually of decreased SI on T1-weighted images and increased SI on T2-weighted images, with variable enhancement patterns (2).

More diffuse processes, such as iron overload and fatty infiltration, can also affect the liver. A number of diseases can cause increased amounts of iron in the body. Patients with iron overload demonstrate decreased hepatic SI on all

sequences due to the magnetic susceptibility effect of the iron products. Gradient-echo (GRE) sequences are the most sensitive for this effect (2). Primary hemochromatosis is a genetic disorder that leads to excess amounts of iron absorption from the gastrointestinal tract. This iron is subsequently deposited in the hepatocytes and eventually in the pancreas and heart. Iron is not deposited in the spleen, because these patients have an abnormal reticuloendothelial system (RES) (2).

Iron overload due to multiple transfusions (greater than approximately 40 U blood) is known as *hemosiderosis* or *secondary hemochromatosis*. The excess iron is accumulated via phagocytosis by the normal RES in these patients, and therefore the liver and spleen have an abnormal appearance (decreased SI relative to skeletal muscle) (2).

MRI is used to confirm the presence of iron overload and to assess for liver disease secondary to the excess iron deposition (cirrhosis, HCC). For a more in-depth discussion of MRI and iron overload states, I recommend references 2, 5, 6, and 7.

A number of conditions can lead to increased lipid deposition in the liver, including steroid use, obesity, diabetes, pregnancy, and alcohol use. Fatty infiltration of the liver can be seen on ultrasound as diffuse or regional increased echogenicity and as diffuse or regional decreased density in

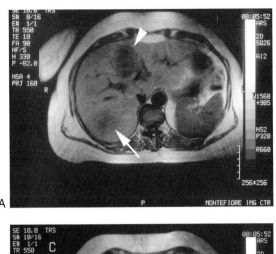
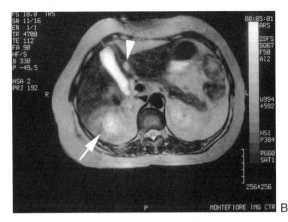
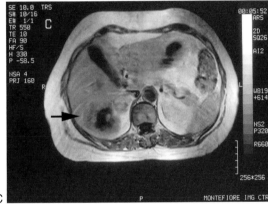
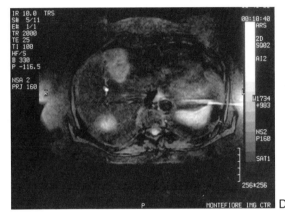

FIG. 21-4. Liver metastases. This patient with colon cancer is being assessed for metastatic disease. Magnetic resonance imaging revealed a number of liver metastases and a right adrenal lesion suspicious for a metastasis. **A:** Large lesions of low signal intensity (SI) are identified in the posterior segment of the right lobe (*arrow*) and medial segment of the left lobe of the liver (*arrowhead*) on this T1-weighted spin-echo (SE) image [repetition time (TR), 500 ms; echo time (TE), 10 ms]. **B:** At another anatomic level, the posterior lesion is of heterogeneous, slightly increased SI (*arrow*) on this T2-weighted fast spin-echo image (TR, 4,700 ms; TE, 112 ms) (*arrowhead*). **C:** The larger lesion (*arrow*) demonstrates heterogeneous enhancement after administration of gadolinium on this T1-weighted SE (TR, 550 ms; TE, 10 ms). **D:** This short tau inversion recovery image (TR, 2,000 ms; TE, 25 ms; inversion time, 100 ms) at a slightly different level demonstrates the two lesions seen in **A** to be of heterogeneous, increased SI.

the liver on computed tomography (CT). When fatty infiltration is present, chemical shift imaging (see Adrenal Glands, later in this chapter) can demonstrate loss of SI in the liver on the out-of-phase images relative to the in-phase images (Fig. 21-5).

Magnetic Resonance Cholangiopancreatography

Magnetic resonance cholangiopancreatography (MRCP) has requirements similar to those of MR urography (see Magnetic Resonance Urography, under Kidneys, later in this chapter). A heavily T2-weighted sequence is used to obtain source images that can then be used to generate max-

TABLE 21-1. *Magnetic resonance imaging signal characteristics of nodules in cirrhotic livers*

Lesion type	T1-weighting	T2-weighting
Regenerative nodule	Decreased SI	Decreased SI
Adenomatous hyperplasia	Increased SI	Decreased SI
Early hepatocellular carcinoma	Increased SI	Increased SI
Hepatocellular carcinoma	Intermediate to low SI	Increased SI

SI, signal intensity.
From Kressel HY. *Magnetic resonance imaging of the liver. Hospital of the University of Pennsylvania 19th Annual Diagnostic Imaging Seminar Syllabus.* Martha's Vineyard, MA. July 1997.

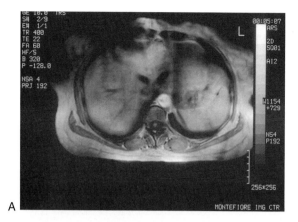

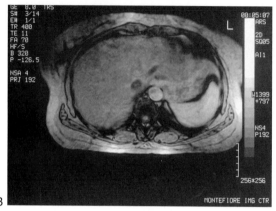

FIG. 21-5. Fatty infiltration of the liver. **A:** In this gradient-echo (GRE) in-phase image [repetition time (TR), 400 ms; echo time (TE), 22 ms; flip angle, 60 degrees], the liver is isointense relative to the spleen. **B:** In this GRE out-of-phase image (TR, 400 ms; TE, 11 ms; flip angle, 70 degrees), the liver is of decreased signal intensity relative to the spleen.

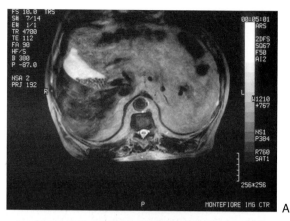

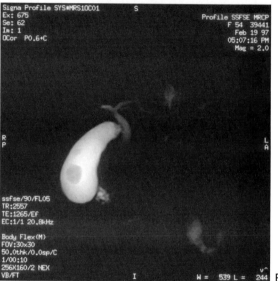

FIG. 21-6. Gallstones. Filling defects, representing gallstones, are noted in the gallbladder of two different patients. **A:** T2-weighted fast spin-echo (FSE) image [repetition time (TR), 4,700 ms; echo time (TE), 112 ms]. **B:** In this maximum intensity projection from a magnetic resonance cholangiopancreatography (single-shot FSE with TR, 2,557 ms; TE, 1,265 ms), portions of the common and right and left hepatic ducts are visualized. From a General Electric Signa Profile, 0.2 T system, courtesy of General Electric Medical Systems, Milwaukee, WI.

imum intensity projection images. The aqueous nature of bile and pancreatic secretions yields signal with these heavily T2-weighted sequences so that the biliary and pancreatic ductal systems can be assessed (1). This technique can be used to detect ductal stones, tumors, or strictures, as well as other processes involving the pancreaticobiliary system. Conventional endoscopic retrograde cholangiopancreatography (ERCP) has the advantage of making it possible to offer therapy at the time of imaging. MRCP is valuable in a variety of patients, such as those who cannot tolerate or have failed conventional ERCP or are of low clinical suspicion for requiring endoscopic therapy. Conventional MR images can supplement the MRCP by assessing the extraductal structures (8). Although MRCP is typically used to assess the pancreatic and biliary tree, this technique, or even routine T2-weighted images, can be used to evaluate the gallbladder and its contents (Fig. 21-6). For greater detail about MRCP technique and interpretation, refer to references 8, 9, and 10.

Contrast Agents

Commonly used intravenous contrast agents include gadolinium chelates and iron oxide–based agents. Gadolinium is administered intravenously and diffuses rapidly through the extracellular space. The paramagnetic nature of gadolinium causes T1 shortening and therefore increased SI on T1-weighted images. Precontrast images are obviously important to obtain for comparison to the postcontrast images. The normal liver derives most of its blood supply from the portal venous system, whereas most liver lesions derive their blood supply from the hepatic artery. The timing of imaging after the injection of gadolinium to correspond to the hepatic arterial phase and portal venous phase is important and can be quite difficult. Ideally, the entire liver can be imaged in a breath-hold. This can then be repeated to image the liver in the various phases of enhancement. If this is not possible, sequential images should be obtained in a focal region of interest as determined by the precontrast images.

If images are obtained in the arterial phase, hypervascular metastases (i.e., renal cell cancer, thyroid cancer, melanoma) are hyperintense relative to the normal liver parenchyma. Metastases characteristically demonstrate rim enhancement, which may become hypointense on subsequent images, representing the so-called peripheral washout (2,11).

Because normal liver enhances more than most neoplasms during the portal venous phase, most metastases are less intense than liver during this phase of the bolus (11). Most tumors have a large interstitial space. Therefore, a greater accumulation of extracellular space agents (i.e., gadolinium) may occur in tumors, relative to normal liver, on delayed imaging (11).

Ferumoxide (Feridex, Berlex Laboratories, Wayne, NJ) is an intravenous agent composed of iron oxide particles. Due to the superparamagnetic nature of this agent, local field inhomogeneities occur causing T2 shortening (10). The iron oxide particles are taken up by normal RES cells found in the liver (Kupffer cells), spleen, and marrow. Kupffer cells are found in normal liver as well as FNH and regenerating nodules. Metastatic lesions and most HCCs lack Kupffer cells. SI is lost where iron oxide particles are distributed, and SI is retained at foci lacking RES cells (i.e., metastases and most HCCs). The maintained SI of metastases and most HCCs becomes more conspicuous against the blackened background of "normal liver" (11,12). Ferumoxide has also been used to help characterize certain lesions. Signal decrease occurs in lesions that contain Kupffer cells or a significant blood pool (i.e., hemangiomas) (12,13). The ferumoxide dose is infused intravenously over approximately 30 minutes. Postcontrast images may be obtained up to 3.5 hours after injection, and therefore "dynamic scanning" is not necessary.

Essentially all abdominal and pelvic MRI examinations require T1- and T2-weighted images in some form. T1-weighted spin-echo (SE) sequences take longer than GRE sequences; however, in my experience at 0.3 T, I have found better contrast and less motion artifact with SE sequences. Fast spin-echo (FSE) sequences offer adequate T2 weighting with reduced scan times relative to SE. A T1-weighted SE sequence of the entire liver can be performed in just under 6 minutes [example values for the Hitachi Airis: repetition time (TR), 550 ms; echo time (TE), 10 ms; 16 slices; number of signals averaged, 4; 10 mm slice thickness; 2 mm gap; scan time, 5 minutes 52 seconds]. The T1 values of most tissues approximately double, from 0.15 to 1.5 T (14). Therefore, at lower field strengths, shorter TR values should be used for T1WI. Shorter TR values help reduce scan time,

allowing one to use a greater number of acquisitions. Increasing the number of acquisitions helps reduce motion artifact and can boost SNR, whereas the shorter TR improves liver-lesion contrast (15). Less slices are available with a shorter TR; therefore, reducing the TR to 300 mSec and increasing the number of acquisitions to eight typically requires that two series of images be obtained. This effectively doubles the amount of time to obtain T1WI of the entire liver to approximately 12 to 13 minutes instead of approximately 6 to 6.5 minutes (example values for the Hitachi Airis: repetition time, 300 ms; TE, 10 ms; 8 slices; number of signal averages, 8; 10 mm slice thickness; 2 mm gap; scan time, 6 minutes 24 seconds). A T2-weighted FSE sequence of the liver can be performed in approximately 5 minutes (example values for the Hitachi Airis: repetition time, 3,450 ms; TE, 120 ms; 18 slices; number of signal averages, 2; 8 mm slice thickness; 2 mm gap; scan time, 5 minutes 4 seconds). STIR images may be helpful to further assess focal liver lesions. T2-weighted FSE images in the sagittal plane may be helpful to assess the dome of the liver. Contrast agents can be helpful to further characterize and detect lesions.

Adrenal Glands

The adrenal gland is the site of production of a number of hormones. If a patient has a hyperfunctioning adenoma (a benign adrenal tumor that produces an excess amount of a particular hormone) the patient will have symptoms related to the excess of the particular hormone (e.g., cortisol in Cushing's syndrome, aldosterone in Conn's syndrome). A noncontrast CT scan is often adequate to localize an adrenal nodule to direct surgery in these cases.

Nonhyperfunctioning adrenal adenomas (benign adrenal tumors that do not produce excess hormone) are almost always incidental findings. These are quite common and occur in approximately 3% of the general population (5).

The adrenal gland is a very common site for metastatic disease (most commonly from lung or breast tumors). In an autopsy series of 1,000 cadavers with a primary epithelial malignancy, 27% of the cadavers had adrenal metastases (5,16). However, many patients with a primary malignancy have benign adrenal masses. In general, in a patient with a primary malignancy and no other site of disease, an adrenal mass is more likely to be an adenoma. However, if that person has known metastases elsewhere, the adrenal lesion is more likely to be a metastasis (5).

MRI is valuable in distinguishing nonhyperfunctioning adenomas from other lesions of the adrenal gland (i.e., metastatic disease or pheochromocytoma). Adrenal adenomas tend to be of decreased SI on T1-weighted images relative to the liver and isointense to slightly hyperintense relative to liver on T2-weighted images. Adrenal metastases tend to be hypointense on T1-weighted images and hyperintense on T2-

weighted images relative to liver. Studies have shown a 20% to 30% overlap in signal characteristics between benign and malignant adrenal lesions on SE imaging. Some researchers have looked at enhancement features to attempt to differentiate these lesions. Nonhyperfunctioning adenomas typically have mild enhancement with rapid washout, whereas malignant lesions and pheochromocytomas have greater initial enhancement and a more delayed washout (5).

Chemical shift imaging (also known as *opposed phase imaging* or *in- and out-of-phase imaging*) is believed to be more reliable. In one study using a 1.5-T system, 19 of 20 adenomas demonstrated signal loss on out-of-phase images relative to in-phase images when comparing the lesion to skeletal muscle or liver. In this study, none of the 12 malignant lesions lost signal from in to out of phase (16).

So what is chemical shift imaging? First, a discussion of basic MRI physics is in order. Typically, MRI analyzes hydrogen protons (^{1}H). Hydrogen protons are found in many human substances, such as fat and water. Hydrogen protons are affected by their surrounding electron environment. Depending on the environment, shielding or deshielding may occur. Electrons circulate around each nucleus and induce a magnetic field that shields the nucleus from the applied magnetic field, which causes the nucleus to precess more slowly. Electrons from other nuclei may oppose or augment the proton's local magnetic field. If the field is augmented, it is considered deshielded, and the nucleus precesses more quickly. Changes from shielding and deshielding are called *chemical shift*. Chemical shift is measured in parts per million (ppm), relative to the precession of hydrogen nuclei in tetramethylsilane. Protons in water have a chemical shift of 4.7 ppm, and those in fat have a chemical shift of approximately 1.2 ppm, for a difference of 3.5 ppm (14).

The Larmor equation states the following:

$$\omega = \gamma B_o$$

where γ is the gyromagnetic frequency and is specific for each type of nucleus, and B_o is the magnetic field strength. For ^{1}H, the gyromagnetic frequency is 42.5 MHz per T. Therefore, at 1.5 T:

The precession frequency = 1.5 T $\times$ 42.5 MHz/T = 64 MHz

The precession frequency difference between ^{1}H of water and fat is as follows:

$$(4.7 \text{ ppm} - 1.5 \text{ ppm}) \times 64 \text{ MHz} = 224 \text{ Hz}$$

Therefore, at 1.5 T, the period of the alternation between ^{1}H of fat and water being in phase is $\frac{1}{224}$ Hz, or 4.4 ms (period = 1/frequency). So at 1.5 T, approximately every 4.4 ms, ^{1}H in fat and water are in phase. Halfway to being in phase, or at approximately 2.2 ms, ^{1}H of fat and water are 180 degrees out of phase (14). Therefore, at 1.5 T, every 4.4 ms, 8.8 ms, 13.2 ms, and so forth, ^{1}H of fat and water are in phase, whereas every 2.2 ms, 6.6 ms, 11 ms, and so forth, they are out of phase. As was noted earlier, this is dependent on field strength. At 0.3 T (one-fifth the field strength of a 1.5-T sys-

tem), the period of alternation is 22 ms. So, the TE for in-phase images at 0.3 T should be approximately 22 ms, and out-of-phase images require a TE of approximately 11 ms.

To obtain out-of-phase images, the TE does not have to be set perfectly when fat and water are 180 degrees out of phase but can be close enough to this calculated time (i.e., out-of-phase images can be obtained at 0.3 T at a TE of 15 ms, which is closer to 11 ms than 22 ms) (Fig. 21-7). Opposed phase images are typically achieved using a GRE sequence. SE sequences have a 180-degree refocusing pulse, and ^{1}H of fat and water therefore are put back into phase, whereas GRE sequences do not have this 180-degree refocusing pulse and are therefore in or out of phase as a function of TE (14,17).

Table 21-2 demonstrates the dependence of TE on field strength for protons of fat and water being in or out of phase. At 1.0 T, a TE of 6.6 ms is in phase, whereas at 1.5 T, a TE of 6.6 ms is out of phase. At both 0.3 and 1.5 T, a TE of 11 ms is out of phase.

Let's apply these physics principles to clinical situations. If fat and water are in the same pixel, the signal will "drop out" on the out-of-phase images relative to the in-phase images. Adrenal adenomas have a relatively high amount of intracellular water and lipid (due to the presence of steroid precursors used in hormone synthesis). Metastases to the adrenal gland typically do not have a significant fatty component (certain tumors, such as some sarcomas, may have a fatty component that can lead to errors; however, these tumors are quite rare) (16,18). Therefore, adrenal adenomas typically drop out (i.e., lose signal) on the out-of-phase images relative to the in-phase images (Fig. 21-8), whereas metastatic lesions maintain their signal on both in- and out-of-phase images.

Although most adrenal adenomas drop out on the out-of-phase images, some adenomas, so-called atypical adenomas, do not behave in this manner. This may occur due to inadequate amounts of intracellular lipid ("lipid-poor adenomas"), or the atypical appearance may be caused by the presence of hemorrhage, calcification, or necrosis (19).

These principles also explain the black line that occurs at fat/water interfaces in the body (i.e., kidney/retroperitoneal fat interface) on out-of-phase images. If a pixel contains just fat (i.e., isolated portion of retroperitoneal fat, lipoma, adrenal myelolipoma), signal is maintained on the in- and out-of-phase images in that pixel (see Fig. 21-7), because no chemical shift difference is occurring (very little water present).

Other Adrenal Lesions

Pheochromocytomas typically occur in the adrenal gland but may arise outside the adrenals. The excess secretion of catecholamines by pheochromocytomas results in hypertension (19). On T1-weighted images, pheochromocytomas are usually hypointense and become very intense on T2-weighted images.

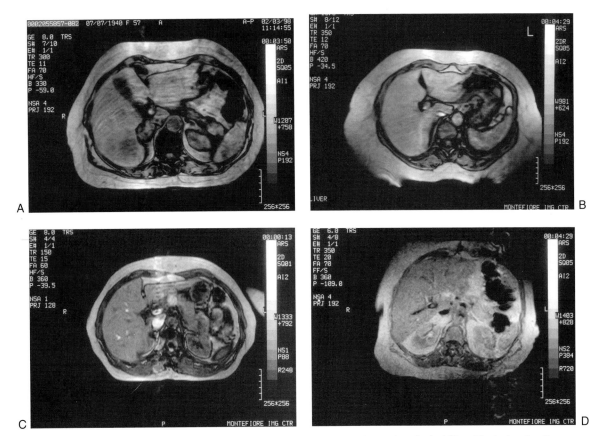

FIG. 21-7. Gradient-echo images from four different patients show chemical shift artifact at echo time 11 ms **(A)**, 12 ms **(B)**, and 15 ms **(C)** but not at 20 ms **(D)**. **A:** Repetition time (TR), 300 ms; flip angle (FA), 70 degrees. **B:** TR, 350 ms; FA, 70. **C:** TR, 150 ms; FA, 60. **D:** TR, 350 ms; FA, 70.

Myelolipomas are benign masses that contain fat and myeloid elements. The MRI appearance varies depending on the amount of fat present. STIR images can demonstrate signal loss when prominent fat is present. If prominent fat is present, out-of-phase images may show chemical shift artifact at the interface of fat and "normal" adrenal tissue (20).

Primary adrenal carcinoma often presents as a large mass. The ability of MRI to scan in multiple planes is valuable in establishing whether the lesion is adrenal in origin or arising from another structure in the region, such as the kidney. Variable signal on T1- and T2-weighted images may be seen depending on the degree of hemorrhage and necrosis present.

Adrenal cysts may be posttraumatic, postinfectious, or congenital. As expected, they are typically of decreased SI on T1-weighted images and increased SI on T2-weighted images without enhancement. They may have a variable MRI appearance due to the presence of blood product or calcification (1).

T1-weighted SE, T2-weighted FSE, and in- and out-of-phase images in the axial plane make up the basic evaluation

of the adrenal glands on an open MRI. Sagittal or coronal images and STIR images may be helpful depending on the size, orientation, and makeup of the lesion.

Kidneys

Although ultrasound and CT are the major imaging modalities for evaluating the kidneys, MRI plays a valuable role in renal imaging. On T1-weighted images, corticomedullary differentiation is seen in normal kidneys (the cortex being of higher SI than the medulla). On T2-weighted

TABLE 21-2. *Dependence of echo time on field strength for in and out of phase images*

Field strength (T)	Echo time in phase (ms)	Echo time out of phase (ms)
0.3	22, 44	11, 33
1.0	6.6, 13.2	3.3, 9.9
1.5	4.4, 8.8, 13.2	2.2, 6.6, 11

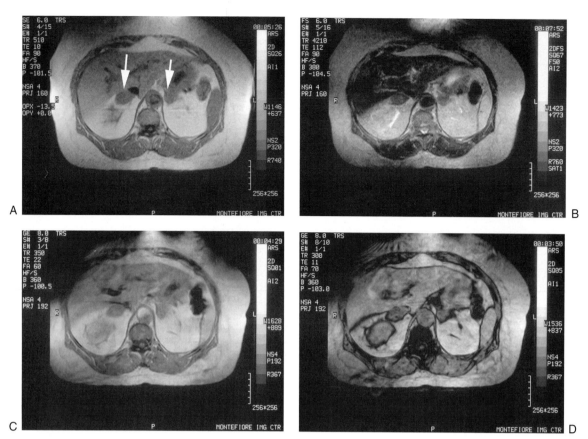

FIG. 21-8. Adrenal adenoma. A computed tomographic scan revealed bilateral adrenal nodules in a patient with hypertension. Magnetic resonance imaging (MRI) was requested to rule out pheochromocytoma. MRI demonstrates bilateral adrenal nodules that are of decreased signal intensity on T1-weighted spin-echo (*arrows*) [repetition time (TR), 510 ms; echo time (TE), 10 ms] **(A)** and T2-weighted fast spin-echo (TR, 4,210 ms; TE, 112 ms) **(B)** images (not consistent with a pheochromocytoma). The lesions are isointense to the liver and slightly hypointense to the spleen on in-phase gradient-echo (GRE) images [TR, 350 ms; TE, 22 ms; flip angle (FA), 60 degrees] **(C)** and become hypointense to liver and spleen on out-of-phase GRE images (TR, 300 ms; TE, 11 ms; FA, 70 degrees) **(D)**—consistent with adrenal adenomas. These lesions were stable in size for 15 months.

images, normal kidneys are typically of fairly homogeneous intermediate SI (Fig. 21-9).

The potential nephrotoxicity of iodinated contrast used in CT and intravenous urograms may be of concern in a patient with compromised renal function. Iodinated contrast may be contraindicated for other reasons, such as allergies or patient dependence on certain medications (e.g., metformin). MRI has superior contrast resolution relative to noncontrast CT. MRI may also be used to further evaluate questionable findings on CT (i.e., possible invasion or degree of invasion of the inferior vena cava by a renal cell carcinoma).

Renal cysts are very common benign processes: More than half of individuals older than 50 years have at least one (21). Renal cysts are typically well circumscribed and show decreased SI on T1-weighted images, increased SI on T2-weighted images, and no enhancement on MRI (Fig. 21-10). Cysts may show increased SI on T1-weighted images when

hemorrhage is present. Small septations or calcifications may complicate their appearance.

Angiomyolipomas are benign tumors composed of variable amounts of fat, smooth muscle, and blood vessels (21). These are often well-circumscribed masses that may cause hematuria. Depending on the degree of fat present in the lesion, opposed phase images or STIR can be helpful. It may be difficult to distinguish angiomyolipomas that contain only very small amounts of fat from other solid lesions by imaging alone.

MRI is limited in its evaluation of calculi, but secondary changes such as hydronephrosis are well imaged.

Renal malignancies are not uncommon. These are typically renal cell carcinomas; however, other tumors, such as lymphoma and metastatic disease, may involve the kidneys. In patients with renal cell carcinoma, MRI is excellent for assessing the size and extent of the primary mass as well as

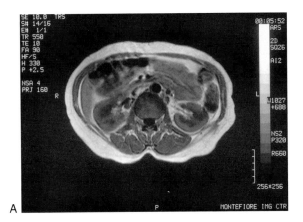

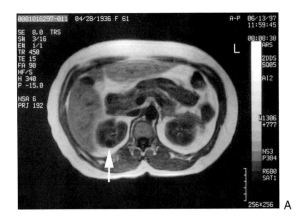

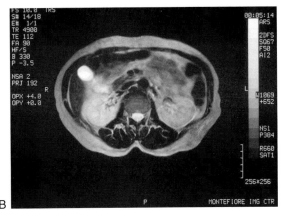

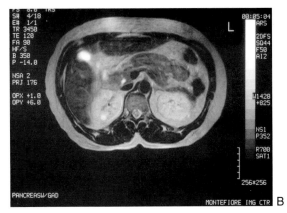

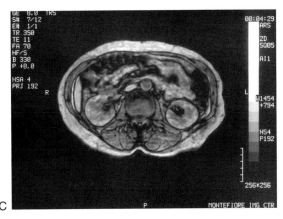

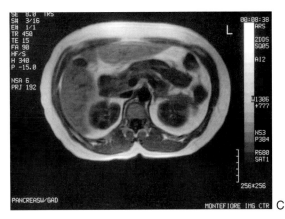

FIG. 21-9. Normal kidneys. **A:** Corticomedullary differentiation is seen on this T1-weighted spin-echo image [repetition time (TR), 550 ms; echo time (TE), 10 ms]. **B:** The kidneys are fairly homogeneous and of intermediate signal intensity on this T2-weighted fast spin-echo image (TR, 4,900 ms; TE, 112 ms). **C:** Out-of-phase image (TR, 350 ms; TE, 11 ms; flip angle, 70 degrees) demonstrates chemical shift artifact at the interface of retroperitoneal fat and kidney parenchyma.

FIG. 21-10. Renal cyst. A small cyst present in the posterior aspect of the right kidney demonstrates decreased signal intensity (SI) on a T1-weighted spin-echo (*arrow*) [repetition time (TR), 450 ms; echo time (TE), 15 ms] image **(A)** and increased SI on a T2-weighted fast spin-echo (TR, 3,450 ms; TE, 120 ms) image **(B)**. **C:** No enhancement is present after administration of gadolinium on this gradient-echo (TR, 150 ms; TE, 15 ms; flip angle, 60 degrees) image.

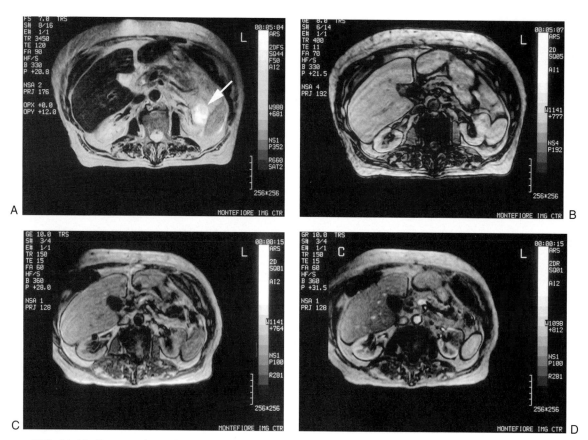

FIG. 21-11. Presumed renal cell carcinoma. A noncontrast computed tomographic scan of the chest revealed a left renal mass. **A:** A 3 cm × 2 cm mass of heterogeneous increased signal intensity (*arrow*) is present on this T2-weighted fast spin-echo image [repetition time (TR), 3,450 ms; echo time (TE), 120 ms]. **B:** This out-of-phase image (TR, 400 ms; TE, 11 ms; flip angle, 70 degrees) demonstrates the contour-deforming left renal mass. Pre– **(C)** and Post–gadolinium administration **(D)** gradient-echo images (TR, 150 ms; TE, 15 ms; FA, 60) show slight enhancement in the mass. Although this mass is consistent with a renal cell carcinoma, surgery was not performed due to the patient's medical condition.

the presence of adenopathy, vascular invasion, and distant metastases. Renal cell carcinoma may be solid, cystic, or both, with areas of necrosis or hemorrhage and therefore can be quite variable in appearance on MRI (Fig. 21-11). Renal cell carcinoma typically enhances, but some may show little or no enhancement. The size at presentation varies from those that are small (less than approximately 3 cm) and are discovered incidentally to very large lesions that present with various symptoms.

Magnetic Resonance Urography

MR urography uses a very heavily T2-weighted sequence with a long TE that essentially eliminates all signal from anything but water (i.e., urine, bile, cerebrospinal fluid). A large field of view is used to allow inclusion of the kidneys, ureters, and bladder. Thin slices (≤3 mm) with no gap are used to obtain the source images in the coronal plane, which are then used to create MIP images. Because the signal received

comes from urine, some degree of distention of the collecting system is necessary. MR urography optimally involves high-resolution images to help evaluate for the presence of small tumors, stones, or strictures. The degree and location of hydronephrosis can readily be evaluated (19) (Fig. 21-12).

T1-weighted SE and T2-weighted FSE images in the axial plane make up the basic evaluation of the kidneys in open MRI. At lower field strengths, out-of-phase images help better define the renal border against the retroperitoneal fat and help evaluate for contour-deforming masses. Sagittal or coronal (or both), STIR, and postgadolinium images may be helpful depending on the size, orientation, and makeup of the lesion.

Pancreas

Ultrasound and CT are the primary imaging modalities used in evaluating the pancreas. MRI is helpful in evaluating for the presence and extent of adenocarcinoma and other

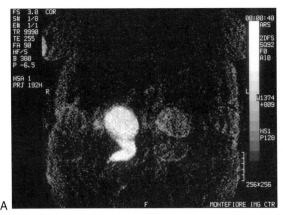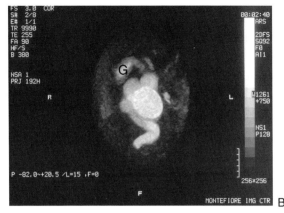

FIG. 21-12. Magnetic resonance urography (MRU) of hydronephrosis. **A:** Coronal T2-weighted fast spin-echo source image (repetition time, 9,990 ms; echo time, 255 ms). **B:** Maximum intensity projection. Marked right-sided hydroureteronephrosis is noted to the level of the midureter. A very large fibroid was the cause of the obstruction. Three sets of eight source images were obtained. Each set of eight images was obtained over 40 seconds for a total scan time of 2 minutes for the MRU. *G* marks the gallbladder.

solid masses of the pancreas, as well as for assessing cystic masses. Ideally, thin-section T1-weighted images with fat suppression are obtained.

The pancreatic parenchyma is typically bright on T1-weighted images. The pancreas is of variable SI on T2-weighted images, and solid tumors can be difficult to detect on T2-weighted images. T2-weighted images are helpful in assessing ducts, fluid collections, and cystic masses. The SI of most pancreatic tumors (adenocarcinoma) is low on T1-weighted images, offering a large degree of contrast between normal pancreas and tumor. Pancreatitis can also cause decreased SI on T1-weighted images. Fat-suppressed T1-weighted images increase the tissue contrast between normal pancreas and surrounding fat. The high SI of normal pancreas relative to the decreased SI of tumor is also better appreciated with the application of fat suppression (5).

Pancreatic cancer is typically hypovascular and therefore is of low SI on the initial postgadolinium images. Considerable enhancement may occur on later images (5). Islet cell tumors of the pancreas typically demonstrate marked increased SI on T2-weighted images and are hypervascular.

Benign and malignant cystic neoplasms of the pancreas can occur. The cystic component demonstrates increased SI on T2-weighted images. Variable amounts of septations may lead to a very complex appearance. The distinction between benign and potentially malignant cystic lesions is often impossible.

Spleen

CT is still the primary imaging modality of the spleen. Neoplastic processes, such as lymphoma and metastatic disease and, quite rarely, primary splenic tumors such as angiosarcoma, may involve the spleen. Benign masses, such as hamartomas and hemangiomas, can also be found in the

spleen. Patients who have undergone excessive blood transfusions may demonstrate changes in the spleen due to iron overload (see discussion under Liver, earlier in this chapter). MRI determination of splenic involvement or lack thereof is helpful in determining the cause of iron overload. Changes in the spleen may occur in patients with portal hypertension, such as splenomegaly, and the presence of Gamna-Gandy bodies (10). The spleen can be the site of infection including *Pneumocystis carinii* pneumonia, fungus, and bacteria. Benign splenic cysts may occur secondary to prior echinococcal infection or trauma or as a developmental anomaly. As expected, splenic cysts exhibit decreased SI on T1-weighted images, increased SI on T2-weighted images, and no enhancement. The spleen is normally of lower SI than the liver on T1-weighted images and of higher SI than the liver on T2-weighted images. Enhancement in the normal spleen can be quite heterogeneous and irregular in the early phase of contrast injection but becomes homogeneous later in the phase of contrast injection.

PELVIS

MRI of the pelvis has numerous applications in women and men.

Adnexae

Ultrasound and CT are commonly used for evaluating patients with adnexal pathology. MRI can demonstrate the typically irregular complex cystic masses of ovarian cancer, as well as the ascites, adenopathy, or peritoneal disease that may be associated with ovarian cancer (Fig. 21-13).

Ovarian dermoids are usually unilateral and typically benign (3). These usually contain fatty and calcified compo-

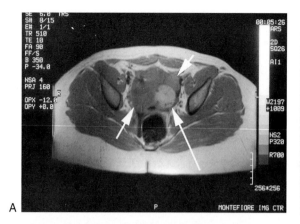

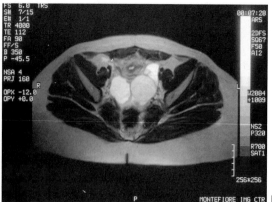

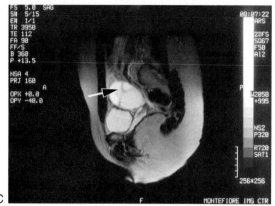

FIG. 21-13. Ovarian cancer. T1-weighted spin-echo axial [repetition time (TR), 510 ms; echo time (TE), 10 ms] **(A)**, T2-weighted fast spin-echo (FSE) (TR, 4,000 ms; TE, 112 ms) **(B)**, and T2-weighted FSE sagittal **(C)** images demonstrate a large complex cystic mass (*arrows*) between the rectum and uterus. Nodular septations are best seen on the sagittal image (*arrow*). Increased signal intensity in the middle component (*long arrow*) on the T1-weighted image is due to hemorrhagic material. Surgery revealed a low-grade cystadenocarcinoma.

nents as well as cystic components. STIR can help confirm the presence of a fatty component (Fig. 21-14). Interpretation of STIR images should be made with caution, as STIR does not selectively suppress fat but instead suppresses signal from substances with a relatively short T1. Therefore, a hemorrhagic ovarian cystic lesion may demonstrate signal loss on STIR related to the presence of blood product (methemoglobin) and be misinterpreted as a dermoid (22).

Endometriosis is defined as the presence of functioning endometrial glands and stroma in locations other than in the endometrial cavity of the uterus. It commonly involves the ovaries, fallopian tubes, and other para-uterine structures.

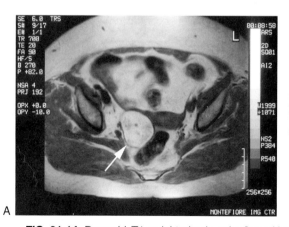

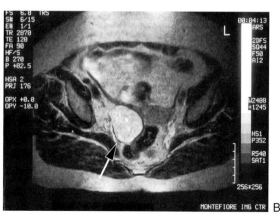

FIG. 21-14. Dermoid. T1-weighted spin-echo [repetition time (TR), 700 ms; echo time (TE), 20 ms] **(A)** and T2-weighted fast spin-echo (TR, 2,870 ms; TE, 120 ms) **(B)** images reveal a 5 cm × 4 cm right adnexal mass with signal intensity similar to fat (*arrows*). The patient could not tolerate further images, and therefore short tau inversion recovery images could not be obtained. Surgery confirmed the diagnosis of an ovarian dermoid.

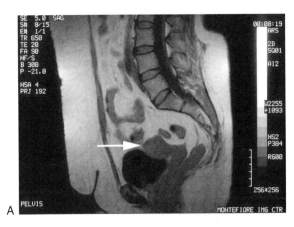

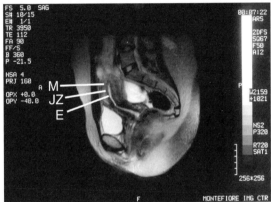

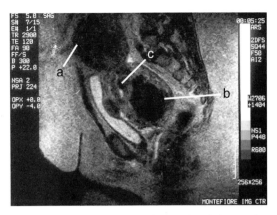

FIG. 21-16. Fibroids. Sagittal T2-weighted fast spin-echo image (repetition time, 2,900 ms; echo time, 120 ms) in a patient with numerous masses of decreased signal intensity consistent with fibroids. The locations of these fibroids are also demonstrated, including (*a*) a large subserosal fundal fibroid, (*b*) a large posterior intramural fibroid, and (*c*) a smaller submucosal fibroid abutting the posterior aspect of the endometrium.

FIG. 21-15. Normal uterus. A: This T1-weighted spin-echo image [repetition time (TR), 650 ms; echo time (TE), 20 ms] demonstrates the uterus (*arrow*) to be of homogeneous low to intermediate signal intensity. B: This sagittal T2-weighted fast spin-echo image (TR, 3,950 ms; TE, 112 ms) in a different patient demonstrates the normal zonal anatomy of the uterus (*E*, endometrium; *JZ*, junctional zone; *M*, myometrium). A cystic adnexal mass is identified posterior to the uterus. Notice the marked difference in the uterine axis between these two patients.

images, the uterus is fairly homogeneous and of intermediate SI (Fig. 21-15).

Leiomyomas (fibroids) are common benign neoplasms of the uterus occurring in 20% to 40% of women of reproductive age (22). The size, number, and location of fibroids can be assessed by MRI. Fibroids are of low SI on T1- and T2-weighted images. Increased SI may be seen with degeneration (22) (Fig. 21-16).

Adenomyosis is another common disease affecting the uterus. In adenomyosis, endometrial tissue extends into the myometrium. Patients with adenomyosis may have symp-

Hemorrhage into an endometrial implant can produce an endometrioma, complex cystic structures that have variable appearances on T1- and T2-weighted images depending on the chronicity of the hemorrhagic material. Other lesions, such as hemorrhagic ovarian cysts, pelvic inflammatory disease, and ovarian neoplasms, may resemble endometriosis (1).

Uterus

Ultrasound is the primary imaging modality for uterine pathology. However, due to the multiplanar capabilities and excellent intrauterine contrast on T2-weighted images, MRI is an excellent modality for evaluating uterine pathology. The normal zonal anatomy of the uterus is demonstrated on T2-weighted images, delineating the centrally located hyperintense endometrium from the hypointense junctional zone and the more peripheral myometrium. On T1-weighted

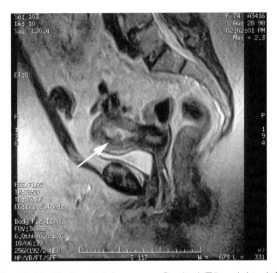

FIG. 21-17. Endometrial cancer. Sagittal T2-weighted fast spin-echo image (repetition time, 3,650 ms; echo time, 90 ms; General Electric Signa Profile 0.2 T) through the uterus demonstrates a markedly irregular endometrial cavity (*arrow*). Biopsy revealed endometrial cancer. Case courtesy of Dr. Peter A. Rothschild.

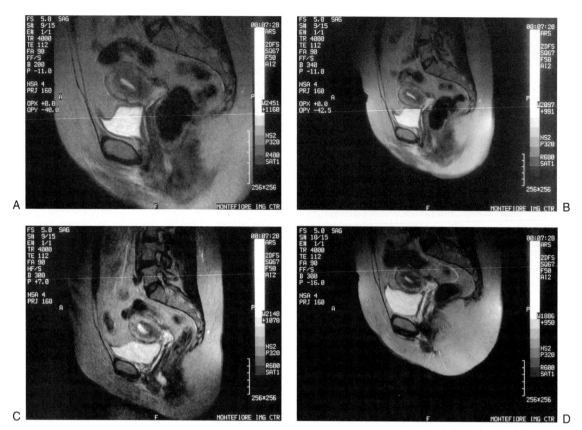

FIG. 21-18. Four sagittal T2-weighted fast spin-echo images (repetition time, 4,000 ms; echo time, 112 ms) on the same volunteer patient demonstrate the differences between a small field of view (FOV) (20 cm) **(A)** and large FOV (34 cm) **(B)** with a pelvic coil and between a pelvic coil **(C)** and a body coil **(D)** with the same FOV (30 cm). The signal to noise ratio is better with the larger FOV, but uterine detail is better seen with the smaller FOV. The pelvic coil image is superior to the body coil image.

toms similar to those seen with fibroids; however, therapy is very different. Hysterectomy is the definitive treatment for adenomyosis, whereas focal myomectomies may be attempted with fibroids. Adenomyosis is demonstrated on MRI as an enlarged, irregular junctional zone. On T2-weighted images, scattered high-SI foci may be seen in the junctional zone corresponding to the ectopic portions of endometrium. Increased SI can be seen on corresponding T1-weighted images, representing hemorrhage within the ectopic endometrium (22).

Endometrial cancer often presents with postmenopausal bleeding. With the presence of cancer, the endometrium is usually irregular and enlarged and an accumulation of material may be present within the endometrial cavity (Fig. 21-17). Myometrial invasion can be evaluated by MRI. It can be difficult to distinguish endometrial cancer from cervical cancer that has extended superiorly. Endometrial polyps and hyperplasia may also be difficult to distinguish from endometrial cancer.

MRI is valuable in assessing the uterus for congenital anomalies. The septate and bicornuate forms are two of the more common congenital anomalies of the uterus. These entities can be detected and distinguished from one another by MRI. A septate uterus has a portion of fibrous tissue extending inferiorly from the fundus. The fibrous tissue is of intermediate to decreased SI. In addition, the fundal contour is fairly normal. A bicornuate uterus has myometrium (which is of greater SI on T2-weighted images than fibrous tissue) extending between the two horns and an inward cleft at the fundus. Although septate uterus and bicornuate uterus are causes for early miscarriages, therapy for each entity differs, and accurate characterization is therefore important. In the case of a septate uterus, a hysteroscopic resection of the fibrous septum can be performed. A bicornuate uterus requires an open pelvic surgical procedure with a metroplasty to repair the anomaly (22). A high association of renal anomalies exists when uterine anomalies are present, and at least a cursory evaluation of the kidneys (number and location) should therefore be performed in these patients (22).

The normal uterine cervix is homogeneously hypointense on MRI. Cervical cancer is of increased SI on T2-weighted images. MRI can evaluate the extent of tumor and assess for spread of disease to regional nodes.

T1-weighted SE and T2-weighted FSE axial images are used in scanning the adnexae. STIR images can be helpful by

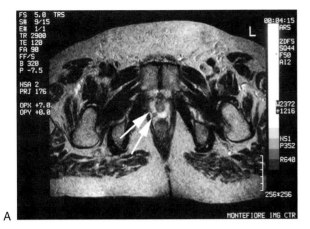

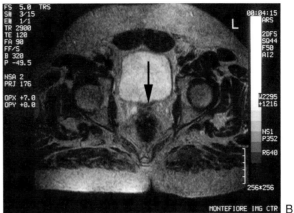

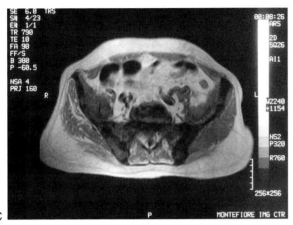

FIG. 21-19. Prostate cancer. Axial T2-weighted image [repetition time (TR), 2,900 ms; echo time (TE), 120 ms] in a patient with prostate cancer. **A:** Areas of decreased signal intensity (SI) in the peripheral zone (*arrows*) are consistent with foci of tumor. **B:** Area of decreased SI in the seminal vesicles (*arrow*) is with invasion by prostate cancer. **C:** T1-weighted image (TR, 790 ms; TE, 10 ms) in a different patient with prostate cancer. Heterogeneous decreased SI in the pelvic bones is consistent with metastatic disease.

suppressing the signal of pelvic fat and thereby increasing the range of contrast in other pelvic structures. Sagittal and coronal images and postgadolinium images may be helpful. T2-weighted images in planes orthogonal to the uterine axis are needed to best evaluate the outer contour of the uterus and the contents of the endometrial cavity and to delineate the zonal anatomy. The axis of the uterus is extremely variable from patient to patient (see Fig. 21-15). Therefore, the scout images play an important role in setting up the remainder of the study. A smaller field of view for the uterus is desirable but must be weighed against potential signal loss. Therefore, the appropriate field of view varies from patient to patient. If the patient can fit into a dedicated pelvis coil, this should be used instead of a body coil, because the pelvis coil offers a better signal-to-noise ratio (Fig. 21-18).

Prostate and Bladder

MRI of the prostate is best suited as a staging tool for prostate cancer. The zonal anatomy of the prostate is fairly well delineated on T2-weighted images. The peripheral zone is of high SI on T2-weighted images. This zone is the site of most prostate cancer, which is hypointense on T2-weighted images. Extension of tumor through the prostatic capsule and into the seminal vesicles can be seen by MRI. However, MRI is not reliable at detecting microscopic capsular invasion (1,23). Those patients believed to have disease contained within the prostatic capsule are potential surgical candidates (1,23). The seminal vesicles contain fluid and therefore are typically of increased SI on T2-weighted images. Decreased SI on T2-weighted images in the seminal vesicles is seen with tumor invasion (Fig. 21-19). On T1-weighted images, increased SI may be seen in the seminal vesicles from foci of hemorrhage if the patient is imaged after a biopsy has been performed (23). MRI can also assess for pelvic adenopathy and osseus metastases. The central and transitional zones make up the central gland, where benign prostatic hypertrophy occurs (23).

Diseases of the bladder may also be assessed by MRI, facilitated by the inherent contrast differences between the bladder wall and urine (Fig. 21-20). For a more detailed discussion of prostate and bladder MRI, I recommend reference 23.

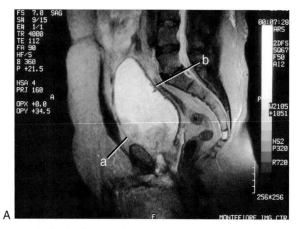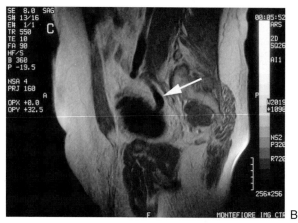

FIG. 21-20. Bladder cancer (transitional cell cancer). **A:** Sagittal T2-weighted image [repetition time (TR), 4,000 ms; echo time (TE), 112 ms] demonstrates (*a*) a large mass at the inferior aspect of the bladder and (*b*) a second smaller lesion posteriorly. **B:** Sagittal T1-weighted image (TR, 550 ms; TE, 10 ms) demonstrates dilatation of the right ureter (*arrow*) extending from the bladder superiorly, caused by the large bladder mass involving the trigone.

REFERENCES

1. Brown JJ, Wippold FJ Jr. *Practical MRI: a teaching file*. Philadelphia: Lippincott–Raven Publishers, 1996.
2. Ros PR, ed. *MRI clinics of North America. MR imaging of the liver*. Philadelphia: WB Saunders, May 1997.
3. Rumack CM, Wilson SR, Charboneau JW, eds. *Diagnostic ultrasound*. St. Louis: Mosby, 1991.
4. Semelka RC, Brown ED, Ascher SM, et al. Hepatic hemangiomas: a multi-institutional study of appearance on T2-weighted and serial gadolinium-enhanced gradient-echo MR images. *Radiology* 1994;192:402–406.
5. Mirowitz SA, ed. *MRI clinics of North America. Extrahepatic abdominal MR imaging*. Philadelphia: WB Saunders, February 1995.
6. Siegelman ES, Mitchell DG, Semelka RC. Abdominal iron deposition: metabolism, MR findings and clinical importance. *Radiology* 1996;199:13–22.
7. Siegelman ES, Mitchell DG, Outwater E, Munoz SJ, Rubin R. Idiopathic hemochromatosis: MR imaging findings in cirrhotic and precirrhotic patients. *Radiology* 1993;188:637–641.
8. Barish MA, Soto JA. MR cholangiopancreatography: techniques and clinical applications. *AJR Am J Roentgenol* 1997;169:1295–1303.
9. Fulcher AS, Turner MA, Capps GW. MR cholangiography: technical advances and clinical applications. *Radiographics* 1999;19:25–41.
10. Fulcher AS, Turner MA. MR pancreatography: a useful tool for evaluating pancreatic disorders. *Radiographics* 1999;19:5–24.
11. Rofsky NM, ed. *MRI clinics of North America. Contrast agents for body MR imaging*. Philadelphia: WB Saunders, February 1996.
12. Vogl TJ, Hammersting R, Schwarz W. Superparamagnetic iron oxide-enhanced versus gadolinium-enhanced MR imaging for differential diagnosis of focal liver lesions. *Radiology* 1996;198:881–887.
13. Reimer P, Tomach B. Hepatic MRI with SPIO: detection and characterization of focal liver lesions. *Eur Radiol* 1998;8(7):1198–1204.
14. Elster AD. *Questions and answers in magnetic resonance imaging*. St. Louis: Mosby, 1994.
15. Mattrey R, Trambert M, Edelman RR. MR Imaging of the Upper Abdomen and Adrenal Glands. In: Edelman R, et al., eds. *Clinical magnetic resonance imaging*. Philadelphia: WB Saunders, 1990.
16. Abrams HL, Spiro R, Goldstein N. Metastases in carcinoma: analysis of 1000 autopsied cases. *Cancer* 1950;3:74–85.
17. Mitchell DG, Crovello M, Matteucci T, Petersen RD, Miettinen MM. Benign adrenocortical masses: diagnosis with chemical shift MR imaging. *Radiology* 1992;185:345–351.
18. Tsushima Y, Ishizaka H, Matsumoto M. Adrenal masses: differentiation with chemical shift, fast low angle shot MR imaging. *Radiology* 1993;186:705–709.
19. Brown JJ, ed. *MRI clinics of North America. Genitourinary MR imaging*. Philadelphia: WB Saunders, February 1997.
20. Mirowitz SA. Diagnostic pitfalls and artifacts in abdominal MR imaging: a review. *Radiology* 1998;208:577–589.
21. Amis ES Jr, et al. *Essentials of uroradiology*. Boston: Little, Brown and Company, 1991.
22. Mezrich R, ed. *MRI clinics of North America. The female pelvis*. Philadelphia: WB Saunders, May 1994.
23. Tempany MC, ed. *MRI clinics of North America. The male pelvis*. Philadelphia: WB Saunders, August 1996.

Open MRI,
edited by Peter A. Rothschild and Debra Reinking Rothschild.
Lippincott Williams & Wilkins. Philadelphia © 2000.

CHAPTER **22**

Kinematic Magnetic Resonance Imaging of the Joints

Frank G. Shellock

A functional assessment of the joints is accomplished using kinematic magnetic resonance imaging (MRI) techniques (1–4). *Kinematic* is a biomechanical term that describes the movement of a body without reference to force or mass (5). Kinematic MRI involves evaluation of joint function with respect to the various interactions of the soft tissue and osseous anatomic features that the joint comprises. Typically, the relative alignment of anatomic structures is studied through a given range of motion (ROM) for the joint to determine the existence of an abnormality (1–4).

Kinematic MRI techniques were developed in recognition of the fact that certain pathologic conditions that affect the joints depend on the specific positions of the joints (e.g., flexion or extension), are related to reactions to stressed or "loaded" conditions, or both. Conventional, static-view MRI examinations may miss abnormal findings because the joint is not assessed through a ROM or during a loaded condition (e.g., in cases of patellar subluxation, peroneal tendon subluxation, carpal instability) (1–4). The functional information obtained using kinematic MRI often is used to definitively identify and characterize the underlying abnormality or to supplement the information acquired with standard MRI techniques. Combining kinematic MRI with the routine examination of the joint provides a means of conducting a more thorough examination and improves the diagnostic yield of the imaging procedure.

Kinematic MRI techniques have been developed and applied to assess the ankle, cervical spine, patellofemoral joint, shoulder, wrist, and temporomandibular joint (1–4,6–65). All forms of MRI systems have been used for kinematic MRI examinations of the joints, including high-field, tunnel-shaped MRI systems; low- or midfield, open MRI systems;

low-field, C-shaped magnet MRI systems; and low-field, dedicated-extremity MRI systems (1–4,6–65). MRI systems with open configurations offer the desirable advantages of being able to accomplish greater incremental movements for certain joints (e.g., the shoulder and cervical spine) and are inherently more comfortable for patients during kinematic MRI scanning.

This chapter discusses the basic kinematic MRI protocols used for functional imaging of the joints (with the exception of the temporomandibular joint), describes the various clinical applications and indications for kinematic MRI, and illustrates the usefulness of these techniques for diagnosis or elucidation of pathologic conditions. Table 22-1 provides a summary of the proposed indications for kinematic MRI of the joints.

GENERAL PRINCIPLES OF KINEMATIC MAGNETIC RESONANCE IMAGING

Protocols and Techniques

Protocols for kinematic MRI have used a variety of pulse sequences and joint positioning strategies. In general, kinematic MRI methods are divided into four primary types: (a) the incremental, passive positioning technique; (b) the cine-cyclic technique; (c) the active movement (i.e., dynamic) technique; and (d) the active movement against resistance technique (3,4).

The incremental, passive positioning technique involves the gradual movement of the joint through a specific ROM. MR images are obtained at each position using a T1-weighted spin-echo (SE), fast spin-echo (FSE), or gradient-echo (GRE) pulse sequence (3,4).

The cine-cyclic method (also known as *motion-triggered MRI*) is similar to a gated MRI procedure, such as that used for cardiac studies. During this type of kinematic MRI, physical movement of the joint is repeated for several min-

F. G. Shellock: Department of Radiology, University of Southern California School of Medicine, Los Angeles, California; R & D Services, Inc., Los Angeles, California

TABLE 22-1. *Indications for kinematic magnetic resonance imaging (MRI) of the joints*

Ankle
  Differentiates partial- from full-thickness tears of
    ligaments and tendons
  Identifies position-dependent pathologic findings
  Determines occult subluxation of the peroneal tendons
  Identifies subtalar instability syndrome
  Supplements diagnostic information provided by routine
    MRI of the ankle
Cervical spine
  Identifies position-dependent pathologic findings
  Supplements diagnostic information provided by routine
    MRI of the cervical spine
Patellofemoral joint
  Defines patellofemoral joint anatomy
  Identifies and characterizes patellar alignment and
    tracking abnormalities
  Guides and evaluates treatment techniques
Shoulder
  Evaluates abnormalities of the anterior glenoid labrum
  Supplements diagnostic information provided by routine
    MRI of the shoulder
Wrist
  Identifies position-dependent pathologic findings
  Determines and characterizes carpal instability
  Differentiates partial- from full-thickness tears of the
    intercarpal ligaments
  Supplements diagnostic information provided by routine
    MRI of the wrist

utes while MR images are obtained, usually using a T1-weighted SE pulse sequence (3,4,28,29).

The active movement technique uses a GRE pulse sequence or echo-planar imaging (EPI) to rapidly obtain MR images during active or dynamic motion of the joint. A temporal resolution of one image per second or less is typically required for this form of kinematic MRI procedure (3,4,32,36,41).

The active movement against resistance method is similar to the active movement technique with respect to the MRI protocol requirements. However, this form of kinematic MRI also imposes a resistive load to stress the joint during dynamic movement using a special positioning device (3,4,42,43).

Positioning Devices

Positioning devices are necessary accessories for the performance of kinematic MRI examinations (3,4). These devices maintain and guide the joint in a specific plane for imaging and through a specific ROM. Kinematic MRI positioning devices must be constructed from components that are compatible with the electromagnetic fields used during MRI (e.g., plastic, wood, nonferromagnetic metals).

Kinematic MRI positioning devices must be designed with a thorough understanding of the biomechanical aspects of the joint. For example, positioning devices designed for the

patellofemoral joint should permit unrestricted rotational movements of the lower extremity while the joint moves from approximately 45 degrees of flexion to extension (i.e., the ROM for the patellar articulation with the femoral trochlear groove that is necessary to accurately visualize patellar tracking abnormalities) (1–4). This movement of the patellofemoral joint can only be accomplished with the patient in a prone or supine position. Placement of the patient on his or her side in a lateral position for kinematic MRI of the patellofemoral joint prevents rotational movements of the lower extremity and adversely influences patellofemoral joint kinematics (3,5). Accordingly, the diagnostic capability of the kinematic MRI examination is impaired.

Positioning devices used for kinematic MRI may also apply a resistance to the joint during movement using various mechanisms, including resistive rubber bands, vacuum techniques, or pneumatically driven methods. Positioning devices typically have component parts that permit incorporation of surface coils to facilitate MRI. Surface coils are especially crucial for MRI examinations of the smaller joints, such as the ankle and wrist. Several commercially available positioning devices have been developed in consideration of the above-mentioned factors and principals, including those sold by Chamco (Cocoa Beach, FL), General Electric Medical Systems (Milwaukee, WI), and Captain Plastic (Seattle, WA).

Visualization of Kinematic Magnetic Resonance Images

The MR images obtained using kinematic MRI techniques may be visualized as individual, static images or displayed as a cine-loop. Visualization of the MR images as a cine-loop involves using the software provided with the MRI system to produce a forward-and-backward "paging" format of the multiple images obtained at a single section location. Display of the images acquired in this manner facilitates rapid viewing of the multiple images that are usually obtained at the different section locations of the joint being evaluated.

Compared with viewing individual static images of the kinematic MRI study, the cine-loop display is considered to provide the best diagnostic information regarding the joint with respect to the various patterns of normal or abnormal motions that may exist. This is particularly important for cases in which the kinematic abnormality may be subtle. Furthermore, making videotapes of the kinematic MRI cine-loops enables the examinations to be easily maintained as permanent records for the imaging facility and to be sent to the referring physicians so that they can view the studies and share the findings with their patients.

The kinematic MRI examination is usually evaluated using qualitative criteria developed and applied in consideration of the specific biomechanical aspects of the joint with regard to the interactions between soft tissue structures and osseous anatomy that occur during a given ROM. This information is described herein for the various joints.

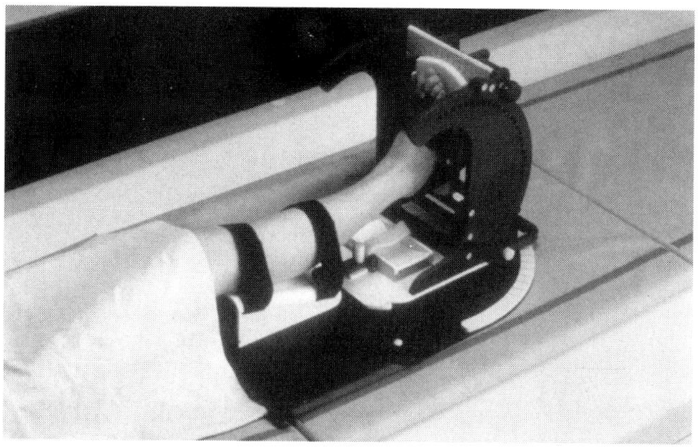

FIG. 22-1. Positioning device for kinematic magnetic resonance imaging examination of the ankle. This positioning device allows the ankle to be placed into incremental, passive positions of dorsiflexion, neutral, and plantarflexion as well as in inversion and eversion.

ANKLE

Kinematic MRI of the ankle continues to evolve with respect to its clinical applications (1–4,6–8). Using a combination of standard, high-resolution static MRI methods and kinematic MRI, a variety of pathologic conditions that affect this joint have been studied. Investigations indicate that kinematic MRI studies provide a more thorough examination of the ankle, particularly in cases conducted to assess subluxation of osseous anatomy, to determine the presence of loose bodies, to identify impingement syndromes, and to evaluate soft tissue abnormalities (1–4,6–8).

Some of the specific clinical applications for kinematic MRI of the ankle includes assessment of tibiotalar rotation, evaluation of subtalar instability, characterization of the loading area of the talar dome, and determination of conditions that affect the tendons and ligaments (1–4,6–8). More recently, an important kinematic MRI of the ankle application has been developed for the assessment of subluxation of the peroneal tendons (7).

Protocol

The small size and complex anatomy of the ankle make high-resolution kinematic MRI views essential for the optimal examination of this joint (1–4). Therefore, an apparatus that incorporates a surface coil should be used for this procedure (Fig. 22-1). This type of positioning device permits high-resolution imaging for static and kinematic MRI studies (4,6).

For the kinematic MRI examination, the patient is typically placed on the MRI system table in a supine position. The foot and ankle are fixed to the positioning device using Velcro straps, foam pads, or other means. Kinematic MRI is performed using an incremental, passive positioning technique

with the ankle positioned in dorsiflexion and then progressively moved through an ROM to full plantarflexion, while sagittal or axial (depending on the anatomy of interest) T1-weighted SE or GRE images are acquired at each increment.

In other cases, incremental, passive positioning of the ankle may be performed with the ankle placed in inversion, neutral, and eversion positions (e.g., if the intent is to assess subtalar instability or the lateral and medial soft tissue structures), while coronal MR images are obtained. Again, T1-weighted SE or GRE images are typically acquired at each increment. Section thickness should be 5 to 7 mm, using a 10- to 16-cm field of view. Either individual, static MR images or a cine-loop format can be used to evaluate the multiple images obtained at different section locations for the kinematic MRI study of the ankle.

Normal Kinematics

The movement of the ankle joint occurs primarily in the sagittal plane, which permits dorsiflexion (i.e., flexion) and plantarflexion (i.e., extension) as the talus rotates beneath the tibia and fibula (5) (Fig. 22-2). The stability of the ankle is preserved mainly by the configuration of the talus and its conformation to the shapes of the tibia and fibula (4,5,66,67). Primary soft tissue stabilizing structures include the anterior talofibular and calcaneofibular ligaments on the lateral aspect of the joint and the deltoid ligament on the medial side. The various musculotendinous structures that encompass the ankle are involved in stabilization of the joint to a lesser degree.

Abnormalities of the osseous anatomy and alterations of the soft tissue restraints (e.g., overstretched, partially torn, or ruptured ligaments) markedly affect the stability of the ankle and can produce substantial malalignment or subluxation of joint surfaces (5,66,67). These changes are typically manifested as a loss of ROM and pain-related symptoms, particularly with the ankle in a dorsiflexed position (66,67). Furthermore, slight displacements of the tibiotalar or fibulotalar articulations can produce dramatic changes in the loading stresses on the ankle and create severe pathologic conditions (66,67).

Pathokinematics

Because of the relatively limited experience with kinematic MRI of the ankle, the examples in the following sections represent only a partial compilation of the potential uses of this diagnostic imaging technique when imaging this joint in the sagittal plane.

Position-Related Impingement

Evaluation of patients with chronic ankle pain is difficult, because a variety of possible mechanisms, including

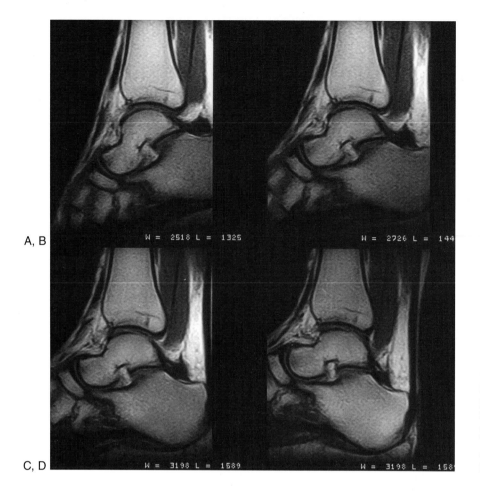

A, B

C, D

FIG. 22-2. Kinematic magnetic resonance imaging examination of the ankle in full plantarflexed **(A)**, partial plantarflexed **(B)**, neutral **(C)**, and dorsiflexed **(D)** positions (sagittal T1-weighted spin-echo image). This normal kinematic study shows smooth, even movement as the talus rotates beneath the tibia.

impingement of osseous anatomy (Fig. 22-3), impingement of soft tissue structures, osteochondritis dissecans, or loose bodies, are potentially responsible for the symptoms. Kinematic MRI combined with high-resolution, static-view MRI of the ankle provides diagnostic information that permits differentiation and characterization of these various conditions (1–4,6).

Osseous or soft tissue impingement syndromes that affect the ankle typically cause pain and inhibit motion during dorsiflexion (66,67). In the past, it was thought that impingement syndromes of the ankle were simply caused by osseous structures, such as an osteophyte on the anterior aspect of the tibia that impacts the talus during dorsiflexion (Fig. 22-4). However, soft tissue impingement syndromes associated with inversion injuries of the ankle have since been described (66,67). After tears of the lateral ankle ligaments—usually the talofibular ligament, the calcaneofibular ligament, or both—the healing process may be accompanied by scarring and capsular hypertrophy predominantly found in the antero-lateral space. This finding can produce a soft tissue impingement during dorsiflexion of the ankle. In these cases,

kinematic MRI can demonstrate impingement of the soft tissue mass during movements of the ankle.

Kinematic MRI of the ankle has also been used to evaluate conditions that affect the Achilles tendon. For example, kinematic MRI may be used to differentiate between partial- and full-thickness tears and to study the Achilles tendon after surgical restoration (Fig. 22-5).

Subluxation of the Peroneal Tendons

Ankle injuries may result in subluxation of the peroneal tendons, which is often unrecognized and frequently misdiagnosed as an ankle sprain, such that the appropriate initial management of the patient is delayed (7,68,69). Chronic subluxation of the peroneal tendons can be disabling, particularly if tendon pathology is also present.

The incidence of peroneal tendon subluxation is on the rise owing to an increase in recreational sports activities and in awareness of the abnormality. Although lateral joint pain and tenderness are characteristic signs of peroneal tendon abnor-

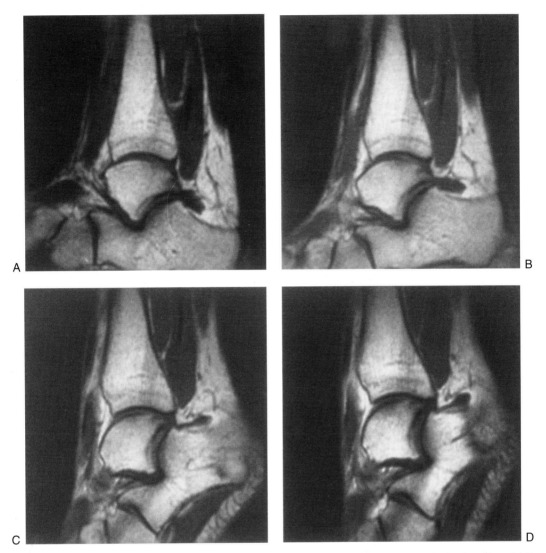

FIG. 22-3. Kinematic magnetic resonance imaging (MRI) examination of the ankle in dorsiflexed **(A)**, neutral **(B)**, partial plantarflexed **(C)**, and full plantarflexed **(D)** positions (sagittal gradient-echo image). An osseous impingement prevents proper movement into the dorsiflexed position. There is an anterior shift of the talus relative to the tibia. This disorder would go undetected by routine MRI of the ankle because it is position dependent.

malities, other associated lesions may produce identical symptoms (7,68,69).

In the acute injury, clinical evaluation of the peroneal tendons may be hindered by associated swelling and tenderness, which can be partially attributed to disruption of neighboring ligaments or osseous structures (68,69). Additionally, pain over the calcaneofibular ligament with peroneal tendon subluxation can confuse the presenting symptomatology. Chronic, recurrent subluxation is also difficult to detect clinically, especially if the displacement is subtle or the tendons spontaneously move back into position. Therefore, the identification of peroneal tendon subluxation by physical examination is frequently a problematic task because the clinical

signs may mimic other forms of ankle injuries and coexisting abnormalities may be present.

Various biomechanical mechanisms of injury are postulated to be responsible for subluxation of the peroneal tendons, including violent or forced dorsiflexed or plantarflexed positions of the ankle (68,69). In consideration of the pathokinematics of this abnormality, it is helpful to visualize the peroneal tendons during dorsiflexed and plantarflexed ankle movements using kinematic MRI (7,68,69). Doing so allows direct identification of subluxation of the peroneal tendons and provides the ability to determine occult displacements, because spontaneous reduction of subluxated tendons is known to occur (7,69).

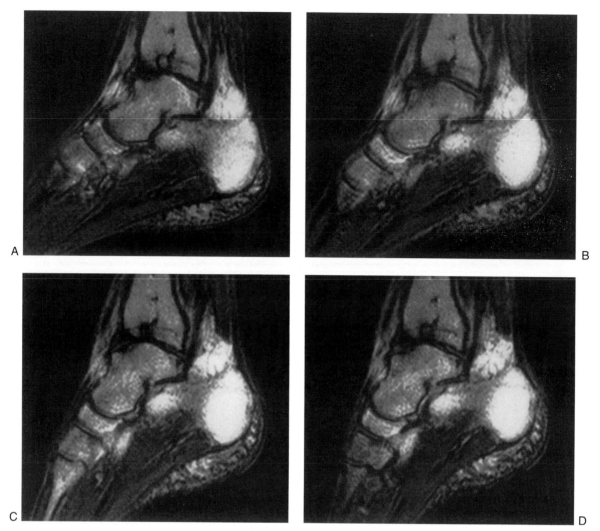

FIG. 22-4. Kinematic magnetic resonance imaging examination of the ankle in dorsiflexed **(A)**, neutral **(B)**, partial plantarflexed **(C)**, and full plantarflexed **(D)** positions (sagittal T1-weighted spin-echo image). The osseous impingement that prevents movement into the dorsiflexed position was caused by a relatively large osteophyte on the talus. Sclerotic osseous changes are also seen in the tibia. This patient had a prior traumatic injury.

Peroneal tendon subluxation is often associated with serious sequelae. A patient who has subluxation of the peroneal tendons that is not repaired or treated in the early stages after injury typically has a poor prognosis (68,69). Therefore, a timely and accurate diagnosis of this abnormality is critical for appropriate patient management. Kinematic MRI of the ankle performed in the axial plane using the aforementioned positioning device to move the joint in incremental, passive positioning has been reported to be a useful means of identifying subluxation of the peroneal tendons (7).

Peroneal Tendons

Normal Kinematics

The normal kinematics of the peroneal tendons is dependent on the integrity of several elastic structures: the superior peroneal retinaculum and the inferior peroneal tendon retinaculum. In addition, the retromalleolar groove must be shaped to facilitate retention of the peroneal tendons during movements of the ankle (68,69).

The peroneal tendon complex is comprised of the peroneus longus and brevis tendons, which are ensheathed by a common synovial membrane. The tendon and sheath bundle course through a fibro-osseous canal composed primarily of the superior peroneal retinaculum and the undersurface of the distal fibular tip. These structures, along with the retromalleolar groove, maintain the peroneal tendons in a constant position during movements of the ankle. Therefore, the normal kinematic study of the peroneal tendons shows these structures in a fixed position relative to the retromalleolar groove of the lateral malleolus during dorsiflexed, neutral, and plantarflexed positions of the ankle (7). In addition, at the level of the calcaneus, the peroneal tendons should be positioned parallel relative to the lateral border of the calca-

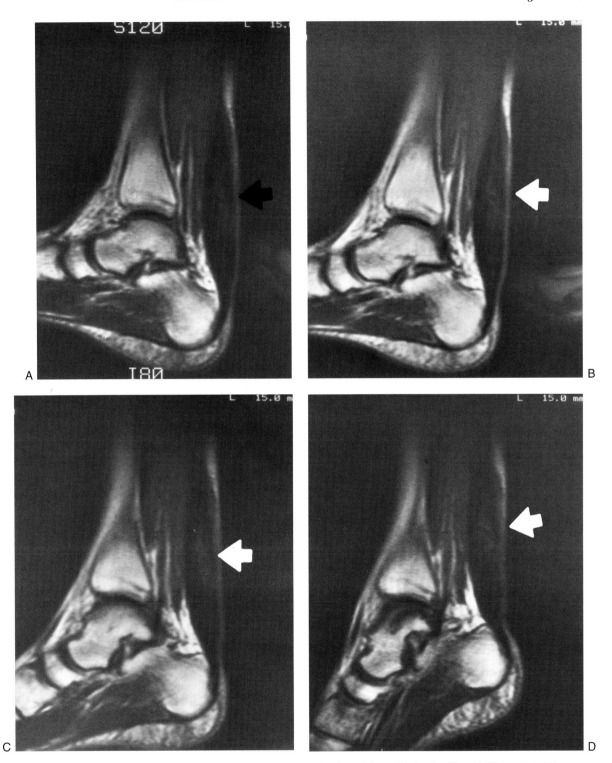

FIG. 22-5. Kinematic magnetic resonance imaging examination of the ankle in dorsiflexed **(A)**, neutral **(B)**, partial plantarflexed **(C)**, and full plantarflexed **(D)** positions (sagittal T1-weighted spin-echo image). This study was performed to assess the Achilles tendon after a surgical repair. Note the site of the musculotendinous junction where the tendon was repaired (*arrows*).

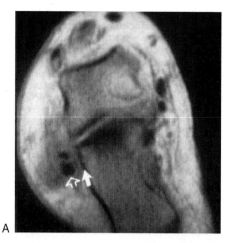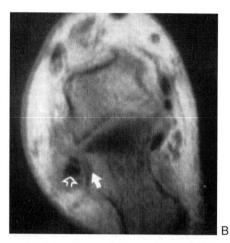

A

B

FIG. 22-6. Kinematic magnetic resonance imaging examination of the ankle in dorsiflexed **(A)** and fully plantarflexed **(B)** positions using incremental, passive positioning technique (axial fast spoiled gradient-echo image). Image of the peroneal tendons (*white arrows*) obtained at the level of the calcaneous shows lateral subluxation relative to the lateral border of the calcaneous (*clear arrows*). The peroneal longus tendon is displaced laterally relative to the calcaneus and becomes distorted in this position.

neus during dorsiflexed, neutral, and plantarflexed movements of the ankle.

Pathokinematics

Subluxation of the peroneal tendons occurs when the tendons move laterally over the lateral malleolus. This condition may occur with varying degrees of severity, from subtle displacements relative to the retromalleolar groove associated with dorsiflexed or plantarflexed movements of the ankle to constant displacement of the peroneal tendons unrelated to the position of the ankle (i.e., the peroneal tendons remain in a displaced position irrespective of the position of the ankle) (7,68,69). When an abnormality is present, the kinematic MR images obtained in the axial plane show the peroneal tendons displaced relative to the retromalleolar groove or relative to the lateral aspect of the calcaneus, or both, in association with changes in the position of the ankle (Fig. 22-6). In rare cases, medial subluxation of the peroneal tendons occurs.

The primary causes of peroneal tendon subluxation include those associated with predisposing anatomy, such as a shallow, flat, or convex retromalleolar groove, and a weakened, overstretched, or torn peroneal retinaculum. Various forms of retinacular pathology may be responsible for subluxation of the peroneal tendons, including congenital absence of the retinaculum, laxity of the retinaculum in a paralyzed extremity or an extremity in chronic pronation, or retinacular hyperelasticity (68,69).

CERVICAL SPINE

Functional assessment of the cervical spine may be performed using kinematic MRI techniques. The kinematic MRI examination of the cervical spine is capable of showing the relationship between the odontoid, foramen magnum, and cervical spinal cord as the patient's neck is moved through an ROM (1–4,9–18). Frequently, abnormalities that affect the cervical spine go undetected using routine MRI with the patient's cervical spine in a neutral position because the pathology or condition is position dependent (1–4,9–18). Kinematic MRI examinations contribute to a more thorough evaluation of the anatomy of the cervical spine, with indications that include the assessment of the rheumatoid cervical spine, cervical spondylitic myelopathy, cervical spondylosis, and other conditions (9–18). Furthermore, the kinematic MRI examination provides critical information for staging disorders and

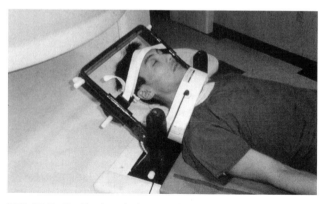

FIG. 22-7. Positioning device used to perform kinematic magnetic resonance imaging (MRI) examination of the cervical spine. The positioning device permits incremental, passive movements of the cervical spine into flexed, neutral, and extended positions. Midsagittal images are usually obtained to assess the cervical spine using the kinematic MRI technique. Note the surface coil that facilitates the kinematic MRI examination.

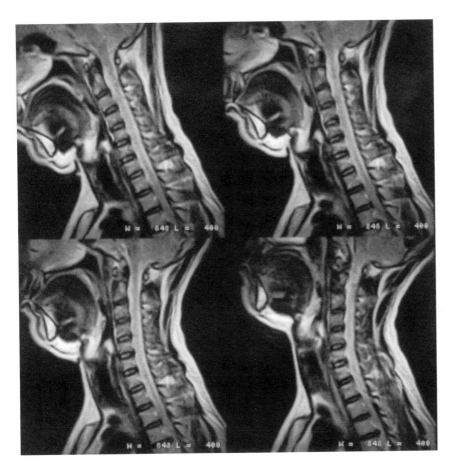

FIG. 22-8. Kinematic magnetic resonance imaging examination of the cervical spine shows extended, neutral, and flexed positions using the incremental, passive positioning technique (sagittal fast spoiled gradient-echo image). This is a normal kinematic examination of the cervical spine.

planning conservative or surgical treatments of the cervical spine (9–13,16–18).

Muhle et al. (14) indicated that kinematic MRI of the cervical spine gave additional noninvasive data concerning physiologic changes of the cervical subarachnoid space and the cervical cord during flexion and extension in healthy individuals. Muhle et al. (13) further reported that kinematic MRI of the cervical spine identified a high percentage of cases with increased spinal stenosis at flexion and extension that were not observed in the neutral position. They concluded that this technique is capable of demonstrating dynamic factors responsible for the pathogenesis of cervical spondylotic myelopathy (13).

Allmann et al. (18) studied patients with rheumatoid arthritis of the cervical spine using kinematic MRI. The kinematic MRI procedure provided good differentiation of the extension of pannus tissue cranial, ventral, and dorsal of the dens with displacing and impinging effects on the spinal cord during the associated movements. Allmann et al. (18) reported that fusion, instabilities, and compressions of the bone marrow often can only be detected with the aid of the kinematic MRI procedure.

Protocol

Kinematic MRI of the cervical spine is performed using a positioning device that incorporates a flexible surface

coil or other similar coil configuration to facilitate imaging using an incremental, passive positioning technique or active movement (i.e., dynamic) technique (1–4,9–18) (Fig. 22-7). For the kinematic MRI procedure, midsagittal images are usually obtained with the cervical spine in extended, neutral, and flexed positions (Fig. 22-8). If an abnormality is seen on the midsagittal images, oblique axial images may be obtained through the area of affected anatomy. T1-weighted, T2-weighted SE, FSE, and GRE pulse sequences have all been reportedly used for kinematic MRI procedures. T2-weighted FSE imaging parameters selected to produce a myelographic effect are considered optimal for the kinematic MRI examination of the cervical spine.

Evaluation of Kinematic Magnetic Resonance Imaging of the Cervical Spine

The midsagittal images obtained through the cervical spine are typically assessed using the same qualitative criteria applied to MR images acquired using routine imaging techniques (1–4,9–18). Attention is directed toward evaluation of position-dependent occipita-cervical changes, cord narrowing, subluxation, or other form of functional pathology (Fig. 22-9).

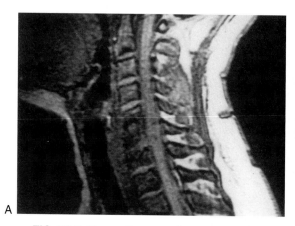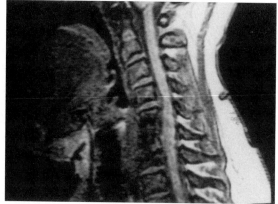

A   B

FIG. 22-9. Kinematic magnetic resonance imaging examination of the cervical spine shows neutral **(A)** and flexed **(B)** positions using the incremental, passive positioning technique (sagittal fast spoiled gradient-echo image). A narrowing of the cord seen during flexion is not apparent with the cervical spine in a neutral position.

PATELLOFEMORAL JOINT

Disorders of the patellofemoral joint are a primary source of anterior knee pain and occur with a frequency comparable to that of meniscal lesions (70–76). Patellar malalignment and abnormal tracking are typically produced by incongruence between the patella and femoral trochlear groove, resulting in instability of the patellofemoral joint. Malalignment and maltracking of the patellar are believed to produce substantial shearing forces and excessive contact stresses that develop lesions and eventual degeneration of the articular cartilage (70–76). A chronically malaligned patella may also change the load distribution in the patellofemoral joint and cause clinical symptoms in the absence of a detectable cartilage defect (70–76). Other possible causes of anterior knee pain that are less prevalent but should be considered in the differential diagnosis include overstretching of retinacular structures, reflex sympathetic dystrophy, bursitis, plica syndrome, hyperplasia of the peripatellar fat pad, and synovitis.

The detection of patellofemoral joint abnormalities solely by physical examination is often a formidable task, because the clinical signs may mimic other forms of internal derangements of the knee, and coexisting abnormalities are common (70–73). In addition, patients with persistent symptoms after patellar realignment surgery present a particular diagnostic challenge (24,27). Proper classification of abnormal patellar alignment and tracking is crucial for determination of the most appropriate treatment for these conditions (70,71,73).

Abnormal conditions of patellar alignment and tracking typically exist during the earliest portion of the ROM of this joint, as the patella enters and articulates with the femoral trochlear groove (71–73,77,78). As flexion of the joint increases, the patella moves deeper into the femoral trochlear groove. At this point, patellar displacement is less likely to occur, because the femoral trochlear groove buttresses and stabilizes the patella (71–73).

Because patellofemoral incongruence is most likely to occur during the initial degrees of joint flexion, diagnostic imaging techniques that show the joint during this portion of the ROM are best suited for the identification of abnormalities (1–4,73,77). Imaging the patellofemoral joint at 25 degrees or more of flexion frequently causes clinically important information to be overlooked. Studies have shown that patellar malalignment and abnormal tracking are not consistently or reliably identified by imaging techniques that image the joint at flexion angles of larger than 30 degrees (i.e., most plain radiographic methods) (1–4,73,77).

Kinematic MRI was first used for the evaluation of the patellofemoral joint in 1988 (19). Many studies have demonstrated that kinematic MRI is a useful and sensitive means of evaluating patellar alignment and tracking in patients with patellofemoral joint abnormalities (1–4,20–51,54,55,79). In fact, kinematic MRI has been reported to be more effective than physical examination alone in detecting patellofemoral incongruence (47).

Although conventional computed tomography and cine computed tomography have been used to perform kinematic studies of the patellofemoral joint (55,71–73,77,78), kinematic MRI has the advantage of showing the various soft tissue components (i.e., medial and lateral retinacula, patellar tendon, quadriceps muscles) involved in the stability and function of the patellofemoral joint (1–4). This information is frequently useful, because irregularities of one or more of these soft tissue structures are typically responsible for patellofemoral abnormalities (1–4,73,80).

Protocols

Each of the previously described kinematic MRI techniques has been used to evaluate the patellofemoral joint.

Incremental, Passive Positioning Technique

The first applications of kinematic MRI of the patellofemoral joint used an incremental, passive positioning technique (1–4,19–27,30,35,37). This technique involves obtaining multiple axial images at different section locations as one or both patellofemoral joints (patellofemoral joint abnormalities tend to be bilateral, so both joints should be evaluated) are passively flexed into incremental positions using a patient-activated positioning device. The use of this device is crucial because it suspends the patient's patellofemoral joints above the MRI system table with the patient in a prone position. With the patient placed in a prone position, direct anterior or lateral pressure may occur that is frequently sufficient to move the patella and give an erroneous appearance of patellar subluxation (F. G. Shellock, *unpublished observation*, 1987).

The MR images are obtained using a T1-weighted SE pulse sequence at several different section locations while the joint is flexed at 5-degree increments from 5 to 30 degrees. Because the patella and femoral trochlear groove are relatively large structures, comparatively low-resolution imaging parameters can be used for kinematic MRI of the patellofemoral joint (e.g., the body coil may be used for radiofrequency transmission and reception while T1-weighted SE images are obtained with one excitation, 256×128 acquisition matrix, 34- to 40-cm field of view, and a 5-mm section thickness).

When the patient is placed prone on the positioning device, special care should be taken to maintain the individual's lower-extremity alignment pattern (i.e., observed with the patient upright). Furthermore, it is crucial to use a positioning scheme (e.g., prone or supine) that allows rotational movements of the lower extremities to occur during flexion and extension of the patellofemoral joint (1–4). This is important because excessive internal or external rotation of the lower extremities may be partially responsible for abnormal patellar alignment and tracking (71–73). The kinematics of the patellofemoral joint have been shown to be the same with prone and supine positioning of the patient (1–3). Kinematic MRI of the patellofemoral joint using the incremental, passive positioning technique is an acceptable and sensitive means of evaluating patellar alignment and tracking (1–4).

Active Movement Techniques

Faster MRI techniques using fast GRE pulse sequences or EPI provide substantial improvements in temporal resolution, allowing MR images to be obtained during active movement of the patellofemoral joint (1–4,32,36,41,43). The primary advantage of using active movement kinematic MRI techniques is that the patellofemoral joint may be examined in terms of the influence of the activated muscles and other related soft tissue anatomy on patellar alignment and tracking (1–4,80,81). In addition, no sophisticated positioning device is needed, which further reduces the overall examination time.

When performing the active movement technique, a positioning device is used that suspends the patient's patellofemoral joints above the MRI system table, with the patient in a prone position. The patient is instructed to move from approximately 45 degrees of flexion (i.e., the maximum amount of joint flexion that can be achieved within the confines of the MRI system) to extension, while multiple MR images are obtained at a single section location. The patient should begin moving the patellofemoral joint(s) approximately 1 second after hearing the gradient noise that indicates MRI has begun, moving slowly to a fully extended position.

MRI should be conducted by selecting parameters that allow four to six images to be obtained at a single section location at the rate of approximately 1 image per second. Additionally, MR images should be obtained at three to four different section locations to evaluate the entire excursion of the patella as it articulates with the femoral trochlear groove. Compared to the incremental, passive positioning technique, a more physiologic examination is obtained and, in certain instances, abnormal patellar tracking is more apparent during active movement, kinematic MRI studies of the patellofemoral joint (41).

Cine-Cyclic Technique

Another active movement, kinematic MRI technique for imaging the patellofemoral joint uses a special positioning device that incorporates a trigger system, which senses the motion of the patellofemoral joint (28,29,44). The patellar alignment and tracking may then be assessed during active movement in a manner similar to the MRI technique used for cardiac gated studies. The patient is placed supine on the positioning device, and a single patellofemoral joint is flexed and extended repeatedly while GRE images are obtained using a circular surface coil (28,29,44). Compared to an incremental, passive positioning technique, motion-triggered cine kinematic MRI of the patellofemoral joint has been reported to show different patellar tracking patterns (28,29). This kinematic MRI technique supports the benefits of using an active movement method for evaluation of the patellofemoral joint.

Active Movement against Resistance Technique

Kinematic MRI of the patellofemoral joint has evolved so that the examination may be conducted during active movement against an externally applied resistance (3,4,42). The primary intent of developing this particular form of kinematic MRI was to stress the quadriceps and other associated soft tissues to displace the patella in the presence of any imbalances in these anatomic structures (42).

A major determinant of the effective function of the patellofemoral joint is the tolerance displayed in reaction to

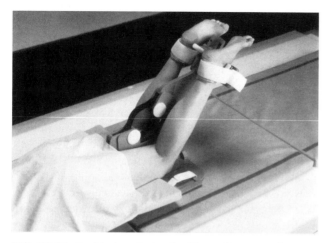

FIG. 22-10. Positioning device for kinematic magnetic resonance imaging examination of the patellofemoral joints using the active movement against resistance technique. The patient is placed on this device in a prone position. Velcro straps are applied loosely near the ankles to maintain the relative alignment of the lower extremities without impairing lower-extremity rotational movements during joint flexion. The patellofemoral joints are suspended over the table to permit uninhibited and unrestricted movement during flexion of the joints. A resistive band is used to apply a load during the examination.

external forces or stresses encountered during weight-bearing or movement (34,80,81). Patients with derangements of the patellofemoral joint usually experience pain or increased symptoms (usually instability) during activities (70–75). These findings are postulated to result from the high magnitude of quadriceps muscle force that occurs during physical actions associated with flexion of the patellofemoral joint (80,81). As the quadriceps muscle force rises, so does the reaction force imposed on the patellofemoral joint.

The active movement against resistance kinematic MRI examination is performed using a positioning device that incorporates a mechanism to apply resistance to the patellofemoral joint in the sagittal plane (Fig. 22-10). With the patient in a prone position, the movement against this resistance primarily requires activation of the extensor mechanism of the knee (42). The design of this device is such that a unilateral or bilateral examination may be accomplished as the patellofemoral joints move through an ROM from approximately 45 degrees of flexion to extension (42).

The loaded conditions of the active movement, kinematic MRI technique are imposed during the earliest increments of joint flexion when the muscle force required and the associated patellofemoral joint reaction forces are the greatest (42,80,81). Imaging parameters similar to previously described active movement technique are used for the active movement against resistance kinematic MRI examination.

The application of resistance to stress the patellofemoral joint during kinematic MRI has been shown to elicit patellar malalignment and tracking abnormalities that may not be observed during unloaded examinations (3,4,42,43). There-

fore, use of this kinematic MRI technique for evaluation of the patellofemoral joint represents an improved diagnostic means for identifying aberrant positions of the patella in relation to the femoral trochlear groove. Accordingly, the active movement against resistance kinematic MRI examination is considered the state-of-the-art method for diagnostic assessment of abnormal movement-related conditions.

Anatomy

Because the patella articulates with the femoral trochlear groove during knee flexion, congruent shapes of the patella and femoral trochlear groove are important for the proper function of the patellofemoral joint (71–76). Dysplastic osseous anatomy, abnormal soft tissue structures, or both are commonly observed in conjunction with patellofemoral instability (1–4,71–76). Careful inspection of the shapes of the patella and femoral trochlear groove often provides additional evidence concerning the presence of a patellofemoral joint disorder. However, the existence of abnormal morphology does not preclude normal patellar alignment and tracking (72,73).

Evaluation of the anatomic features of the patellofemoral joint is best accomplished by obtaining sequential axial images with the joint extended (1–4). Additionally, these axial MR images are useful for determining the position of the inferior pole of the patella relative to the femoral trochlear groove to identify patella alta (i.e., the patella in an excessive superior position) or patella infera (i.e., the patella in an excessive inferior position) (3,4).

Evaluation of Kinematic Magnetic Resonance Imaging

To properly assess patellar alignment and tracking, three to four different section locations through the femoral trochlear groove or femoral trochlea (depending on the position of the patella) should be evaluated during the initial increments of flexion to extension to thoroughly evaluate the kinematic aspects of this joint. The images obtained during the kinematic MRI examination of the patellofemoral joint can be qualitatively analyzed individually or as a cine-loop display (i.e., by making a cine-loop of the four to six MR images obtained at a given section location). The cine-loop display of the acquired images facilitates viewing of multiple images obtained at different section locations. Compared with the static images of patellar alignment and tracking, the cine-loop display is believed to provide the best qualitative information regarding the patellofemoral joint with respect to the pattern of patellar motion.

Limitations of Previously Used Methods

A variety of techniques have been suggested for identifying patellofemoral incongruence (71,73,82,85). The majority were designed for use with plain radiographs obtained at a single increment of joint flexion, usually larger than 30 degrees. These measurements are not practical or helpful for use with the kinematic MRI examination of the patellofemoral joint. The multiple images obtained during kinematic MRI at different increments of joint flexion provide more relevant information insofar as the overall pattern of patellar motion is demonstrated (1–4,47). Furthermore, no agreement has been reached on the usefulness of any particular quantification technique for determining patellar malalignment (1–4,71–73,82–85).

Abnormal patellofemoral joints often have associated anatomic irregularities (e.g., dysplastic patellae, dysplastic osseous anatomy, patella alta, patella infera), and these conditions preclude an accurate assessment of patellar alignment using quantification schemes, because no consistent landmarks exist for proper measurement of congruent patellofemoral anatomy (1–4,47). The quantitative assessment of patellofemoral incongruence has never been used by orthopedists to guide surgical or rehabilitative treatment of patellofemoral joint abnormalities.

Given the various problems associated with performing quantitative measurements of patellofemoral interactions, investigators and clinicians believe it is more appropriate and practical to use qualitative criteria to describe the patella relative to the femoral trochlear groove (or femoral trochlea) for the assessment of the MR images obtained during the kinematic MRI study (1–4,47). The severity of the alignment problem is demonstrated by the movements of the patella over the ROM examined, such that it is easy to determine whether the abnormal patellar movement patterns are improving, staying the same, or worsening during movements of the joint from flexion to extension.

With minor patellar malalignment and abnormal tracking, the displacement of the patella may be transient, as the patella centralizes or moves into a more normal position during increasing increments of joint flexion. Even minor patellofemoral joint incongruence may cause significant symptoms (75,76). With more severe patellar motion abnormalities, the patella is either maintained in its displaced position or further displaced (i.e., progressive subluxation) with increasing increments of joint flexion (1–4,47).

Normal Kinematics

During extension of the patellofemoral joint, essentially no forces are acting on the patella and, therefore, the patella may be situated medially, laterally, or in a centralized position relative to the femoral trochlear groove. Observing a "pseudosubluxation" of the patella during extension is considered a normal variant, because it may be found in any of the aforementioned positions. As previously indicated, images obtained with the patellofemoral joint extended are primarily useful for determining the position of the patella as it enters the femoral trochlear groove for identifying

patella alta or infera as well as to assess the anatomy of the patella and femoral trochlear groove.

During flexion, forces from various sources act on the patella (73,80,81). Normal alignment and tracking of the patella during flexion of the patellofemoral joint are dependent on the interaction of the dynamic stabilizers (i.e., primarily the quadriceps muscles), static stabilizers (i.e., the patellar tendon, lateral patellofemoral ligament, lateral patellar ligament, medial retinaculum, lateral retinaculum, and fascia lata), osseous structures (i.e., congruency between the shapes of the patella and femoral trochlear groove), and alignment of the femur and tibia (5,73,80,81). The disruption of one or more of the above is typically responsible for patellofemoral joint dysfunction.

Normal patellar alignment and tracking are displayed when the ridge of the patella is positioned directly in the center of the femoral trochlear groove and this orientation is maintained throughout the early and later increments of joint flexion, as the patella moves in a vertical plane (Fig. 22-11). Abnormalities of patellar alignment and tracking, which are usually transverse displacements, are apparent on the kinematic MRI examination when any deviation of this normal pattern of patellar movement is exhibited on one or more section locations at five degrees of joint flexion or greater (1–4,47).

Pathokinematics

Lateral Subluxation of the Patella

Lateral subluxation of the patella is a form of patellar malalignment in which the central ridge of the patella is laterally displaced relative to the femoral trochlear groove (or the center-most part of the femoral trochlea in cases of patella alta) and the lateral facet of the patella overlaps the lateral aspect of the femoral trochlea (Figs. 22-12, 22-13, and 22-14). Lateral subluxation is the most common form of patellar malalignment and abnormal tracking and occurs with varying degrees of severity (1–4).

Imbalanced forces from lateral soft tissue structures possibly combined with insufficient counterbalancing forces from medial soft tissue structures are typically the cause of lateral subluxation of the patella. A dysplastic patella, dysplastic femoral trochlear groove, or patella alta may also be partially responsible for this patellofemoral joint abnormality.

A redundant lateral retinaculum is sometimes associated with lateral subluxation of the patella in cases of lateral subluxation of the patella. This is an especially important finding that may be identified by kinematic MRI techniques and indicates that the subluxated patella is not caused by excessive force from the lateral retinaculum (1–4). Therefore, surgical release of the lateral retinaculum (a procedure frequently performed to realign a laterally subluxated patella) is unlikely to be the appropriate treatment for this type of patellar malalignment and abnormal tracking.

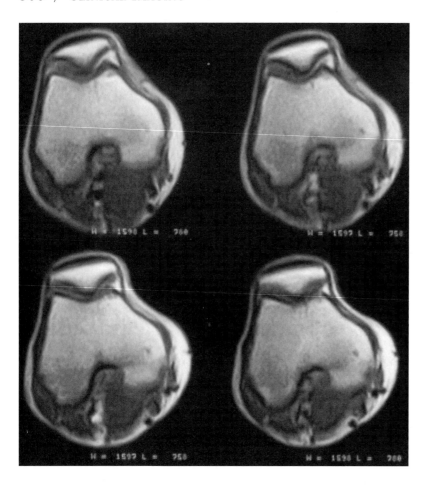

FIG. 22-11. Kinematic magnetic resonance imaging examination of the patellofemoral joint obtained using the active movement against resistance technique (axial fast spoiled gradient-echo image). This normal kinematic study demonstrates the patella in centralized positions relative to the femoral trochlear groove throughout the range of motion studied.

Lateral Patellar Tilt (Excessive Lateral Pressure Syndrome)

Lateral patellar tilt, or excessive lateral pressure syndrome (ELPS), was first described by Ficat and Hungerford (71). This form of patellar malalignment is a clinico-radiologic entity that is clinically characterized by anterior knee pain and radiologically characterized by tilting of the patella with functional patellar lateralization, usually onto a dominant lateral facet (71). A small amount of lateral displacement of the patella may or may not be present during joint flexion as increasing tension from one or more overly taut soft tissue structure(s) tilts the patella in a lateral fashion. Tilting of the patella onto the lateral aspect of the femoral trochlear groove often shifts the patellar ridge medially, and this may be designated *medial subluxation of the patella*, as opposed to ELPS (3,4). Several factors indicate that the main pathologic component of ELPS is excessive force from the lateral retinaculum (1–4,71). Because the patellar tilting that occurs with ELPS may be transient (i.e., centralization or correction of the patellar malalignment occurs during joint flexion) or progressive (i.e., additional patellar tilting is seen with increasing increments of joint flexion), kinematic MRI of the patellofemoral joint is particularly useful for identifying and characterizing this abnormality (1–4).

Medial Subluxation of the Patella (Patella Addentro)

Medial subluxation of the patella is distinguished by medial displacement of the patellar ridge relative to the femoral trochlear groove or the centermost part of the femoral trochlea (Figs. 22-15 and 22-16). Medial subluxation of the patella (patella addentro) has been characterized and studied extensively by clinical and diagnostic imaging techniques (23,24,86,87). This type of abnormal patellar alignment and tracking is frequently found in patients after surgical patellar realignment procedures in which overcompensation of the lateral tethering or stabilizing mechanisms of the patellofemoral joint has occurred (1–4,86,87). For example, the lateral soft tissue structures of the patellofemoral joint may be excessively released during a lateral retinacular release procedure, causing a patella that was laterally subluxated to become medially displaced.

Medial subluxation of the patella may also be found in patients without previous patellar realignment surgery (1–4,23,24). Various factors, singly or in combination, may be responsible for producing this type of aberrant patellar alignment and tracking, including an excessively tight medial retinaculum, insufficient lateral retinaculum, abnormal patellofemoral anatomy, and an imbalance of the

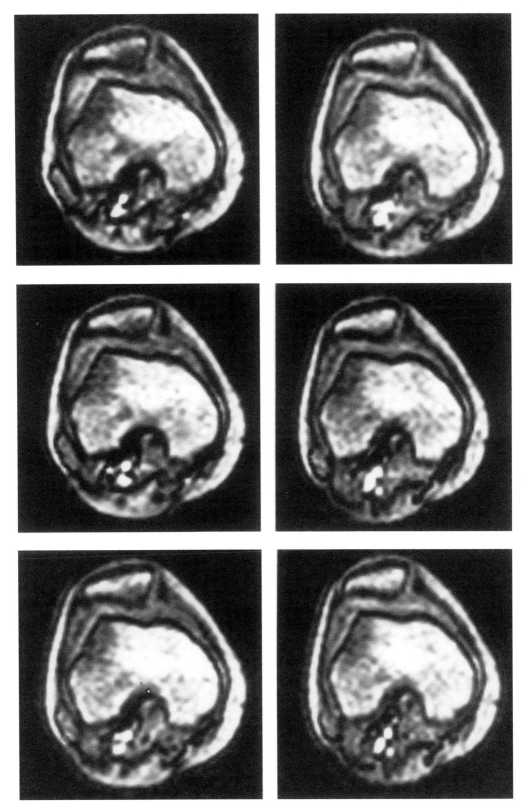

FIG. 22-12. Kinematic magnetic resonance imaging examination of the patellofemoral joint obtained using the active movement against resistance technique (axial fast spoiled gradient-echo image). This patient has lateral subluxation of the patella. Additionally, areas of decreased signal intensity in the lateral femoral condyle and median ridge of the patella are indicative of bone contusions. These findings are suggestive of a prior traumatic lateral dislocation of the patella.

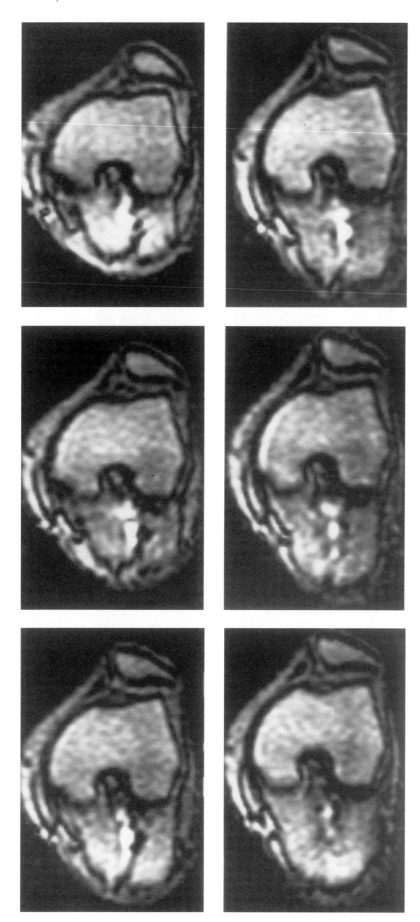

FIG. 22-13. Kinematic magnetic resonance imaging examination of the patellofemoral joint obtained using the active movement against resistance technique (axial fast spoiled gradient-echo image). This patient has lateral subluxation and lateral tilting of the patella.

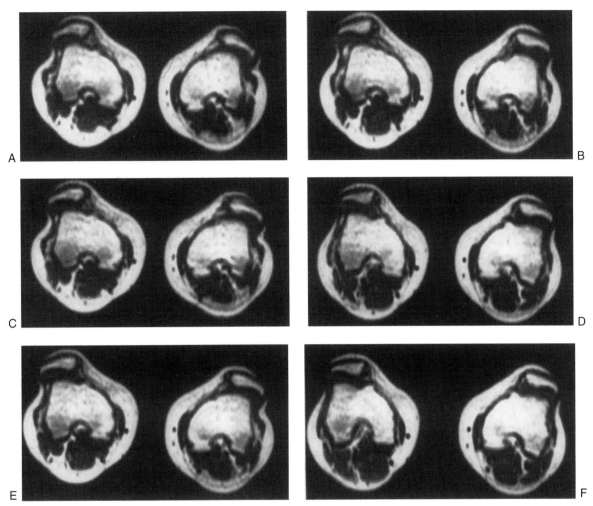

FIG. 22-14. Kinematic magnetic resonance imaging examination of the patellofemoral joint obtained using incremental, passive positioning technique (axial T1-weighted spin-echo image). This patient has bilateral lateral subluxation of the patellae. Laxity of the lateral retinacular structures on both joints suggests that a lateral release may not be an appropriate surgical treatment for these abnormal patellar positions: **(A)** 5 degrees, **(B)** 20 degrees, **(C)** 10 degrees, **(D)** 25 degrees, **(E)** 15 degrees, **(F)** 30 degrees.

quadriceps muscles. Extreme internal rotation of the lower extremities and atrophy of the vastus lateralis are common clinical findings in patients with medially subluxated patellae (Fig. 22-17). Determination of medial subluxation of the patella and distinguishing this particular form of patellar malalignment and abnormal tracking from lateral subluxation are crucial for the selection of the proper rehabilitative therapy or surgical treatment (86,87).

Lateral-to-Medial Subluxation of the Patella

Lateral-to-medial subluxation of the patella is a pattern of abnormal patellar alignment and tracking whereby the patella is positioned in a slight lateral subluxation during the initial increments of joint flexion (i.e., 5 to 10 degrees), moves into and across the femoral trochlear groove or femoral trochlea as flexion increases, and displaces medially during the higher increments of flexion. This relatively uncommon abnormality is typically found in association with patellofemoral joints that have patella alta, dysplastic osseous anatomy, or both, because insufficient stabilization is provided by the femoral trochlear groove (1–4). In addition, lateral-to-medial subluxation of the patella may occur in patellofemoral joints in which surgical attempts at patellar realignment have been unsuccessful.

The biomechanical factors responsible for lateral-to-medial subluxation of the patella are quite complicated. Various disordered or uncoordinated forces that act on the patella during joint flexion cause this pattern of abnormal patellar tracking and alignment. Kinematic MRI of the patellofemoral joint is particularly suited for determining the lateral-to-medial subluxation because it demonstrates the various positions of the patella at several different increments of joint flexion (1–4).

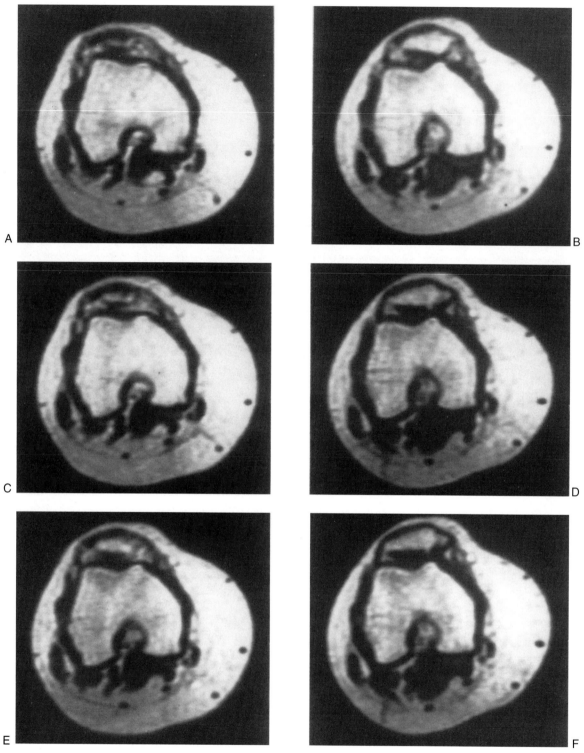

FIG. 22-15. Kinematic magnetic resonance imaging examination of the patellofemoral joints obtained using the incremental, passive positioning technique (axial T1-weighted spin-echo image). This patient has severe medial subluxation of the patella. A thickened lateral retinaculum is noted secondary to two prior lateral release surgeries: **(A)** 5 degrees, **(B)** 20 degrees, **(C)** 10 degrees, **(D)** 25 degrees, **(E)** 15 degrees, **(F)** 30 degrees.

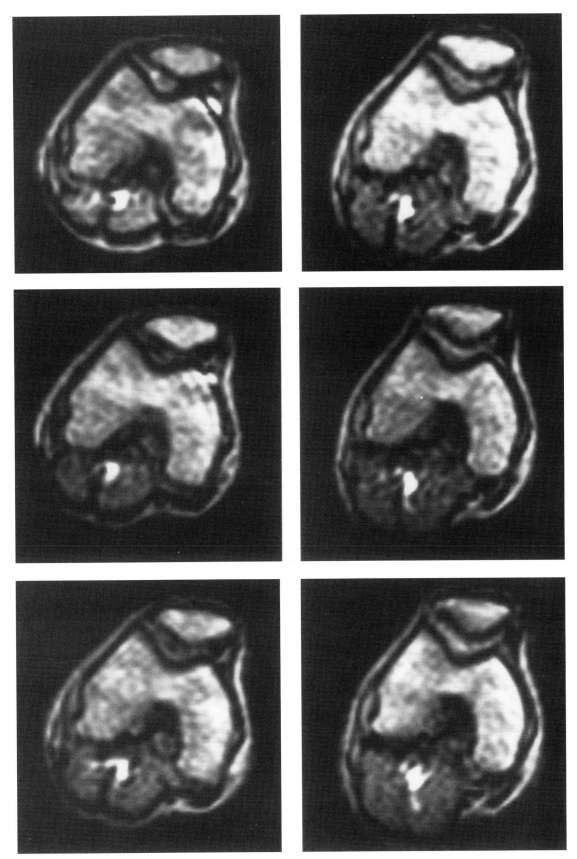

FIG. 22-16. Kinematic magnetic resonance imaging examination of the patellofemoral joint obtained using the active movement against resistance technique (axial fast spoiled gradient-echo image). This patient has medial subluxation of the patella. The patient did not have a prior surgery performed on this joint.

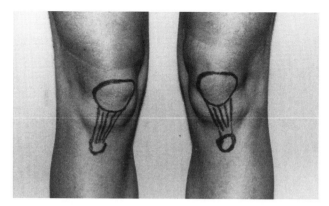

FIG. 22-17. Bilateral internal rotation of the lower extremities is commonly found in association with medial subluxation of the patella.

Evaluation of Treatment Techniques

In addition to obtaining diagnostic information for the patellofemoral joint, kinematic MRI has been used successfully to assess conservative methods of treatment, including taping and bracing methods (1–4,37,45,46,49,51) (Fig. 22-18).

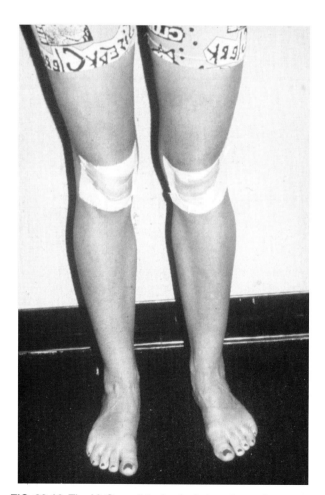

FIG. 22-18. The McConnell taping technique is used as a conservative technique to treat patellofemoral joint abnormalities.

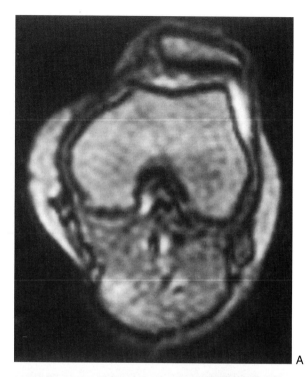

A

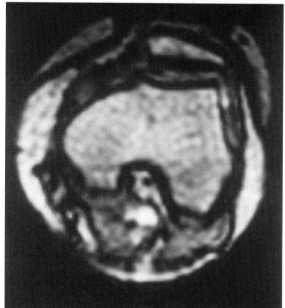

B

FIG. 22-19. Kinematic magnetic resonance imaging examination used to assess the affect of a conservative treatment technique: treatment of lateral subluxation before **(A)** and after **(B)** application of a brace (axial fast spoiled gradient-echo image). Note that the application of the brace centralized the patella relative to the femoral trochlear groove.

For example, kinematic MRI of the patellofemoral joint has been used to determine the effects of a brace designed to correct patellar malalignment and abnormal tracking by imaging patients with and without the brace applied (Figs. 22-19 and 22-20).

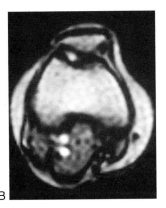 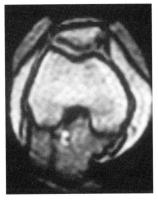

A, B

FIG. 22-20. Kinematic magnetic resonance imaging examination used to assess the affect of a conservative treatment technique: treatment of medial subluxation before **(A)** and after **(B)** application of a brace (axial fast spoiled gradient-echo image). Note that the application of the brace centralized the patella relative to the femoral trochlear groove.

SHOULDER

Kinematic MRI of the shoulder has been conducted using low-field, midfield, high-field and, most recently, a midfield, double-doughnut interventional MRI system (56–59). An investigation assessing the use of kinematic MRI of the shoulder during internal and external rotation movements of this joint exhibited good visualization of the anterior glenoid labrum (AGL) and demonstrated the role of the AGL in stabilizing the glenohumeral joint anteriorly, in conjunction with the capsular ligaments (56). Accordingly, kinematic MRI of the shoulder may be used to demonstrate the AGL limiting the ROM of the shoulder by becoming entrapped at the extremes of motion (56). Avulsions of the AGL may also be better characterized using a kinematic MRI study of the shoulder. The distance between the lesser tuberosity and coracoid process can be measured to quantify the degree of subcoracoid impingement seen on the kinematic MR images of the shoulder (56).

A study conducted by Allmann et al. (59) examined shoulder lesions in a variety of positions using kinematic MRI techniques in an open 0.2-T MRI system and a conventional 1.0-T MRI system. Spoiled GRE, T1-weighted SE, and T1- and T2-weighted FSE images were obtained during these examinations with the studies placed in a cine-loop for interpretation. The investigators reported that normal variations of the glenohumeral joint were easy to recognize. Subluxations of the humeral head and rupture of the labrum were well demonstrated along abnormal distances between osseous structures during dynamic movements. Accordingly, the authors concluded that kinematic MRI studies appear to be useful in visualizing the capsular ligament complex of the glenohumeral joint in impingement and instability syndromes. Kinematic MRI of the shoulder also provides information on dynamic changes and, thus, may prove to be an important diagnostic tool for the overall assessment of the shoulder (59). With additional experience, the role of kinematic MRI of the shoulder will be further refined.

WRIST

Kinematic MRI has been applied in a variety of manners to examine the wrist. To date, this MRI technique has been reported to be useful for detection of subtle abnormalities of carpal motion, instability patterns, transitory subluxation, and tears of the intercarpal ligaments that are not easily evaluated by routine MRI techniques (1–4,60–64).

Kinematic MRI of the wrist offers several advantages over standard wrist fluoroscopy. For example, kinematic MRI can provide tomographic information and direct visualization of the interosseous ligaments (1–4,60–68). Idiopathic pain syndromes related to motion are often not sufficiently characterized by static-view MRI techniques, especially if transitory subluxations are present. Kinematic MRI examinations of the wrist provide enhanced imaging of the muscles, tendons, ligaments, hyaline, and fibrocartilaginous structures during controlled motion. This kinematic MRI technique is believed to be useful in the assessment of impingement syndromes or other abnormalities related to movements or different positions of the wrist (1–4).

One investigation indicated that kinematic MRI using a positioning device to hold the wrist in "radial-stressed" and "ulnar-stressed" positions while obtaining coronal images was useful for the detection of interosseous ligament defects, especially those involving the scapholunate and lunotriquetral ligaments (63). This simple kinematic method appears to improve the diagnostic accuracy of MRI for identification of abnormalities considered particularly challenging to evaluate using conventional MRI techniques (63).

Protocol

The small size of the wrist necessitates use of a receive-only or transmit-receive surface coil to obtain high-resolution images for the kinematic MRI study (1–4). This surface coil configuration may also be used to obtain high-resolution static MRI views of the wrist for the routine MRI examination. For

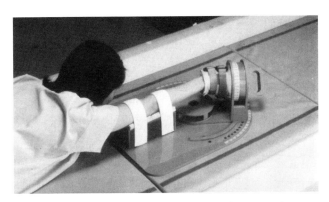

FIG. 22-21. Positioning device for kinematic magnetic resonance imaging examination of the wrist. Using an incremental, passive positioning technique, the wrist can be placed in ulnar, neutral, and radial deviated positions and flexion, neutral, and extension positions for the examination.

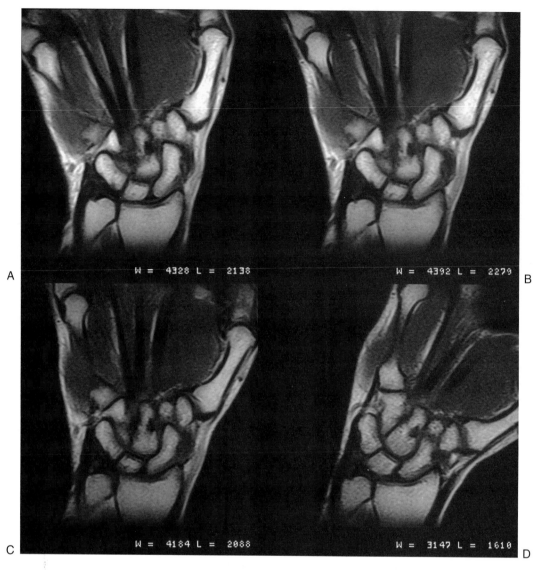

FIG. 22-22. Kinematic magnetic resonance imaging examination of the wrist in ulnar **(A)**, neutral **(B)**, and radial **(C,D)** deviated positions (coronal T1-weighted spin-echo image). In this normal kinematic study the carpal bones move in a smooth arc formed and bordered by the radius and ulna. No abnormal widening of any of the intercarpal spaces is seen, and no distal or proximal displacements of the carpal bones are seen with the wrist in these positions. Additionally, no evidence of positive or negative ulnar variance is present.

the kinematic MRI study, the wrist is typically placed in radial, neutral, and ulnar deviated positions using an incremental, passive positioning technique. T1- and T2-weighted SE, FSE, or GRE pulse sequences may be used to obtain images in the coronal plane, with an 8- to 12-cm field of view to assess carpal translation of the intercarpal ligaments. T1-weighted pulse sequences are typically used for the kinematic MRI examinations of the wrist in the sagittal plane in flexed, neutral, and extended positions for evaluation of volar or dorsal intercalated segmental instability (1–4).

A positioning device is used to incrementally position the wrist through the desired ROM (Fig. 22-21). The patient is typically placed in a prone position with the hand and wrist

in the positioning device. The elbow is extended, and foam padding is placed at various sites under the patient's axilla, arm, and elbow for support and comfort. Similar to other types of kinematic MRI studies, multiple static images or a cine-loop format may be used to view the acquired images. However, the cine-loop display is best for demonstrating subtle instability patterns of the carpal bones.

Normal Kinematics

The normal kinematic MRI examination of the wrist in the coronal plane with the wrist positioned in radial, neutral,

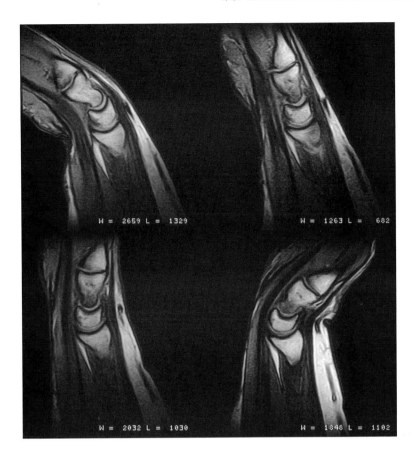

FIG. 22-23. Kinematic magnetic resonance imaging examination of the wrist in flexed, neutral, and extended positions (sagittal T1-weighted spin-echo image). This normal kinematic study shows no evidence of carpal instability.

and ulnar positions shows the carpal bones bordered by the radius and ulna, moving in a smooth, symmetric manner (62,89–92) (Figs. 22-22 and 22-23). Any deviation from a symmetric pattern of movement of the carpal bones is indicative of an abnormality or instability.

The normal carpal relationships have been classically described by Gilula (89) as three separate arcs: Arc I follows the main convex curvatures of the proximal surfaces of the scaphoid, lunate, and triquetrum carpal bones; arc II outlines the distal concave curvatures of these three bones; and arc III traces the main proximal curvatures of the hamate and capitate. Any disruption of these arcs suggests an abnormality at the respective site. Abnormalities may be caused by laxity of the ligament, a tear of the ligament, or a fracture of one of the carpal bones (62,89–92).

Careful assessment of intercarpal spacing may also provide evidence of an abnormality (62,89–92). Spacing should be evenly distributed between the carpal bones, without any significant or uneven intercarpal widening, proximal or distal movement, or anterior or posterior displacement of the carpal bones. The normal intercarpal space is approximately 1 to 2 mm wide. Increased joint space is suggestive of an abnormal ligament, increased joint fluid, synovial hypertrophy, or other forms of pathokinematics. Decreased joint space may be caused by an abnormal ligament, loss of cartilage, carpal coalition, or dislocation or subluxation of the carpal bones (62,89–92).

The presence of ulnar variance, positive or negative, should also be noted on the kinematic MRI study of the wrist, because it may be an indication of the mechanism responsible for the abnormality (62). For example, positive ulnar variance has been associated with tears of the triangular fibrocartilage complex and articular erosions of the lunate and triquetrum (Fig. 22-24). Negative ulnar variance is often seen with Kienbock's disease or avascular necrosis of the lunate.

Pathokinematics

Carpal Instability

Carpal bone instability is typically caused by a hyperextension impact injury (62,89–92). The specific carpal site of the instability depends on the position of the hand (i.e., flexed or extended, or in ulnar or radial deviation) at the time of contact. Early detection and treatment of carpal bone dissociations are crucial for a satisfactory clinical outcome. Conventional plain film x-rays, computed tomography, or static-view MRI may be inconclusive in identifying carpal bone instability because the abnormality may be so subtle that it escapes detection unless the wrist is manipulated such that asynchronous motion of the carpals, widening of the joint space, or both may be appreciated. Kinematic MRI of

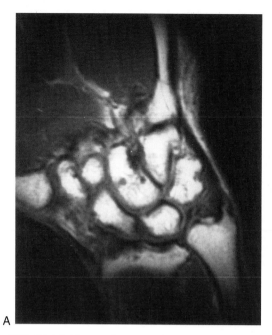 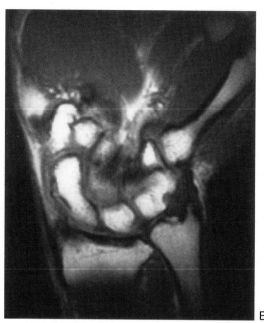

FIG. 22-24. Kinematic magnetic resonance imaging examination of the wrist in radial **(A)** and ulnar **(B)** deviated positions (coronal T1-weighted spin-echo image). This study shows cystic degeneration in the triquetrum. Positive ulnar variance is also seen. Signal changes noted in the triangular fibrocartilage complex are compatible with a tear **(A)**. Impingement between the distal ulna and triquetrum occurs during ulnar deviation **(B)**.

the wrist provides an adequate depiction of the pathokinematic aspects of carpal instability (1–4).

Position-Related Impingement

Kinematic MRI of the wrist may also furnish additional useful diagnostic information related to osseous and soft tissue pathologic changes that occur in conjunction with motion-related impingement syndromes (1–4,62). In positive ulnar variance, for example, kinematic MRI of the wrist can not only identify the impingement during wrist movement—in this case, ulnar deviation—but can also characterize other existing abnormalities. This imaging technique offers many aspects of pertinent diagnostic information.

FUTURE DIRECTIONS

The implementation of fast GRE pulse sequences has led to increased temporal resolution capabilities, thus permitting rapid imaging of the joints during active motion for kinematic MRI examinations (4). This development has been a significant improvement for kinematic MRI of joints because a more physiologic and functional assessment can be achieved. With the widespread use of other fast pulse sequence techniques, additional applications of kinematic MRI are being defined and used in the clinical setting.

EPI has been installed on many clinical MRI systems. The imaging speed of these MRI systems has been exploited to facilitate kinematic MRI examination of the joints. How-

ever, specific protocols need to be further developed for the appropriate clinical applications. EPI has thus far shown encouraging results for the kinematic MRI examination of the patellofemoral joint (32).

Open MRI systems have undergone several technological improvements that enable these devices to attain image quality that lends itself to MRI examinations of the joints. Because the patient is more accessible in these MRI systems and increased area is available for movement, it will be possible to perform MRI-guided physical examinations of the joints. This evolution of kinematic MRI is presently under development at a number of research centers. MRI systems designed for mini-

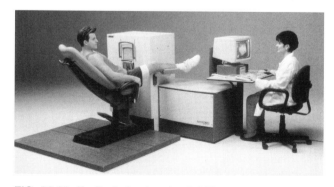

FIG. 22-25. Dedicated extremity, 0.2-T magnetic resonance imaging (MRI) system (Artoscan; available from Lunar, Madison, WI, and Esaote, Milan, Italy). This uniquely designed MRI system has been used successfully to perform kinematic MRI examinations of the patellofemoral joint and wrist.

mally invasive interventional procedures are now being used for kinematic MRI procedures (57,58). Several preliminary studies have been conducted using these highly sophisticated MRI systems to examine the patellofemoral joint, shoulder, and lumber spine.

Low-cost, niche, or dedicated extremity MRI systems developed for musculoskeletal applications have been used to perform kinematic MRI studies (Fig. 22-25). These examinations have been successfully performed on the wrist to assess carpal instability and patellofemoral joint to determine patellar tracking abnormalities (64,65).

PRACTICAL CONSIDERATIONS

Kinematic MRI procedures enhance the ability to evaluate joints and, therefore, should be used on a routine basis whenever pertinent indications are noted. Specialized training for MRI technologists and radiologists is necessary to ensure that kinematic MRI procedures are performed and interpreted properly. In addition, the appropriate MRI center staff member (usually the radiologist) should inform and educate referring physicians (e.g., orthopedic surgeons, physiatrists, neurologists) about the availability of kinematic MRI examinations. Referring physicians must be advised with respect to the advantages and indications for ordering kinematic MRI examinations for their patients.

REFERENCES

1. Shellock FG, Mandelbaum B. Kinematic MRI of the joints. In: Mink JH, Deutsch A, eds. *MRI of the musculoskeletal system: a teaching file.* New York: Raven Press, 1990.
2. Shellock FG, Mink JH, Deutsch A, Pressman B. Kinematic MRI of the joints: techniques and clinical applications. *Magn Reson Q* 1991;7:104–135.
3. Shellock FG. Kinematic MRI of the joints. In: Stoller DW, ed. *Magnetic resonance imaging in orthopaedics and rheumatology*, 2nd ed. Philadelphia: Lippincott–Raven Publishers, 1996.
4. Shellock FG. Kinematic MRI of the joints. Seminars in musculoskeletal radiology. *Magn Reson Imag Sports Med* 1997;1:143–173.
5. Nordin M, Frankel VH. *Basic biomechanics of the musculoskeletal system*, 2nd ed. Philadelphia: Lea & Febiger, 1989.
6. Shellock FG, Mink JH, Sullenberger P. High-resolution static and kinematic MRI of the ankle. *Magn Reson Med* 1990;2:766.
7. Shellock FG, Feske W, Frey C, Terk M. Peroneal tendons: use of kinematic MR imaging to determine subluxation. *J Magn Reson Imag* 1997;7:451–454.
8. Muhle C, Brinkmann G, Brossman J, Wesner F, Heller M. Kinematic MR imaging of the ankle: initial results with ultra-fast imaging. *Acta Radiologica* 1997;38:885–889.
9. Bell GR, Stearns KL. Flexion-extension MRI of the upper rheumatoid cervical spine. *Orthopedics* 1991;14:969–973.
10. Shellock FG, Sullenberger P, Mink JH, et al. MRI of the cervical spine during flexion and extension: development and implementation of a new technique. *J Magn Reson Imag* 1994;S21.
11. Naegele M, Kaden B, Koch FW, Kunze V, Woell B, Bruening R. Dynamic functional MR imaging of the cervical spine. *Radiology* 1992;185(P):219.
12. Weidenmaier W, Schnarkowski P, Haeussler MD, Friedrich JM. Dynamics of the cervical spine: functional MR imaging in 50 patients after distention injury. *Radiology* 1992;85(P):219.
13. Muhle C, Weinert D, Falliner A, et al. Dynamic changes of the cervical spinal canal in patients with cervical spondylosis at flexion and extension using magnetic resonance imaging. *Invest Radiology* 1998;33:444–449.
14. Muhle C, Wiskirchen J, Weinert D, et al. Biomechanical aspects of the subarachnoid space and cervical cord in healthy individuals examined with kinematic magnetic resonance imaging. *Spine* 1998;23:556–567.
15. Muhle C, Bischoff L, Weinert D, et al. Exacerbated pain in cervical radiculopathy at axial rotation, flexion, extension, and coupled motions of the cervical spine: evaluation by kinematic magnetic resonance imaging. *Invest Radiology* 1998;33:279–288.
16. Muhle C, Metzner J, Weinert D, et al. Classification system based on kinematic MR imaging in cervical spondylitic myelopathy. *AJNR Am J Neuroradiol* 1998;19:1763–1771.
17. Muhle C, Metzner J, Weinert D, et al. Kinematic MR imaging in surgical management of cervical spine disc disease, spondylosis, and spondylotic myelopathy. *Acta Radiologica* 1998;40:146–153.
18. Allmann KH, Schafer O, Uhl M, et al. Kinematic versus static MRI study of the cervical spine in patients with rheumatoid arthritis. *Rofo Fortscher Geb Rontgenstr Neuen Bildgeb Verfahr* 1999;170:22–27.
19. Shellock FG, Mink JH, Fox JM. Patellofemoral joint: kinematic MRI to assess tracking abnormalities. *Radiology* 1988;168:551–553.
20. Shellock FG, Mink JH, Deutsch AL, Fox JM. Evaluation of patellar tracking abnormalities using kinematic MRI: clinical experience in 130 patients. *Radiology* 1989;172:799–804.
21. Kujala UM, Osterman K, Kormano M, Komu M, Schlenzka D. Patellar motion analyzed by magnetic resonance imaging. *Acta Orthop Scand* 1989;60:13–16.
22. Shellock FG, Mink JH, Deutsch AL, Fox JM. Kinematic magnetic resonance imaging for evaluation of patellar tracking. *Phys Sports Med* 1989;17:99–108.
23. Shellock FG, Mink J, Deutsch A, Fox J. High incidence of medial subluxation of the patella identified by kinematic MR imaging. *Med Sci Sports Exerc* 1989;21:S90.
24. Shellock FG, Mink JH, Deutsch AL, Fox JM, Ferkel RD. Evaluation of patients with persistent symptoms after lateral retinacular release by kinematic magnetic resonance imaging of the patellofemoral joint. *Arthroscopy* 1990;6:226–234.
25. Kujala UM, Osterman K, Kormano M, Nelimarkka O, Hurme M, Taimela S. Patellofemoral relationships in recurrent patellar dislocation. *J Bone Joint Surg [Br]* 1989;71:788–792.
26. Kujala UM, Osterman K, Kormano M, Komu M, Schlenzka D. Patellar motion analyzed by magnetic resonance imaging. *Acta Orthop Scand* 1989;60:13–16.
27. Shellock FG, Mink JH, Fox JM, Ferkel RD, Friedman M, Molnar T. Kinematic MRI evaluation of symptomatic patients following two or more patellar realignment surgeries. *J Magn Reson Imag* 1991;1:175.
28. Brossman J, Muhle C, Schroder C, Melchert UH, Spielmann RP, Heller M. Motion-triggered cine MR imaging: evaluation of patellar tracking patterns during active and passive knee extension. *Radiology* 1993;187:205–212.
29. Brossman J, Muhle C, Bull CC, et al. Evaluation of patellar tracking in patients with suspected patellar malalignment: cine MR imaging vs. arthroscopy. *AJR Am J Roentgenol* 1993;162:361–367.
30. Koskinen SK, Hurme M, Kujala UM, Kormano M. Effect of lateral release on patellar motion in chondromalacia: an MRI study of 11 knees. *Acta Orthop Scand* 1990;61:311–312.
31. Shellock FG, Mink JH, Deutsch A, Meeks T, Fox J, Molnar T. Axial loaded stress views and kinematic MRI evaluation of patellar alignment and tracking: results in 98 patellofemoral joints. *Radiology* 1990;177(P):263.
32. Shellock FG, Cohen MS, Brady T, Mink JH, Pfaff JM. Evaluation of patellar alignment and tracking: comparison between kinematic MRI and "true" dynamic imaging by hyperscan MRI. *J Magn Reson Imag* 1991;1:148.
33. Shellock FG, Fox JM, Deutsch A, Mink JH. Medial subluxation of the patella: radiologic and physical findings. *Radiology* 1991;181(P):179.
34. Shellock FG, Mink JH, Fox JM. Identification of medial subluxation of the patella in a dancer using kinematic MRI of the patellofemoral joint: a case report. *Kinesiol Med Dance* 1991;13:1–9.
35. Shellock FG. Patellofemoral joint abnormalities in athletes: evaluation by kinematic MRI. *Top Magn Reson Imag* 1991;3:1–30.
36. Shellock FG, Foo TKF, Deutsch A, Mink JH. Patellofemoral joint: evaluation during active flexion with ultrafast spoiled GRASS MR imaging. *Radiology* 1991;180:581–585.
37. Koskinen SP, Kujala UM. Effect of patellar brace on patellofemoral relationships. *Scand J Med Sci Sports* 1991;1:119–122.
38. Koskinen SK, Hurme M, Kujala UM. Restoration of patellofemoral congruity by combined lateral release and tibial tuberosity transpo-

sition as assessed by MRI analysis. *Int Orthopedics* 1991;15: 363–366.

39. Koskinen SK, Kujala UM. Patellofemoral relationships and distal insertion of the vastus medialis muscle: a magnetic resonance imaging study in nonsymptomatic subjects and in patients with patellar dislocation. *Arthroscopy* 1992;8:865–868.

40. Shellock FG, Kim S, Mink J, Deutsch A, Fox J. "Functional" patella alta determined by axial plane imaging of the patellofemoral joint: association with abnormal patellar alignment and tracking. *J Magn Reson Imag* 1992;2(P):93.

41. Shellock FG, Mink JH, Deutsch AL, Foo TKF. Kinematic MR imaging of the patellofemoral joint: comparison between passive positioning and active movement techniques. *Radiology* 1992;84:574–577.

42. Shellock FG, Mink JH, Deutsch AL, Foo TKF, Sullenberger P. Patellofemoral joint: identification of abnormalities using active movement, "unloaded" vs "loaded" kinematic MR imaging techniques. *Radiology* 1993;88:575–578.

43. Shellock FG, Mink JH, Deutsch AL. Patellofemoral joint: advanced kinematic MRI techniques. *Appl Radiology* 1994;23:23–32.

44. Brossmann J, Muhle C, Bull CC, et al. Evaluation of patellar tracking in patients with suspected patellar malalignment: cine MR imaging vs arthroscopy. *AJR Am J Roentgenol* 1994;162:361–367.

45. Shellock FG, Mink JH, Deutsch AL, Fox J, Molnar T, Kvitne R. Effect of a patellar realignment brace on patellofemoral relationships: evaluation using kinematic MR imaging. *J Magn Reson Imag* 1994;4:590–594.

46. Worrell TW, Ingersoll CD, Farr J. Effect of patellar taping and bracing on patellar position. An MRI study. *J Sports Rehabil* 1994;3:146–153.

47. Brown SM, Bradley WG. Kinematic magnetic resonance imaging of the knee. *MRI Clin North Am* 1994;2:441–449.

48. Brossmann J, Muhle C, Bull CC, et al. Cine MR imaging before and after realignment surgery for patellar tracking: comparison with axial radiographs. *Skeletal Radiol* 1995;24:191–196.

49. Shellock FG, Mink JH, Deutsch DL, Molnar T. Effect of a newly-designed patellar realignment brace on patellofemoral relationships: a case report. *Med Sci Sports Exerc* 1995;27:469–472.

50. Shellock FG, Deutsch A, Mink JM. MR imaging assessment of internal derangement of the knee and patellar tracking abnormalities: high incidence of combined abnormalities. *Radiology* 1996;201(P):170.

51. Worrell T, Ingersoll CD, Brockrath-Pugliese K, Minis P. Effect of patellar taping and bracing on patellar position as determined by MRI in patients with patellofemoral pain. *J Athletic Training* 1998;33:16–20.

52. Powers CM, Pfaff M, Shellock FG. Active movement, loaded kinematic MRI of the patellofemoral joint: reliability of quantitative measurements. *J Magn Reson Imag* 1998;8:724–732.

53. Powers CM, Shellock FG, Perry J. The influence of bony stability on patellar tracking. American Academy of Orthopedic Surgeons, 65th Annual Meeting Program; 4 February 1999; Anaheim, CA.

54. Witonski D, Goraj B. Patellar motion analyzed by kinematic and dynamic axial magnetic resonance imaging in patients with anterior knee pain syndrome. *Arch Orthop Trauma Surg* 1999;119:46–49.

55. Muhle C, Brossman J, Heller M. Kinematic CT and MR imaging of the patellofemoral joint. *Europ Radiol* 1999;9:508–518.

56. Bonutti PM, Norfray JF, Friedman RJ, Genez BM. Kinematic MRI of the shoulder. *J Comput Assist Tomogr* 1993;17:666–669.

57. Bergman AG, Beaulieu CF, Butts K, et al. Shoulder impingement: motion evaluation of abduction in 10 normal volunteers using a 0.5 T MRT system. *Magn Reson Med* 1997;2:1006.

58. Beaulieu CF, Bergman AG, Butts K, et al. Dynamic MR imaging of glenohumeral stability in normal volunteers. *Magn Reson Med* 1997;1:28.

59. Allmann KH, Uhl M, Gufler H, et al. Cine-MR imaging of the shoulder. *Acta Radiologica* 1997;38:1043–1046.

60. Fulmer JM, Harms SE, Flamig DP, Guerdon G, Machek J, Dolinar J. High-resolution cine MR imaging of the wrist. *Radiology* 1989;173:26.

61. Bergey PD, Zlatkin MB, Dalinka M, Osterman AL, Machek J, Dolinar J. Dynamic MR imaging of the wrist: early results with a specially designed positioning device. *Radiology* 1989;73:26.

62. Reicher MA, Kellerhouse LE. Normal wrist anatomy, biomechanics, basic imaging protocol, and normal multiplanar MRI of the wrist. In: Reicher MA, Kellerhouse LE, eds. *MRI of the hand and wrist.* New York: Raven Press, 1990.

63. Tjin A, Ton ER, Pattynama PMT, Bloem JL, Obermann WR. Interosseous ligaments: device for applying stress in wrist MR imaging. *Radiology* 1995;196:863–864.

64. Mastantuono M, Larciprete M, Argento G, et al. Wrist dynamic MR imaging with a dedicated magnetic in the study of carpal instability: a new technique. *Magn Reson Med* 1995;3:1530.

65. Shellock FG, Stone KR, Crues JV. Development and clinical application of kinematic MRI of the patellofemoral joint using an extremity MR system. *Med Sci Sports Exerc* 1999;31:788–791.

66. Perlman M, Leveille D, DeLeonibus J, et al. Inversion lateral ankle trauma: differential diagnosis, review of the literature, and prospective study. *J Foot Surg* 1987;26:95.

67. Bassett FH, Gates HS, Billys JB, Morris HB, Nikolaou PK. Talar impingement by anteroinferior tibiofibular ligament. *J Bone Joint Surg [Am]* 1990;72:55–65.

68. Butler BW, Lanthier J, Wertheimer SJ. Subluxing peroneals: a review of the literature and case report. *J Foot Surg* 1992;32:134–139.

69. Geppert MJ, Sobel M, Bohne WH. Lateral ankle instability as a cause of superior peroneal retinacular laxity: an anatomic and biomechanical study of cadaveric feet. *Foot Ankle* 1993;14:330–334.

70. Kummel BM. The diagnosis of patellofemoral derangements. *Prim Care* 1980;7:199.

71. Ficat RF, Hungerford DS. *Disorders of the patello-femoral joint.* Baltimore: Williams & Wilkins, 1977.

72. Larson RL. Subluxation-dislocation of the patella. In: Kennedy JC, ed. *The injured adolescent knee.* Baltimore: Williams & Wilkins, 1979.

73. Fulkerson JP, Hungerford DS. *Disorders of the patellofemoral joint,* 2nd ed. Baltimore: Williams & Wilkins, 1990.

74. Insall J, Falvo KA, Wise DW. Patellar pain and incongruence. II: clinical application. *Clin Orthop* 1983;176:225–232.

75. Moller BN, Krebs B, Jurik AG. Patellofemoral incongruence in chondromalacia and instability of the patella. *Acta Orthop Scand* 1986;57:232–234.

76. Moller BN, Moller-Larsen F, Frich LH. Chondromalacia induced by patellar subluxation in the rabbit. *Acta Orthop Scand* 1989;60:188–191.

77. Schutzer SF, Ramsby GR, Fulkerson JP. Computed tomographic classification of patellofemoral joint pain patients. *Orthop Clin North Am* 1986;17:235–248.

78. Stanford W, Phelan J, Kathol MH, et al. Patellofemoral joint motion: evaluation by ultrafast computed tomography. *Skeletal Radiol* 1988;17:487–492.

79. Conway WF, Hayes CW, Loughran T, et al. Cross-sectional imaging of the patellofemoral joint and surrounding structures. *Radiographics* 1991;11:195–211.

80. Kaplan E. Some aspects of functional anatomy of the human knee joint. *Clin Orthop* 1962;23:18–32.

81. Otis JC, Gould JD. The effect of external load on torque production by knee extensors. *J Bone J Surg [Am]* 1986;68:65–70.

82. Insall J. Chondromalacia patellae: patellar malalignment syndrome. *Orthop Clin North Am* 1979;10:117–127.

83. Laurin CA, Dussault R, Levesque HP. The tangential X-ray investigation of the patellofemoral joint: X-ray technique, diagnostic criteria and their interpretation. *Clin Orthop* 1979;144:16–26.

84. Merchant AC, Mercer RL, Jacobsen RH, Cool CR. Roentgenographic analysis of patellofemoral congruence. *J Bone Joint Surg [Am]* 1974;56:1391–1396.

85. Carson WG, James SL, Larson RL, Singer KM, Winternitz WW. Patellofemoral disorders: physical and radiographic evaluation. Part II: radiographic examination. *Clin Orthop Rel Res* 1984;185:178–186.

86. Eppley RA. Medial patellar subluxation. In: Fox J, Del Pizzo W, eds. *The patellofemoral joint.* New York: McGraw-Hill, 1993.

87. Hughston JC, Deese M. Medial subluxation of the patella as a complication of lateral release. *Am J Sports Med* 1988;16:383.

88. Molnar TJ. Patellar rehabilitation. In: Fox J, Del Pizzo W, eds. *The patellofemoral joint.* New York: McGraw-Hill, 1993.

89. Gilula LA. Carpal injuries: analytic approach and case exercises. *AJR Am J Roentgenol* 1977;133:503.

90. Culver JE. Instabilities of the wrist. *Clin Sports Med* 1986;5:725.

91. Lichtman DM, Noble WH, Alexander CE. Dynamic triquetrolunate instability. *J Hand Surg* 1984;9:185.

92. Linscheid RL, Dobyns H, Beabout JW, Bryan RS. Traumatic in stability of the wrist. *J Bone Joint Surg [Am]* 1972;540:1612–1618.

SECTION IV

Future Directions

Open MRI,
edited by Peter A. Rothschild and Debra Reinking Rothschild.
Lippincott Williams & Wilkins. Philadelphia © 2000.

CHAPTER 23

Interventional Magnetic Resonance Imaging

Jack Chen, Kim Nguyen, Shantanu Sinha, Yoshimi Anzai, Usha Sinha, and Robert Lufkin

The use of magnetic resonance imaging (MRI) to guide biopsy or aspiration cytology was first reported in the mid-1980s. Since then, the equipment, instruments, and interventional techniques have undergone further development. Despite the pressure resulting from health care reform and managed care in the United States in the early 1990s, new MRI scanners with an open design were introduced by almost every major MRI manufacturer. Along with the magnet design, an array of support workstations, in-room image monitors, and MRI-compatible needles and trackers has been developed for MRI-guided procedures.

The use of MRI-guided therapeutic procedures has been largely limited to small series in research centers and is only now beginning to receive mainstream clinical validation. MRI interventional applications currently include aspiration cytology, stereotactic depth electrode placement for electroencephalography, focused ultrasound (US), cryosurgery, chemo-ablation, thermal ablation using a laser, and radiofrequency (RF) ablation.

EQUIPMENT

Open Magnetic Resonance Imaging Systems

Current designs of interventional MRI scanners emphasize direct access to patients, in an effort to facilitate therapy, monitoring, and anesthesia (1–3). All systems have a similar design that allows improved access to the patient.

J. Chen, S. Sinha, U. Sinha, R. Lufkin: Department of Radiological Sciences, University of California, Los Angeles, UCLA School of Medicine, Los Angeles, California

K. Nguyen: Department of Radiology, University of California, San Francisco, Medical Center, San Francisco, California

Y. Anzai: Department of Radiological Sciences, University of Michigan Medical School, Ann Arbor, Michigan

Open magnets create more space for the patient's body but sacrifice magnetic energy efficiency when compared with traditional closed magnets. The magnet openings disrupt the natural flow of magnetic flux through the field, which increases the difficulties in homogenizing the field. As magnetic field strength increases, this problem becomes more prominent, resulting in a larger magnet and excessive weight and costs. Thus, most open MRI scanners operate at low- and midfield strength, whereas closed MRI scanners operating at high-field strength are widely available.

Three types of magnets are available: resistive electromagnets, permanent magnets, and superconducting magnets. Resistive magnets are relatively inexpensive to build, weigh less, and can be switched off; however, the disadvantages include field instability caused by the dependence on a continuous electrical power supply and the requirement for cooling facilities. Permanent magnets are most promising. Open permanent magnets have been built up to 0.35 T for a 16- to 18-in. magnet gap by using ferrite or rare earth magnetic materials. Exceeding 0.35 T is difficult because of weight and costs. The advantages of permanent magnets are low fringe field (no need for magnet shielding), minimal maintenance requirement, and minimal electrical power consumption. The disadvantages are the relatively poor field homogeneity and heavy weight. Superconducting magnets possess the highest field stability, the least eddy current effect, and a field uniformity that cannot be achieved by electromagnets or permanent magnets.

Magnetic Resonance Imaging–Compatible Instruments

The first step toward practical interventional MRI is the development of instruments that can function safely and satisfactorily in the strong magnetic fields of clinical MRI scanners. One major area of concern is the properties of instruments constructed from materials with high magnetic susceptibility, such as standard surgical stainless steel. Such ferromagnetic objects may experience significant force when positioned near the MRI scanner. The potential for accidents due to the magnetically induced force on surgical instruments or monitoring equipment cannot be ignored.

Two levels of MRI compatibility should be considered: instruments and devices that can be used near the magnet (level 1) and devices that are fully MRI compatible and can be used in the image plane and during image acquisition (level 2). The following principles of MRI compatibility are incomplete and reflect only initial experiences with MRI guidance:

- Any instrument moved into the MRI suite should be nonmagnetic and not attracted by the magnetic field.
- Two levels of MRI compatibility can be recognized: level 1, nonmagnetic, and level 2, MRI compatible.
- All instruments and devices to be used in an MRI suite should be classified as level 1 or 2 and approved according to the magnet type.
- Level 2 devices can be used in the RF cabin during acquisition. They are nonmagnetic but can cause limited susceptibility artifacts when used within the image plane.
- MRI-compatible instruments should ideally be labeled according to the MRI system for which they can be used. The label should include the brand name, the manufacturer of the magnet, and the sequence type with the respective artifact size.
- An instrument used near the magnet but not during acquisition should be nonmagnetic.
- An implant present in the magnetic field during acquisition should not cause major artifacts that alter the images.
- An instrument in the image plane but outside the body should not cause distortion of the magnetic field.
- An implant that is in the image plane and the field of view (FOV) should not cause relative distortion of the magnetic field and should feature an adequate visualization of artifact.

Material, magnet field strength, angle of instrumentation to the magnetic field, and sequence type are key factors in determining artifact size. Ferromagnetic material cannot be used for MRI instruments. The magnetic field distortion is so extensive that imaging is impossible. Stainless steel has the best mechanical properties for most interventional instruments. Alloys with high nickel content and nonmagnetic characteristics are appropriate for smaller interventional instruments of up to 1 mm in diameter.

Image artifacts may result from large magnetic susceptibility differences between introduced instruments and the diamagnetic patient. Susceptibility artifacts also depend on the pulse sequence applied. For example, spin-echo sequences are less sensitive to time-independent local magnetic field variations, whereas gradient-echo sequences are sensitive to time-dependent and time-independent local field changes. The degree of image distortion also depends on the strength of the main magnetic field and increases with higher field strengths.

Since the first MRI-compatible needles were developed, a variety of MRI-compatible instruments have become available (4,5). Induced force on interventional equipment and associated artifacts can be minimized by optimizing pulse sequences, by using a shorter echo time, thinner slice, smaller FOV, and higher readout gradient; by replacing standard medical grade stainless steel with higher nickel content stainless steel or other nonferrous alloys or ceramics; and so forth. MRI-compatible needles, forceps, scissors, cannulas, and other instruments (Daum Inc., Germany; Cook Inc., Indianapolis, IN; EFMT, Bochum, Germany; EZ-EM, Westbury, NY; Nicromed Inc., Bochum, Germany; Radionics, Inc., Burlington, MA) are manufactured at reasonable prices. Similar modifications have been made with other support instrumentation such as anesthesia monitoring equipment, lasers, RF generators, and tracking systems.

Another major concern is the electrical conductivity of metal devices. The fluctuating gradient field generated by the MRI scanner to form images induces voltage and current in a closed conducting loop according to Faraday's law of magnetic induction. The induced current may cause resistive heating of the metal device and pose a hazard to the patient and attending medical personnel. If two metal objects are placed near each other, the hazard of electrical arcing also becomes a factor. In addition, the eddy currents induced in metal objects have long decay times and may distort the imaging field, causing artifacts. To ensure safety and reduce artifacts, the design of interventional devices must avoid closed or nearly closed metal loops and incorporate minimal bulk metal.

A third area of concern is the electromagnetic interference between the MRI scanner and interventional electronics. For example, the RF generator used in RF thermal ablation may emit electromagnetic radiation, which interferes with the scanner's reception of MRI signal from the patient's body, causing imaging artifacts. Conversely, the fluctuating magnetic field used in MRI may interfere with the operation of some monitoring equipment. Although MRI-compatible monitoring devices are now commercially available from some manufacturers, all electronic equipment must be tested for electromagnetic interference in the MRI scanner room before being used in an interventional procedure.

In-Room Video Display

Interventional MRI requires an MRI-compatible in-room monitor with standard image quality. Cathode ray tube monitors cannot be used near the magnetic field because of distortion. Analog thin-film active matrix monitors provide excellent resolution.

Localization Systems

Frame-based stereotactic MRI has been implemented for guiding biopsies, tumor resections, tumor ablations, deep electroencephalogram electrode placement, and functional target localization for functional ablation (6,7). In addition to helping localize the coordinates of the target area, the stereotactic frame also serves as a fixation device during imaging and as a probe carrier during surgery. In an open scanner, images are not necessarily acquired preoperatively, because the patient with the frame can be positioned during the entire procedure within the scanner without needing to be removed from the gantry. The accuracy of stereotactic MRI guidance is limited by various factors: susceptibility artifacts at interventional probe-tissue or tissue-air interfaces; the linearity and calibration of magnetic field gradients, and eddy currents of the pulsed gradients excited in the cryo-shield. Because MRI is more prone to potentially greater geometric distortion than is computed tomography (CT), meticulous quality control is essential.

Frameless stereotactic localization further reduces patient discomfort and makes the therapeutic procedure less invasive. Furthermore, stereotactic frames can be used only when rigidity and immobility of the organ with respect to the frame have been accomplished. These prerequisites are satisfied only for brain and bone surgery; they are not satisfied for most organs or soft tissue (8). An MRI-compatible arm enables frameless targeting even in regions that are flexible and mobile. The operating arm can supply information about its location and orientation, thus eliminating the need for preoperative imaging (9).

Passive Tracking

In the passive tracking method, the device is visualized by the signal void it creates and by its susceptibility artifact (10,11). The MRI-compatible needles introduce only a local signal loss of a linear shape, which allows visualization without entirely obscuring the underlying anatomic structure. The location of the needle is updated at a frequency limited by the time required for image acquisition, reconstruction, and display. Image acquisition times are usually reduced through the use of gradient-echo sequences. However, such sequences may produce unacceptably large artifacts at high-field strength. Fast spin-echo sequences with a scan time of 4 seconds have been used for breast lesion localization at 1.5 T (12). A rapid gradient-echo sequence with an acquisition time of 800 ms and an interleaved gradient-echo planar sequence with an acquisition time of 350 to 400 ms have been investigated as ultrafast sequences for guidewire placement for vascular interventions under MRI visualization (13).

Active Tracking

In active tracking, real-time tracking with the position of the device tip updated 20 times per second is possible. In this

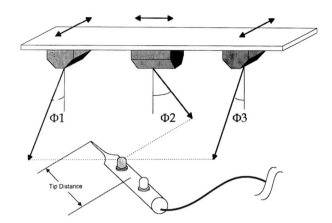

FIG. 23-1. An optical tracking system uses three linear detectors spaced apart on a bar suspended over the work area. Infrared light-emitting diodes (LEDs) on a probe sequentially light up and are detected by the sensors. The three measured angles—ϕ1, ϕ2, and ϕ3—are sufficient to locate the LED in three-dimensional space. When the location of the second LED is measured, the orientation of the probe can be determined and the location of the probe tip calculated. Image courtesy of CL Domoulin.

technique, a small RF coil, consisting of an untuned single loop of less than 1 mm in diameter, is attached to the tip of the interventional device (14) (Fig. 23-1). Such a coil is insensitive to signal coming from more than 1 or 2 mm away. Because only four excitations with a short repetition time (12 to 20 ms) are required to update the position of the coil, temporal resolutions of 20 frames per second can be easily achieved. The positional accuracy of the RF coil can be found at a resolution of less than 1 mm, which is typically the in-plane resolution of MR images. The position of the coil, updated 20 times per second, is superposed on a previously acquired MR image. This technique has been verified *in vitro* and *in vivo* when used with intravascular catheters (15).

Schemes for Reduction of Scan Time

The development of ultrafast pulse sequences for rapid acquisition and reconstruction is another challenge. To approximate real-time imaging (fluoroscopic mode), not only image acquisition but also image reconstruction must be very high speed. Spatial and temporal resolution are trade-offs for a given signal-to-noise ratio.

Many recent studies have focused on the development of sequences with very short repetition times. Several promising approaches have been taken, including echo-planar imaging (EPI), a hybrid of EPI and spin-echo methods, keyhole imaging, local look (LOLO) techniques, striped k-space techniques, and wavelet-encoded data acquisition (16–18).

EPI provides the shortest scan time. It requires substantial hardware modifications, as a series of fast frequency and phase-encoding gradients are required to generate a train of gradient-echoes after a single RF excitation. EPI suffers from a low signal to noise ratio and is very sensitive to local field changes.

Other rapid imaging strategies involve selective filling of the raw data matrix (k-space). Such restricted FOV imaging focuses on continually updating the lower frequency domains of the k-space, while acquiring only a subset of the higher frequency domain. "Keyhole" imaging and LOLO techniques each use these subsampling methods to significantly shorten the imaging time (19).

The reduction of scan speed by imaging a reduced FOV is applicable to MRI therapeutic intervention in which dynamic changes are limited to a small portion of the total FOV. To prevent aliasing in the reduced FOV images is to excite a strip rather than the entire slice as proposed in the LOLO method (20). The LOLO technique uses a single-shot turbo spin-echo and can acquire a real-time 128×128 image matrix in 50 to 150 ms.

The simplest keyhole strategy is to acquire a reference image at full resolution and only the central k-space line for the dynamic images. The dynamic images are then reconstructed after substituting the higher k-space lines from the reference high-resolution image. The stripe k-space data acquisition strategy is an extension of the keyhole technique (21). By rotating each new raw data set, the entire k-space is updated after a few keyhole cycles, resulting in improved image quality without lengthening the keyhole acquisition time.

Wavelet encoding is an alternative to phase encoding that reduces acquisition times by a factor of up to 10 (22). In contrast to the Fourier transform, the wavelet transform is localized in space. Only those regions of an image that are mainly affected by the movement of the interventional device are updated. A limitation of this method is that it is based on spatially selective excitations and is thus extremely sensitive to the calculation and excitation of RF profile.

Thermal Monitoring

MRI-guided thermal ablation therapy would be greatly aided by the development of accurate MR thermal monitoring. Although tissue heating may be monitored by implanted transducers, such as thermocouples or thermistors, this technique is invasive and potentially hazardous and can yield temperature measurement at only a few points because of the limited number of probes. A high temporal resolution is required to monitor RF and high-intensity focused US ablation procedures, whereas the requirement for laser-induced thermotherapy and hyperthermia applications is more relaxed. The temperature dependency of three MRI tissue parameters has been used for MR thermometry: T1 relaxation (23–26), the diffusion coefficient D (27), and the chemical shift of the water peak (28,29). Each of these parameters has merits and drawbacks when used for MR thermometry.

The temperature sensitivity of the diffusion coefficient is 2.4% per 1°C, which is higher than the temperature sensitivities of T1 (0.8% to 2.0% per 1°C) and proton resonance frequency (–0.0107 ppm per 1°C for pure water, –0.007 to –0.009 ppm per 1°C for *in vitro* muscle and other organ tissue) (30–32). The T1 dependence on temperature varies in different tissue, and tissue physiologic and metabolic changes during thermal therapy cause deviations from linear behavior. The temperature sensitivity of the diffusion coefficient is high, but diffusion imaging requires large applied magnetic field gradients for rapid imaging. Recent trends in investigations at high-field strengths have established that the proton resonance frequency method is more suitable for MR thermometry than is the measurement of diffusion and T1.

Of the various parameters, changes in T1 relaxation with thermal changes were first studied *in vitro* and seemed to provide a good correlation. The studies suggested a slight rise in T1 with heating and a signal decrease in T1-weighted images over a limited range (28° to 43°C). However, *in vivo* temperature measurement based on T1 changes showed that these changes can be influenced by tissue perfusion and proton density variation (33). A significant hysteresis exists between signal intensity and temperature (34). Another concern is that at high-energy depositions during thermal ablation, the induced T1 changes may be irreversible and unpredictable (35). Moreover, recent *ex vivo* studies using brain and muscle demonstrated that the slope of relaxation time was positive for muscle but negative for brain, so that the signal level may increase or decrease with heating, depending on the tissue (34). Thus, T1 temperature monitoring cannot yield unambiguous result in all situations despite the use of currently available technique.

Another parameter for MR temperature mapping is the diffusion coefficient of water, D. In the physiologic temperature range, the sensitivity of diffusion to temperature is approximately 2.4%, which is about twice as high as that of the T1 relaxation time (27). The drawback of the measurement of the diffusion coefficient *in vivo* is that because diffusion imaging is very sensitive to bulk motion and tissue anisotropy, it requires ultrafast acquisition schemes such as EPI to avoid motion artifacts.

MR thermometry using water proton chemical shift imaging (28,29) is of growing interest. The temperature dependency of the water proton chemical shift has been measured using the phase difference of a dynamic, multiplanar RF-spoiled fast field echo sequence (29). Chemical shift imaging seems to be a potentially robust technique. The accuracy and efficacy of water proton chemical shift imaging, such as *in vivo* MR thermometry, need to be validated in further investigations.

TREATMENT TECHNIQUES

Cryoablation

Cryosurgery is a therapeutic method that involves ablation of tissue by freezing via direct contact with a cryoprobe. A cryogen, typically liquid nitrogen, is circulated through the probe, which is thermally insulated along its length except at the tip. Thermal exchange occurs between the probe and the tissue, and a frozen region gradually extends outward from the probe tip.

In experiments on rabbit brain, 8 to 10 minutes of freezing was required to create a lesion 5 mm deep (36). Thawing of the frozen tissue also required approximately 8 minutes.

With recent advances in imaging, hope prevails that cryoablation may play a role in the treatment of tumors (36,37).

Advantages of cryosurgery include the following:

- Cryosurgery is an intrinsically focal therapy. Cryoprobes of various sizes are available, ranging from small, thin probes approximately 3 mm in diameter to probes with diameters larger than 1 cm.
- Larger tissue volumes can be treated cryosurgically than can be safely resected. Tumor margin that extends beyond an organ boundary can be treated.
- No dose limitation exists with cryosurgery, unlike radiotherapy.
- Cryosurgery produces sharp margins of destruction, allowing minimal damage of surrounding healthy tissue.
- Minimal blood loss is associated with cryosurgery.
- Large vessels are protected from freezing by the internal flow of warm blood.

Recently, intraoperative US has been used to guide cryoablative surgery in the prostate and the liver (38). Advances in MRI, and in the field of interventional MRI in particular, now make MRI a potential powerful tool for directing the cryoablation of deep tumors (39). The factors that make focal cryosurgical ablation particularly well suited to interventional MRI guidance include (a) the ability of MRI to image the entire volume of tissue during freezing with high accuracy and in real time; (b) the easy direction of the freezing boundary under MRI; (c) the sharp, definable margin of necrosis that cryosurgical freezing produces; (d) the ability to detect and stage cancers using combined MRI and magnetic resonance spectroscopic imaging and use this information for planning focal treatment and follow-up; (e) the ability of MRI to assess the effectiveness of treatment immediately after thawing; and (f) the possibility of controlling the freezing process automatically. Previous animal experiments have demonstrated the ability of MRI to monitor the extent of the frozen region during surgery. Recently, MRI-compatible cryoprobes have been developed and thorough investigation of MRI-guided cryosurgery has been conducted on the rabbit brain (37).

The frozen region is apparent for all MRI pulse sequences as a well-defined area of signal void, with a sharp interface to nonfrozen tissue, which can be tracked in time during the freezing process. The signal void of the frozen area is presumably due to a significant decrease in the spin-spin relaxation rates as liquid water transitions to ice, rendering the water protons invisible to MRI.

T1-weighted images, although less accurate for dynamic monitoring, display the interesting feature of a bright band at the boundary of the freeze front. This represents nonfrozen cooled tissue adjacent to the freeze front. Early results indicate that after freezing, gadolinium enhancement at the margin of the frozen region correlates with vascular damage and ischemic necrosis at the center of the lesion (Fig. 23-2).

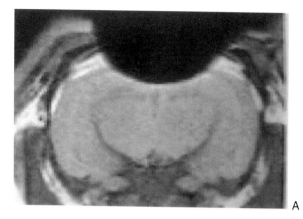

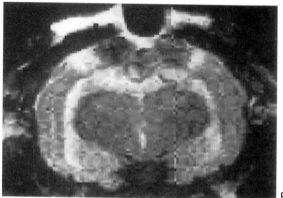

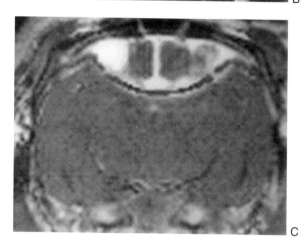

FIG. 23-2. Spin-echo (SE) images during and after cryosurgery of rabbit brain. **A:** T1-weighted SE at the end of freezing. **B:** T2-weighted SE 13 minutes after the onset of thawing. **C:** T1-weighted SE 31 minutes after the onset of thawing and 9 minutes after injecting a single dose of gadolinium diethylene-triamine penta–acetic acid (Gd-DTPA) to monitor blood–brain barrier damage. At 31 minutes, enhancement was first seen at the margin of the cryoablation lesion and the cingulate gyrus. The central portion of the lesion was not as bright as the margin, probably because Gd-DTPA could not reach the center of the lesion through the heavily damaged vasculature. The field of view was 3.0 cm × 3.5 cm. Images courtesy of J. C. Gilbert.

MR images provide adequate spatial and temporal resolution of the expanding frozen lesion, as well as delineation of brain edema and blood–brain barrier breakdown after thawing. Because the freezing interface moves through the tissue at velocities in the range of millimeters per minute, image updates at 30-second intervals are adequate to monitor the freezing front in quasi real time.

Although MRI-guided focal cryoablation is still at the research stage, only a few technical details remain to be solved before this technique can be applied in a clinical setting. Most of these details involved developing MRI-compatible devices (e.g., cryoprobes, freezing devices, patient-positioning equipment, and accessory hardware). The development of an MRI-compatible cryosurgical system is currently under way. Imaging sequences must also be optimized for lower field interventional magnet systems, but MRI-guided cryosurgical ablation has great potential to improve patient care as this minimally invasive therapy evolves.

Laser Therapy

Interstitial laser thermotherapy (ILT) is a new therapeutic technique that offers the advantage of transmitting energy directly into deep tumors through a fiberoptic probe. ILT causes thermal tissue injury due to laser energy deposition, resulting in coagulative necrosis. Unlike traditional hyperthermia, in which the tissue is heated to 43° to 45°C for more than 10 minutes, usually to augment some other therapy, in thermal ablation using laser or RF, the temperature is raised to above 65°C to produce protein denaturation. ILT may result in coagulative necrosis of tissue wherever enough energy is delivered through the fiberoptic probe. Hence, accurate localization of the laser fiberoptic within a target tumor and careful monitoring with MRI are essential for successful treatment.

ILT is one of the most promising thermal ablation techniques available (40–44). The Nd:YAG (neodymium:yttrium aluminum garnet) laser is most commonly used for interstitial applications. The major advantages of ILT as a thermal ablation technique are as follows:

1. ILT creates a powerful heat source that is potentially capable of destroying a large volume of tissue.
2. Few artifacts by laser and fiber are seen on MRI.
3. The small caliber of the laser fiber does not require large-bore needle insertion.
4. The technique is independent of radiation wavelength sensitivity (nonspecific thermal injury).
5. Tissue damage to adjacent normal structures is minimal.

MRI allows detection of tumor, localization of an instrument within the target tumor, and demonstration of thermal tissue injury. Over a limited temperature range, an approximately linear change in tissue T1 relaxation time with temperature provides the basis for the MRI signal reduction upon heating (45). Above temperatures 20°C higher than body temperature, nonlinear behavior induces measurement

errors. Because true temperature calibration cannot easily be achieved, it is essential to correlate thermal changes on the images with histopathologic results so that a marker of adequate management can be obtained (46). The MRI sequence should have two-dimensional fast low-angle shot sequences demonstrating increased signal within brain tumor as the temperature increases during ILT. T2-weighted images of an acute ILT lesion show low signal coagulative necrosis, with or without a central cavity, surrounded by high signal edema. Histopathologic correlation in animal models has shown that lesion size increases for up to 1 week after laser treatment and then gradually decreases by infiltration of phagocytotic cells from adjacent vital tissue. Granulation tissues then form around the lesion, which eventually progresses to a residual fibrotic scar.

Typical treatment of a large liver metastasis requires 10,000 to 20,000 J of energy at 805 nm delivered into the lesion over 500 seconds (Fig. 23-3). Shorter duration, high-power treatments have been tried, but they result in vaporization of tissue and intense charring of the local vicinity of the probe tissue, which reduces the overall lesion size produced. Vaporization can also cause a small explosion, which may be dangerous in closed space such as brain (47).

Radiofrequency Ablation

RF thermal ablation is a technique for tissue destruction by resistive heating using an RF (approximately 500 kHz) alternating current (48,49). Unlike earlier antenna-based methods of RF (and microwave heating), direct interstitial methods at low frequency (<1 MHz) avoid limitations of differential effects across changing dielectric properties in tissue (e.g., hot spots). A probe system, usually consisting of an active and a dispersive electrode, is connected to the patient to complete an electrical circuit. The uninsulated tip of the active electrode or RF probe is placed at the center of the target tissue, and an alternating current is conducted through the probe. Because of the impedance (resistance of tissue surrounding the probe), ionic agitation causes frictional heating, which results in tissue damage secondary to coagulation necrosis. The size of the RF lesion produced is a function of the length and diameter of the exposed electrode tip and the energy delivered. The power deposition is proportional to the square of the local E field (or current density), whereas the actual temperature change is a function of tissue parameters, including thermal conductivity, electrical conductivity, perfusion, and local heat sinks, such as large vessels.

RF has been used in the neurosurgical field for more than 3 decades and has proved to be a safe thermal ablation technique. The central temperature adjacent to the RF probe can be raised to 80°C to create coagulative necrosis so that overheating of tissue (vaporization or charring) can easily be avoided.

Recent reports show various applications in which RF energy deposition, via direct interstitial electrode placement,

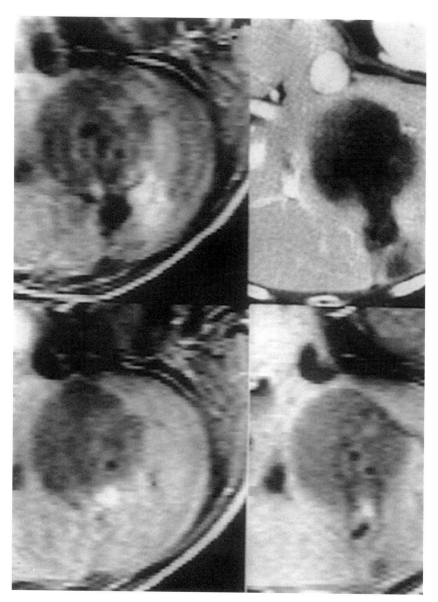

FIG. 23-3. Magnetic resonance images acquired at peak burn for laser therapy of a patient with liver metastasis with three pullbacks and 24 hours after procedural computed tomography. From ref. 46, with permission.

has been used successfully in curative and palliative treatment of cancer patients. The feasibility of the use of MRI-guided RF ablation for treatment of brain lesions was demonstrated in 1995 (50). Abdominal tumors have also been treated with RF thermal therapy. These efforts have primarily been directed toward the treatment of liver metastases (51). More recently, this treatment method was extended to use in MRI for localization and treatment monitoring (52).

One challenge for the use of RF electromagnetic energy for thermal ablation of tumors is minimization of its interaction with the MRI scanner. After all, the scanner is designed to detect extremely small time-varying magnetic fields and, as such, may detect any spurious fields generated in the frequency range of the imager, thus reducing image quality. For example, a 500-kHz RF generator has its seventeenth harmonic at 8.5 MHz (approximately 0.2 T), the

forty-second harmonic at approximately 21 MHz (approximately 0.5 T), the eighty-fifth harmonic at 42.5 MHz (1.0 T), and the one hundred twenty-eighth harmonic at 64 MHz (1.5 T). Distortions to the waveform resulting from imperfections in generating a pure sine wave may broaden the spectrum around these harmonics and lead to spurious interference on scanners operating near these frequencies. RF ablation systems that operate at other frequencies will likely have similar problems, particularly because higher power levels are being used.

The MRI appearance of the RF lesion is similar to that produced by laser: a well-defined ellipsoidal area of coagulative necrosis surrounded by edema. MRI is sensitive enough to detect the acute thermal injury that can be missed by other imaging modalities. MRI studies indicate that the lesions are well delineated from surrounding normal tissue.

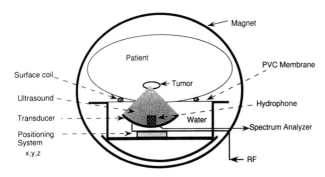

FIG. 23-4. A clinical prototype magnetic resonance imaging–guided focused ultrasound system. PVC, polyvinyl chloride; RF, radiofrequency. Image courtesy of K. Hynynen.

With the availability of accurate stereotactic techniques and the recent development of an MRI-compatible RF unit, the use of dynamic MRI to monitor the ablation of deep lesions in the body has become a potentially useful application of interventional MRI.

Focused Ultrasound Ablation

The only noninvasive imaging method that allows highly localized tissue destruction deep in the body is US. Use of US in focal tissue coagulation dates back to the 1940s, but early experience did not lead to the use of US in routine practice because of the lack of image guidance and the complexity of the procedure. By using high-intensity focused ultrasound (HIFU), focal hyperthermia can be induced to destroy lesions in soft tissue and cause direct thermal coagulation necrosis and cavitation (30,53).

HIFU (frequency, 0.5 to 10.0 MHz) beams are generated by piezoceramics and focused using lenses and a reflecting surface (Fig. 23-4). For therapeutic purposes, the transducer is driven at the frequency that maximizes power output. A typical transducer converts 50% to 90% of the RF power to acoustic power. The beam emitted converges at the focal zone, in which the lesion is located, and then dissipates. The relative US power disposition is highest at the focal zone and decreases significantly in the near and far fields. With sufficient intensity, very sharp temperature profiles can be produced so that an intense rise of temperature causing accurately targeted tissue destruction is attainable within a few seconds in the focal zone. Furthermore, unlike other energy delivery systems such as RF and lasers, the location of ablation can easily be removed and the focus of destruction made very small.

Destruction of tissues is achieved by two major mechanisms: (a) rapid increase of temperature locally, causing coagulation and denaturation of the cellular protein and (b) generation of microbubbles, similar to that of boiling water, which disrupt the cellular structure mechanically.

Histologic studies of HIFU ablation of the brain, liver, and kidneys have shown that it is possible to produce a well-localized and well-demarcated necrotic lesion. Numerous studies and phase 1 clinical trials have been performed under US guidance for the treatment of breast, liver, and prostate tumors.

The main advantages of using HIFU are that it is noninvasive and can be focused. These advantages allow deep targets to be precisely destroyed without damaging overlying or surrounding tissues. These characteristics also make it possible to deliver the energy quickly, thus reducing undesirable effects such as perfusion or thermal conduction and motion artifacts on MRI. The disadvantages of US are its need for an acoustic window and its small focal size. The strong attenuation in bones and reflection from gas interfaces limit the use of US to sites that offer a soft tissue window for the beam propagation. US propagation through overlying tissues limits the amount of energy transfer to deep tissues and allows only target volumes up to 3 to 4 cm to be coagulated in a 1- or 2-hour treatment session (54). This size is larger if the target volume is more superficial. Large tumors can be treated in multiple settings or by extending the treatment time. The tissue destruction profile depends on the applied power, duration of sonication, tissue type, and vascularity and must be closely monitored. Because MRI can provide excellent tissue contrast and possibly temperature monitoring, MRI may be able to guide noninvasive, well-controlled US surgery.

US-induced lesions are not only visible in MRI, but the dimensions of the destroyed lesion also correlate well with T2-weighted images. Direct near-real-time imaging of tissue destruction is possible.

Chemoablation

Percutaneous ethanol injection is one example of chemoablation. Ethanol enters cell by diffusion, producing cell dehydration and protein denaturation, which lead to coagulation necrosis. The broadest application of percutaneous ethanol injection has been for management of liver tumors. The choice of management depends on several factors, including the severity of underlying liver disease and the number, size, and location of the lesions (55). A more predictable ablation can be attained in encapsulated lesions because ethanol infusion tends to follow anatomic tissue planes. The hydrophilic nature of ethanol makes it difficult to produce a well-controlled, uniform, reproducible lesion size and shape. MRI is used to guide the placement of needles and cannulas for the instillation of chemotherapeutics. For example, hepatocellular carcinoma is a soft tumor typically surrounded by hard cirrhotic parenchyma, which allows selective diffusion of ethanol into the neoplastic tissue. Once recurrence occurs, percutaneous ethanol injection can be used repeatedly without increased risk. However, the efficacy of ethanol ablation in liver metastases is much lower than that in primary tumors. This difference appears to

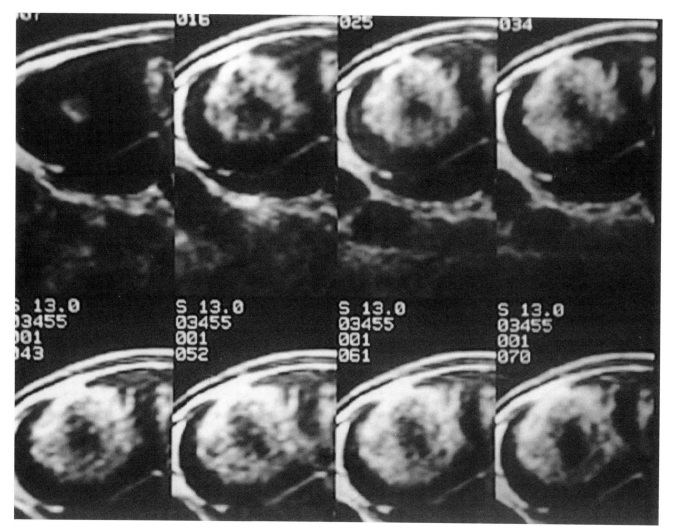

FIG. 23-5. Sequential T2-weighted spin-echo images of the paraspinal muscles in a New Zealand rabbit *in vivo* (from left to right and top to bottom, the images were obtained at 2-minute intervals during and after ethanol injection). The initial region of hyperintensity corresponds to the presence of the injected fluid, and the subsequent growing area of hypointensity corresponds to cellular dehydration in the early stages and to coagulative necrosis in the latter stages.

be caused by the irregularity of ethanol diffusion in metastatic lesions, which have more heterogeneous architecture and a firmer consistency.

In ethanol ablation, MRI has been shown to be useful for assessing proper delivery by indirectly imaging ethanol in the interstitium. This assessment is done by using the minimal chemical shift of ethanol from water. The water signal is selectively suppressed using a fast inversion recovery sequence with water suppression. On T2-weighted fast spin-echo images, initial hyperintensity at the site of injection progressively enlarged but was followed in minutes by a zone of hypointensity, which enlarged over the subsequent hours, surrounded by a hyperintense rim (Fig. 23-5). It was thought that the initial hyperintensity represented the ethanol, whereas the subsequent hypointensity represented the ensuing dehydration in the eventual coagulative necrosis (56).

CLINICAL APPLICATIONS

Brain

Image-Guided Neurosurgery

Intraoperative MRI has been integrated into management of neurosurgical disease in the following areas: stereotactic brain biopsy and electrode placement, image-guided tumor resection, and image-guided tumor ablation. Using MRI as a road map, tools such as MRI-compatible neuroendoscopy may have a dramatic effect on minimally invasive neurosurgery.

Brain Biopsy

MRI is now recognized as the best imaging technique for the detection of most intracranial pathologies. With the

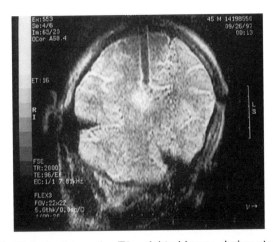

FIG. 23-6. An interactive T2-weighted image during stereotactic brain biopsy of a small deep lesion. The needle is seen in the lesion. EC, echo; FOV, field of view; FSE, fast spin-echo; TE, echo time; TR, repetition time. Image courtesy of T. M. Moriarty.

development of the MRI-compatible stereotactic frame, stereotactic brain biopsy is now routinely performed based on MRI data in many institutions (Fig. 23-6). Stereotactic coordinates and the optimum angle of the probe insertion are calculated with high accuracy based on MRI. New interventional MRI magnets with an open design and in-room monitors now allow frameless stereotactic brain biopsy and possible treatment.

Stereotactic Depth Electrode Placement for Electroencephalography

Intracerebral electroencephalography is sometimes used to localize medically intractable epilepsy to define the site and extent of the epileptogenic focus. Until recently, the most widely used method was stereoscopic angiography, and a double-grid system was used to place the electrodes. Stereoscopic angiography with digital subtraction provides a safe trajectory for the electrode and avoids intracranial vessels such as the sylvian vessels and the vein of Labbe during temporal lobe electrode placement. This method, however, limits the working space available for implantation.

Given the ability of MRI to provide detailed anatomic and angiographic information, interventional MRI may provide not only real-time feedback during insertion, noninvasive localization, and assessment of position accuracy but also the freedom to choose the target and the entry point (57,58). In the future, once a seizure focus is localized, it is hoped that treatment can be performed by interventional MRI using, for example, RF or laser ablation rather than a large partial lobectomy.

Magnetic Resonance Imaging–Guided Open Surgical Procedures

With appropriately equipped open design MRI systems, some groups are using MRI during surgical procedures such as craniotomy. This new application is being explored at centers in Heidelberg, Zurich, Los Angeles, Boston, Minneapolis, and Erlangen. The ultimate value and indications of the technique remain to be defined.

Magnetic Resonance Imaging–Guided Brain Tumor Ablation

MRI-guided thermal ablation of brain tumors thus far appears to be a safe, minimally invasive treatment that deserves further study. Unlike radiation, it is not contraindicated by a cumulative toxicity, and it may serve as a palliative alternative for end-stage patients who do not wish to undergo open craniotomy.

Advantages of MRI-guided brain tumor ablation include the following:

1. Minimally invasive
2. Minimal adjacent vital tissue damage
3. May be repeated as often as necessary
4. Can be performed after whole-brain radiation
5. Less costly than open craniotomy

Trials are currently ongoing to assess the use of MRI-guided thermal ablation of brain tumors. The Düsseldorf group performed a clinical pilot study of MRI-guided Nd-YAG laser ablation on 31 patients with brain tumor (59). Three-dimensional turbo FLASH sequences were used to determine the position of light guide. The time of irradiation varied from 10 to 20 minutes. Phase-sensitive two-dimensional FLASH and echo-shifted turbo FLASH were used to generate a color-coded heat map. The results are summarized in the table below:

Study population	31
Neurologic deterioration during ablation	2
Transient deficit after ablation (vasogenic edema)	4
Persistent deficit after ablation	1
Patients with astrocytoma grade II	24
Neurologic status unchanged after ablation	6
Neurologic status improved after ablation	18

The study demonstrated that MRI is well suited to monitor laser-induced thermotherapy. A typical laser lesion comprised a central and peripheral zone that formed the total lesion size, which is circumscribed by an enhancing rim demarcating the outer border of the irreversibly damaged lesion (Fig. 23-7) (59).

At the University of California, Los Angeles, ablation of brain tumor is under investigation using RF ablation (50). The technique is as follows:

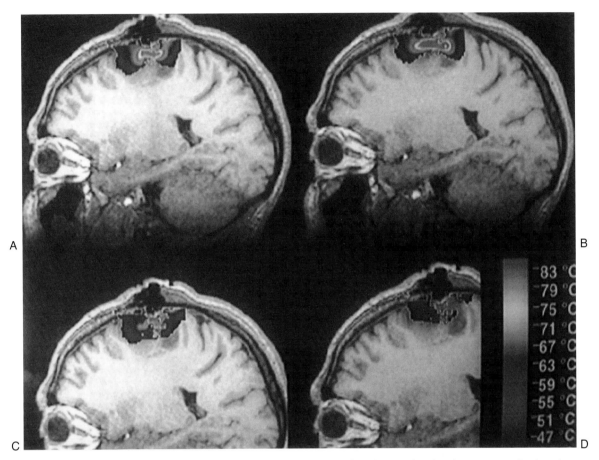

FIG. 23-7. Postprocessed phase-sensitive two-dimensional fast low-angle shot images acquired and displayed during and after laser-induced thermotherapy (LITT). The calculated temperatures are color-coded (bottom right), gradually increasing the heat-affected zone with increasing maximum temperatures. **A–D:** Images acquired during LITT 1, 4, 8, and 10 minutes after starting the laser therapy. The temperature returned to baseline values. However, some scattered pixels remain unchanged during cooling. Images courtesy of T Kahn. In Lufkin R, ed. *Interventional MRI*. St. Louis: Mosby, 1999.

1. Pretreatment MRI stereotaxis for localization of brain tumor.
2. Place biopsy needle if necessary or RF probe (Radionics) into the tumor through a 3-mm twist-drill hole (Fig. 23-8).
3. Apply RF power to achieve an intratumoral temperature of 80°C for 1 minute.
4. Repeat this 1-minute treatment until MRI demonstrates that the entire tumor volume and a small rim of normal tissue has been destroyed.

The RF brain lesion appears as a central focus of high signal on noncontrast T1-weighted images. This presumably represents a heat-induced methemoglobin effect, surrounded by a low signal ring. Postgadolinium T1-weighted images demonstrate a rim of enhancement peripheral to a low signal ring seen on noncontrast T1-weighted images.

This represents the acute thermal lesion. As the lesion matures (3 to 7 days), a peripheral low signal area of hemosiderin is also noted on T2-weighted images. The RF lesion and adjacent edema increase in size for up to 1 week after RF therapy and then gradually decrease unless local recurrence occurs.

Spine

Acute and chronic back pain with or without disc herniation is one of the major medical problems in health care worldwide. Acute and chronic lower back pain may be due to a variety of causes. Radicular pain caused by herniations, pseudoradicular pain in the facet joints, or local pain in the iliosacral joints may all require treatment.

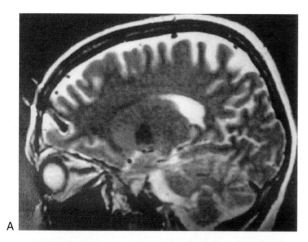

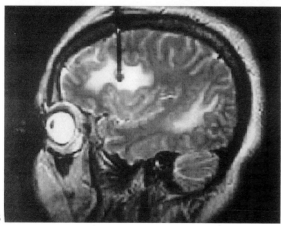

FIG. 23-8. Radiofrequency (RF) electrodes and ablation. **A:** T2-weighted fast spin-echo image of a patient with an anterior RF electrode in place. **B:** T2-weighted fast spin-echo image of another patient with a more posterior RF electrode in place confirms the location of the electrode within the tumor.

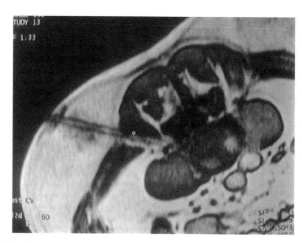

FIG. 23-9. Magnetic resonance–guided periradicular therapy for management of a disc herniation in level L4-5 on the right. The needle tip is advanced directly to the nerve root in the foramen. The double line artifact shows that the center of the needle is in the next plane. If the needle is within the plane, only one black artifact is present. Image courtesy of RMM Seibel.

A number of microinvasive techniques have been developed for these treatments, including CT-guided techniques for microinvasive periradicular therapy, mechanical percutaneous nucleotomy, and percutaneous laser nucleotomy, as well as CT-guided facet joint therapy and iliosacral joint therapy (3,60–62). Microinvasive interventional MRI is a new tool in spinal guidance technology (2). Most of the treatment can be performed without general anesthesia and on an outpatient basis.

Periradicular therapy was developed for patients with failed back surgery syndromes. Using MRI guidance, a 22-gauge coaxial needle is advanced through the lower third of the foramen to cross the nerve root (Fig. 23-9). Injection of long-acting anesthesia (Bupivacaine) and steroid (Triamcinolone) is performed. Also, injection at the facet and iliosacral joints can be performed to relieve pseudoradicular pain. Preliminary results have shown a response rate of greater than 90% for the relief of pain (63).

Grönemeyer et al. treated 110 patients with percutaneous nucleotomy and showed that 82% experienced complete pain relief and 92% had improved neurologic findings immediately after percutaneous nucleotomy (64). All nucleotomies can be combined with flexible microendoscopy (2). For these procedures, an MRI-compatible endoscopy system must be installed near the gantry (a portable system is available from Micromed, Winston-Salem, NC). Lower field strength MRI systems are advantageous because they allow some conventional electronic equipment to be positioned inside the MRI suite.

Head and Neck

Head and Neck Biopsy

MRI is rapidly replacing CT in aspiration for head and neck lesions, because MRI permits precise needle placement into comparatively inaccessible areas, such as the skull base and submandibular region, in which beam-hardening artifacts limit the effectiveness of CT (65–67). Another advantage is the superior tip localization of MRI by obtaining an oblique or orthogonal image along the course of the needle, similar to that of US.

By using MRI-compatible needles of variable length and curvature with coaxial 26-gauge sampling needles, lesions in this small and closely spaced area can be accessed in different ways:

- The subzygomatic/infratemporal approach can be performed to access lesions in the parapharyngeal space, skull base, and infratemporal fossa (Fig. 23-10). The patient's mouth is held open during the insertion. The triangle outlined by the zygoma, coronoid process, and mandibular condyle forms the landmark for needle insertion.

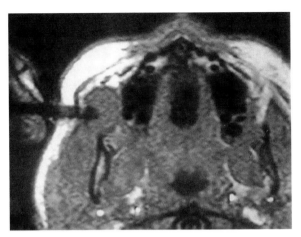

FIG. 23-10. A direct anterior subzygomatic approach to an anterior soft tissue mass was used to diagnose hemangioma.

- The retromandibular approach is useful for accessing the paraoropharyngeal, parotid, and the lower masticator spaces. The needle is placed just posterior to the angle of the mandible and more than 1 cm below the tragus to avoid damaging the facial nerve.
- The submastoid approach can be used to access lesions in the skull base. The needle is inserted 1 cm inferior to the mastoid tip along the anterior aspect of the sternocleidomastoid muscle.
- A direct approach is also possible.

Therapy

Palliative management options for recurrent head and neck cancer are limited by the proximity of vital vascular and neural structures and the aggressive nature of these tumors. Wide local resection of these lesions may result in functional and cosmetic deformities. Most head and neck tumors are treated by surgery, radiation therapy, or both. MRI-guided minimally invasive thermal ablation could be another alternative, if thermal energy delivery can be controlled accurately by MRI. Although the efficacy of interstitial laser therapy needs to be demonstrated further in larger series, preliminary clinical trials at the University of California, Los Angeles, and in Berlin showed promising results (68–70).

Breast

Breast Biopsy

Breast carcinoma is a leading cause of death for women in the United States and Europe. Because of high soft tissue contrast, MRI has been able to detect breast carcinomas that are not visible with the usual mammographic techniques. The most common clinical scenario leading to MRI-guided breast biopsy is the detection of additional enhancing lesions on breast MRI performed for the local staging of breast cancer (71). In this setting, MRI localization wires may be placed so that these lesions can be excised during excision of primary lesions. This technique may also be used to clearly define the margins of abnormal enhancement so that a lesion and its surrounding intraductal component may be excised in one sitting. With the recent development of breast biopsy surface coils, the breast can now be compressed and stabilized while the patient is in a prone position. Although experience is limited thus far, successful biopsy under MRI guidance has been performed in lesions that are not detectable or easily localized by other modalities (72).

Breast Treatment

Management of breast cancer has moved toward breast conservation, with the goal of maximized cosmesis without compromising overall survival. Several ablation techniques have been investigated for the treatment of breast tumors. A preliminary clinical trial of interstitial laser photocoagulation for breast cancer followed by surgery has recently been presented; it showed excellent correlation of MRI appearance and pathology. The study suggests that MRI-guided interstitial laser photocoagulation for breast cancer is a potentially useful tool (73). Another study of MRI-guided HIFU therapy for breast fibroadenomas is currently under way (74). Several issues should be addressed before ablation techniques can replace lumpectomy. One reservation is the loss of material for histopathologic examination when the whole tumor is ablated, because future treatment options may depend on the histologic information. Additionally, the residual enhancing material seen on MRI 48 to 72 hours after ablation may be caused by inflammatory response or residual tumor, thus necessitating multiple biopsies of the treated margin.

Abdomen and Pelvis

Percutaneous interventional procedures in the abdomen and pelvis are primarily performed for biopsies but are also done for sympathectomies and drainages. CT-, fluoroscopically, and US-guided punctures have been reported in the literature for nearly 30 years. In 1967, Nordenstrom reported the first series of percutaneous fluoro-guided lymph node biopsies (75). Different approaches, such as transperitoneal, translumbar, and transvascular procedures using different imaging modalities, are described.

Fine-needle biopsies are most often performed for cytologic and histologic diagnosis in the abdomen, retroperitoneum, pelvis, lymph nodes, bones, and joints. In general, the results with percutaneous aspiration techniques are very good. Success rates of greater than 80% have been reported for cytologic diagnosis.

Sonographic and CT-guided biopsies are established diagnostic techniques. However, US-guided methods have been replaced increasingly by CT guidance (76). MRI techniques for clinical treatments in the abdomen are new (77). Although they have the potential to replace a large number of conventional techniques, they should be used carefully to minimize possible injury to vital structures (78). Biopsies of large tumor masses or abscesses are possible as is percutaneous tumor therapy with ethanol ablation, RF, lasers, or cryotherapy.

In the near future, more treatments in the abdomen and pelvis will be performed. RF, cryosurgical, and laser techniques have great potential for treatment of prostate tumors, and MRI-guided drainage of large cysts and abscesses in the liver, pancreas, and retroperitoneum is an area of active investigation currently. Eleven tumors (refractory to conventional treatment) in seven patients were treated during 13 ablations using MRI-guided RF ablation between 1996 and 1997 as a part of a phase I clinical trial (79). Treatment sites included the liver, retroperitoneum, abdominal wall, and pelvis. No morbidity or toxicity has been encountered, although postablation MRI showed small amounts of fluid adjacent to liver in two patients after liver ablation, without symptoms or a drop in hematocrit.

MRI-guided laser ablation of liver tumors was investigated by Vogl's group in phase I (20 patients with 49 treated lesions) and phase II studies (105 patients with 306 lesions) (80). The phase II study demonstrated an overall cumulative survival rate of 86% after 12 months and 63% after 28 months, both of which are comparable with data obtained from the literature regarding patients who underwent hepatic resections; these data are better than data obtained from patients who received chemotherapy or no management.

In the future, combined MRI and endoscopic therapy especially for obstetrics, gallbladder, urinary tract, colon, and sympathectomy at all levels of the spines may be used routinely if endocoils, MRI-compatible endoscopic systems, or both are developed.

REFERENCES

1. Anzai Y, Desalle A, Black K, et al. Interventional MRI imaging. *Radiographics* 1993;13:897–990.
2. Grönemeyer DHW, Seibel RMM, Melzer A, Schmidt A. Image guided access technique. *Endosc Surg Allied Technol* 1995;3:69–75.
3. Grönemeyer DHW, Seibel RMM, Melzer A, et al. Future of advanced guidance techniques by interventional CT and MR. *Min Invasive Ther* 1995;4:251–259.
4. Mueller P, Stark D, Simeone J, et al. MR-guided aspiration biopsy: needle design and clinical trials. *Radiology* 1986;161:605–607.
5. Lufkin R, Teresi L, Hanafee W. New needle for MR guided aspiration cytology of the head and neck. *AJR Am J Roentgenol* 1987;149:380–382.
6. Kondziolka D, Dempsey PK, Lunsford LD, et al. A comparison between MRI and computed tomography for stereotactic coordinate determination. *Neurosurgery* 1992;30:402.
7. Maciunas RJ, Kessler RM, Maurer C, Mandava V, Watt G, Smith G. A universal system for interactive image-directed neurosurgery. *Sterotactic Funct Neurosurg* 1992;58:108.
8. Gybels J, Suetens P. Image-guided surgery. *Verh K Acad Geneeskd Belg* 1997;59:35.
9. Williams ML. Graphics workstations for therapy of the brain. In: De Salles A, Lufkin R, eds. *Minimally invasive therapy of the brain*. New York: Thieme Medical Publishers, 1997.
10. Bakker CJG, Hoogeveen RM, Weber J, van Vaals JJ, Viergever MA, Mali WP. Visualization of dedicated catheters using fast scanning techniques with potential for MR-guided vascular interventions. *Magn Reson Med* 1996;36:816.
11. Bakker CJG, Hoogeveen RM, Weber J, van Vaals JJ, Viergever MA, Mali WP. MR-guided endovascular interventions: susceptibility-based catheter and near-real-time imaging technique. *Radiology* 1997;202:273.
12. Daniel BL, Ikeda DM, Glover GH, Herfkens RJ. Interactive MR-guided breast lesion localization: a phantom study. Proceedings from the Fourth Annual Meeting of International Society for Magnetic Resonance Medicine. New York, 1996.
13. Köchli VD, McKinnon GC, Hofmann E, von Schulthess G. Vascular interventions guided by ultrafast MR imaging: evaluation of different materials. *Magn Reson Med* 1994;31:309.
14. Dumoulin CL, Souza SP, Darrow RD. Real time monitoring of invasive devices using magnetic resonance. *Magn Reson Med* 1993;29:411.
15. Leung DA, Debatin JF, Wildermuth S, et al. Intravascular MR tracking catheter: preliminary experimental evaluation. *AJR Am J Roentgenol* 1995;164:1265.
16. Busch M, Bornstedt A, Wendt M, Duerk JL, Lewin JS, Grönemeyer DHW. Fast "real time" imaging with different k-space. Update of strategies for interventional procedures. *J Magn Reson Imaging* 1998;8: 944–954.
17. Wendt M, Lenz G, Batz L, Busch M, Bornstedt A, Grönemeyer DHW. Dynamic tracking algorithm for interventional MRI using wavelet-encoding. *Proc Soc Magn Reson* 1995;2:1162.
18. Busch M, Grönemeyer DHW, Seibel RMM. Keyhole sequences for interventional procedures. Proceedings of interventional MRI workshop. Marina Del Rey, CA, 1994:106–107.
19. Van Vaals J, Brummer M, Dixon W, et al. "Keyhole" method for accelerating imaging of contrast agent uptake. *J Magn Reson Imaging* 1993;3:671–675.
20. Van Vaals J, van Yperen G, de Boer R. Real-time MR imaging using the LoLo method for interactive and interventional MRI at 0.5 T and 1.5 T. Proceedings of the Second Annual Meeting of the Society for Magnetic Resonance Medicine. San Francisco, 1994.
21. Duerk JL, Lewin JS, Wu DH. Application of keyhole imaging to interventional MRI: a simulation study to predict sequence requirements. *J Magn Reson Imaging* 1996;6:918.
22. Weaver JB, Xu Y, Healy DM, Driscoll JR. Wavelet-encoded MR imaging. *Magn Reson Med* 1992;24:257.
23. Parker DL, Smith V, Sheldon P, Crooks LE, Fussell L. Temperature distribution measurements in two-dimensional NMR imaging. *Med Phys* 1983;10:321–325.
24. Hall A, Prior M, Hand J, et al. Observation by MR imaging of *in vivo* temperature changes induced by radiofrequency hyperthermia. *J Comput Assist Tomogr* 1990;14:430–436.
25. Hall L, Talagala S. Mapping of pH and temperature distribution using chemical-shift-resolved tomography. *J Magn Reson* 1985;65:501–505.
26. Ebner FRS. Temperature monitoring for tissue ablation by means of MRI. Proceedings of interventional MRI workshop. Marina Del Rey, CA, 1994:119.
27. LeBihan D, Delannoy J, Levin R. Temperature mapping with MR imaging of molecular diffusion: application to hyperthermia. *Radiology* 1989;171:853–857.
28. Hindeman JC. Proton resonance shift of water in the gas an liquid states. *J Chem Phys* 1966;44:4582.
29. Stollberger R. Thermal monitoring using the water proton chemical shift. Proceedings of interventional MRI workshop, Boston, 1994:12.
30. Cline HE, Hynynen K, Hardy C, et al. MR temperature mapping of focused ultrasound surgery. *Magn Reson Med* 1994;31:628–636.
31. Chung AH, Hynynen K, Colucci V, Oshio K, Cline HE, Jolesz FA. Optimization of spoiled gradient-echo phase imaging for *in vivo* localization of a focused ultrasound beam. *Magn Reson Med* 1996;36:745.
32. De Poorter J, De Wagter C, De Deene Y, et al. The proto-resonance-frequency-shift method compared with molecular diffusion for quantitative measurement of two-dimensional time-dependent temperature distribution in a phantom. *J Magn Reson* 1994;103:234.
33. Young I, Hand J, Oatridge A, et al. Further observations on the measurement of tissue T1 to monitor temperature *in vivo* by MRI. *Magn Reson Med* 1994;31:342–345.
34. Goldhaber DM, Deli M, Grönemeyer DHW, et al. Measurement of tissue temperature by MRI. *IEEE Nucl Sci Med Imaging* 1993;3:1702–1705.

35. Lewa C, Majewska Z. Temperature relationships of proton spin-lattice relaxation time T1 in biological tissues. *Bull Cancer (Paris)* 1980;67:525–530.

36. Gilbert J, Rubinsky B, Roos M, et al. MRI-monitored cryosurgery in the rabbit brain. *Magn Reson Imaging* 1993;11:1155–1164.

37. Vining E, Duckwiler G, Udkoff R, et al. MRI of the thalamus following cryothalamotomy for Parkinson's disease and dystonia. *J Neuroimaging* 1991;1:146–147.

38. Onik G, Gilbert J, Hoddick W, et al. Ultrasonic monitoring of hepatic cryosurgery: preliminary report on an animal model. *Cryobiology* 1992;21:715.

39. Matsumoto R, Oshiro K, Jolesz F. Monitoring of laser and freezing-induced ablation in the liver with T1-weighted MR imaging. *J Magn Reson Imaging* 1992;2:555–562.

40. Jolesz FA, Bleier AR, Jakab P, Ruenzel PW, Huttl K, Jako GJ. MR imaging of laser tissue interactions. *Radiology* 1988;168:249–253.

41. Gatenby RA, Hartz WH, Engstro PF, et al. CT-guided laser therapy in resistive human tumor: phase I clinical trials. *Radiology* 1987;163:172–175.

42. Anzai Y, Lufkin RB, Hirshowitz, et al. MR imaging-histopathologic correlation of thermal injuries induced with interstitial Nd:YAG laser irradiation in the chronic model. *J Magn Reson Imaging* 1992;2:671–678.

43. Anzai Y, Lufkin RB, Saxton RE, et al. Nd:YAG interstitial laser phototherapy guided by magnetic resonance imaging in an *ex vivo* model: dosimetry of laser-MR-tissue interaction. *Laryngoscope* 1991;101(7 Pt 1):755–760.

44. Anzai Y, Lufkin RB, Castro DJ, et al. MR imaging-guided interstital Nd:YAG laser phototherapy: dosimetry study of acute tissue damage in an *in vivo* model. *J Magn Reson Imaging* 1991;1:553–559.

45. Dickinson RJ, Hall AS, Hind AJ, Young IR. Measurement of changes in tissue temperature using MR imaging. *J Comput Assist Tomogr* 1986;10:468.

46. Roberts HS, et al. Magnetic resonance imaging control of laser destruction of hepatic metastases: correlation with post-operative dynamic helical CT. *J Min Invasive Ther All Tech* 1997;6:53.

47. Paley M, Hall-Craggs MA, Bown SG Principles of MR-guided laser therapy. In: Lufkin R, ed. *Interventional MRI*. St. Louis: Mosby, 1998:221.

48. Siegfried J. 500 percutaneous thermocoagulation of the gasserian ganglion of trigeminal pain. *Surg Neurol* 1997;8:126–131.

49. Matsumoto SS, Shima F, Hasuo K, et al. MR imaging of stereotactic thalamotomy using radiofrequency methods. *Nippon Igaku Hoshasen Gakkai Zashi* 1992;52:1559–1564.

50. Anzai Y, Lufkin R, DeSalles A, et al. Preliminary experience with MR guided thermal ablation of brain tumors. *AJNR Am J Neuroradiol* 1995;16:39–45.

51. Rossi S, Di Staci M, Buscarini, et al. Percutaneous RF interstitial thermal ablation in treatment of liver cancer. *AJR Am J Roentgenol* 1996;167:759.

52. Lewin JS, Connell CF, Duerk JL, et al. Interactive MR-guided radiofrequency interstitial thermal ablation of abdominal tumors: clinical trial for evaluation for safety and feasibility. *J Magn Reson Imaging* 1998;8:40–47.

53. Hynynen K, Darkazanli A, Unger E, et al. MRI-guided noninvasive ultrasound surgery. *Med Phys* 1993;20:107–115.

54. Fan X, Hynynen K. Ultrasound surgery using multiple sonications: treatment time considerations. *Med Biol* 1996;22:471.

55. Liu CL, Fan S. Nonresectional therapies for hepatocellular carcinoma. *Am J Surg* 1997;173:358.

56. Adam G, Neuerburg J, Bücker A, et al. Interventional magnetic resonance: initial clinical experience with a 1.5-tesla magnetic resonance system combined with c-arm fluoroscopy. *Invest Radiol* 1997;32:191.

57. Lufkin R, Jordan S, Vinuela F, et al. MR imaging with topographic EEG electrodes in place. *AJNR Am J Neuroradiol* 1988;9:953–954.

58. Kelly P, Sharbrough F, Kall B, et al. Magnetic resonance imaging-based computer-assisted stereotactic resection of the hippocampus and amygdala in patients with temporal lobe epilepsy. *Mayo Clin Proc* 1987;62:103–108.

59. Khan T, Harth T, Kiwit JC, Schwarzmaier HJ, Wald C, Mödder U. *In vivo* MR thermometry using phase-sensitive sequences: preliminary experience during MRI-guided laser-induced interstitial thermotherapy of brain tumors. *J Magn Reson Imaging* 1998;8:160.

60. Grönemeyer DHW, Seibel RMM, Busch M, et al. Interventional magnetic resonance imaging. In: Siebel RMM, Grönemeyer DHW, eds. *Interventional computed tomography*. Oxford: Blackwell, 1990:289–305.

61. Seibel RMM, Grönemeyer DH, Sorensen RA, et al. Percutaneous nucleotomy with CT and fluoroscopic guidance. *J Vasc Interv Radiol* 1992;3:571–576.

62. Seibel RMM, Grönemeyer DH. Microinvasive CT guided dissection technique in the spinal canal. *End Sur All Tech* 1994;12:313–321.

63. Grönemeyer DHW, Seibel RMM. MRI and CT-scopic microsurgery and drug instillation for outpatient treatments. In: Lemke HU, Inamura K, Jaffe C, Vannier MW, eds. *Computer assisted radiology*. New York: Springer, 1995:1384–1392.

64. Grönemeyer DHW, Seibel RMM, Schmidt A, Kremer G, Vanleeuwen P. Atraumatic CT-controlled percutaneous laser nucleotomy. *Min Invasive Ther* 1994;2:247.

65. Wenokur R, Andrew J, Abemeyor E, et al. Magnetic resonance imaging-guided fine needle aspiration for the diagnosis of skull base lesions. *Skull Base Surg* 1992;2:167–170.

66. Trapp T, Lufkin R, Abemayor E, Layfield L, Hanafee W, Ward P. MR guided aspiration cytology for the head and neck. *Laryngoscope* 1989;99:105–108.

67. Lufkin RB. MR guided needle biopsy with a high-field-strength MR system. *AJNR Am J Neuroradiol* 1991;12:1268.

68. Castro D, Lufkin R, Saxton RE, et al. Metastatic head and neck malignancy treated with MR guided laser therapy: an initial case report. *Laryngoscope* 1992;102:26–32.

69. Castro D, Saxton RE, Lufkin R. Interstitial photoablative laser therapy guided by magnetic resonance imaging for the treatment of deep tumors. *Semin Surg Oncol* 1992;8:233–241.

70. Vogl TJ, Mack MG, Muller P, et al. Recurrent nasopharyngeal tumors: preliminary clinical results with interventional MR imaging-controlled laser-induced thermotherapy. *Radiology* 1995;196:725–733.

71. Orel SG, Schnall MD, Powell CM, et al. Staging of suspected breast cancer: effect of MR imaging and MR-guided biopsy. *Radiology* 1995;196:115.

72. Orel SG, Schnall MD, Newman RW, et al. MR imaging guided localization and biopsy of breast lesions: initial experience. *Radiology* 1994;193:97–102.

73. Hall-Craggs MA, Paley WM, Mumtaz H, et al. Laser therapy of breast carcinomas: MR/histopathological correlation. Proceedings of interventional MRI workshop. Boston, 1994:61.

74. Pomeroy O, et al. MR guided treatment of breast fibroadenomas by high intensity focused ultrasound. Proceedings of interventional MRI workshop. Boston, 1994:62.

75. Nordenstrom B. Paraxiphoid approach to the mediastinum for mediastinography and mediastinal needle biopsy: a preliminary report. *Invest Radiol* 1967;2:141.

76. Grönemeyer DHW, Seibel RMM, Arnold WH, Kramann B, Stark E. Atlas of CT-guided biopsies. In: Seibel RMM, Grönemeyer DHW, eds. *Interventional computed tomography*. Oxford: Blackwell, 1990:3–5.

77. Grönemeyer DHW, Seibel RMM, Kaufman L, et al. Interventional MRI cracks device and design barriers. *Diagn Imaging Int* 1990;11/12:32–36.

78. Grönemeyer D, Seibel RMM, Melzer A, et al. Equipment configuration and procedures—preferences for interventional microtherapy. *J Digital Imaging* 1996;9:81–86.

79. Lewin JS. Interactive MR-guided radiofrequency interstitial thermal ablation of abdominal tumors: clinical trial for evaluation of safety and feasibility. *J Magn Reson Imag* 1998;8:40.

80. Vogl TJ, Mack MG. Clinical uses of MR-guided laser ablation of liver. In: Lufkin R, ed. *Interventional MRI*. St. Louis: Mosby, 1998:356–365.

Open MRI,
edited by Peter A. Rothschild and Debra Reinking Rothschild.
Lippincott Williams & Wilkins. Philadelphia © 2000.

CHAPTER 24

Magnetic Resonance Angiography of the Head and Neck in an Open Scanner

Joy D. Foster and John Koveleski

In the open magnetic resonance imaging (MRI) setting, the extent to which a practice performs magnetic resonance angiography (MRA) is influenced by the following factors: the comfort and knowledge of the radiologist and technologist with vascular anatomy of the head and neck, the level of education of the technologist and radiologist in the different open MRI techniques used in MRA and the indications for their usage, and the scan time required for the examination. The radiologist should take the lead in educating the technologists and referring doctors to generate and maintain referrals for MRA. In our current medical environment, radiologists have a responsibility to direct referring clinicians to the correct and most accurate imaging modality appropriate for the patient's diagnosis. This holds true for MRA: Radiologists must know the indications for the MRI examination on an open MRI scanner. Should the diagnosis not "fit" the indications for MRA, a brief telephone conversation with the referring clinician saves time, helps avoid lost revenues, and cements a good referral pattern.

In the ideal world, patients referred for MRA would weigh no more than 170 lb and would never be claustrophobic. However, we are rarely presented with ideal patients. Open MRA is often the only modality available for many patients before subjecting them to conventional cerebral angiography. Although this fact may change in the near future, with the advent of computed tomographic angiography (1), MRA is currently the only noninvasive imaging modality capable of generating an image similar to conventional contrast angiography with a high degree of sensitivity and variable specificity.

The goals of this chapter are to explore the current indications for MRA of the head and neck and types of imaging techniques used along with suggested indications for their

use specifically related to open MRI. Pitfalls of certain imaging techniques and examples of normal and abnormal vascular anatomy are also discussed. A brief comparison of mid versus high-field MRI is first necessary.

MID VERSUS HIGH-FIELD MAGNETIC RESONANCE ANGIOGRAPHY

Comparison of current mid- and low-field MRI with high-field MRI must be evaluated. Korogi et al. (2) compared the sensitivity of diagnosing intracranial aneurysms at 0.5 and 1.5 T. They found a slightly greater sensitivity (75%) in detection of aneurysms larger than 5 mm at 1.5 T compared with 56% at 0.5 T. Grandin et al. (3) performed a retrospective analysis of the accuracy of a 0.5-T unit in the detection of intracranial aneurysms. They had a cohort of 140, compared to Korogi et al.'s study of 31, and they combined spin-echo images with MRAs to evaluate the sensitivity of MRA compared to cerebral angiography. Grandin et al.'s group concluded that a mid-field system was not a limiting factor in the diagnosis of intracranial aneurysms. More comparison studies clearly are needed with current state-of-the-art open MRI.

INDICATIONS

MRA of the neck is indicated in the evaluation of carotid bifurcation disease. Patients with carotid bifurcation disease often have symptoms that suggest a transient ischemic attack and an audible bruit on physical examination. The request for the MRA is often preceded by a carotid ultrasound with color Doppler capability, which has demonstrated a hemodynamically significant region of stenosis. MRA offers a highly accurate noninvasive means of detecting significant stenosis at or near the carotid bifurcation (Figs. 24-1 and 24-2) (4,5). The North American Symp-

J. D. Foster: Open MRI, Hayward, California; Open MRI, Louisville, Kentucky

J. Koveleski: Magnetic Imaging Center, Mechanicsburg, Pennsylvania

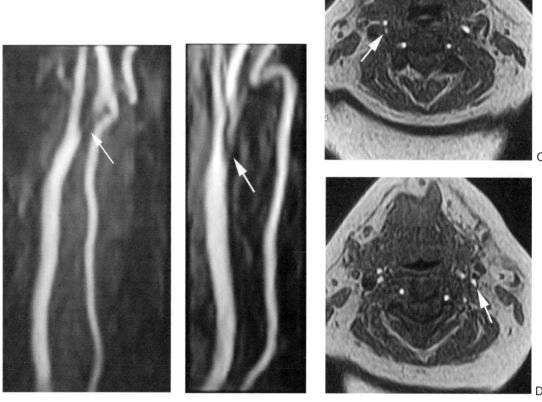

A, B
C
D

FIG. 24-1. A: Two-dimensional (2D) time of flight (TOF) angiogram of the left carotid bifurcation demonstrates stenosis of the left proximal internal carotid artery in a 55-year-old woman (*arrow*). The stenosis is overestimated on the maximum intensity projection (MIP) image (compare to **D**). Image courtesy of Ocean Medical Imaging Center, Toms River, NJ. **B:** 2D TOF angiogram at the level of the right carotid bifurcation demonstrates a region of stenosis involving the origin of the right internal carotid artery (*arrow*). **C:** Source axial image more clearly demonstrates the stenosis in the right proximal internal carotid artery (*arrow*). The left common carotid artery is seen in this slice owing to a higher bifurcation in comparison to the right. **D:** Mild stenosis of the left proximal internal carotid artery is also demonstrated (*arrow*). Note that the MIP images overestimate the degree of stenosis.

tomatic Carotid Endarterectomy Trial (6) showed a significant reduction in strokes in patients with a 70% or greater stenosis who underwent carotid endarterectomy.

The advantage of MRA is that it is noninvasive and can be performed in a relatively short time compared to conventional contrast angiography. Similar to MRI of other anatomic regions, MRA of the neck offers a high degree of sensitivity (Fig. 24-3). The specificity—that is, the accurate determination of the degree of stenosis of the vessel—is variable but has improved with the combined use of source partition images and maximum intensity projections (MIPs) (7,8) (Fig. 24-4; see also Figs. 24-1 and 24-2).

Although small carotid and vertebral artery dissections have been demonstrated with MRA (9), the utility of open MRI scanners with regard to this diagnosis is uncertain. More research with extensive comparison studies needs to be performed.

MRA of the intracranial circulation usually focuses on the circle of Willis and is indicated for the evaluation of aneurysms (>5 mm), arteriovenous malformations, intracranial occlusions (arterial and venous sinus thrombosis), and in the workup of subarachnoid hemorrhage (2,3,10,11). This last group of patients is often seen in an outpatient environment after initial hospital workup and discharge.

Patients referred for workup of possible aneurysm may have a family history, and therefore the MRA can serve as a screening examination. Patients with polycystic kidney disease and coarctation of the aorta have an increased incidence of developing aneurysms and are often referred for screening MRA. The noninvasiveness of the MRI examination and its relative rapidity make it preferable to conventional contrast angiography and ideal for screening.

Some studies have shown that the accuracy of MRA is enhanced by evaluation of the source images and the MIPs

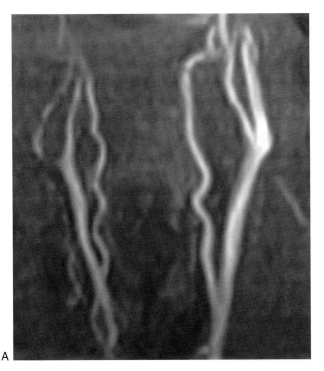

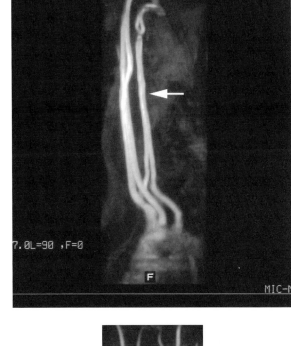

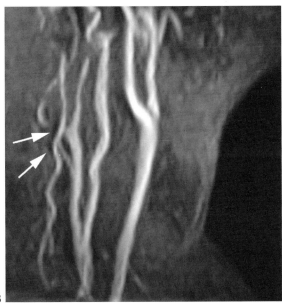

FIG. 24-2. A: Two-dimensional (2D) time of flight (TOF) angiogram at the level of the carotid bifurcation. Frontal projection. A marked contrast is seen between the normal left carotid bifurcation and the abnormal right carotid bifurcation. Multiple regions of stenosis are demonstrated within the proximal right internal carotid artery. Image courtesy of Ocean Medical Imaging Center, Toms River, NJ. **B:** 2D TOF angiogram, right to left rotation. The region of stenosis in the proximal right internal carotid artery is obscured by overlap of the right vertebral artery (*arrows*).

FIG. 24-3. Two-dimensional time of flight angiogram of the carotid arteries from the level of the aortic arch using a quad coil. **A:** Demonstration of the common carotid arteries and carotid bifurcations from a sagittal projection. The vertebral arteries (*arrow*) are demonstrated posterior to the common carotid arteries. **B:** Coronal projection demonstrates the origin of the common carotid arteries and vertebral arteries from the aortic arch. The vertebral arteries are visualized distally to the level of origin of the basilar artery.

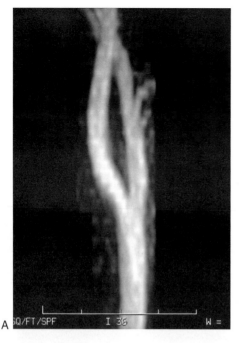

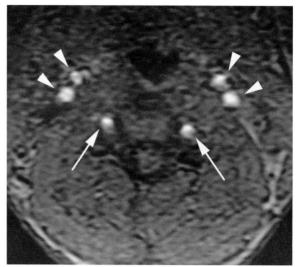

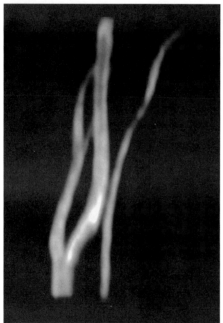

FIG. 24-4. A: Two-dimensional (2D) time of flight (TOF) angiogram at the level of the carotid bifurcation in a normal volunteer. The vertebral artery has been selectively omitted from the maximum intensity projection image. **B:** Source images clearly identify the level of the carotid bifurcation bilaterally (*arrowheads*) and flow within the vertebral arteries (*arrows*). **C:** 2D TOF angiogram at the level of the carotid bifurcation in a different patient. This image demonstrates artificial reduction in the width of the internal carotid artery at the level of the bifurcation secondary to eddy currents. Images courtesy of Toshiba America Medical Systems, South San Francisco, CA.

(7,12). Often, the intracranial MRA is accompanied by routine brain imaging. T2-weighted brain images should be included in the interpretation of the MRA.

IMAGING TECHNIQUES

The two imaging parameters most commonly used in open MRA are time of flight (TOF) and phase contrast. Both of these techniques use a gradient-echo pulse sequence. Both techniques generate a bright blood angiographic image (13,14). As a result, the imaged vessels have a similar appearance to conventional angiographic images. Either

technique can be applied to a two- (2D) or three-dimensional (3D) format. 2D imaging requires the acquisition of multiple thin slices, which are stacked postacquisition to create a volumetric image. In contrast, 3D imaging involves acquisition of an entire volume of data or multiple sets of volume data that are stacked to create an angiographic image.

Time of Flight

In TOF imaging, the area to be examined (e.g., carotid bifurcation in the neck) is subjected to multiple radiofrequency (RF) pulses, which cause stationary tissue within the area to lose longitudinal magnetization and signal. The tissues become saturated and appear dark on the MR image because of this loss of longitudinal magnetization (14,15). Blood flowing into the imaging plane is unsaturated and appears bright. The signal intensity of the blood vessel is affected by the course of the vessel through the imaging volume and the length of time the blood within the vessel remains in the imaging volume. Blood vessels perpendicular to the imaging volume are not subjected to as many RF pulses as is blood in tortuous vessels. Blood in the tortuous vessels, therefore, experiences more RF pulses and potentially becomes saturated, resulting in signal loss or "drop out." This phenomenon is known as *in-plane saturation* (16). A simple way to remember this concept is that the more horizontal component of the vessel becomes saturated and appears darker than the brighter, vertical component. Similarly, slower flowing blood due to stenosis, turbulence, or slower flow rates also becomes saturated, owing to prolonged exposure to the multiple RF pulses, and appears dark or at least less bright than in the rest of the vessel. Thicker imaging slabs also subject blood vessels to prolonged RF pulsation. As a result, blood exiting the plane is not as bright as incoming blood (15,16).

Repetition Time and Flip Angle

The amount of tissue saturation is determined by the time interval between the RF pulses (TR) and the intensity of the RF pulse (flip angle). The longer the TR, the less likely the blood vessels will be affected by saturation. Prolongation of the TR results in improved angiographic contrast at the expense of poor background suppression and in increased scan time. Background suppression is dependent on loss of longitudinal magnetization. The time necessary to recover longitudinal magnetization is the T1 value of the tissue. Tissues with short T1 values, such as fat or methemoglobin, have time to recover with longer TR intervals and appear bright. Improved background suppression can be achieved with shorter TR intervals and larger flip angles. The flip angle must also be carefully chosen, because too large a flip angle results in saturation of blood flow within the imaging plane. Varying the flip angle within the imaging plane is another means of improving angiographic contrast. To lessen the saturation effects on blood vessels at the end of the imaging slab, the flip angle across the slab can be gradually increased. Doing so results in greater background suppression at the end of the imaging slab and improved angiographic contrast. Commonly known as *tilted optimized nonsaturating excitation* (TONE) or *ramped flip angle excitation*, this technique is used in 3D volumetric angiography as a means of contrast improvement across the imaging slab (15,16).

Echo Time

The echo time (TE) is also an important factor in determining image contrast. In regions of turbulent flow, mixing of saturated and unsaturated spins occurs. This is often seen distal to a region of stenosis. The longer the TE, the greater the degree of mixing resulting in signal loss. A loss of signal could result in inaccurate depiction of the lumen size, potentially causing an overestimation in the degree of stenosis. To maximize signal, short TEs are used (13–16).

Saturation Bands

Improvement in angiographic contrast can also be achieved by application of multiple RF pulses outside the imaging plane or slab. Doing so results in localized tissue saturation. Saturation bands can be effectively used to saturate blood flow outside the area of interest and improve image contrast. For example, in the evaluation of the carotid arteries, placement of a saturation band superior to the imaging slab causes a loss of longitudinal magnetization (no signal) in venous structures flowing down and into the imaging plane. In the evaluation of the circle of Willis, saturation bands can be applied superiorly, over the sagittal sinus, to diminish overlap of deep venous anatomy. A simple means to remember where saturation bands should be placed is based on direction of flow. Venous flow is directed toward the heart. In imaging arterial vessels in the head or neck, the goal is to suppress venous return by placement of a saturation band above (superior to) the arterial vessels of interest. In arterial evaluation below the heart, venous return flows inferiorly to superiorly. Thus, saturation bands are placed below the arterial region of interest. For venous angiography, the saturation band should be placed to best suppress arterial flow (15,16).

Magnetization Transfer

Magnetization transfer is another means of background suppression in 3D TOF imaging. A high-frequency RF pulse out of resonance with unbound hydrogen protons is applied to selectively saturate bound hydrogen protons found primarily in tissues containing protein, such as muscle and gray and white matter in the brain, and not in flowing blood.

Role of Gadolinium

In an attempt to improve the sensitivity and specificity of MRA, recent research has focused on the use of intravenous gadolinium–enhanced MRA. The T1 shortening effects of gadolinium allow visualization of arterial and venous flow. Vessel visualization with TOF techniques is less dependent on in-plane saturation and saturation related to slab thickness. The disadvantage of gadolinium lies in its enhancement of background tissues. Early reports by Runge and coworkers (17) demonstrated improved visualization of aneurysms, arterial occlusions, and arteriovenous malformations in post–contrast-enhanced 3D TOF MRA compared to unenhanced 3D TOF MRA. Jung et al. (18) evaluated the optimal dose range of intravenous gadopentetate dimeglumine in intracranial MRA using a 3D TOF technique. They concluded that 5 to 10 mL was an optimal dose range allowing improved evaluation of stenotic vessels and venous drainage in arteri-

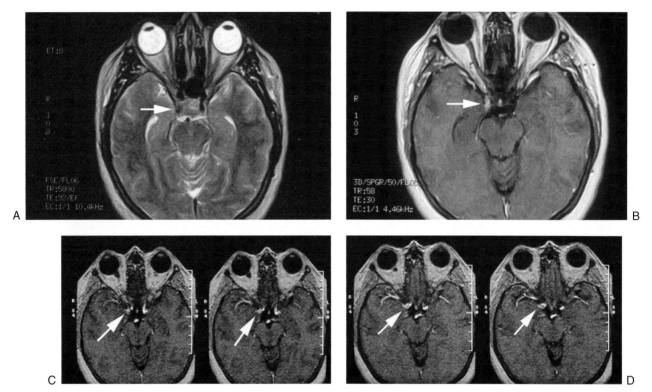

FIG. 24-5. Fifty-two-year-old woman referred for suspected aneurysm. **A:** Axial T2-weighted fast spin-echo image demonstrated mildly increased signal intensity in the region of the right cavernous sinus (*arrow*). **B:** Postcontrast T1-weighted volumetric axial image demonstrates abnormal enhancement (*arrow*). **C,D:** Axial source images obtained from a three-dimensional time of flight angiogram clearly demonstrate the presence of a small aneurysm arising from the right posterior communicating artery (*arrows*).

ovenous malformations. Other authors (19,20) evaluated the possible role of intravenous gadolinium in improving the specificity of MRA of the neck. The potential for improved sensitivity of the diagnosis of small aneurysms and specificity of diagnosing vascular stenosis at lower field strengths used in open MRI is encouraging. Assessment of the benefits versus the risks of contrast administration, particularly in patients referred for screening MRA, must be considered before changing to invasive-type protocols (Fig. 24-5).

Phase Contrast

Phase contrast techniques do not rely on saturation effects to generate an angiographic image and are not affected by T1 values of surrounding tissues. A gradient-echo sequence is still used. The difference is the application of a bipolar gradient pulse, which causes a shift or change in moving spins parallel to the direction of the gradient. The bipolar gradient is applied twice along each orthogonal axis, changing the polarity (positive/negative) of the gradient with each pulse application. Stationary spins or tissue is nullified by this change. Moving spins generate an echo based on the amount of phase shift. The phase shift depends on the strength of the applied gradient, velocity of flow, and direction of flow. Therefore, bipolar gradients must be applied in all three axes to accurately identify flow direction. Doing so results in longer scan times compared to TOF techniques (9,15). One of the advantages of phase contrast angiography is the ability to detect slow flow, which is important for the evaluation of partially thrombosed aneurysms and venous flow abnormalities. Equally important attributes are the relative insensitivity to saturation effects, the ability to determine flow direction and speed, and excellent background subtraction.

Phase contrast techniques require selection by the technologist of a velocity encoding (VENC) value specific for the region of interest. Phase contrast angiography allows quantitative and directional analysis, because the phase shift is directly related to the velocity of blood flow (13,15). Selection of VENC values is required to specify the velocities that will generate a phase shift and an angiographic image. If vessels in the region of interest possess higher flow rates than the selected VENC value, they will be incorrectly depicted, both in direction of flow and in magnitude. This phenomenon is known as *aliasing* (9,13,15,21). In general, arterial structures have higher VENC values than do slower, venous structures.

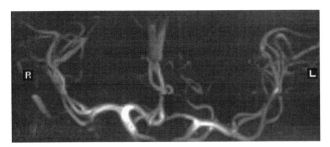

FIG. 24-6. Three-dimensional time of flight angiogram of the circle of Willis obtained using a multiple overlapping thin slab acquisition technique. Frontal projection demonstrates faint artifactual dark bands throughout the image that can be seen using this technique.

Two-Dimensional versus Three-Dimensional Imaging

Phase contrast and TOF can be used with 2D and 3D techniques. A variation of the 3D slab technique uses multiple overlapping thin slab acquisition rather than a single slab acquisition. This multiple slab acquisition technique improves flow-related enhancement due to diminished saturation effects at the expense of longer scan time (22) (Fig. 24-6). 3D TOF imaging has a higher signal-to-noise ratio, allowing higher resolution and the ability to reconstruct thinner slices in comparison to 2D imaging, especially at lower field strength. 3D TOF is less susceptible to in-plane saturation resulting from vessels coursing parallel within the imaging slab in comparison to 2D imaging. Tortuous vessels are, therefore, better visualized with 3D techniques (Figs. 24-7 and 24-8). Regions of tight stenosis with associated turbulent flow can be overestimated with 2D techniques because of the requirement for longer TEs with resultant turbulent dephasing (15,21). 2D techniques are preferable to 3D TOF in the evaluation of slow-flowing blood because of decreased satu-

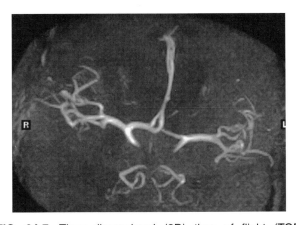

FIG. 24-7. Three-dimensional (3D) time of flight (TOF) angiogram looking down on the circle of Willis in a 35-year-old normal man. Note that the posterior communicating arteries are not generally identified on the maximum intensity projection image using a 3D TOF technique due to their slower flow rates. These must be evaluated on the source images.

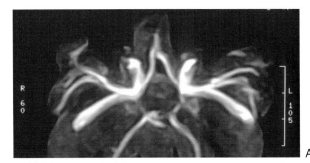

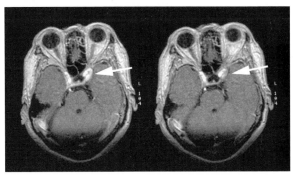

FIG. 24-8. A: Three-dimensional time of flight angiogram of the circle of Willis in a normal volunteer. The image is rotated in a head to foot direction. Tortuosity of the intracavernous portion of the internal carotid arteries is often seen on the maximum intensity projection image. **B:** The source image clearly demonstrates the presence of a tortuous left internal carotid artery rather than an aneurysm (*arrows*).

ration effects (9,21) (Fig. 24-9; see also Fig. 24-3). Patient cooperation is another consideration when deciding which technique to use. Movement affects an entire 3D slab, possibly rendering the examination nondiagnostic. 2D techniques are less susceptible to patient motion. This factor is very important with open MRI because of the longer imaging times when compared to high-field closed MRI (Table 24-1).

3D phase contrast and 3D TOF can be used in the evaluation of arteriovenous malformations. The use of multiple VENC values allows the differentiation of feeding arteries from draining veins with 3D phase contrast. Phase contrast techniques are better for distinguishing regions of thrombus from slow flow in aneurysms (21). However, because of the gradient strength required for phase contrast angiography, this technique is not currently available on all open magnets. Because of the complexity and requirements for prescan selection of VENC values, aneurysms may not be seen (23). Turtz et al. (24) described a case report of an 11-mm pericallosal arterial aneurysm not demonstrated on a 3D phase contrast angiogram.

PROCESSING AND PITFALLS

Processing (reconstruction) and interpretation of the MRA are as, if not more, important as the choice of imaging protocol. Both techniques generate source images. The original

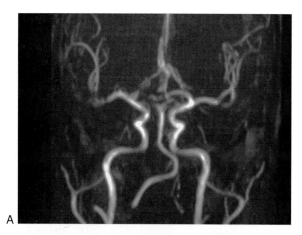

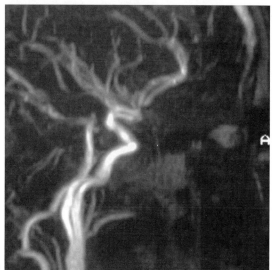

FIG. 24-9. Two-dimensional (2D) time of flight (TOF) angiogram of the circle of Willis in coronal **(A)** and sagittal **(B)** projections. With 2D TOF imaging, slower venous flow is also visualized. The degree of resolution is not as great as that obtained with three-dimensional imaging techniques. Greater coverage of the vasculature is also achieved with 2D TOF techniques.

data are also processed using an MIP algorithm, which selectively retains the regions of highest intensity and discards lower background intensity, resulting in a 3D image similar to a conventional angiogram. MIP images, although visually attractive, have been shown to erroneously reduce the width of vessels owing to the occurrence of eddy currents along the wall (25). These may result in a decrease in signal along the vessel wall, relative to the vessel lumen, because regions of decreased intensity have been subtracted out of the MIP image (see Fig. 24-4). Therefore, an MIP image can potentially result in exaggeration of true stenosis. In addition to eddy currents, saturation effects can occur at or near the end of an imaging volume and in association with slow flow seen in arteriovenous malformations (Fig. 24-10). Both cases can result in signal loss and nonvisualization on the MIP image. Regions of increased signal on the MIP image do not always originate from blood vessels. TOF techniques are sensitive to

TABLE 24-1. *Comparison of three- and two-dimensional time of flight imaging*

Three-dimensional time of flight	Two-dimensional time of flight
Volumetric acquisition	Thin slice acquisition better for venous and slower flow evaluation
Better for evaluation of stenosis	Can overestimate stenosis
Saturation at the end of the imaging slab	In-plane saturation of tortuous vessels
More susceptible to motion artifact	Less susceptible to motion artifact

T1 (longitudinal magnetization recovery) values. Tissues with short T1 values, such as fat, methemoglobin in subacute thrombus, and enhancing with paramagnetic MRI contrast agents, could potentially be seen on the MIP image (26). Due to these limitations, MRA interpretation should be based on evaluation of the source images in concert with the MIP

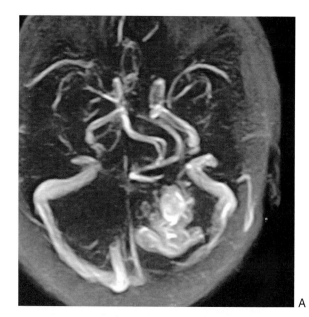

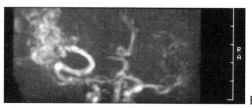

FIG. 24-10. A: Two-dimensional (2D) time of flight (TOF) angiogram in a 45-year-old woman with an arteriovenous malformation (AVM). The 2D TOF image better demonstrates slower flow within the nidus and venous drainage of the AVM. **B:** Angiogram of the same patient rotated in a left to right direction. The slower flow within the nidus is not as well visualized in the maximum intensity projection images.

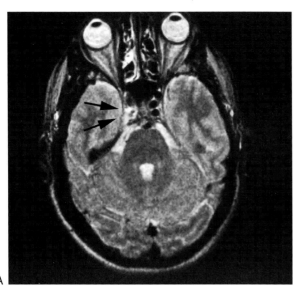

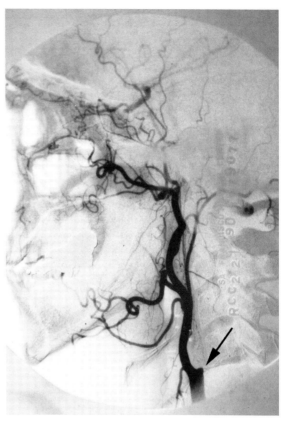

FIG. 24-11. A: Axial T2-weighted image at the level of the cavernous sinus. This case demonstrates the utility of combining interpretation of magnetic resonance angiograms with axial T2-weighted images. High-grade occlusion of the right internal carotid artery can be diagnosed (*arrows*). B: Conventional angiogram in the same patient (lateral projection) demonstrates complete occlusion of the right internal carotid artery at the level of the carotid bifurcation (*arrow*).

reconstructions and axial spin-echo images, if available (7,12,25,26) (Fig. 24-11; see also Figs. 24-4, 24-5, and 24-8). Such an approach results in increased diagnostic accuracy, greater confidence from referring physicians, and an increase in patient referrals to open MRI facilities.

CONCLUSION

MRA in open scanners is in its infancy in comparison to high-field strength closed scanners. Similar to the evolution of other aspects of open MRI, the advance of MRA will be determined by many factors, including improvement in the strength of the gradients, rise times, coil design, and image resolution and reduction in scan time. Research in open MRI, especially related to the indications and accuracy of MRA, has to be embraced by radiologists in outpatient imaging centers and supported by the administrators of those centers. Doing so allows validation of the technique with resultant expansion in the number of examinations performed and anatomic regions evaluated. Finally, an understanding of the type of angiographic techniques and their limitations and mechanisms for improvement is critical before MRA can become a substantial part of the outpatient imaging repertoire in an open MRI center. Future improvements in open MRI technology will have many benefits; one of the most important of which will be MRA and the indi-

cations for the examination. Newer open MRI scanners and techniques with substantially improved gradients, slew rates, and MRA sequences will allow greater sensitivity and a shift toward parity with closed high-field MRI. As open MRI technology improves at its current rapid pace, vast improvements in MRA will be evident in the future.

REFERENCES

1. Schwartz RB, Tice HM, Hooten SM, et al. Evaluation of cerebral aneurysms with helical CT: correlation with conventional angiography and MR angiography. *Radiology* 1994;192:717–722.
2. Korogi Y, Takahashi M, Mabuchi N, et al. MR angiography of intracranial aneurysms: a comparison of 0.5 T and 1.5 T. *Comput Med Imaging Graph* 1997;21:111–116.
3. Grandin CB, Mathurin P, Duprez T, et al. Diagnosis of intracranial aneurysms: accuracy of MR angiography at 0.5 T. *AJNR Am J Neuroradiol* 1998;19:245–252.
4. Heiserman JE, Drayer BP, Fram EK, et al. Carotid artery stenosis: clinical efficacy of two-dimensional time-of-flight MR angiography. *Radiology* 1992;182:761–768.
5. Litt AW, Eidelman EM, Pinto RS, et al. Diagnosis of carotid artery stenosis: comparison of 2DFT time-of-flight MR angiography with contrast angiography in 50 patients. *AJNR Am J Neuroradiol* 1991;12:149–154.
6. NASCET Collaborators. Beneficial effect of carotid endarterectomy in symptomatic patients with high-grade carotid stenosis. *N Engl J Med* 1991;325:445–453.
7. Anderson CM, Lee RE, Levin DL, et al. Measurement of internal carotid artery stenosis from source MR angiograms. *Radiology* 1994;193:219–226.

8. Pavone P, Marsili L, Catalano C, et al. Carotid arteries: evaluation with low-field-strength MR angiography. *Radiology* 1992;184:401–404.

9. Edelman R. MR angiography: present and future. *AJR Am J Roentgenol* 1993;161:1–11.

10. Zamani A. MRA of intracranial aneurysms. *Clin Neurosci* 1997;4: 123–129.

11. Wilcock D, Jaspan T, Holland I, et al. Comparison of magnetic resonance angiography with conventional angiography in the detection of intracranial aneurysms in patients presenting with subarachnoid haemorrhage. *Clin Radiol* 1996;51:330–334.

12. Korogi Y, Takahashi M, Mabuchi N, et al. Intracranial aneurysms: diagnostic accuracy of MR angiography with evaluation of maximum intensity projection and source images. *Radiology* 1996;199:199–207.

13. Edelman R, Mattle H, Atkinson D, Hoogewoud H. MR angiography. *AJR Am J Roentgenol* 1990;154:937–946.

14. Pavone P, Laghi A, Catalano C. Flow phenomena. In: Arlart IP, Bongartz GM, Marchal G, eds. *Magnetic resonance angiography*. Germany: Springer-Verlag, 1996:23–34.

15. Kanal E. Overview of MR angiography. From course syllabus, Advances in Mid and Low Field MRI; October 15–18, 1998; Tampa, FL.

16. Anderson CM, Lee RE. Time-of-flight techniques. In: Finn JP, ed. *Magnetic resonance imaging clinics of North America*. Philadelphia: WB Saunders, 1993:217–227.

17. Runge VM, Kirsch JE, Lee C. Contrast-enhanced MR angiography. *J Magn Reson Imaging* 1999;3:233–239.

18. Jung HW, Chang KH, Choi DS, et al. Contrast-enhanced MR angiography for the diagnosis of intracranial vascular disease: optimal dose of gadopentetate dimeglumine. *AJR Am J Roentgenol* 1995;165: 1251–2155.

19. Slosmman F, Stolpen AH, Lexa FJ, et al. Extracranial atherosclerotic carotid artery disease: evaluation of non-breath-hold three-dimensional gadolinium-enhanced MR angiography. *AJR Am J Roentgenol* 1998;170:489–495.

20. Enochs WS, Ackerman RH, Kaufman JA, Candia M. Gadolinium-enhanced MR angiography of the carotid arteries. *J Neuroimaging* 1998;8:185–190.

21. Huston J III, Ehman RL. Comparison of time-of-flight and phase-contrast MR neuroangiographic techniques. *Radiographics* 1993;13:5–19.

22. Parker DL, Yuan C, Blatter DD. MR angiography by multiple thin slab 3D acquisition. *Magn Reson Med* 1991;17:434–451.

23. Araki Y, Kahmura E, Tsukaguchi I. A pitfall in detection of intracranial unruptured aneurysm on three-dimensional phase contrast MR angiography. *AJNR Am J Neuroradiol* 1994;15:1618–1623.

24. Turtz A, Allen D, Koenigsberg R, Goldman HW. Nonvisualization of a large cerebral aneurysm despite high-resolution magnetic resonance angiography. Case report. *J Neurosurg* 1995;82:294–295.

25. Anderson CM, Saloner D, Tsuruda JS, et al. Artifacts in maximum-intensity-projection display of MR angiograms. *AJR Am J Roentgenol* 1990;154:623–629.

26. Wilcock DJ, Jaspan T, Worthington BS. Problems and pitfalls of 3-D TOF magnetic resonance angiography of the intracranial circulation. *Clin Radiol* 1995;50:526–532.

Open MRI,
edited by Peter A. Rothschild and Debra Reinking Rothschild.
Lippincott Williams & Wilkins. Philadelphia © 2000.

CHAPTER 25

Advances in Neuroimaging: Clinical Diffusion Imaging in Open Magnetic Resonance Imaging

Lawrence N. Tanenbaum

Diffusion-weighted magnetic resonance imaging (MRI) techniques have had a formidable effect on clinical neuroimaging, affecting the evaluation of cerebral ischemia as well as the characterization and differentiation of nonspecific focal brain lesions. Diffusion-weighted imaging (DWI) facilitates early detection of ischemia and reduces the cost and morbidity of diagnosis of a number of disease states. The recent availability of diffusion techniques on open MRI systems brings this powerful technology to patients who face challenges that prevent access to closed high-field systems, such as size or claustrophobia.

DIFFUSION TECHNIQUES

With diffusion techniques, MRI is sensitized to the random microscopic motion of water molecules in tissues. Symmetric bipolar diffusion gradients impart and then reverse phase modulations of protons in tissues. Protons with restricted motion are rephased by the second gradient pulse and thus exhibit relatively high signal. Randomly diffusing spins experience an additional phase shift due to motion in the graded magnetic field and thus remain out of phase and relatively low in signal.

Although water diffusion in gray matter is relatively random (isotropic), in white matter, motion is anisotropic, with free movement *along* fiber tracts and restricted *across* tracts. The brain's structural anisotropy contributes to a complex appearance on images sensitized to diffusion in a single direction (anisotropic images) with restricted regions of white matter motion brighter than those with free motion in the white matter and cortex.

L. N. Tanenbaum: Department of Neuroscience, Seton Hall School of Graduate Medical Education, South Orange, New Jersey; Departments of Neuroradiology, Magnetic Resonance Imaging, and Computed Tomography, New Jersey Neuroscience Institute at John F. Kennedy Medical Center, Edison, New Jersey

At high field, echo-planar imaging techniques are typically used to perform DWI. These ultrafast techniques obtain diffusion information sensitized to multiple directions in a rapid, clinically feasible time frame. Isotropic, or trace-weighted, images can be created by a mathematical combination of these images. Trace-weighted images eliminate signal from structures that are not bright on all diffusion directions and highlight pathologic changes that alter diffusion from the normal in all directions. The degree of diffusion weighting, or B value, used for clinical purposes is typically between 800 and 1,000 seconds per mm^2. A 30-slice study on a typical high-performance, high-field magnet with images sensitized to diffusion in three orthogonal (x, y, and z) directions, along with a data set obtained without diffusion weighting (B value = 0) requires less than 40 seconds. Obtaining images at at least two different levels of diffusion weighting (B values) allows calculation of maps of the apparent diffusion coefficient (ADC map). Whereas trace-weighted images combine T2 and diffusion effects, ADC maps are specific for diffusion alterations. This differentiation can be useful in characterizing nonspecific brain lesions.

On open low-field (0.2-T) systems, diffusion is performed using line-scan techniques. In contrast to typical MRI acquisitions that use a two- or three-dimensional Fourier transformation of a plane or volume of tissue, line scanning involves a one-dimensional Fourier transformation of an excited column of tissue (Fig. 25-1). Typical parameters on an open MRI system (General Electric Medical Systems, Milwaukee, WI, 0.2 Tesla Profile) are 7.5-mm slice thickness, 0-mm gap, 64 × 64 matrix, and 30-cm field of view with a B value of 800. An 18-slice study requires just over 10 minutes for a single direction acquisition. Because scanning is performed in a column-by-column, slice-by-slice fashion, the images are relatively resistant to macroscopic motion despite long overall scan times. The time required to acquire images in three orthogonal directions limits the clinical utility of trace-weighted or anisotropic techniques and ADC mapping on open systems. Although

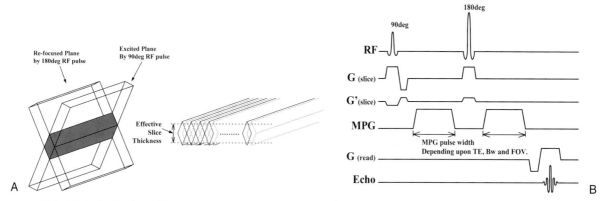

FIG. 25-1. A: Basics of line-scan imaging. Line-scan spin-echo techniques involve a one-dimensional Fourier transform of an excited column of tissue. **B:** Line-scan diffusion pulse sequence diagram. FOV, field of view; G, gradient; MPG, multiplanar gradient; RF, radiofrequency; TE, echo time.

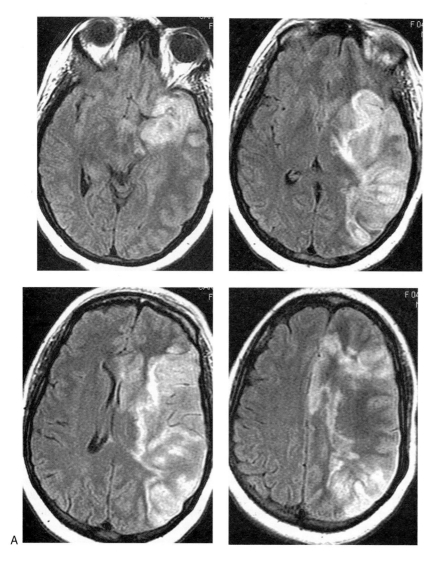

FIG. 25-2. Recent infarction. **A:** High-field fluid attenuated inversion recovery images demonstrate an infarction of the middle cerebral artery (MCA) territory. *Continued.*

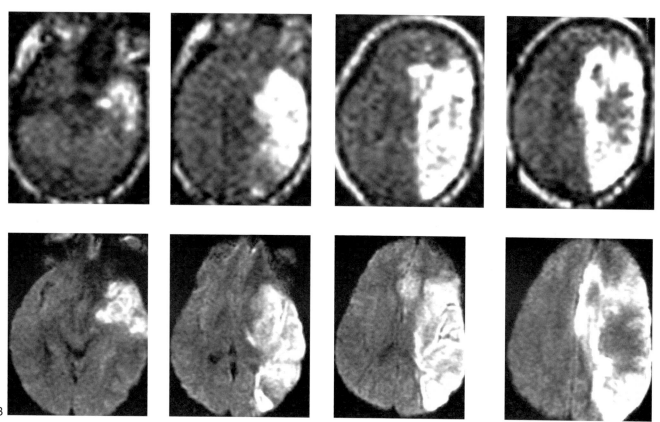

FIG. 25-2. *Continued.* **B:** Studies, 0.2 T (*top*) and 1.5 T (*bottom*), confirm the presence of recent MCA infarction.

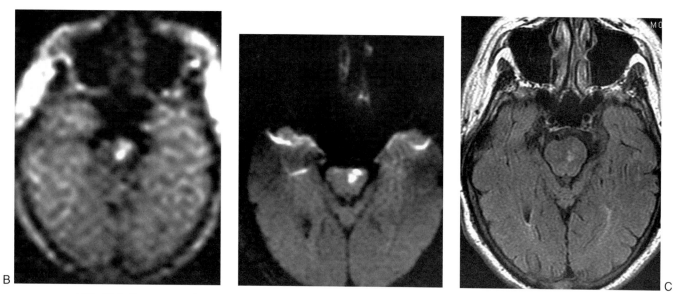

FIG. 25-3. Recent pontine infarction. **A:** 0.2-T diffusion-weighted imaging (DWI) line scan. **B:** 1.5-T DW echo-planar imaging (EPI). **C:** 1.5-T fluid attenuated inversion recovery images demonstrate a recent left pontine infarction. Note the presence of susceptibility artifact distorting the appearance of the ventral pons on the high-field EPI scan, absent on the 0.2-T spin-echo line-scan study.

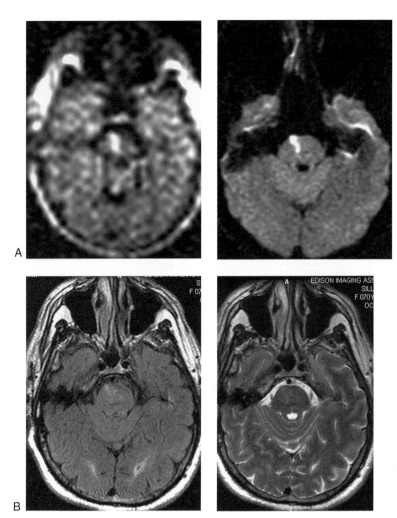

FIG. 25-4. Acute pontine infarction. **A:** Left to right: 0.2-T diffusion-weighted imaging (DWI) line scan and 1.5-T DW echo-planar imaging. **B:** Left to right: 1.5-T fluid attenuated inversion recovery and fast spin-echo images. Both DW studies readily demonstrate acute right pontine ischemic changes that are subtle on the high-field conventional images.

lower in resolution, spin-echo line-scan techniques compare favorably with high-field echo-planar imaging–based techniques (1) (Fig. 25-2), providing less geometric distortion and magnetic susceptibility effect sensitivity important in imaging structures about the skull base (Fig. 25-3).

TENSOR DIFFUSION

Recent advances provide diffusion acquisitions sensitized to motion in six diagonal directions, allowing measurement of the diffusion tensor and creation of maps of relative brain anisotropy (2). Anisotropy maps depict the normal patterns of water motion restriction in highly ordered white matter. Brain derangements too subtle to be detected by structural MRI techniques may be revealed in regional breakdown in water motion restriction (loss of signal) on anisotropy images. This promising technique may have clinical utility in the evaluation of patients with psychiatric disorders, traumatic brain injury, epilepsy, and dementia (3).

CLINICAL UTILITY

Infarction

The primary utility of DWI is in the detection of brain infarction. DWI techniques are more sensitive than conventional MRI techniques and are extraordinarily sensitive in detecting clinically evident ischemia, even when imaging is obtained immediately after the onset of ischemic symptomatology (4) (Fig. 25-4). DWI techniques are also sensitive to the presence of silent ischemia in patients who present with clinically transient ischemic attacks.

The pathophysiologic changes detectable by DWI, although not definitively understood, likely involve the onset of cytotoxic edema with a net bulk motion of water from the free extracellular space to the restricted motion environment of the intracellular space. Cell swelling also reduces the volume of the extracellular compartment that may also contribute to signal changes. The signal intensity changes associated with acute ischemia typically remain evident for approximately 5 to 7 days on trace and individ-

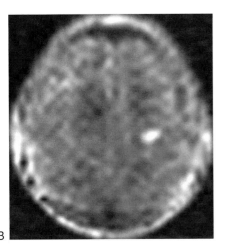
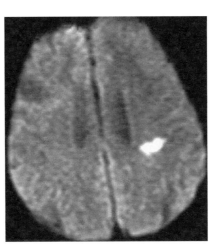
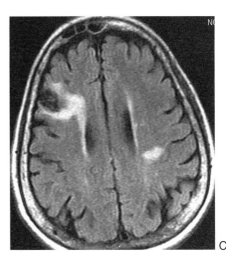

A, B   C

FIG. 25-5. Infarction—recent and old. **A:** 0.2-T diffusion-weighted imaging (DWI) line scan. **B:** 1.5-T DW echo-planar imaging. **C:** 1.5-T fluid attenuated inversion recovery images. Recent left frontal white matter infarction is conspicuous on all techniques. Note that the old right frontal infarction no longer manifests a restriction in diffusion and is not bright on DWI.

ual direction images, with a shorter period of conspicuity on ADC maps.

In clinical practice, the impact of DWI is felt in acute and subacute stroke. Although DWI techniques are sensitive by the time a patient can present for scanning, offering near perfect sensitivity in hyperacute stroke and potentially affecting brain preservation and thrombolytic therapy, these cases are relatively uncommon in clinical practice. More often, in the clinical setting, patients present for MRI somewhat later (18 to 36 hours) after the onset of ischemic symptoms. Signal changes due to infarction are typically present on MRI by this time, using traditional techniques such as fluid attenuated inversion recovery fast spin-echo, but may not be recognized as distinct

from a background of chronic ischemia (Fig. 25-5). The ability of DWI to differentiate between recent and remote infarction provides a significant boost in the practical sensitivity of MRI in the subacute setting (5). Improving the sensitivity and specificity of MRI in this setting can have a favorable impact on the cost-effectiveness and morbidity of treatment and perhaps improve patient outcome.

Demyelinating Disease

Conventional methods of differentiating active demyelination from chronic, inactive lesions in multiple sclerosis is via use of gadolinium-enhanced conventional imaging sequences.

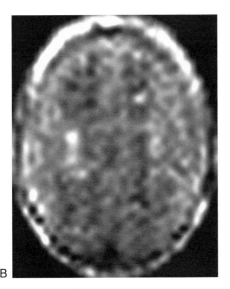
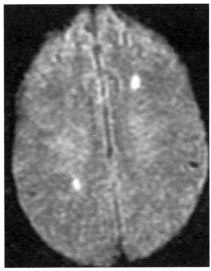
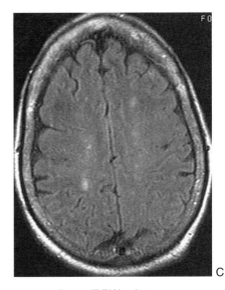

A, B   C

FIG. 25-6. Multiple sclerosis (MS). **A:** 0.2-T diffusion-weighted imaging (DWI) line scan. **B:** 1.5-T DW echo-planar imaging. **C:** 1.5-T fluid attenuated inversion recovery (FLAIR) images. Cerebrospinal fluid–suppressed FLAIR studies are well suited to the depiction of MS plaques. Active plaques are bright on DWI, whereas chronic plaques can demonstrate an increase in the apparent diffusion coefficient (low signal).

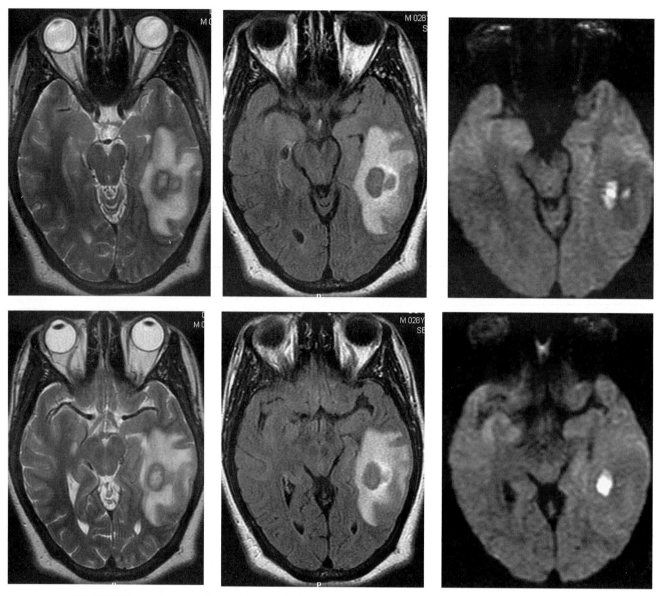

FIG. 25-7. Pyogenic brain abscess. Left to right: 1.5-T T2-weighted fast spin-echo, fluid attenuated inversion recovery, and diffusion-weighted imaging (DWI). Double-ring lesion surrounded by vasogenic edema. Note the characteristic appearance on DWI with hypointense edema and a hyperintense lesion.

Active lesions demonstrate contrast enhancement, with an increasing sensitivity at higher doses of contrast (0.1 to 0.3 mmol per kg) (6,7). DWI appears to offer similar information with active lesions demonstrating increased signal and potentially avoiding the need for routine contrast use in these situations (Fig. 25-6).

Mass Lesion Characterization

DWI techniques can yield powerful characterization information about focal brain lesions.

Tumor versus Abscess

Neoplastic lesions have a varied appearance on DWI but are typically unimpressive without striking areas of high signal associated with the lesion itself, even when necrotic. Nonspecific perilesional vasogenic edema is typically hypointense on DWI (and hyperintense on ADC maps). Abscesses can have a characteristic appearance with hyperintensity on DWI associated with the lesion itself, surrounded by hypointense edema (8,9) (Fig. 25-7). This noninvasive differentiation of tumor from abscess can be critical in reducing the cost and morbidity of treatment in these patients.

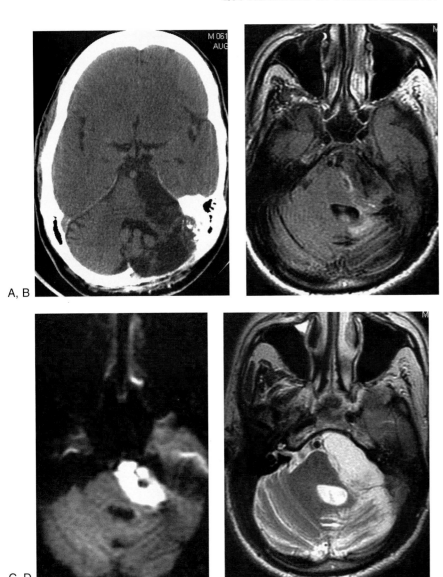

FIG. 25-8. Residual epidermoid cyst. **A:** Unenhanced computed tomography (CT). **B:** 1.5-T fluid attenuated inversion recovery (FLAIR). **C:** Diffusion-weighted imaging (DWI). **D:** T2-weighted fast spin-echo (FSE). Note the difficulty in differentiating the operative changes from residual tumor on CT and T2-weighted FSE. High signal gliosis is distinguished from low-signal cerebrospinal fluid and encephalomalacia on FLAIR. Heterogeneous signal in the cerebellopontine angle cistern is a hint of the presence of a lesion. The residual epidermoid cyst is very high in signal on the DW images, thus simplifying diagnosis.

Tumor versus Infarction

Although DWI can readily differentiate neoplastic lesions and recent infarction, the appearance of tumor and stroke can overlap in the subacute setting. Subacute infarctions may be only slightly hyperintense as they fade in conspicuity on DWI and may not be distinguishable from some neoplasms at any given point in their evolution. Whereas signal intensity on trace-weighted and individual direction DWI represents a combination of diffusion and T2 effects, ADC maps depict diffusion alterations only and are free from so-called T2 shine-through, which can complicate lesion characterization. Because most neoplasms manifest an increase in diffusion coefficient, ADC maps

readily differentiate these lesions from acute and subacute infarction (low to normal ADC).

Arachnoid versus Epidermoid Cyst

Although extraaxial cystic lesions may have signal intensity patterns that are similar on conventional T1- and T2-weighted imaging sequences, the behavior of these lesions on DWI is strikingly different. The signal intensity of an arachnoid cyst is similar to that of cerebrospinal fluid, whereas an epidermoid cyst demonstrates striking increased signal on DWI (10). Diffusion properties therefore allow ready differentiation of an epidermoid cyst from an arach-

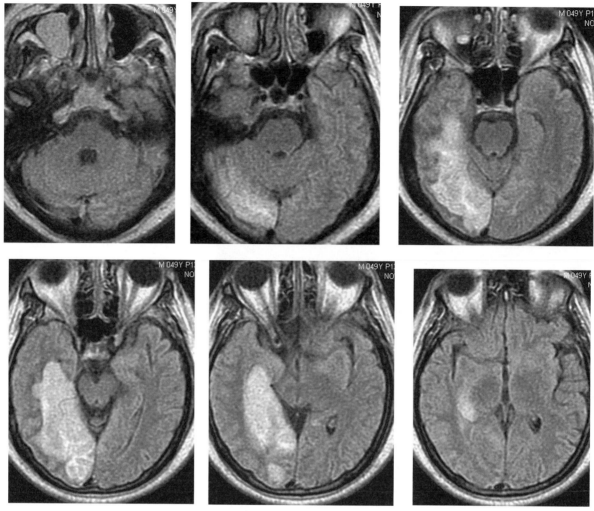

FIG. 25-9. Case study. 0.2-T fluid-attenuated inversion recovery images from a patient with a lesion suspicious for a tumor of the right temporal lobe. See text and Fig. 25-10.

noid cyst and, after partial resection, from adjacent cerebrospinal fluid (Fig. 25-8).

CASE STUDY

A 49-year-old patient is referred to the office of a neuro-oncologist with a 1.5-T scan demonstrating a lesion thought to be suspicious for a tumor of the right temporal lobe. A fol-low-up study was undertaken to characterize the lesion and clarify the diagnosis.

Multiple 0.2-T fluid attenuated inversion recovery images are presented for review (Fig. 25-9). What is your differential diagnosis? What would you do next to confirm your impression or differentiate between possibilities?

A 0.2-T DWI study (Fig. 25-10) shows striking increased signal within the right temporal lobe consistent with a recent infarction. What confirms the diagnosis?

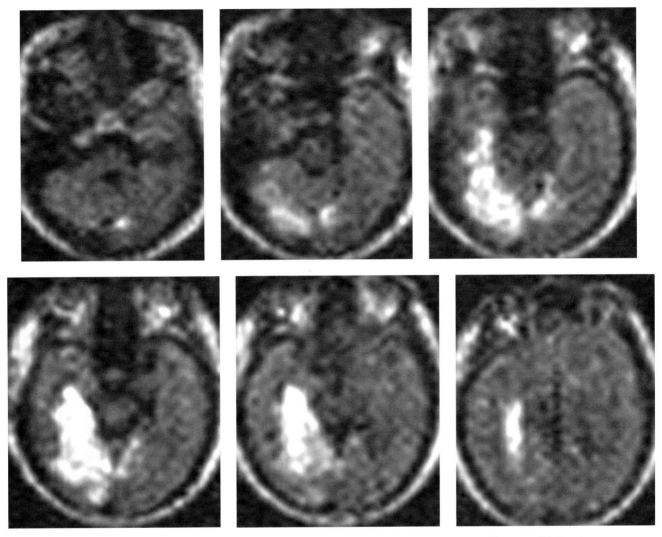

FIG. 25-10. Case study (continued). 0.2-T DWI study on the same patient as in Fig. 25-9. Notice the striking increased signal within the right temporal lobe.

The telltale involvement of the left temporal lobe seals the diagnosis of a bilateral posterior cerebral artery infarction.

REFERENCES

1. Tanenbaum LN, Borden N, Eshkar NE, et al. Open MR diffusion imaging: comparison of line scan diffusion imaging at 0.2T with diffusion weighted EPI at 1.5T in patients with recent infarction. Presented at the American Society of Neuroradiology, San Diego, CA, May 1999.
2. Peled S, Gudbjartsson H, Westin CF, et al. Magnetic resonance imaging shows orientation and asymmetry of white matter fiber tracts. *Brain Res* 1998;780(1):27–33.
3. Buchsbaum MS, Tang CY, Peled S, et al. MRI white matter diffusion anisotropy and PET metabolic rate in schizophrenia. *Neuroreport* 1998;9(3):425–430.
4. Barest GD, Sorenson AG, Gonzalez RG. Magnetic resonance imaging of cerebral infarction. *Top Magn Reson Imaging* 1998;9(4):199–207.
5. Tanenbaum LN, Johnson BA, Drayer BP, et al. Comparison of diffu-

sion weighted single shot EPI and fast FLAIR in the evaluation of patients with subacute ischemic symptoms. Presented at the Annual Meeting of the Eastern Society of Neuroradiology, Tarrytown, NY, September 1997 and the Annual Meeting of the Western Neuroradiology Society, Palm Springs, CA, October 1997.
6. Clanet M, Berry I. Magnetic resonance imaging in multiple sclerosis. *Curr Opin Neurol* 1998;11(4):299–303.
7. McFarland HF. The lesion in multiple sclerosis: clinical, pathological, and magnetic resonance imaging considerations. *J Neurol Neurosurg Psychiatry* 1998;64(Suppl 1):S26–S30.
8. Kim YJ, Chang KH, Song IC, et al. Brain abscess and necrotic or cystic brain tumor: discrimination with signal intensity of diffusion weighted MR imaging. *AJR Am J Roentgenol* 1998;171:1487–1490.
9. Tsuchiya KI, Yamakami N, Hachiya J, et al. Multiple brain abscesses: discrimination from cerebral metastases by diffusion weighted magnetic resonance imaging. *Int J Neuroradiol* 1998;4(4):258–262.
10. Tsuruda JS, Chew WM, Moseley ME, Norman D. Diffusion-weighted MR imaging of the brain: value of differentiating between extraaxial cysts and epidermoid tumors. *AJR Am J Roentgenol* 1990;155(5):1059–1065.

Open MRI,
edited by Peter A. Rothschild and Debra Reinking Rothschild.
Lippincott Williams & Wilkins. Philadelphia © 2000.

CHAPTER 26

Teleradiology in Open Magnetic Resonance Imaging

R. Craig Platenberg and V. G. Raaj Prasad

Teleradiology and open magnetic resonance imaging (MRI) are complementary technologies that form a natural fit in today's environment. In addition to their more traditional role as a supplement to high-field systems, open MRI systems are increasingly being used as the sole MRI system in small community hospitals and free-standing imaging centers. Open systems were initially used for large or obese patients and for patients with claustrophobia or severe anxiety. With improvements in hardware and software, open systems have become capable of high-quality imaging for the vast majority of clinical indications. Improvements in gradient strength, coil design, and sequence optimization have made open MRI systems clinically viable in many scenarios. Furthermore, these systems fit well with the economics of far-flung and rural areas. As more and more open MRI systems are being located in remote and rural areas, the role of teleradiology assumes greater significance.

Teleradiology is the use of electronic information and communications technologies to transfer digital electronic images so that radiologists may provide diagnostic services from locations separated by distance. In the broader context of telemedicine, telecommunications technology has many implications for improving patient care, public health, access, patient education, physician education, research, administration, and data management (1). Many branches of medicine are now using telemedicine tools (2). Approximately 50% of all radiology practices use some form of teleradiology. In fact, the first and most important medical use of telecommunications technology is so commonplace that it is frequently overlooked. Virtually every radiology practice uses telephone and facsimile communications in its daily practice. Radiology is a specialty that uses advanced telecommunications technologies in many clinical settings. A wide range of teleradiology applications, from on-call coverage and consultation–second opinion overreads to remote primary diagnosis, use filmless technology. Defining the need for services, identifying the existing telecommunications infrastructure, and assessing the speed of transmission and the cost of providing services are important steps in establishing a successful teleradiology endeavor.

For any teleradiology application to be viable, it must be accessible, accountable, and affordable. Present constraints of infrastructure limitations, reimbursement, licensure issues, telecommunications regulations, malpractice insurance, and confidentiality must be addressed and overcome.

HISTORICAL PERSPECTIVE

As advances in telecommunication technologies have occurred, the medical use of these technologies has followed. As early as the Civil War, medical information was transmitted from one location to another. The numbers of people wounded and orders for medical supplies were communicated between Baltimore and Washington using public telegraph in 1844 (1). Alexander Graham Bell patented the telephone in 1876, and in 1906 the first electrocardiographic (ECG) transmissions by phone were performed. The first experimental television transmissions were undertaken in 1927. In 1949, the Jean-Talon Hospital in Montreal used a television to perform x-ray data transmissions (3). The Psychiatric Institute of the University of Nebraska was one of the first facilities to use closed-circuit television monitoring in 1955. In 1959, the University used video links to transmit neurologic examinations across campus for medical student teaching. The first radiotelemetry for monitoring patients in an intensive care unit was described in the *Journal of Anesthesiology* in 1961 (4). In 1963, Kenneth T. Bird established

R. C. Platenberg: Wide Open MRI, Med-Ted International Corporation, McLean, Virginia

V. G. R. Prasad: Image Enhancement System, Inc., Hayward, California

an interactive television link between a clinic at Logan International Airport and Massachusetts General Hospital. Boland cites this as the first example of teleradiology as an entity in and of itself in his review (5). In 1967, the University of Miami and the City of Miami Fire Department used radio channels to transmit ECG data to Jackson Memorial Hospital for patients in extremis. In 1968, Massachusetts General Hospital added interactive television microwave links for ECG, voice, stethoscope, and macroscopy and developed a telepsychiatry link with the local Veterans Administration.

Between 1960 and 1970, the National Aeronautics and Space Administration (NASA) played a crucial role in the development of telemedicine. The need to monitor astronauts in space led to an infusion of funds and interest in telemedicine. The Department of Health Education and Welfare also participated in telemedicine projects with NASA, Lockheed, and the Indian Health Service. These entities combined to provide health care to astronauts in space and to the Papago Indian reservation in Arizona. Space Technology Applied to Rural Papago Advanced Health Care was the result of the combined efforts of these organizations (6). The program ran from 1972 to 1975 and consisted of a van linked to a Public Health Service hospital by two-way microwave telemedicine and audio transmission providing ECG, x-ray, and other medical services. In 1971, 26 sites in Alaska used the ATS-1, the first NASA series of applied technology satellites, to provide health care to remote locations in Alaska. This was a field trial that determined that satellite systems could be used effectively by health care providers and could be useful for most medical conditions except for emergency care. In 1989, NASA established a SpaceBridge to Armenia to extend medical consultation for the victims of a massive earthquake in the Soviet Republic of Armenia (1). This program was later extended to Ufa to assist burn victims after a railway accident. Telemedicine consults using video, voice, and fax occurred between Armenia and four U.S. medical centers.

Since the early 1980s, radiologists have been using teleradiology techniques to provide on-call coverage to hospital-based radiology practices. A corresponding growth in telemedicine literature has taken place and is clearly evidenced by the Internet search results for the topic "telemedicine." The number of telemedicine projects has exploded since the deregulation of the telecommunications industry in the United States in the 1970s. Teleradiology techniques have led the way with other specialties of medicine now taking telemedicine techniques from research and academic centers into pilot projects phases and clinical use.

TELERADIOLOGY COMPONENTS

A teleradiology implementation consists of three components: data acquisition, data transfer, and data display. Data acquisition may be performed by direct image capture or by secondary image capture methods. *Direct capture* occurs when the image data produced by the digital modality, in terms of matrix size and pixel bit depth, is transferred to a teleradiology system. Video frame grabbing and film digitizing fall under the category of secondary capture. Of the two methods, the American College of Radiology (ACR) standard for teleradiology states that the direct capture method is desirable for primary diagnosis and further recommends that the digital imaging and communications in medicine (DICOM) standard be used. In the case of secondary image capture, the ACR standard states that the image should be digitized to a matrix size as large or larger than that of the original image. The images should be digitized to a bit depth of at least 8 bits per pixel.

The ACR guidelines for data transmission for purposes of official interpretation state that the digital data received must have no loss of clinically significant information. It further states that the transmission system should have error-checking capability.

The ACR guidelines (7) for display systems used for official interpretation are as follows:

1. Gray-scale monitor luminance of at least 50 foot-lamberts
2. Accurate association of patient and demographic data with the images
3. Window width and level adjustments
4. Pan and zoom functions
5. Image rotation and flipping functions with correct labeling of patient orientation
6. Display of matrix size, bit depth, and compression ratio

In recent times, desktop computer monitors have become capable of accurately reproducing and rendering medical images.

Network Technologies

Any discussion of teleradiology would be incomplete without at least a brief description of the telecommunications technologies that enable modern teleradiology. Therefore, we overview some basic network concepts and enumerate the choices available today.

Networks effect data transfers over long distances. A network may be of two basic types: local area network (LAN) and wide area network (WAN). An LAN is generally restricted to a small local area or a building. A WAN covers large geographic distances and therefore is significant for teleradiology applications. A typical teleradiology network includes WAN and LAN components.

Ethernet, developed by Xerox's Palo Alto Research Center, is the most popular network standard. Three different Institute of Electrical and Electronic Engineers Ethernet standards for LAN communication have been defined: standard Ethernet [10 megabits per second (Mbps)], fast Ethernet (100 Mbps), and gigabit Ethernet (1 gigabit per second).

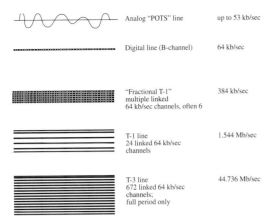

Analog "POTS" line	up to 53 kb/sec
Digital line (B-channel)	64 kb/sec
"Fractional T-1" multiple linked 64 kb/sec channels, often 6	384 kb/sec
T-1 line 24 linked 64 kb/sec channels	1.544 Mb/sec
T-3 line 672 linked 64 kb/sec channels; full period only	44.736 Mb/sec

FIG. 26-1. Circuit-switched and full-period services. POTS, plain old telephone service. Modified with permission from ref. 9.

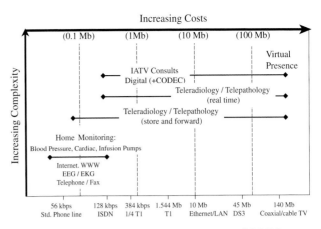

FIG. 26-2. Effects of increasing bandwidth. CODEC, compression/decompression (scheme); EEG, electroencephalography; EKG, electrocardiogram; IATV, interactive television; ISDN, integrated services digital network; LAN, local area network; WWW, World Wide Web. Modified with permission from ref. 1.

Different Ethernet implementations use different types of cabling including coaxial, unshielded twisted pair, and fiberoptic cabling. A detailed discussion of the different telecommunications technologies that enable WANs is beyond the scope of this chapter. However, a brief mention of the common ones is in order (Fig. 26-1). Most developed countries have telephone lines placed throughout their countries. These standard voice telephone lines are capable of transmitting at a rate of 56 kilobits per second (kbps) data rate. However, Federal Communication Commission regulations limit transmission rates to 53 kbps. Integrated services digital network (ISDN) allows up to 128 kbps over two 64-kbps channels using the basic rate interface. Speeds of 1.5 Mbps are possible with an ISDN prime rate interface. T1 lines are also capable of 1.5 Mbps. Fractional T1 lines with reduced bandwidths and thereby reduced costs are also available. Increased bandwidth is usually coupled with increased capabilities and costs (Fig. 26-2). Other higher speed technologies are available but are rarely needed for teleradiology applications. Satellite and wireless telecommunication technologies are worth mentioning because of their special significance to teleradiology services to remote areas that are not connected in other ways. Digital wireless radiology consults have been studied using portable laptop computers (8).

Digital Imaging and Communications in Medicine Standard

The DICOM standard, created by the ACR and National Electric Manufacturers Association (NEMA), is an attempt to provide a platform to ensure interoperability among image-generating modalities, postprocessing workstations, diagnostic display workstations, and image archival systems in a multivendor environment. The previous lack of such a standard posed difficulties. Proprietary transmission and data

formats, requiring dedicated workstations linked to various imaging modalities, did not offer user flexibility and interoperability between different devices and interpretation software. The DICOM standard is comprised of 14 parts (Table 26-1) at the time of this writing, with part 15 expected in the near future. The different parts provide descriptions of the information model, object and data definitions, information exchange protocols, and storage media formats. Nevertheless, the selection and integration of DICOM conformant

TABLE 26-1. *Parts of the digital imaging and communications in medicine (DICOM) v3.0 standard*

Part	Original standard #	Title
1	PS 3.1-1998	Introduction and Overview
2	PS 3.2-1998	Conformance
3	PS 3.3-1998	Information Object Definitions
4	PS 3.4-1998	Service Class Specifications
5	PS 3.5-1998	Data Structure and Semantics
6	PS 3.6-1998	Data Dictionary
7	PS 3.7-1998	Message Exchange
8	PS 3.8-1998	Network Communication Support for Message Exchange
9	PS 3.9-1998	Point-to-Point Communication
10	PS 3.10-1998	Support for Message Exchange for Media Interchange
11	PS 3.11-1998	Media Storage Application Profiles
12	PS 3.12-1998	Media Formats and Physical Media for Media Interchange
13	PS 3.13-1998	Print Management Point-to-Point Communication Support
14	PS 3.14-1998	Grayscale Standard Display Function

Used with permission from ref. 9.

TABLE 26-2. *Lossless versus lossy (LS) compression*

Parameter	Lossless	Lossy
Data degradation	No	Yes, varies with the compression ratio
Compression ratio	Up to 3 or 4:1	Usually 10 to 20:1; appropriate amount varies from modality to modality
Types	Lossless JPEG; JPEG-LS; entropy encoding techniques such as run-length, Hoffman, and arithmetic coding; and certain wavelet techniques	Baseline JPEG, other forms of JPEG, certain wavelet techniques
Utility	Typically not enough compression for an economical or practical advantage for some aspects of telemedicine	Provides adequate compression for telemedicine

JPEG, joint photographic experts group.
Modified with permission from ref. 9.

products for your practice are not without pitfalls. Not all vendors have interpreted the standard in exactly the same manner. In fact, the DICOM standard may be more appropriately termed a *DICOM suggestion*. Various open, low-field magnets are capable of transmitting a DICOM image to a workstation. However, not all workstations have robust, user-friendly cut-line display, three-dimensional representations of maximum intensity projection images, or the display of all scan data present on film. Not all proprietary software for transmission and DICOM formats is available on all modalities. Different workstation interfaces with various vendors' equipment may lead to frustration on the radiologist's part in implementing a teleradiology system.

To implement a successful DICOM application, it is important to distinguish DICOM connectivity from true interoperability. *Connectivity* simply means that two systems can exchange data. *Interoperability* means that these data exchanges are performed in a way that ensures full functionality (as related to image manipulation) is preserved across the connection. DICOM conformance and DICOM connectivity do not ensure complete interoperability, and the current scenario is far from "plug and play."

The DICOM conformance statement, which is required of every DICOM conformant product, serves as a starting point in the consideration of a DICOM product. An examination of the conformance statement shows whether the necessary DICOM services have been implemented to enable your desired connection. For example, a DICOM archive should be a storage service class provider and an MRI system that sends data to this archive should be a storage service class user. Further careful evaluation is necessary to ensure that the full capability of the product is realizable on the DICOM data received from the imaging modalities. This is especially important because many vendors implement user-friendly features based on certain optional information that may not be provided by the DICOM data source. Therefore, the right question to ask is not whether a particular product is DICOM conformant but whether it is compatible with the other DICOM-conformant products that you may have purchased or are considering purchasing for your practice.

Data Compression

The speed of image transmission may be improved in two ways: by increasing the bandwidth of the communication channel or by reducing the actual amount of data transmitted. Here, we present a brief discussion of the latter. Bandwidth considerations were discussed in conjunction with the telecommunications infrastructure earlier.

Reducing the amount of data may be accomplished by the following:

1. Video frame grabbing 8-bit images instead of using full 16-bit images, as in the case of direct capture
2. Formatting multiple images per frame capture
3. Data compression

Of the above three methods, data compression is significant because of its application to direct captured images. Compression schemes fall under two categories: lossless and lossy. In the case of lossless compression, it is possible to decompress the data and obtain the original image, whereas this is not possible in the case of lossy schemes. Truly lossless algorithms produce compression ratios of only up to 3:1. The resulting compression ratio is data dependent, and the user does not specify the compression ratio in the case of lossless algorithms. Lossy schemes, in general, produce better compression ratios than do lossless schemes (Table 26-2). The user may specify the compression ratio, but the exact ratio is rarely achieved. However, the lossy algorithms typically produce a compression ratio very close to the specified one. Although the term *lossless* provides a feeling of comfort in the context of medical diagnostic images, it has been found that lossy schemes are capable of compressing data with no loss in diagnostic quality. This has led to U.S. Food and Drug Administration approval of teleradiology systems using lossy methods.

The two most common compression schemes in use for medical images are JPEG (Joint Photographic Experts Group) compression and wavelet compression. Of the two, JPEG has been in longer use and enjoys many years of standardization and support. Certain other advantages are as follows:

1. Both lossless and lossy JPEG algorithms are available.
2. Application-specific extensions such as 12-bit extension for medical imaging are available.

Wavelet compression is relatively new but has gained a lot of momentum because of the following advantages:

1. It offers the best rate to distortion ratios.
2. Unlike JPEG, wavelet compression produces no block artifacts, even at higher compression ratios.
3. It better represents abrupt transitions in image data.

Many different wavelet transformations have been described; the Daubechies wavelet filter is the most popular. Newer variations, such as the compression with reversible embedded wavelets system developed by Ricoh (Tokyo, Japan), has been submitted to the ACR–National Electric Manufacturers Association and International Standards Organization as a lossless and lossy still image compression standard.

For small field-of-view and large-matrix MR images, the use of lossy compression may have a negligible effect on image quality. According to Thrall, lossy wavelet compression with ratios approaching 30:1 can be performed with no loss of diagnostic quality (3). High compression ratios may be acceptable for plain film digitization, but digital data tolerates lesser degrees of compression.

CASE STUDY

The following is a real-life example of a teleradiology link implementation and how a change in clinical need and usage necessitated an infrastructure change to remain cost effective.

In early 1998, a teleradiology link was established between an open MRI center in the Midwest (source) and another in California (destination). Initially, an occasional need to transmit one or two patient studies to California existed. However, a quick report (within 1 hour of the scan) was expected on those cases.

The implementation is presented below. Your particular situation may be different, and some extrapolation may be necessary.

Data Size and Bandwidth Calculations

Average number of images per study at this site = 100
Average stored matrix size of each image = 256 × 256
Number of pixels per image = 256 × 256 = 65,536 pixels
Number bytes per pixel = 2 bytes
Number of bytes per image = 65,536 × 2 = 131,072 bytes
   = 128 kilobytes (1 kilobyte = 1,024 bytes)
Average data size per study (100 images) = 128 × 100 = 12,800 kilobytes
Estimated header size per image = 1 kilobyte
Estimated total data size = 12,800 + (1 × 100) = 12,900 kilobytes

This is approximately 12.6 megabytes (1 megabyte = 1,024 kilobytes). To be able to transmit this data within 20 minutes, the required bandwidth is calculated as follows:

Average data size per study = 12,900 kilobytes
Data rate to transmit in 20 minutes = 12,900/20 = 645 kilobytes per minute
   = 645/60 = 10.75 kilobytes per second
   = 10.75 × 8 = 86 kilobits per second (1 byte = 8 bits)

The value of 86 kbps falls well within the bandwidth offered by a two-channel basic rate interface ISDN (128 kbps). Clearly, a 56-kb analog modem would not suffice for this purpose.

The reader may notice that in these calculations, we have used the following conversions:

1 kilobyte = 2^{10} bytes = 1,024 bytes
1 megabyte = 1,024 kilobytes

This is in accordance with strict technical conventions. You may find that metric conversions are also commonly used. Therefore, a word of caution is in order. Comparing the actual performance of your teleradiology application with the theoretical expectation is confusing if vendors use different conventions. This difference should be kept in mind when communicating with vendors and other service providers.

Implementation

Based on the need and the previous calculation, a dial-up ISDN connection was selected as the communication link, with Pipeline (Lucent Technologies, Murray Hill, NJ) ISDN routers on both ends. The transmitting and receiving machines were connected to the routers at the respective ends. The transmitting machine implemented a DICOM storage service class user, and the receiving machine implemented a DICOM storage service class provider. The transmitting machine used the direct capture method to acquire images from the MRI system. The source router automatically dialed the destination router and established a Transmission Control Protocol/Internet Protocol (TCP/IP) network connection over the ISDN lines whenever the source machine attempted to send data. The telephone connection was automatically closed after the transmission was completed. One may wonder why a smaller bandwidth along with data compression was not chosen. Lossless JPEG compression was, in fact, used in this application. However, because lossless compression is data-dependent and a particular compression ratio is not guaranteed, the worst-case scenario of no compression was used for this design.

Change in Clinical Need

The recurring cost associated with the above implementation was the nominal fixed fee for ISDN service and variable connection time charges. Because the usage was low, this proved to be cost effective. However, the need for transmitting cases over the teleradiology link increased over the year and, by the end of 1998, almost all cases were transmitted over the teleradiology link, which increased the charges significantly and made this implementation quite expensive.

Please note that the key cost element in this case is the variable connection cost, which is directly proportional to the usage. Therefore, any attempt to change the infrastructure should address this issue and possibly eliminate the correlation. The Internet was our chosen solution. Instead of initiating a call directly to the destination, we established connections to the Internet on both ends that did not incur any usage-based charges. Local Internet service providers established connections that were available 24 hours a day for a flat monthly fee at the two locations. For the same bandwidth, the flat fee of a few hundred dollars has proven much less expensive than the telephone charges incurred earlier.

Because the Internet is a shared medium, the transmission speed may be influenced, to an extent, by the Internet traffic. Thus, it is important to select an Internet service provider whose infrastructure is sufficient to meet your requirements. Temporary bottlenecks may occur owing to the inherent nature of the Internet, but this solution has proven effective in our experience. We have found it to be stable enough to serve our practice in a cost-effective manner.

PRACTICAL ISSUES

For a teleradiology practice to be successful, one must assess the clinical need and purpose of the teleradiology application, the existing infrastructure, the required speed of transmission, and the cost of establishing and maintaining a network. Teleradiology programs are designed to provide evening coverage for emergency and immediate reads, consultation and second opinion reads by specialists assisting radiologists in rural areas or where subspecialists are not represented, and for remote primary diagnosis. Clinical needs may also change over time, and the teleradiology application should be modified to suit current needs.

Certain practical constraints should also be considered. Not all technologies are universally available. Therefore, the existing telecommunications infrastructure frequently determines your range of choices. Satellite communications to otherwise unconnected remote and rural areas may be a possibility, but the costs may be prohibitive.

Data security and patient confidentiality issues must be seriously addressed, especially when using the Internet as the transmission medium. The deregulation of the telecommunications industry in the United States enabled the lowering of costs to establish high-speed networks. Telecommunications regulations in other countries may be restrictive to the growth of teleradiology.

Reimbursements for teleradiology consultations are not as problematic as reimbursement for telemedicine consultations in general, but attention to regional reimbursements for

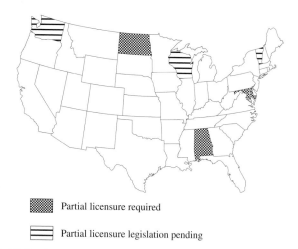

Partial licensure required

Partial licensure legislation pending

FIG. 26-3. States requiring partial licensure of out-of-state telemedicine providers. Modified with permission from ref. 9.

radiology services is important. Licensing and credentialing issues are critical. Although not all states mandate full licensure, many providers of teleradiology are licensed in the state in which they interpret images and in the states in which the images are obtained (Figs. 26-3 and 26-4) (9). Development of national licensure for the United States seems to be a rational alternative to obtaining multiple licenses in different jurisdictions. Maintaining credentials in hospitals and with insurance companies may require a significant amount of effort in developing teleradiology practices. Local physician attitudes, threat of lost income, malpractice, safety, and efficacy issues must be addressed. Medical regulations and certificates of need are also barriers to establishing a teleradiology MRI system in a regulated certificates of need environment.

Marketing a teleradiology practice is not without challenges. The patients and the referring physicians must be convinced that the teleradiology link is sufficiently reliable

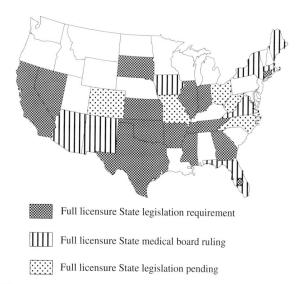

Full licensure State legislation requirement

Full licensure State medical board ruling

Full licensure State legislation pending

FIG. 26-4. States requiring full licensure of out-of-state telemedicine providers. Modified with permission from ref. 9.

to enable timely reads and reports. To be a successful global service provider, the services rendered must be accessible. Networks must become universally available for the benefit of patients and providers. This requires cooperation between industry and local governments. In addition, accountability on the part of the medical profession is absolutely necessary. Physicians must be willing and able to expand their practices using advanced telecommunications tools. Medical school training and continued medical education for doctors out of training will help change physicians' attitudes. Cooperation between the business sector and the medical system is necessary.

Finally, for a provider to be successful, his or her services must be affordable. Economies of scale and control issues become important as does determining the cost of the infrastructure needed to provide services. It is essential to develop a multidisciplinary team of physicians, MRI technologists, telecommunications personnel, finance, MRI service engineers, lawyers, and transcriptionists when designing a freestanding open MRI center in the teleradiology environment.

CONCLUSION

The use of electronic information and communications technologies to provide professional radiologic diagnostic services allows the radiologist to assist in patient care even when the location of care is separated by distance. This possibility is significant in the context of open MRI systems, which are imminently suitable for far-flung and rural areas. Teleradiology overcomes geographic barriers to medical diagnostic image interpretation. Each individual practice must assess the needs of its referring population to determine the optimum combination of infrastructure and data compression relative to the cost of establishing and maintaining the teleradiology application. Properly identifying the clinical need, evaluating the necessary infrastructure, understanding its strengths and limitations, defining the acceptable speed criteria, determining the cost, and balancing all of the foregoing ultimately determine the success of a teleradiology endeavor.

REFERENCES

1. Field MJ, ed. *Telemedicine: a guide to assessing telecommunications in health care*. Committee on Evaluating Clinical Applications of Telemedicine. Division of Health Care Services, Institute of Medicine Washington: National Academic Press, 1996.
2. Dakins DR. The envelope, please: top 10 telemedicine programs for 1998. *TeleHealth Mag* 1998;4:32–48.
3. Jaffe C, Harle T. *Handbook of teleradiology applications*. Radiological Society of North America Monograph. St. Joseph, MI: IPC Communications Services, 1997.
4. Davis DA, Thornton W, Grosskreutz DC, et al. Radiotelemetry in patient monitoring. *Anesthesiology* 1961;22(6):1010–1013.
5. Boland GWL. Teleradiology: another revolution in radiology? *Clin Radiol* 1998;53:547–553.
6. Space Technology Applied to Rural Papago Advanced Health Care (STARPAHC) project. On-line description at Telemedicine Information Exchange. http://tie.telemed.org.
7. *ACR standard for teleradiology: diagnostic radiology standard no 2*. Reston, VA: American College of Radiology, 1998.
8. Repponen J, Iikko E, Jyrkinen L, et al. Digital wireless radiology consultation with a portable computer. *J Telemed Telecare* 1998;4: 201–205.
9. Mulloy J, Pomeranz SJ. *Teleradiology: step by step*. Cincinnati: MRI EFI Publications, 1998.

SECTION V

Appendix

Open MRI,
edited by Peter A. Rothschild and Debra Reinking Rothschild.
Lippincott Williams & Wilkins. Philadelphia © 2000.

Responsibilities of the Open Magnetic Resonance Imaging Medical Director

Peter A. Rothschild

The medical director at an open magnetic resonance imaging (MRI) facility can make or break the center. The ideal medical director for an open MRI center is a radiologist who is a "true believer" in open MRI. This individual should have extensive experience with open magnets and detailed knowledge of their advantages and disadvantages. An empathetic medical director who understands the psychological issues facing claustrophobic and obese patients is a necessity. The medical director's treatment of MRI patients should set an example for the entire staff.

The more involved the medical director is in the marketing efforts of the center, the better. As a physician, the medical director has better access to referring doctors, on a doctor-to-doctor basis, than the marketing director does. Telephoning positive findings, turning around reports in 24 hours, offering tours of the facility, and sitting down to go over results with referring physicians are all ways the medical director can participate in the marketing of an open MRI center. Hospital rounds and in-service seminars are also opportunities to educate referring physicians about the capabilities of open MRI.

The medical director must be willing to undertake certain administrative responsibilities. Above all, he or she must know open MRI inside and out. Ideally, the medical director will be a specialist in MRI or at least have a very strong interest in MRI. The medical director must have intimate knowledge of the workings of the magnet in use at the imaging center. Each magnet model has certain unique characteristics, which can be used to the center's advantage. The medical director should understand these characteristics well enough to be able to push the envelope and maximize the scanner's capabilities, especially regarding protocol and coil solutions. Many MRI manufacturers offer physician and

> ### Qualities Sought in an Open MRI Director
>
> - Extensive experience with open MRI
> - Detailed knowledge of open MRI's advantages and disadvantages
> - Willingness to learn
> - Friendly, empathetic personality
> - Sensitivity to overweight and claustrophobic patients
> - Enthusiastic involvement in marketing efforts

technologist courses on their specific open magnet; the medical director and, ideally, all the radiologists and technologists who work with the scanner should attend these courses.

Many MRI centers or departments have a parade of radiologists who rotate through and read. To run efficiently and effectively, however, one physician—the medical director—must assume responsibility for the center's radiology and ensure that all radiologists are working toward the same goal. Creating an optimal environment requires that the medical director be aware of and involved in the day-to-day running of the center and that the director work well with the center manager to achieve common goals. For example, the medical director should be involved in the scheduling process, to help devise procedures to ensure that only appropriate candidates are scheduled for MRI. Ideally, the medical director is responsible for at least some training of front-desk personnel to ensure that the correct questions are asked during the scheduling process. Front-desk personnel must be thoroughly trained in order to guarantee that patients are scheduled for the appropriate examinations and that patients with contraindications for MRI are properly screened out. Although it may not, at first blush, seem appropriate to involve the medical director with scheduling, improper scheduling will result in lost time slots and inappropriate studies and will reflect poorly on the MRI center and the radiologists associated with the center.

P. A. Rothschild: Department of Radiology, University of California at San Francisco, San Francisco, California; Open MRI, Hayward, California; Open MRI, Louisville, Kentucky

Administrative Responsibilities

- Leadership with a vision of providing the best possible diagnostic services to patients and referral doctors
- Development of protocols to ensure that only appropriate patients are scheduled for MRI
- Development of procedures and assistance in training for scheduling process
- Communication with radiologic technologists regarding sequence and protocol selection
- Establishment of emergency plans and maintenance of equipment to handle medical emergencies, such as contrast reactions
- Assumption of overall responsibility for patients and medical records including follow-up and its documentation
- Assumption of overall responsibility for radiology reports, their timeliness, accuracy, clarity, and conciseness

Another duty of the medical director is to ensure that a radiologist is always available for communication with the radiologic technologists regarding clinical issues, such as sequences for specific patients, whether specific patients are candidates for MRI, and so forth. The medical director should also ensure that the imaging center has emergency procedures and equipment in place for handling any life-threatening events, such as contrast reactions.

The medical director is responsible for verifying that all radiology reports are completed in a timely fashion and that the referring doctor's questions are thoroughly answered. It is critical that a mechanism is in place to ensure that radiologists calls referring doctors directly to report urgent findings, especially if the findings were unexpected. The medical director should work with others to develop and implement procedures to ensure that follow-up phone calls have been made and that proper documentation is completed.

In conclusion, the medical director must not restrict his or her activity to merely reading films but to truly being a consultant: a consultant for referring doctors, for MRI technologists, the center manager, the marketing manager, and the clerical personnel who schedule patients. The medical director should lead and inspire the entire center staff to provide superb service to patients and referring doctors.

SUGGESTED READING

Adult learning principles key to staff training. *Physician Relat Update* 1998;7:99.

Asante E. Beyond culture and regular staff meetings. *Radiol Manage* 1999;21:29.

Ayers J, Bonhag R. Work performance follows human enhancement. *Adm Radiol J* 1998;17:27.

Bee J, Denning JJ. Seven practice-management tips to increase productivity. *Conn Med* 1992;56:302.

Cohen KR. Playing for keeps. For a lasting relationship, apply matchmaking techniques when hiring. *Contemp Longterm Care* 1999;22:28,32,34.

Flanagan L. How does your practice sound on the phone? *Fam Pract Manage* 1999;6:45.

Index